Springer Series in Statistics

More information about this series at http://www.springer.com/series/692

Brajendra C. Sutradhar

Longitudinal Categorical Data Analysis

Springer

Brajendra C. Sutradhar
Department of Mathematics and Statistics
Memorial University of Newfoundland
St. John's, NL, Canada

ISSN 0172-7397 ISSN 2197-568X (electronic)
ISBN 978-1-4939-2136-2 ISBN 978-1-4939-2137-9 (eBook)
DOI 10.1007/978-1-4939-2137-9
Springer New York Heidelberg Dordrecht London

Library of Congress Control Number: 2014950422

Printed on acid-free paper

Springer is part of Springer Science+Business Media (www.springer.com)

To Bhagawan Sri Sathya Sai Baba
my Guru

for teaching me over the years to do my works with love. Bhagawan Baba says that the works done with hands must be in harmony with sanctified thoughts and words; such hands, in fact, are holier than lips that pray.

Preface

Categorical data, whether categories are nominal or ordinal, consist of multinomial responses along with suitable covariates from a large number of independent individuals, whereas longitudinal categorical data consist of similar responses and covariates collected repeatedly from the same individuals over a small period of time. In the latter case, the covariates may be time dependent but they are always fixed and known. Also it may happen in this case that the longitudinal data are not available for the whole duration of the study from a small percentage of individuals. However, this book concentrates on complete longitudinal multinomial data analysis by developing various parametric correlation models for repeated multinomial responses. These correlation models are relatively new and they are developed by generalizing the correlation models for longitudinal binary data [Sutradhar (2011, Chap. 7), *Dynamic Mixed Models for Familial Longitudinal Data,* Springer, New York]. More specifically, this book uses dynamic models to relate repeated multinomial responses which is quite different than the existing books where longitudinal categorical data are analyzed either marginally at a given time point (equivalent to assume independence among repeated responses) or by using the so-called working correlations based GEE (generalized estimating equation) approach that cannot be trusted for the same reasons found for the longitudinal binary (two category) cases [Sutradhar (2011, Sect. 7.3.6)]. Furthermore, in the categorical data analysis, whether it is a cross-sectional or longitudinal study, it may happen in some situations that responses from individuals are collected on more than one response variable. This type of studies is referred to as the bivariate or multivariate categorial data analysis. On top of univariate categorical data analysis, this book also deals with such multivariate cases, especially bivariate models are developed under both cross-sectional and longitudinal setups. In the cross-sectional setup, bivariate multinomial correlations are developed through common individual random effect shared by both responses, and in the longitudinal setup, bivariate structural and longitudinal correlations are developed using dynamic models conditional on the random effects.

As far as the main results are concerned, whether it is a cross-sectional or longitudinal study, it is of interest to examine the distribution of the respondents (based on their given responses) under the categories. In longitudinal studies, the possible change in distribution pattern over time is examined after taking the correlations of the repeated multinomial responses into account. All these are done by fitting a suitable univariate multinomial probability model in the cross-sectional setup and correlated multinomial probability model in the longitudinal setup. Also these model fittings are first done for the cases where there is no covariate information from the individuals. In the presence of covariates, the distribution pattern may also depend on them, and it becomes important to examine the dependence of response categories on the covariates. Remark that in many existing books, covariates are treated as response variables and contingency tables are generated between response variable and the covariates, and then a full multinomial or equivalently a suitable log linear model is fitted to the joint cell counts. This approach lacks theoretical justification mainly because the covariates are usually fixed and known and hence the Poisson mean rates for joint cells should not be constructed using association parameters between covariates and responses. This book avoids such confusions and emphasizes on regression analysis all through to understand the dependence of the response(s) on the covariates.

The book is written primarily for the graduate students and researchers in statistics, biostatistics, and social sciences, among other applied statistics research areas. However, the univariate categorical data analysis discussed in Chap. 2 under cross-sectional setup, and in Chap. 3 under longitudinal setup with time independent (stationary) covariates, is written for undergraduate students as well. These two chapters containing cross-sectional and longitudinal multinomial models, and corresponding inference methodologies, would serve as the theoretical foundation of the book. The theoretical results in these chapters have also been illustrated by analyzing various biomedical or social science data from real life. As a whole, the book contains six chapters. Chapter 4 contains univariate longitudinal categorical data analysis with time dependent (non-stationary) covariates, and Chaps. 5 and 6 are devoted to bivariate categorical data analysis in cross-sectional and longitudinal setup, respectively. The book is technically rigorous. More specifically, this is the first book in longitudinal categorical data analysis with high level technical details for developments of both correlation models and inference procedures, which are complemented in many places with real life data analysis illustrations. Thus, the book is comprehensive in scope and treatment, suitable for a graduate course and further theoretical and/or applied research involving cross-sectional as well as longitudinal categorical data. In the same token, a part of the book with first three chapters is suitable for an undergraduate course in statistics and social sciences. Because the computational formulas all through the book are well developed, it is expected that the students and researchers with reasonably good computational background should have no problems in exploiting them (formulas) for data analysis.

The primary purpose of this book is to present ideas for developing correlation models for longitudinal categorical data, and obtaining consistent and efficient estimates for the parameters of such models. Nevertheless, in Chaps. 2 and 5, we consider categorical data analysis in cross-sectional setup for univariate and bivariate responses, respectively. For the analysis of univariate categorical data in

Chap. 2, multinomial logit models are fitted irrespective of the situations whether the data contain any covariates or not. To be specific, in the absence of covariates, the distribution of the respondents under selected categories is computed by fitting multinomial logit model. In the presence of categorical covariates, similar distribution pattern is computed but under different levels of the covariate, by fitting product multinomial models. This is done first for one covariate with suitable levels and then for two covariates with unequal number of levels. Both nominal and ordinal categories are considered for the response variable but covariate categories are always nominal. Remark that in the presence of covariates, it is of primary interest to examine the dependence of response variable on the covariates, and hence product multinomial models are exploited by using a multinomial model at a given level of the covariate. Also, as opposed to the so-called log linear models, the multinomial logit models are chosen for two main reasons. First, the extension of log linear model from the cross-sectional setup to the longitudinal setup appears to be difficult whereas the primary objective of the book is to deal with longitudinal categorical data. Second, even in the cross-sectional setup with bivariate categorical responses, the so-called odds ratio (or association) parameters based Poisson rates for joint cells yield complicated marginal probabilities for the purpose of interpretation. In this book, this problem is avoided by using an alternative random effects based mixed model to reflect the correlation of the two variables but such models are developed as an extension of univariate multinomial models from cross-sectional setup. With regard to inferences, the likelihood function based on product multinomial distributions is maximized for the case when univariate response categories are nominal. For the inferences for ordinal categorical data, the well-known weighted least square method is used. Also, two new approaches, namely a binary mapping based GQL (generalized quasi-likelihood) and pseudo-likelihood approaches, are developed. The asymptotic covariances of such estimators are also computed.

Chapter 3 deals with longitudinal categorical data analysis. A new parametric correlation model is developed by relating the present and past multinomial responses. More specifically, conditional probabilities are modeled using such dynamic relationships. Both linear and non-linear type models are considered for these dynamic relationships based conditional probabilities. The models are referred to as the linear dynamic conditional multinomial probability (LDCMP) and multinomial dynamic logit (MDL) models, respectively. These models have pedagogical virtue of reducing to the longitudinal binary cases. Nevertheless, for simplicity, we discuss the linear dynamic conditional binary probability (LDCBP) and binary dynamic logit (BDL) models in the beginning of the chapter, followed by detailed discussion on LDCMP and MDL models. Both covariate free and stationary covariate cases are considered. As far as the inferences for longitudinal binary data are concerned, the book uses the GQL and likelihood approaches, similar to those in Sutradhar (2011, Chap. 7), but the formulas in the present case are simplified in terms of transitional counts. The models are then fitted to a longitudinal Asthma data set as an illustration. Next, the inferences for the covariate free LDCMP model are developed by exploiting both GQL and likelihood approaches; however, for simplicity, only likelihood approach is discussed for the covariate free MDL model.

In the presence of stationary covariates, the LDCMP and MDL regression models are fitted using the likelihood approach. As an illustration, the well-known Three Miles Island Stress Level (TMISL) data are reanalyzed in this book by fitting the LDCMP and MDL regression models through likelihood approach. Furthermore, correlation models for ordinal longitudinal multinomial data are developed and the models are fitted through a binary mapping based pseudo-likelihood approach.

Chapter 4 is devoted to theoretical developments of correlation models for longitudinal multinomial data with non-stationary covariates, whereas similar models were introduced in Chap. 3 for the cases with stationary covariates. As opposed to the stationary case, it is not sensible to construct contingency tables at a given level of the covariates in the non-stationary case. This is because the covariate levels are also likely to change over time in the non-stationary longitudinal setup. Consequently, no attempt is made to simplify the model and inference formulas in terms of transitional counts. Two non-stationary models developed in this chapter are referred to as the NSLDCMP (non-stationary LDCMP) and NSMDL (non-stationary MDL) models. Likelihood inferences are employed to fit both models. The chapter also contains discussions on some of the existing models where odds ratios (equivalent to correlations) are estimated using certain "working" log linear type working models. The advantages and drawbacks of this type of "working" correlation models are also highlighted.

Chapters 2 through 4 were confined to the analysis of univariate longitudinal categorical data. In practice, there are, however, situations where more than one response variables are recorded from an individual over a small period of time. For example, to understand how diabetes may affect retinopathy, it is important to analyze retinopathy status of both left and right eyes of an individual. In this problem, it may be of interest to study the effects of associated covariates on both categorical responses, where these responses at a given point of time are structurally correlated as they are taken from the same individual. In Chap. 5, this type of bivariate correlations is modeled through a common individual random effect shared by both response variables, but the modeling is confined, for simplicity, to the cross-sectional setup. Bivariate longitudinal correlation models are discussed in Chap. 6. For inferences for the bivariate mixed model in Chap. 5, we have developed a likelihood approach where a binomial approximation to the normal distribution of random effects is used to construct the likelihood estimating equations for the desired parameters. Chapter 5 also contains a bivariate normal type linear conditional model, but for multinomial response variables. A GQL estimation approach is used for the inferences. The fitting of the bivariate normal model is illustrated by reanalyzing the well-known WESDR (Wisconsin Epidemiologic Study of Diabetic Retinopathy) data.

In Chap. 6, correlation models for longitudinal bivariate categorical data are developed. This is done by using a dynamic model for each multinomial variables conditional on the common random effect shared by both variables. Theoretical details are provided for both model development and inferences through a GQL estimation approach. The bivariate models discussed in Chaps. 5 and 6 may be extended to the multivariate multinomial setup, which is, however, beyond the scope of the present book. The incomplete longitudinal multinomial data analysis is also beyond the scope of the present book.

St. John's, Newfoundland, Canada Brajendra C. Sutradhar

Acknowledgements

It has been a pleasure to work with Marc Strauss, Hannah Bracken, and Jon Gurstelle of Springer-Verlag. I also wish to thank the production manager Mrs. Kiruthiga Anand, production editor Ms. Anitha Selvaraj, and their production team at Springer SPi-Global, India, for their excellent production jobs.

I want to complete this short but important section by acknowledging the inspirational love of my grand daughter Riya (5) and grand son Shaan (3) during the preparation of the book. I am grateful to our beloved Swami Sri Sathya Sai Baba for showering this love through them.

Contents

1 Introduction 1
1.1 Background of Univariate and Bivariate Cross-Sectional Multinomial Models 1
1.2 Background of Univariate and Bivariate Longitudinal Multinomial Models 3
References 6

2 Overview of Regression Models for Cross-Sectional Univariate Categorical Data 7
2.1 Covariate Free Basic Univariate Multinomial Fixed Effect Models 7
2.1.1 Basic Properties of the Multinomial Distribution (2.4) 9
2.1.2 Inference for Proportion $\pi_j (j = 1, \ldots, J-1)$ 12
2.1.3 Inference for Category Effects $\beta_{j0}, j = 1, \ldots, J-1$, with $\beta_{J0} = 0$ 15
2.1.4 Likelihood Inference for Categorical Effects $\beta_{j0}, j = 1, \ldots, J-1$ with $\beta_{J0} = -\sum_{j=1}^{J-1} \beta_{j0}$ Using Regression Form 19
2.2 Univariate Multinomial Regression Model 20
2.2.1 Individual History Based Fixed Regression Effects Model 20
2.2.2 Multinomial Likelihood Models Involving One Covariate with $L = p+1$ Nominal Levels 25
2.2.3 Multinomial Likelihood Models with $L = (p+1)(q+1)$ Nominal Levels for Two Covariates with Interactions 53
2.3 Cumulative Logits Model for Univariate Ordinal Categorical Data 63
2.3.1 Cumulative Logits Model Involving One Covariate with $L = p+1$ Levels 64
References 87

3 Regression Models For Univariate Longitudinal Stationary Categorical Data ... 89
3.1 Model Background ... 89
3.1.1 Non-stationary Multinomial Models ... 90
3.1.2 Stationary Multinomial Models ... 91
3.1.3 More Simpler Stationary Multinomial Models: Covariates Free (Non-regression) Case ... 92
3.2 Covariate Free Basic Univariate Longitudinal Binary Models ... 93
3.2.1 Auto-correlation Class Based Stationary Binary Model and Estimation of Parameters ... 93
3.2.2 Stationary Binary AR(1) Type Model and Estimation of Parameters ... 100
3.2.3 Stationary Binary EQC Model and Estimation of Parameters ... 107
3.2.4 Binary Dynamic Logit Model and Estimation of Parameters ... 114
3.3 Univariate Longitudinal Stationary Binary Fixed Effect Regression Models ... 120
3.3.1 LDCP Model Involving Covariates and Estimation of Parameters ... 122
3.3.2 BDL Regression Model and Estimation of Parameters ... 137
3.4 Covariate Free Basic Univariate Longitudinal Multinomial Models ... 144
3.4.1 Linear Dynamic Conditional Multinomial Probability Models ... 145
3.4.2 MDL Model ... 167
3.5 Univariate Longitudinal Stationary Multinomial Fixed Effect Regression Models ... 179
3.5.1 Covariates Based Linear Dynamic Conditional Multinomial Probability Models ... 180
3.5.2 Covariates Based Multinomial Dynamic Logit Models ... 193
3.6 Cumulative Logits Model for Univariate Ordinal Longitudinal Data With One Covariate ... 209
3.6.1 LDCP Model with Cut Points g at Time $t-1$ and j at Time t ... 213
3.6.2 MDL Model with Cut Points g at Time $t-1$ and j at Time t ... 232
References ... 245

4 Regression Models For Univariate Longitudinal Non-stationary Categorical Data ... 247
4.1 Model Background ... 247
4.2 GEE Approach Using 'Working' Structure/Model for Odds Ratio Parameters ... 249
4.2.1 'Working' Model **1** for Odds Ratios (τ) ... 250

4.3 NSLDCMP Model ... 253
4.3.1 Basic Properties of the LDCMP Model (4.20) ... 254
4.3.2 GQL Estimation of the Parameters ... 256
4.3.3 Likelihood Estimation of the Parameters ... 260
4.4 NSMDL Model ... 264
4.4.1 Basic Moment Properties of the MDL Model ... 266
4.4.2 Existing Models for Dynamic Dependence Parameters and Drawbacks ... 270
4.5 Likelihood Estimation for NSMDL Model Parameters ... 272
4.5.1 Likelihood Function ... 272
References ... 280

5 Multinomial Models for Cross-Sectional Bivariate Categorical Data ... 281
5.1 Familial Correlation Models for Bivariate Data with No Covariates ... 281
5.1.1 Marginal Probabilities ... 281
5.1.2 Joint Probabilities and Correlations ... 282
5.1.3 Remarks on Similar Random Effects Based Models ... 283
5.2 Two-Way ANOVA Type Covariates Free Joint Probability Model ... 284
5.2.1 Marginal Probabilities and Parameter Interpretation Difficulties ... 286
5.2.2 Parameter Estimation in Two-Way ANOVA Type Multinomial Probability Model ... 287
5.3 Estimation of Parameters for Covariates Free Familial Bivariate Model (5.4)–(5.7) ... 293
5.3.1 Binomial Approximation Based GQL Estimation ... 294
5.3.2 Binomial Approximation Based ML Estimation ... 304
5.4 Familial (Random Effects Based) Bivariate Multinomial Regression Model ... 309
5.4.1 MGQL Estimation for the Parameters ... 312
5.5 Bivariate Normal Linear Conditional Multinomial Probability Model ... 317
5.5.1 Bivariate Normal Type Model and its Properties ... 317
5.5.2 Estimation of Parameters of the Proposed Correlation Model ... 321
5.5.3 Fitting BNLCMP Model to a Diabetic Retinopathy Data: An Illustration ... 330
References ... 337

6 Multinomial Models for Longitudinal Bivariate Categorical Data ... 339
6.1 Preamble: Longitudinal Fixed Models for Two Multinomial Response Variables Ignoring Correlations ... 339
6.2 Correlation Model for Two Longitudinal Multinomial Response Variables ... 340
6.2.1 Correlation Properties For Repeated Bivariate Responses ... 342

6.3 Estimation of Parameters 348
6.3.1 MGQL Estimation for Regression Parameters 348
6.3.2 Moment Estimation of Dynamic Dependence (Longitudinal Correlation Index) Parameters 360
6.3.3 Moment Estimation for σ^2_ξ (Familial Correlation Index Parameter) 363
References 366

Index 367

Chapter 1
Introduction

1.1 Background of Univariate and Bivariate Cross-Sectional Multinomial Models

In univariate binary regression analysis, it is of interest to assess the possible dependence of the binary response variable upon an explanatory or regressor variable. The regressor variables are also known as covariates which can be dichotomized or multinomial (categorical) or can take values on a continuous or interval scale. In general the covariate levels or values are fixed and known. Similarly, as a generalization of the binary case, in univariate multinomial regression setup, one may be interested to assess the possible dependence of the multinomial (nominal or categorical) response variable upon one or more covariates. In a more complex setup, bivariate or multivariate multinomial responses along with associated covariates (one or more) may be collected from a large group of independent individuals, where it may be of interest to (1) examine the joint distribution of the response variables mainly to understand the association (equivalent to correlations) among the response variables; (2) assess the possible dependence of these response variables (marginally or jointly) on the associated covariates. These objectives are standard. See, for example, Goodman (1984, Chapter 1) for similar comments and/or objectives. The data are collected in contingency table form. For example, for a bivariate multinomial data, say response y with J categories and response z with R categories, a contingency table with $J \times R$ cell counts is formed, provided there is no covariates. Under the assumption that the cell counts follow Poisson distribution, in general a log linear model is fitted to understand the marginal category effects (there are $J-1$ such effects for y response and $R-1$ effects for z response) as well as joint categories effect (there are $(J-1)(R-1)$ such effects) on the formation of the cell counts, that is, on the Poisson mean rates for each cell. Now suppose that there are two dichotomized covariates w_1 and w_2 which are likely to put additional effect on the Poisson mean rates in each cell. Thus, in this case, in addition to the category effects, one is also interested to examine the effect of w_1, w_2, w_1w_2(interaction)

B.C. Sutradhar, *Longitudinal Categorical Data Analysis*, Springer Series in Statistics, DOI 10.1007/978-1-4939-2137-9_1

on the Poisson response rates for both variables y and z. A four-way contingency table of dimension $2 \times 2 \times J \times R$ is constructed and it is standard to analyze such data by fitting the log linear model. One may refer, for example, to Goodman (1984); Lloyd (1999); Agresti (1990, 2002); Fienberg (2007), among others, for the application of log linear models to fit such cell counts data in a contingency table. See also the references in these books for 5 decades long research articles in this area. Note that because the covariates are fixed (as opposed to random), for the clarity of model fitting, it is better to deal with four contingency tables each at a given combined level for both covariates (there are four such levels for two dichotomized covariates), each of dimension $J \times R$, instead of saying that a model is fitted to the data in the contingency table of dimension $2 \times 2 \times J \times R$. This would remove some confusions from treating this single table of dimension $2 \times 2 \times J \times R$ as a table for four response variables w_1, w_2, y, and z. To make it more clear, in many studies, log linear models are fitted to the cell counts in a contingency table whether the table is constructed between two multinomial responses or between one or more covariates and a response. See, for example, the log linear models fitted to the contingency table (Agresti 2002, Section 8.4.2) constructed between injury status (binary response with yes and no status) and three covariates: gender (male and female), accident location (rural and urban), and seat belt use (yes or no) each with two levels. In this study, it is important to realize that the Poisson mean rates for cell counts do not contain any association (correlations) between injury and any of the covariates such as gender. This is because covariates are fixed. Thus, unlike the log linear models for two or more binary or multinomial responses, the construction of a similar log linear model, based on a table between covariates and responses, may be confusing. To avoid this confusion, in this book, we construct the contingency tables only between response variables at a given level of the covariates. Also, instead of using log linear models we use multinomial logit models all through the book whether they arise in cross-sectional or longitudinal setup.

In cross-sectional setup, a detailed review is given in Chap. 2 on univariate nominal and ordinal categorical data analysis (see also Agresti 1984). Unlike other books (e.g., Agresti 1990, 2002; Tang et al. 2012; Tutz 2011), multinomial logit models with or without covariates are fitted. In the presence of covariates product multinomial distributions are used because of the fact that covariate levels are fixed in practice. Many data based numerical illustrations are given. As an extension of the univariate analysis, Chap. 5 is devoted to the bivariate categorical data analysis in cross-sectional setup. A new approach based on random effects is taken to model such bivariate categorical data. A bivariate normal type model is also discussed.

Note however that when categorical data are collected repeated over time from an individual, it becomes difficult to write multinomial models by accommodating the correlations of the repeated multinomial response data. Even though some attention is given on this issue recently, discussions on longitudinal categorical data remain inadequate. In the next section, we provide an overview of the existing works on the longitudinal analysis for the categorical data, and layout the objective of this book with regard to longitudinal categorical data analysis.

1.2 Background of Univariate and Bivariate Longitudinal Multinomial Models

It is recognized that for many practical problems such as for public, community and population health, and gender and sex health studies, it is important that binary or categorical (multinomial) responses along with epidemiological and/or biological covariates are collected repeatedly from a large number of independent individuals, over a small period of time. More specifically, toward the prevention of overweight and obesity in the population, it is important to understand the longitudinal effects of major epidemiological/socio-economic variables such as age, gender, education level, marital status, geographical region, chronic conditions and lifestyle including smoking and food habits; as well as the effects of sex difference based biological variables such as reproductive, metabolism, other possible organism, and candidate genes covariates on the individual's level of obesity (normal, overweight, obese class 1, 2, and 3). Whether it is a combined longitudinal study on both males and females to understand the effects of epidemiological/socio-economic covariates on the repeated responses such as obesity status, or two multinomial models are separately fitted to males and females data to understand the effects of both epidemiological/socio-economic and biological covariates on the repeated multinomial responses, it is, however, important in such longitudinal studies to accommodate the dynamic dependence of the multinomial response at a given time on the past multinomial responses of the individual (that produces longitudinal correlations among the repeated responses) in order to examine the effects of the associated epidemiological and/or biological covariates. Note that even though multinomial mixed effects models have been used by some health economists to study the longitudinal employment transitions in women in Australia (e.g., Haynes et al. 2005, Conference paper available online), and the Manitoba longitudinal home care use data (Sarma and Simpson 2007), and by some marketing researchers (e.g., Gonul and Srinivasan 1993; Fader et al. 1992) to study the longitudinal consumer choice behavior, none of their models are, however, developed to address the longitudinal correlations among the repeated multinomial responses in order to efficiently examine the effects of the covariates on the repeated responses collected over time. More specifically, Sarma and Simpson (2007), for example, have analyzed an elderly living arrangements data set from Manitoba collected over three time periods 1971, 1976, and 1983. In this study, living arrangement is a multinomial response variable with three categories, namely independent living arrangements, stay in an intergenerational family, or move into a nursing home. They have fitted a marginal model to the multinomial data for a given year and produced the regression effects of various covariates on the living arrangements in three different tables. The covariates were: age, gender, immigration status, education level, marital status, living duration in the same community, and self-reported health status. Also home care was considered as a latent or random effects variable. There are at least two main difficulties with this type of marginal analysis. First, it is not clear how the covariate effects from three different years can be combined to interpret the overall effects of the covariates on the responses over the whole duration of the study. This indicates that it is important to develop a general model to find the overall effects of the covariates on the responses as opposed to the marginal effects. Second, this study did not accommodate the possible correlations among the repeated multinomial responses (living arrangements) collected over three time points. Thus, these estimates are bound to be inefficient. Bergsma et al. (2009, Chapter 4) analyze the contingency tables for two or more variables at a given time point, and compare the desired marginal or association among variables over time. This marginal approach is, therefore, quite similar to that of Sarma and Simpson (2007).

Some books are also written on longitudinal models for categorical data in the social and behavioral sciences. See, for example, Von Eye and Niedermeir (1999); Von Eye (1990). Similar to the aforementioned papers, these books also consider time as a nominal fixed covariates defined through dummy variables, and hence no correlations among repeated responses are considered. Also, in these books, the categorical response variable is dichotomized which appears to be another limitation.

Further, there exists some studies in this area those reported mainly in the statistics literature. For a detailed early history on the development of statistical models to fit the repeated categorical data, one may, for example, refer to Agresti (1989); Agresti and Natarajan (2001). It is, however, evident that these models also fail to accommodate the correlations or the dynamic dependence of the repeated multinomial responses. To be specific, most of the models documented in these two survey papers consider time as an additional fixed covariate on top of the desired epidemiological/socio-economic and biological covariates where marginal analysis is performed to find the effects of the covariates including the time effect. For example, see the multinomial models considered by Agresti (1990, Section 11.3.1); Fienberg et al. (1985); Conaway (1989), where time is considered as a fixed covariate with certain subjective values, whereas in reality time should be a nominal or index variable only but responses collected over these time occasions must be dynamically dependent. Recently, Tchumtchoua and Dey (2012) used a model to fit multivariate longitudinal categorical data, where responses can be collected from different sets of individuals over time. Thus, this study appears to address a different problem than dealing with longitudinal responses from the same individual. As far as the application is concerned, Fienberg et al. (1985); Conaway (1989) have illustrated their models fitting to an interesting environmental health data set. This health study focuses on the changes in the stress level of mothers of young children living within 10 miles of the three mile island nuclear plant in USA. that encountered an accident. The accident was followed by four interviews; winter 1979 (wave 1), spring 1980 (wave 2), fall 1981 (wave 3), and fall 1982 (wave 4). In this study, the subjects were classified into one of the three response categories namely low, medium, and high stress level, based on a composite score from a 90-item checklist. There were 267 subjects who completed all four interviews. Respondents were stratified into two groups, those living within 5 miles of the plant and those live within 5–10 miles from the plant. It was of interest to compare the distribution of individuals under three stress levels collected over four different time points. However, as mentioned above, these studies, instead of developing multinomial correlation models, have used the time as a fixed covariate and performed marginal analysis. Note that the multinomial model used by Sarma and Simpson (2007) is quite similar to those of Fienberg et al. (1985); Conaway (1989).

Next, because of the difficulty of modeling the correlations for repeated multinomial responses, some authors such as Lipsitz et al. (1994); Stram et al. (1988); Chen and Kuo (2001) have performed correlation analysis by using certain arbitrary 'working' longitudinal correlations, as opposed to the fixed time covariates based marginal analysis. Note that in the context of binary longitudinal data analysis, it has, however, been demonstrated by Sutradhar and Das (1999) (see also Sutradhar 2011, Section 7.3.6) that the 'working' correlations based so-called generalized estimating equations (GEE) approach may be worse than simpler method of moments or quasi-likelihood based estimates. Thus, the GEE approach has serious theoretical limitations for finding efficient regression estimates in the longitudinal setup for binary data. Now because, longitudinal multinomial model may be treated as a generalization of the longitudinal binary model, there is no reasons to believe that the 'working' correlations based GEE approach will work for longitudinal multinomial data.

This book, unlike the aforementioned studies including the existing books, uses parametric approach to model the correlations among multinomial responses collected over time. The models are illustrated with real life data where applicable. More specifically, in Chaps. 3 and 4, lag 1 dynamic relationship is used to model the correlations for repeated univariate responses. Both conditionally linear and non-linear dynamic logit models are used for the purpose. For the cases, when there is no covariates or covariates are stationary (independent of time), category effects after accommodating the correlations for repeated responses are discussed in detail in Chap. 3. The repeated univariate multinomial data in the presence of non-stationary covariates (i.e., time dependent covariates) are analyzed in Chap. 4. Note that these correlation models based analysis for the repeated univariate multinomial responses generalizes the longitudinal binary data analysis discussed in Sutradhar (2011, Chapter 7). In Chap. 6 of the present book, we consider repeated bivariate multinomial models. This is done by combining the dynamic relationships for both multinomial response variables through a random effect shared by both responses from an individual. This may be referred to as the familial longitudinal multinomial model with family size two corresponding to two responses from the same individual. Thus this familial longitudinal multinomial model used in Chap. 6 may be treated as a generalization of the familial longitudinal binary model used in Sutradhar (2011, Chapter 11). The book is technically rigorous. A great deal of attention is given all through the book to develop the computational formulas for the purpose of data analysis, and these formulas, where applicable, were computed using Fortran-90. One may like to use other softwares such as R or S-plus for the computational purpose. It is, thus, expected that the readers desiring to derive maximum benefits from the book should have reasonably good computing background.

References

Agresti, A. (1984). *Analysis of ordinal categorical data.* New York: Wiley.

Agresti, A. (1989). A survey of models for repeated ordered categorical response data. *Statistics in Medicine, 8,* 1209–1224.

Agresti, A. (1990). *Categorical data analysis,* (1st ed.) New York: Wiley.

Agresti, A. (2002). *Categorical data analysis,* (2nd ed.) New York: Wiley.

Agresti, A., & Natarajan, R. (2001). Modeling clustered ordered categorical data: A survey. *International Statistical Review, 69,* 345–371.

Bergsma, W., Croon, M., & Hagenaars, J. A. (2009). *Marginal models: For dependent, clustered, and longitudinal categorical data.* New York: Springer.

Chen, Z., & Kuo, L. (2001). A note on the estimation of the multinomial logit model with random effects. *The American Statistician, 55,* 89–95.

Conaway, M. R. (1989). Analysis of repeated categorical measurements with conditional likelihood methods. *Journal of the American Statistical Association, 84,* 53–62.

Fader, P. S., Lattin, J. M., & Little, J. D. C. (1992). Estimating nonlinear parameters in the multinomial logit model. *Marketing Science, 11,* 372–385.

Fienberg, S. E. (2007). *The analysis of cross-classified categorical data.* New York: Springer.

Fienberg, S. F., Bromet, E. J., Follmann, D., Lambert, D, & May, S. M. (1985). Longitudinal analysis of categorical epidemiological data: A study of three mile island. *Environmental Health Perspectives, 63,* 241–248.

Goodman, L. A. (1984). *The analysis of cross-classified data having ordered categories.* London: Harvard University Press.

Gonul, F., & Srinivasan, K. (1993). Modeling multiple sources of heterogeneity in multinomial logit models: Methodological and managerial issues. *Marketing Science, 12,* 213–229.

Haynes, M., Western, M., & Spallek, M. (2005). Methods for categorical longitudinal survey data: Understanding employment status of Australian women. *HILDA (Household Income and Labour Dynamics in Australia) Survey Research Conference Paper*, University of Melbourne, 29–30 September. Victoria: University of Melbourne.

Lipsitz, S. R., Kim, K. G., & Zhao, L. (1994). Analysis of repeated categorical data using generalized estimating equations. *Statistics in Medicine, 13,* 1149–1163.

Lloyd, C. J. (1999). *Statistical analysis of categorical data.* New York: Wiley.

Sarma, S., & Simpson, W. (2007). A panel multinomial logit analysis of elderly living arrangements: Evidence from aging in Manitoba longitudinal data, Canada. *Social Science & Medicine, 65,* 2539–2552.

Stram, D. O., Wei, L. J., & Ware. J. H. (1988). Analysis of repeated ordered categorical outcomes with possibly missing observations and time-dependent covariates. *Journal of the American Statistical Association, 83,* 631–637.

Sutradhar, B. C. (2011). *Dynamic mixed models for familial longitudinal data.* New York: Springer.

Sutradhar, B. C., & Das, K. (1999). On the efficiency of regression estimators in generalized linear models for longitudinal data. *Biometrika, 86,* 459–465.

Tang, W., He, H., & Tu, X. M. (2012). *Applied Categorical and Count Data Analysis.* Florida: CRC Press/Taylor & Francis Group.

Tchumtchoua, S., & Dey, D. K. (2012). Modeling associations among multivariate longitudinal categorical variables in survey data: A semiparametric bayesian approach. *Psychometrika, 77,* 670–692.

Tutz, G. (2011). *Regression for categorical data.* Cambridge Series in Statistical and Probabilistic Mathematics. Cambridge: Cambridge University Press.

Von Eye, A. (1990). Time series and categorical longitudinal data, Chapter 12, Section 6, in *Statistical Methods in Longitudinal Research, edited.* (vol 2). New York: Academic Press.

Von Eye, A., & Niedermeir, K. E. (1999). *Statistical analysis of longitudinal categorical data in the social and behavioral sciences: An introduction with computer illustrations.* London: Psychology Press.

Chapter 2
Overview of Regression Models for Cross-Sectional Univariate Categorical Data

2.1 Covariate Free Basic Univariate Multinomial Fixed Effect Models

Let there be K individuals and an individual responds to one of the J categories. For $j = 1,\ldots,J$, let π_j denote the marginal probability that the response of an individual belongs to the jth category so that $\sum_{j=1}^{J}\pi_j = 1$. Suppose that $y_i = [y_{i1},\ldots,y_{ij},\ldots,y_{i,J-1}]'$ denotes the $J-1$ dimensional multinomial response variable of the ith ($i = 1,\ldots,K$) individual such that $y_{ij} = 1$ or 0, with $\sum_{j=1}^{J} y_{ij} = 1$. Further suppose that for a q-dimensional unit vector 1_q, for example,

$$y_i^{(j)} = \delta_{ij} = [01'_{j-1}, 1, 01'_{J-1-j}]'$$

denotes the response of the ith individual that belongs to the jth category for $j = 1,\ldots,J-1$, and

$$y_i^{(J)} = \delta_{iJ} = 01_{J-1}$$

denotes that the response of the ith individual belongs to the Jth category which may be referred to as the reference category. It then follows that

$$P[y_i = y_i^{(j)} = \delta_{ij}] = \pi_j, \text{for all } j = 1,\ldots,J. \qquad (2.1)$$

For convenience of generalization to the covariate case, we consider

$$\pi_j = \begin{cases} \frac{\exp(\beta_{j0})}{1+\sum_{g=1}^{J-1}\exp(\beta_{g0})} & \text{for } j = 1,\ldots,J-1 \\ \frac{1}{1+\sum_{g=1}^{J-1}\exp(\beta_{g0})} & \text{for } j = J, \end{cases} \qquad (2.2)$$

B.C. Sutradhar, *Longitudinal Categorical Data Analysis*, Springer Series in Statistics, DOI 10.1007/978-1-4939-2137-9_2

It then follows that the elements of y_i follow the multinomial distribution given by

$$P[y_{i1},\ldots,y_{ij},\ldots,y_{i,J-1}] = \frac{1!}{y_{i1}!\cdots y_{ij}!\cdots y_{iJ}!}\Pi_{j=1}^{J}\pi_j^{y_{ij}}, \tag{2.3}$$

where $y_{iJ} = 1-\sum_{j=1}^{J-1} y_{ij}$. Now suppose that out of these K independent individuals, $K_j = \sum_{i=1}^{K} y_{ij}$ individuals belong to the jth category for $j = 1,\ldots,J$, so that $\sum_{j=1}^{J} K_j = K$. By an argument similar to that of (2.3), one may write the joint distribution for $\{K_j\}$ with $K_J = K-\sum_{j=1}^{J-1} K_j$, that is, the multinomial distribution for $\{K_j\}$ as

$$\begin{aligned} P[K_1,\, K_2,\ldots,K_j,\, \ldots,K_{J-1}] &= \frac{K!}{K_1!\cdots K_j!\cdots K_J!}\Pi_{j=1}^{J}\pi_j^{\sum_{i=1}^{K} y_{ij}} \\ &= \frac{K!}{K_1!\cdots K_J!}\Pi_{j=1}^{J}\pi_j^{K_j}. \end{aligned} \tag{2.4}$$

In the next section, we provide some basic properties of this multinomial distribution. Inference for the multinomial probabilities through the estimation of the parameters $\beta_{j0}(j=1,\ldots,J-1)$, along with an example, is discussed in Sect. 2.1.2.

A derivation of the multinomial distribution (2.4):
Suppose that

$$K_j \sim Poi(\mu_j),\ j=1,\ldots,J,$$

where $Poi(\mu_j)$ denotes the Poisson distribution with mean μ_j, that is,

$$P(K_j|\mu_j) = \frac{\exp(-\mu_j)\mu_j^{K_j}}{K_j!},\ K_j = 0,1,2,\ldots$$

Also suppose that K_j's are independent for all $j = 1,\ldots,J$ It then follows that

$$K = \sum_{j=1}^{J} K_j \sim Poi(\mu = \sum_{j=1}^{J}\mu_j),$$

and conditional on total K, the joint distribution of the counts $K_1,\ldots,K_j,\ldots,K_{J-1}$, has the form

$$P[K_1,\ldots,K_j,\ldots,K_{J-1}|K] = \frac{\Pi_{j=1}^{J}[\frac{\exp(-\mu_j)\mu_j^{K_j}}{K_j!}]}{\frac{\exp(-\mu)\mu^K}{K!}},$$

where now $K_J = K - \sum_{j=1}^{J-1} K_j$ is known. Now by using $\pi_j = \frac{\mu_j}{\mu}$, one obtains the multinomial distribution (2.4), where $\pi_J = 1 - \sum_{j=1}^{J-1} \pi_j$ is known.

Note that when $K = 1$, one obtains the multinomial distribution (2.3) from (2.4) by using $K_j = y_{ij}$ as a special case.

2.1.1 Basic Properties of the Multinomial Distribution (2.4)

Lemma 2.1.1. *The count variable $K_j (j = 1, \ldots, J-1)$ marginally follows a binomial distribution $B(K_j; K, \pi_j)$, with parameters K and π_j, yielding $E[K_j] = K\pi_j$ and $var[K_j] = K\pi_j(1-\pi_j)$. Furthermore, for $j \neq k, j,k = 1, \ldots, J-1$, $cov[K_j, K_k] = -K\pi_j\pi_k$.*

Proof. Let

$$\xi_1 = \pi_1,\ \xi_2 = [1-\pi_1],\ \xi_3 = [1-\pi_1-\pi_2], \ldots, \xi_{J-1} = [1-\pi_1-\cdots-\pi_{J-2}].$$

By summing over the range of K_{J-1} from 0 to $[K - K_1 - \ldots, K_{J-2}]$, one obtains the marginal multinomial distribution of $K_1, \ldots, K_{J-2}$ from (2.4) as

$$\begin{aligned}
P[K_1, \ldots, K_j, \ldots, K_{J-2}] &= \frac{K!}{K_1! \cdots K_j! \cdots \{K - K_1 - \cdots - K_{J-2}\}!} \Pi_{j=1}^{J-2} \pi_j^{K_j} [\xi_{J-1}]^{\{K-K_1-\cdots-K_{J-2}\}} \\
&\times \frac{\{K-K_1-\cdots-K_{J-2}\}!}{K_{J-1}!\{K-K_1-\cdots-K_{J-2}-K_{J-1}\}!} \sum_{K_{J-1}=0}^{K-K_1-\cdots-K_{J-2}} [\frac{\pi_{J-1}}{\xi_{J-1}}]^{K_{J-1}} [1-\frac{\pi_{J-1}}{\xi_{J-1}}]^{\{(K-K_1-\cdots-K_{J-2})-K_{J-1}\}} \\
&= \frac{K!}{K_1! \cdots K_j! \cdots \{K-K_1-\cdots-K_{J-2}\}!} \Pi_{j=1}^{J-2} \pi_j^{K_j} [\xi_{J-1}]^{\{K-K_1-\cdots-K_{J-2}\}}. \qquad (2.5)
\end{aligned}$$

By summing, similar to that of (2.5), successively over the range of $K_{J-2}, \ldots, K_2$, one obtains the marginal distribution of K_1 as

$$P[K_1] = \frac{K!}{K_1!\{K-K_1\}!} \pi^{K_1} [1-\pi_1]^{K-K_1}, \qquad (2.6)$$

which is a binomial distribution with parameters (K, π_1). Note that this averaging or summing technique to find the marginal distribution is exchangeable. Thus, for any $j = 1, \ldots, J-1$, K_j will have marginally binomial distribution with parameters (K, π_j). This yields the mean and the variance of K_j as in the Lemma.

Next to derive the covariance between K_j and K_k, for convenience we find the covariance between K_1 and K_2. For this computation, following (2.5), we first write the joint distribution of K_1 and K_2 as

$$\begin{aligned}
P[K_1, K_2] &= \frac{K!}{K_1!K_2!\{K-K_1-K_2\}!} \Pi_{j=1}^{2} \pi_j^{K_j} [\xi_3]^{\{K-K_1-K_2\}} \\
&= \frac{K!}{K_1!K_2!\{K-K_1-K_2\}!} \Pi_{j=1}^{2} \pi_j^{K_j} [1-\pi_1-\pi_2]^{\{K-K_1-K_2\}}. \qquad (2.7)
\end{aligned}$$

It then follows that

$$E[K_1K_2] = \sum_{K_1=0}^{K}\sum_{K_2=0}^{\{K-K_1\}} K_1K_2\frac{K!}{K_1!K_2!\{K-K_1-K_2\}!}\Pi_{j=1}^{2}\pi_j^{K_j}[1-\pi_1-\pi_2]^{\{K-K_1-K_2\}}$$

$$= K(K-1)\pi_1\pi_2\sum_{K_1^*=0}^{K-2}\sum_{K_2^*=0}^{\{K-2-K_1^*\}}\frac{\{K-2\}!}{K_1^*!K_2^*!\{K-2-K_1^*-K_2^*\}!}$$

$$\times\Pi_{j=1}^{2}\pi_j^{K_j^*}[1-\pi_1-\pi_2]^{\{K-2-K_1^*-K_2^*\}}$$

$$= K(K-1)\pi_1\pi_2, \quad (2.8)$$

yielding

$$\mathrm{cov}[K_1,K_2] = E[K_1K_2]-E[K_1]E[K_2] = K(K-1)\pi_1\pi_2-K^2\pi_1\pi_2 = -K\pi_1\pi_2. \quad (2.9)$$

Now because the multinomial distribution is exchangeable in variables, one obtains $\mathrm{cov}[K_j,K_k] = -K\pi_j\pi_k$, as in the Lemma.

Lemma 2.1.2. *Let*

$$\begin{aligned}\psi_1 &= \pi_1\\ \psi_2 &= \frac{\pi_2}{1-\pi_1}\\ \cdots &\quad \cdots\cdots\cdots\\ \psi_{J-1} &= \frac{\pi_{J-1}}{1-\pi_1-\cdots-\pi_{J-2}}.\end{aligned} \quad (2.10)$$

Then the multinomial probability function in (2.3) can be factored as

$$B(y_{i1};1,\psi_1)B(y_{i2};1-y_{i1},\psi_2)\cdots B(y_{i,J-1};1-y_{i1}-\cdots-y_{i,J-2},\psi_{J-1}) \quad (2.11)$$

where $B(x;K^*,\psi)$, for example, represents the binomial probability of x successes in K^* trials when the success probability is ψ in each trial.

Proof. It is convenient to show that (2.11) yields (2.3). Rewrite (2.11) as

$$[\frac{1!}{y_{i1}!(1-y_{i1})!}\pi_1^{y_{i1}}(1-\pi_1)^{1-y_{i1}}]$$

$$\times\frac{(1-y_{i1})!}{y_{i2}!(1-y_{i1}-y_{i2})!}[\frac{\pi_2}{1-\pi_1}]^{y_{i2}}[\frac{1-\pi_1-\pi_2}{1-\pi_1}]^{1-y_{i1}-y_{i2}}$$

$$\cdots\cdots\cdots$$

$$\times\frac{(1-y_{i1}-\cdots-y_{i,J-2})!}{y_{i,J-1}!(1-y_{i1}-\cdots-y_{i,J-1})!}[\frac{\pi_{J-1}}{1-\pi_1-\cdots-\pi_{J-2}}]^{y_{i,J-1}}[\frac{1-\pi_1-\cdots-\pi_{J-1}}{1-\pi_1-\cdots-\pi_{J-2}}]^{1-y_{i1}-\cdots-y_{i,J-1}}.$$

By some algebras, this reduces to (2.3).

Lemma 2.1.3. *The binomial factorization (2.11) yields the conditional means and variances as follows:*

$$
\begin{aligned}
E[Y_{i1}] &= \psi_1, \;\; var[Y_{i1}] = \psi_1(1-\psi_1) \\
E[Y_{i2}|y_{i1}] &= (1-y_{i1})\psi_2, \;\; var[Y_{i2}|y_{i1}] = (1-y_{i1})\psi_2(1-\psi_2) \\
\cdots &\quad \cdots\cdots \\
E[Y_{i,J-1}|y_{i1},\cdots,y_{i,J-2}] &= (1-y_{i1}-\cdots-y_{i,J-2})\psi_{J-1} \\
var[Y_{i,J-1}|y_{i1},\cdots,y_{i,J-2}] &= (1-y_{i1}-\cdots-y_{i,J-2})\psi_{J-1}(1-\psi_{J-1}). \qquad (2.12)
\end{aligned}
$$

Example 2.1. Consider the multinomial model (2.4) with $J = 3$ categories. This model is referred to as the trinomial probability model. Suppose that π_1, π_2, and π_3 denote the probabilities that an individual fall into categories 1, 2, and 3, respectively. Also suppose that out of K independent individuals, these three cells were occupied by K_1, K_2, and K_3 individuals so that $K = K_1 + K_2 + K_3$. Let $\psi_1 = \pi_1$ and $\psi_2 = \frac{\pi_2}{1-\pi_1}$. Then, similar to (2.11), it can be shown that the trinomial probability function (2.4) (with $J = 3$) can be factored as the product of two binomial probability functions as given by

$$B(K, K_1; \psi_1)B(K-K_1, K_2; \psi_2).$$

Similar to Lemma 2.1.3, one then obtains the mean and variance of K_2 conditional on K_1 as

$$E[K_2|K_1] = [K-K_1]\psi_2, \text{ and } \mathrm{var}[K_2|K_1] = [K-K_1]\psi_2(1-\psi_2), \qquad (2.13)$$

respectively. It then follows that the unconditional mean and variance of K_2 are given by

$$E[K_2] = E_{K_1}E[K_2|K_1] = E_{K_1}[(K-K_1)\psi_2] = [K-K\psi_1]\psi_2 = K(1-\pi_1)\frac{\pi_2}{1-\pi_1} = K\pi_2, \qquad (2.14)$$

and

$$
\begin{aligned}
\mathrm{var}[K_2] &= E_{K_1}[\mathrm{var}\{K_2|K_1\}] + \mathrm{var}_{K_1}[E\{K_2|K_1\}] \\
&= E_{K_1}[\{K-K_1\}\psi_2(1-\psi_2)] + \mathrm{var}_{K_1}[\{K-K_1\}\psi_2] \\
&= K(1-\pi_1)\frac{\pi_2}{1-\pi_1}[\frac{1-\pi_1-\pi_2}{1-\pi_1}] + K\pi_1(1-\pi_1)\frac{\pi_2^2}{(1-\pi_1)^2} \\
&= \frac{K\pi_2}{1-\pi_1}[1-\pi_1-\pi_2+\pi_1\pi_2] \\
&= K\pi_2(1-\pi_2), \qquad (2.15)
\end{aligned}
$$

respectively. Note that these unconditional mean (2.14) and variance (2.15) are the same as in Lemma 2.1.1, but they were derived in a different way than that of Lemma 2.1.1. Furthermore, similar to that of (2.15), the unconditional covariance between K_1 and K_2 may be obtained as

$$\begin{aligned}
\mathrm{cov}[K_1,K_2] &= E_{K_1}[\mathrm{cov}\{(K_1,K_2)|K_1\}]+\mathrm{cov}_{K_1}[K_1,E\{K_2|K_1\}] \\
&= \mathrm{cov}_{K_1}[K_1,E\{K_2|K_1\}] \\
&= \mathrm{cov}_{K_1}[K_1,(K-K_1)\psi_2] = -\psi_2 \mathrm{var}[K_1] = -K\pi_1\pi_2, \qquad (2.16)
\end{aligned}$$

which agrees with the covariance results in Lemma 2.1.

2.1.2 *Inference for Proportion* $\pi_j(j=1,\ldots,J-1)$

Recall from (2.4) that

$$P[K_1,\,K_2,\ldots,K_j,\,\ldots,K_{J-1}] = \frac{K!}{K_1!\cdots K_J!}\Pi_{j=1}^{J}\pi_j{}^{K_j}, \qquad (2.17)$$

where π_j by (2.2) has the formula

$$\pi_j = \begin{cases} \frac{\exp(\beta_{j0})}{1+\sum_{g=1}^{J-1}\exp(\beta_{g0})} & \text{for } j=1,\ldots,J-1 \\ \frac{1}{1+\sum_{g=1}^{J-1}\exp(\beta_{g0})} & \text{for } j=J, \end{cases}$$

(a) Moment estimation for π_j

When K_j for $j=1,\ldots,J-1$, follow the multinomial distribution (2.17), it follows from Lemma 2.1 that $E[K_j]=K\pi_j$ yielding the moment estimating equation for π_j as

$$K_j - K\pi_j = 0 \text{ subject to the condition } \sum_{j=1}^{J}\pi_j = 1. \qquad (2.18)$$

Because by (2.18), one writes

$$\pi_J = 1-\sum_{j=1}^{J-1}\pi_j = 1-\sum_{j=1}^{J-1}\frac{K_j}{K} = \frac{K-\sum_{j=1}^{J-1}K_j}{K} = \frac{K_J}{K},$$

thus, in general, the moment estimator for π_j for all $j=1,\ldots,J$, has the form

$$\hat{\pi}_{j,MM} = \frac{K_j}{K}. \qquad (2.19)$$

Note however that once the estimation of π_j for $j = 1,\ldots,J-1$ is done, estimation of π_J does not require any new information because $K_J = K - \sum_{j=1}^{J-1} K_j$ becomes known.

(b) Likelihood Estimation of proportion $\pi_j, j = 1,\ldots,J\text{-}1$

It follows from (2.17) that the log likelihood function of $\{\pi_j\}$ with $\pi_J = 1 - \sum_{j=1}^{J-1} \pi_j$ is given by

$$logL(\pi_1,\ldots,\pi_{J-1}) = k_0 + \sum_{j=1}^{J} K_j log(\pi_j), \tag{2.20}$$

where k_0 is the normalizing constant free from $\{\pi_j\}$. It then follows that the maximum likelihood (ML) estimator of π_j, for $j = 1,\ldots,J-1$, is the solution of the likelihood equation

$$\frac{\partial logL(\pi_1,\ldots,\pi_{J-1})}{\partial \pi_j} = \frac{K_j}{\pi_j} - \frac{K_J}{1-\sum_{j=1}^{J-1}\pi_j} = 0, \tag{2.21}$$

and is given by

$$\hat{\pi}_{j,ML} = \hat{\pi}_{J,ML}\frac{K_j}{K_J}. \tag{2.22}$$

But, as $\sum_{j=1}^{J} \hat{\pi}_{j,ML} = 1$, it follows from (2.22) that

$$\hat{\pi}_{J,ML} = \frac{K_J}{K},$$

yielding

$$\hat{\pi}_{j,ML} = \frac{K_j}{K} = \frac{K_j}{\sum_{j=1}^{J} K_j} \text{ for } j = 1,\ldots,J-1.$$

Thus, in general, one may write the formula

$$\hat{\pi}_{j,ML} = \frac{K_j}{K} = \frac{K_j}{\sum_{j=1}^{J} K_j}, \tag{2.23}$$

for all $j = 1,\ldots,J$. This ML estimate in (2.23) is the same as the moment estimate in (2.19).

(c) Illustration 2.1

To illustrate the aforementioned ML estimation for the categorical proportion, we, for example, consider a modified version of the health care utilization data, studied by Sutradhar (2011). This data set contains number of physician visits by 180 members of 48 families over a period of 6 years from 1985 to 1990. Various

Table 2.1 Summary statistics of physician visits by four covariates in the health care utilization data for 1985

		Number of Visits					
Covariates	**Level**	**0**	**1**	**2**	**3–5**	**≥6**	**Total**
Gender	Male	28	22	18	16	12	96
	Female	11	5	15	21	32	84
Chronic Condition	No	26	20	15	16	11	88
	Yes	13	7	18	21	33	92
Education Level	< High School	17	5	11	10	15	58
	High School	6	4	4	8	11	33
	> High School	16	18	18	19	18	89
Age	20–30	23	17	14	15	15	84
	31–40	1	1	3	3	3	11
	41–50	4	4	5	12	8	33
	51–65	10	5	8	5	13	41
	66–85	1	0	3	2	5	11

Table 2.2 Categorizing the number of physician visits

Latent number of visits	**Visit category**	**1985 visit**
0	None	$K_1 = 39$
1–2	Few	$K_2 = 60$
3–5	Not so few	$K_3 = 37$
6 or more	High	$K_4 = 44$

covariates such as gender, age, education level, and chronic conditions for each of these 180 members were also collected. The full data set is available in Sutradhar (2011, Appendix 6A). The primary objective of this study was to examine the effects of these covariates on the physician visits by accommodating familial and longitudinal correlations among the responses of the members. To have a feeling about this data set, we reproduce below in Table 2.1, some summary statistics on the physicians visit data for 1985 only.

Suppose that we group the physician visits into $J = 4$ categories as in Table 2.2. In the same table we also give the 1985 health status for 180 individuals.

Note that an individual can belong to one of the four categories with a multinomial probability as in (2.3). Now by ignoring the family grouping, that is, assuming all 180 individuals are independent, and by ignoring the effects of the covariates on the visits, one may use the multinomial probability model (2.17) to fit the data in Table 2.2.

Now by (2.23), one obtains the likelihood estimate for π_j, for $j = 1,\ldots,4$, as

$$\hat{\pi}_{j,ML} = \frac{K_j}{K},$$

where $K = 180$. Thus, for example, for $j = 1$, since, $K_1 = 39$ individuals did not pay any visits to the physician, an estimate (likelihood or moment) for the probability that an individual in St. John's in 1985 belong to category 1 was

$$\hat{\pi}_{1,ML} = \hat{\pi}_{1,MM} = 39/180 = 0.217.$$

That is, approximately 22 out of 100 people did not pay any visits to the physician in St. John's (indicating the size of the group with no health complications) during that year. Note that these naive estimates are bound to change when multinomial probabilities will be modeled involving the covariates. This type of multinomial regression model will be discussed in Sect. 2.2 and in many other places in the book.

2.1.3 *Inference for Category Effects β_{j0}, $j = 1,\ldots,J-1$, with $\beta_{J0} = 0$*

2.1.3.1 Moment Estimating Equations for $\beta_{j0}(j = 1,\ldots,J-1)$ Using Regression Form

Because

$$E[K_j] = K\pi_j \text{ for } j = 1,\ldots,J-1,$$

with

$$\pi_j = \frac{m_j}{m} = \frac{\exp(\beta_{j0})}{1 + \sum_{j=1}^{J-1}\exp(\beta_{j0})} = \frac{\exp(x_j'\theta)}{\sum_{j=1}^{J}\exp(x_j'\theta)},$$

and π_J has to satisfy the relationship

$$\pi_J = 1 - \sum_{j=1}^{J-1}\pi_j = 1 - \sum_{j=1}^{J-1}\frac{K_j}{K} = \frac{K_J}{K},$$

one needs to solve for $\theta = (\beta_{10},\ldots,\beta_{j0},\ldots,\beta_{J-1,0})'$ satisfying

$$K_j - K\pi_j = 0, \text{ for all } j = 1,\ldots,J.$$

For convenience, we express all π_j as functions of θ. We do this by using

$$x_j = (01'_{j-1}, 1, 01'_{J-1-j})' \text{ for } j = 1,\ldots,J-1, \text{ and } x_J = 01_{J-1},$$

so that

$$\pi_j = \frac{\exp(x'_j\theta)}{\sum_{j=1}^{J}\exp(x'_j\theta)}, \text{ for all } j = 1,\ldots,J. \tag{2.24}$$

Now solving the moment equations $K_j - K\pi_j = 0$ for $\theta = (\beta_{10},\ldots,\beta_{j0},\ldots,\beta_{J-1,0})'$ is equivalent to solve

$$f(\theta) = X'(y - K\pi) = 0, \tag{2.25}$$

for θ, where $y = (K_1,\ldots,K_j,\ldots,K_J)'$, $\pi = (\pi_1,\ldots,\pi_j,\ldots,\pi_J)'$, and

$$X = \begin{pmatrix} x'_1 \\ x'_2 \\ \cdot \\ x'_{J-1} \\ x'_J \end{pmatrix} = \begin{pmatrix} 1\,0 \cdot 0\,0 \\ 0\,1 \cdot 0\,0 \\ \cdot\;\cdot\;\cdot\;\cdot\;\cdot \\ 0\,0 \cdot 0\,1 \\ 0\,0 \cdot 0\,0 \end{pmatrix} : J \times J-1.$$

2.1.3.2 Marginal Likelihood Estimation for β_{j0} ($j = 1,\ldots, J$-1) with $\beta_{J0} = 0$

Note that due to invariance principle of the likelihood estimation method, one would end up with solving the same likelihood estimating equation (2.23) even if one attempts to obtain the likelihood estimating equations for β_{j0}, $j = 1,\ldots,J-1$, directly. We clarify this point through following direct calculations.

Rewrite the multinomial distribution based log likelihood function (2.20) as

$$logL(\pi_1,\ldots,\pi_J) = k_0 + \sum_{j=1}^{J} K_j log(\pi_j),$$

where, by (2.17), π_j has the formulas

$$\pi_j = \begin{cases} \frac{\exp(\beta_{j0})}{1+\sum_{j=1}^{J-1}\exp(\beta_{j0})} & \text{for } j = 1,\ldots,J-1 \\ \frac{1}{1+\sum_{j=1}^{J-1}\exp(\beta_{j0})} & \text{for } j = J. \end{cases}$$

It then follows for $j = 1,\ldots,J-1$, that

$$\frac{\partial logL(\pi_1,\ldots,\pi_J)}{\partial\beta_{j0}} = \sum_{c=1}^{J-1}\left[\frac{K_c}{\pi_c}\right]\frac{\partial\pi_c}{\partial\beta_{j0}} + [\frac{K_J}{\pi_J}]\frac{\partial\pi_J}{\partial\beta_{j0}}, \tag{2.26}$$

where

$$\frac{\partial \pi_c}{\partial \beta_{j0}} = \begin{cases} \frac{\{1+\sum_{c=1}^{J-1}\exp(\beta_{c0})\}\exp(\beta_{j0})-\exp(\beta_{j0})\{\exp(\beta_{j0})\}}{\left[1+\sum_{c=1}^{J-1}\exp(\beta_{c0})\right]^2} = \pi_j(1-\pi_j) & \text{for } c=j \\ \frac{-\exp(\beta_{c0})\{\exp(\beta_{j0})\}}{\left[1+\sum_{c=1}^{J-1}\exp(\beta_{c0})\right]^2} = -\pi_c\pi_j & \text{for } c \neq j,\ c=1,\ldots,J-1. \\ \frac{-\exp(\beta_{j0})}{\left[1+\sum_{c=1}^{J-1}\exp(\beta_{c0})\right]^2} = -\pi_J\pi_j & \text{for } c=J. \end{cases} \tag{2.27}$$

By using (2.27) in (2.26), we then write the likelihood equation for β_{j0} as

$$\frac{\partial logL(\pi_1,\ldots,\pi_J)}{\partial \beta_{j0}} = \sum_{c=1}^{J}[\frac{K_c}{\pi_c}][-\pi_c\pi_j] + \frac{K_j}{\pi_j}[\pi_j] = 0, \tag{2.28}$$

yielding

$$-K\pi_j + K_j = 0, \text{for } j=1,\ldots,J-1, \tag{2.29}$$

which are the same likelihood equations as in (2.23). Thus, in the likelihood approach, similar to the moment approach, one solves the estimating equation (2.25), that is,

$$f(\theta) = X'(y - K\pi) = 0 \tag{2.30}$$

for θ iteratively, so that $f(\hat{\theta}) = 0$.

Further note that because of the definition of π_j given by (2.2) or (2.17), all estimates $\hat{\beta}_{j0}$ for $j=1,\ldots,J-1$ are interpreted comparing their value with $\beta_{J0}=0$.

2.1.3.3 Joint Estimation of $\beta_{10},\ldots,\beta_{j0},\ldots,\beta_{J\text{-}1,0}$ Using Regression Form

The log likelihood function by (2.20) has the form

$$logL(\beta_{10},\ldots,\beta_{(J-1)0}) = k_0 + \sum_{j=1}^{J} K_j log\, \pi_j.$$

We now write $m_j = \exp(\beta_{j0})$ for $j=1,\ldots,J-1$, and $m_J = \exp(\beta_{J0}) = 1$, and $m = \sum_{j=1}^{J} m_j$, and re-express the above log likelihood function as

$$logL(\beta_{10},\ldots,\beta_{(J-1)0}) = k_0 + \sum_{j=1}^{J} K_j[log\, m_j - log\, m]. \tag{2.31}$$

Next for $\theta = (\beta_{10},\ldots,\beta_{j0},\ldots,\beta_{(J-1)0})'$ express $\log m_j$ in linear regression form

$$\log m_j = x_j'\theta \tag{2.32}$$

such that $\log m_j = \beta_{j0}$ for $j = 1,\ldots,J-1$, and $\log m_J = 0$. Note that finding x'_j for all $j = 1,\ldots,J$ is equivalent to write

$$\log \tilde{m} = [\log m_1,\ldots,\log m_j,\ldots,\log m_J]' = X\theta,$$

where the $J \times (J-1)$ covariate matrix X has the same form as in (2.25), i.e.,

$$X = \begin{pmatrix} x'_1 \\ x'_2 \\ \cdot \\ x'_{J-1} \\ x'_J \end{pmatrix} = \begin{pmatrix} 1\,0\cdot 0\,0 \\ 0\,1\cdot 0\,0 \\ \cdot\;\cdot\;\cdot\;\cdot\;\cdot \\ 0\,0\cdot 0\,1 \\ 0\,0\cdot 0\,0 \end{pmatrix} : J \times J-1. \tag{2.33}$$

It then follows from (2.31) and (2.32) that

$$\begin{aligned} f(\theta) = \frac{\partial logL(\theta)}{\partial\theta} &= \frac{\partial}{\partial\theta}[\sum_{j=1}^{J} K_j x'_j\theta - K log\, m] \\ &= \sum_{j=1}^{J} K_j x_j - \frac{K}{m}\frac{\partial}{\partial\theta}[\sum_{j=1}^{J}\exp(x'_j\theta)] \\ &= \sum_{j=1}^{J} K_j x_j - \frac{K}{m}\sum_{j=1}^{J} m_j x_j \\ &= \sum_{j=1}^{J} K_j x_j - K\sum_{j=1}^{J}\pi_j x_j, \end{aligned} \tag{2.34}$$

yielding the likelihood estimating equation

$$f(\theta) = X'(y - K\pi) = 0, \tag{2.35}$$

same as (2.30).

2.1.3.3.1 Likelihood Estimates and their Asymptotic Variances

Because the likelihood estimating equations in (2.35) are non-linear, one obtains the estimate of $\theta = (\beta_{10},\ldots,\beta_{j0},\ldots,\beta_{J-1,0})'$ iteratively, so that $f(\hat{\theta}) = 0$. Suppose that $\hat{\theta}_0$ is not a solution for $f(\theta) = 0$, but a trial estimate and hence $f(\hat{\theta}_0) \neq 0$. Next suppose that $\hat{\theta} = \hat{\theta}_0 + h^*$ is the estimate of θ satisfying $f(\hat{\theta}) = f(\hat{\theta}_0 + h^*) = 0$. Now by using the first order Taylor's expansion, one writes

$$f(\hat{\theta}) = f(\hat{\theta}_0 + h^*) = f(\hat{\theta}_0) + h^* f'(\theta)|_{\theta=\hat{\theta}_0} = f(\theta)|_{\theta=\hat{\theta}_0} + (\hat{\theta} - \hat{\theta}_0) f'(\theta)|_{\theta=\hat{\theta}_0} = 0$$

yielding the solution

$$\hat{\theta} = \hat{\theta}_0 - \left[\{f'(\theta)\}^{-1} f(\theta)\right] |_{\theta=\hat{\theta}_0}. \tag{2.36}$$

Further, because

$$\begin{aligned}
\frac{\partial \pi_j}{\partial \theta'} &= \frac{1}{m^2}[m\frac{\partial m_j}{\partial \theta'} - m_j \frac{\partial m}{\partial \theta'}] \\
&= \frac{1}{m^2}[mm_j x'_j - m_j \sum_{j=1}^{J} m_j x'_j] \\
&= \pi_j x'_j - \pi_j \sum_{j=1}^{J} \pi_j x'_j \\
&= \pi_j x'_j - \pi_j \pi' X,
\end{aligned} \tag{2.37}$$

one obtains

$$K\frac{\partial \pi_j}{\partial \theta'} = K[\pi_j x'_j - \pi_j \pi' X]. \tag{2.38}$$

Consequently, it follows from (2.35) that

$$\begin{aligned}
f'(\theta) = -KX'\frac{\partial \pi}{\partial \theta'} &= -KX'\{\text{diag}[\pi_1, \ldots, \pi_J] - \pi\pi'\}X \\
&= -KX'[D_\pi - \pi\pi']X,
\end{aligned} \tag{2.39}$$

and the iterative equation (2.36) takes the form

$$\hat{\theta}(r+1) = \hat{\theta}(r) + \left[\frac{1}{K}[X'\{D_\pi - \pi\pi'\}X]^{-1}X'(y - K\pi)\right]_{\theta=\hat{\theta}(r)}, \tag{2.40}$$

yielding the final estimate $\hat{\theta}$. The covariance matrix of $\hat{\theta}$ has the formula

$$\text{var}(\hat{\theta}) = \frac{1}{K}\left[X'\{D_\pi - \pi\pi'\}X\right]^{-1}. \tag{2.41}$$

2.1.4 Likelihood Inference for Categorical Effects $\beta_{j0}, j = 1, \ldots, J-1$ with $\beta_{J0} = -\sum_{j=1}^{J-1} \beta_{j0}$ Using Regression Form

There exists an alternative modeling for π_j such that $\hat{\beta}_{j0}$ for $j = 1, \ldots, J-1$ are interpreted by using the restriction

$$\sum_{j=1}^{J} \hat{\beta}_{j0} = 0, \text{ that is, } \hat{\beta}_{J0} = -\sum_{j=1}^{J-1} \hat{\beta}_{j0}.$$

As opposed to (2.17), π_j's are then defined as

$$\pi_j = \begin{cases} \frac{\exp(\beta_{j0})}{\sum_{c=1}^{J-1} \exp(\beta_{c0}) + \exp(-\sum_{c=1}^{J-1} \beta_{c0})} & \text{for} j = 1, \ldots, J-1 \\ \frac{\exp(-\sum_{c=1}^{J-1} \beta_{c0})}{\sum_{c=1}^{J-1} \exp(\beta_{c0}) + \exp(-\sum_{c=1}^{J-1} \beta_{c0})} & \text{for } j = J. \end{cases} \quad (2.42)$$

Now for $m_j = \exp(\beta_{j0})$ for $j = 1, \ldots, J-1$, and $m_J = \exp(-\sum_{c=1}^{J-1} \beta_{c0})$, one may use the linear form $\log m_j = x_j' \theta$, that is,

$$\log \tilde{m} = [\log m_1, \ldots, \log m_j, \ldots, \log m_J]' = X\theta,$$

where, unlike in (2.25) and (2.33), X now is the $J \times (J-1)$ covariate matrix defined as

$$X = \begin{pmatrix} 1 & 0 & \cdot & 0 & 0 \\ 0 & 1 & \cdot & 0 & 0 \\ \cdot & \cdot & \cdot & \cdot & \cdot \\ 0 & 0 & \cdot & 0 & 1 \\ -1 & -1 & \cdot & -1 & -1 \end{pmatrix}. \quad (2.43)$$

Thus, the likelihood estimating equation has the same form

$$f(\theta) = X'(y - K\pi) = 0 \quad (2.44)$$

as in (2.35), but with covariate matrix X as in (2.43) which is different than that of (2.33).

Note that because $\beta_{J0} = 0$ leads to different covariate matrix X as compared to the covariate matrix under the assumption $\beta_{J0} = -\sum_{j=1}^{J-1} \beta_{j0}$, the likelihood estimates for $\theta = (\beta_{10}, \ldots, \beta_{(J-1)0})'$ would be different under these two assumptions.

2.2 Univariate Multinomial Regression Model

2.2.1 *Individual History Based Fixed Regression Effects Model*

Suppose that a history based survey is done so that in addition to the categorical response status, an individual also provides p covariates information. Let $w_i = [w_{i1}, \ldots, w_{is}, \ldots, w_{ip}]'$ denote the p-dimensional covariate vector available from the ith $(i = 1,\ldots,K)$ individual. To incorporate this covariate information, the multinomial probability model (2.1)–(2.2) may be generalized as

$$P[y_i = y_i^{(j)} = \delta_{ij}] = \pi_{(i)j} = \begin{cases} \frac{\exp(\beta_{j0}+\beta_j' w_i)}{1+\sum_{g=1}^{J-1}\exp(\beta_{g0}+\beta_g' w_i)} & \text{for } j = 1,\ldots,J-1 \\ \frac{1}{1+\sum_{g=1}^{J-1}\exp(\beta_{g0}+\beta_g' w_i)} & \text{for } j = J, \end{cases} \tag{2.45}$$

(see also Agresti 1990, p. 343, Exercise 9.22) where $\beta_j = [\beta_{j1},\ldots,\beta_{js},\ldots,\beta_{jp}]'$ for $j = 1,\ldots,J-1$. Let

$$\theta^* = [\beta_1^{*'},\ldots,\beta_j^{*'},\ldots,\beta_{J-1}^{*}{}']', \text{ where } \beta_j^* = [\beta_{j0},\beta_j']'.$$

Then as an extension to (2.4), one may write the likelihood function as

$$L(\theta^*) = L(\beta_1^*,\ldots,\beta_{J-1}^*) = \prod_{i=1}^{K}\prod_{j=1}^{J} \frac{1! \times \{\pi_{(i)j}\}^{y_{ij}}}{y_{ij}!} \tag{2.46}$$

where $y_{iJ} = \left(1 - \sum_{j=1}^{J-1} y_{ij}\right)$ and $\pi_{(i)J} = \left(1 - \sum_{j=1}^{J-1} \pi_{(i)j}\right)$. It then follows that the likelihood estimating equation for $\beta_j^* = \left(\beta_{j0}, \beta_j'\right)'$ for $j = 1,\ldots,J-1$, that is,

$$\begin{aligned} \frac{\partial logL(\theta^*)}{\partial \beta_j^*} &= \frac{\partial}{\partial \beta_j^*}\left[C + \sum_{i=1}^{K}\sum_{g=1}^{J-1} y_{ig}\begin{pmatrix}1\\ w_i\end{pmatrix}'\beta_g^* - \sum_{i=1}^{K} log\left\{1 + \sum_{g=1}^{J-1}\begin{pmatrix}1\\ w_i\end{pmatrix}'\beta_g^*\right\}\right] \\ &= \sum_{i=1}^{K}\left[\begin{pmatrix}1\\ w_i\end{pmatrix} y_{ij} - \begin{pmatrix}1\\ w_i\end{pmatrix}\pi_{(i)j}\right] \\ &= \sum_{i=1}^{K}\begin{pmatrix}1\\ w_i\end{pmatrix}\left[y_{ij} - \pi_{(i)j}\right] = 0, \end{aligned} \tag{2.47}$$

leads to the likelihood equation for θ^* as

$$\frac{\partial logL(\theta^*)}{\partial \theta^*} = \sum_{i=1}^{K}\left[I_{J-1} \otimes \begin{pmatrix}1\\ w_i\end{pmatrix}\right]\left[y_i - \pi_{(i)}\right] = 0 \tag{2.48}$$

where $\pi_{(i)} = \left(\pi_{(i)1},\cdots,\pi_{(i)(J-1)}\right)'$ corresponding to $y_i = (y_{i1},\ldots,y_{i(J-1)})'$; w_i is the $p \times 1$ design vector, I_{J-1} is the identity matrix of order $J-1$, and $\otimes$ denotes the Kronecker or direct product. In (2.47), C is a normalizing constant.

This likelihood equation (2.48) may be solved for θ^* by using the iterative equation

Table 2.3 Snoring and heart disease: A frequency table

	Heart disease	
Snoring	Yes	No
Never	24	1355
Occasionally	35	603
Nearly every night	21	192
Every night	30	224

$$\hat{\theta}^*(r+1) = \hat{\theta}^*(r) + \left[\sum_{i=1}^{K}\left[I_{J-1}\otimes\begin{pmatrix}1\\ w_i\end{pmatrix}\right]\left[\text{diag}[\pi_{i1},\ldots,\pi_{J-1}] - \pi_{(i)}\pi'_{(i)}\right]\left[I_{J-1}\otimes\begin{pmatrix}1\\ w_i\end{pmatrix}\right]'\right]^{-1}_{|\hat{\theta}^*(r)}$$
$$\times\sum_{i=1}^{K}\left[I_{J-1}\otimes\begin{pmatrix}1\\ w_i\end{pmatrix}\right]\left[y_i - \pi_{(i)}\right]_{|\hat{\theta}^*(r)}, \quad (2.49)$$

and the variances of the estimator may be found from the covariance matrix

$$\text{var}[\hat{\theta}^*] = \left[\sum_{i=1}^{K}\left[I_{J-1}\otimes\begin{pmatrix}1\\ w_i\end{pmatrix}\right]\left[\text{diag}[\pi_{i1},\ldots,\pi_{J-1}] - \pi_{(i)}\pi'_{(i)}\right]\left[I_{J-1}\otimes\begin{pmatrix}1\\ w_i\end{pmatrix}\right]'\right]^{-1}. \quad (2.50)$$

Note that in the absence of covariates, one estimates $\theta^* = [\beta_{10},\ldots,\beta_{j0},\ldots,\beta_{J-1.0}]'$. In this case, the estimating equation (2.48) for θ^* reduces to the estimating equation (2.35) for θ, because $\sum_{i=1}^{K} y_{ij} = K_j$ and $\sum_{i=1}^{K}\pi_{(i)j} = \sum_{i=1}^{K}\pi_j = K\pi_j$, for example.

2.2.1.1 Illustration 2.2: Binary Regression Model ($J = 2$) with One Covariate

2.2.1.1 (a) An Existing Analysis (Snoring as a Continuous Covariate with Arbitrary Values)

Consider the heart disease and snoring relationship problem discussed in Agresti (2002, Section 4.2.3, p. 121–123). The data is given in the following Table 2.3.

By treating snoring as an one dimensional ($p = 1$) fixed covariate $w_i = w_{i1}$ for the ith individual with its values

$$w_i \equiv w_{i1} = 0, 2, 4, 5, \quad (2.51)$$

for snoring never, occasionally, nearly every night, and every night, respectively, and treating the heart disease status as the binary ($J = 2$) variable and writing

$$y_i = y_{i1} = \begin{cases} 1 \text{ if } i \in \text{yes} \\ 0 \text{ otherwise,} \end{cases}$$

Agresti (2002, Section 4.2.3, p. 121–123), for example, analyzed this 'snoring and heart disease' data by fitting the binary probability model (a special case of the multinomial probability model (2.45))

$$P[y_i = y_i^{(1)}] = P[y_{i1} = 1] = \pi_{(i)1}(w_i) = \frac{\exp(\beta_{10} + \beta_{11} w_i)}{1 + \exp(\beta_{10} + \beta_{11} w_i)}, \tag{2.52}$$

and

$$P[y_i = y_i^{(2)}] = P[y_{i1} = 0] = \pi_{(i)2}(w_i) = \frac{1}{1 + \exp(\beta_{10} + \beta_{11} w_i)}.$$

The binary likelihood is then given by

$$\begin{aligned} L(\theta^*) = L(\beta_{10}, \beta_{11}) &= \Pi_{i=1}^{K} [\pi_{(i)1}(w_i)]^{y_{i1}} [\pi_{(i)2}(w_i)]^{y_{i2}} \\ &= \Pi_{i=1}^{K} [\pi_{(i)1}(w_i)]^{y_{i1}} [1 - \pi_{(i)1}(w_i)]^{1-y_{i1}}, \end{aligned} \tag{2.53}$$

yielding the log likelihood estimating equations as

$$\frac{\partial log\, L(\theta^*)}{\partial \theta^*} = \frac{\partial log \Pi_{i=1}^{K} \frac{\exp[y_{i1}(w_i^{*\prime}\theta^*)]}{1+\exp(w_i^{*\prime}\theta^*)}}{\partial \theta^*} = 0, \tag{2.54}$$

where

$$w_i^{*\prime} = (1, w_i), \text{ and } \theta^* = \beta_1^* = (\beta_{10}, \beta_{11})'.$$

This log likelihood equations may be simplified as

$$\begin{aligned} \frac{\partial log\, L(\theta^*)}{\partial \theta^*} &= \sum_{i=1}^{K} y_{i1} w_i^* - \sum_{i=1}^{K} \pi_{(i)1} w_i^* \\ &= \sum_{i=1}^{K} w_i^* [y_{i1} - \pi_{(i)1}] \\ &= \sum_{i=1}^{K} \begin{pmatrix} 1 \\ w_i \end{pmatrix} [y_{i1} - \pi_{(i)1}] = 0. \end{aligned} \tag{2.55}$$

Note that the binary likelihood equation (2.45) is a special case of the multinomial likelihood equation (2.48) with $J = 2$. This equation may be solved for $\hat{\theta}^*$ by using the iterative equation

$$\hat{\theta}^*(r+1) = \hat{\theta}^*(r) + \left[\sum_{i=1}^{K} \begin{pmatrix} 1 \\ w_i \end{pmatrix} \left[\pi_{(i)1}(1 - \pi_{(i)}) \right] \begin{pmatrix} 1 \\ w_i \end{pmatrix}' \right]^{-1}_{|\hat{\theta}^*(r)}$$

$$\times \sum_{i=1}^{K} \begin{pmatrix} 1 \\ w_i \end{pmatrix} \left[y_i - \pi_{(i)1} \right]_{|\hat{\theta}^*(r)}, \tag{2.56}$$

and the variances of the estimator may be found from the covariance matrix

$$\text{var}[\hat{\theta}^*] = \left[\sum_{i=1}^{K} \begin{pmatrix} 1 \\ w_i \end{pmatrix} \left[\pi_{(i)1}(1 - \pi_{(i)1}) \right] \begin{pmatrix} 1 \\ w_i \end{pmatrix}' \right]^{-1}. \tag{2.57}$$

For the snoring and heart disease relationship problem, the scalar covariate ($w_i = w_{i1}$) based estimates are given by

$$\hat{\theta}^* = \hat{\beta}_1^* \equiv [\hat{\beta}_{10} = -3.87, \text{ and } \hat{\beta}_{11} = 0.40]'.$$

However using this type of scalar covariate, i.e., $w_i = w_{i1}$ with arbitrary values for snoring levels does not provide actual effects of the snoring on heart disease. Below, we illustrate a categorical covariate based estimation for this problem.

2.2.1.1 (b) A Refined Analysis (Snoring as a Fixed Covariate with Four Nominal Levels)

In the aforementioned existing analysis, the snoring status: never, occasionally, nearly every night, every night, has been denoted by a covariate w with values $0, 2, 4$, and 5, respectively. This is an arbitrary coding and may not correctly reflect the levels. To avoid confusion, in the proposed book, we will represent these $L = 4$ levels of the 'snoring' covariate for the ith individual by three dummy covariates ($p = 3$) w_{i1}, w_{i2}, w_{i3} with values

$$(w_{i1}, w_{i2}, w_{i3}) = \begin{cases} (1,0,0) \text{ for occasionally snoring, level 1 } (\ell{=}1) \\ (0,1,0) \text{ for nearly every night snoring, level 2 } (\ell{=}2) \\ (0,0,1) \text{ for every night snoring, level 3 } (\ell{=}3) \\ (0,0,0) \text{ for never snoring, level 4 } (\ell{=}4). \end{cases}$$

Now for $j = 1, \ldots, J-1$ with $J = 2$, by using $\beta_{j1}, \beta_{j2}, \beta_{j3}$ as the effects of w_{i1}, w_{i2}, w_{i3}, on an individual's ($i = 1, \ldots, K$) heart status belonging to jth category, one may fit the probability model (2.45) to this binary data. For convenience, write the model as

$$\pi_{(i)j} = \begin{cases} \dfrac{\exp(\beta_{j0}+\beta_{j1}w_{i1}+\beta_{j2}w_{i2}+\beta_{j3}w_{i3})}{1+\sum_{g=1}^{J-1}\exp(\beta_{g0}+\beta_{g1}w_{i1}+\beta_{g2}w_{i2}+\beta_{g3}w_{i3})} & \text{for } j = 1 \\ \dfrac{1}{1+\sum_{g=1}^{J-1}\exp(\beta_{g0}+\beta_{g1}w_{i1}+\beta_{g2}w_{i2}+\beta_{g3}w_{i3})} & \text{for } j = J = 2. \end{cases} \tag{2.58}$$

It is of interest to estimate the parameters $\theta^* = \beta_1^* = (\beta_{10}, \beta_{11}, \beta_{12}, \beta_{13})'$.

After a slight modification, we may use the likelihood equation (2.45) to estimate these parameters. More specifically, by (2.45), the likelihood equation for $\theta^* = \beta_1^*$ now has the form

$$\sum_{i=1}^{K} w_i^* [y_{i1} - \pi_{(i)1}] = \sum_{i=1}^{K} \begin{pmatrix} 1 \\ w_{i1} \\ w_{i2} \\ w_{i3} \end{pmatrix} [y_{i1} - \pi_{(i)1}] = 0. \tag{2.59}$$

This equation may be solved for $\hat{\theta}^*$ iteratively by using

$$\hat{\theta}^*(r+1) = \hat{\theta}^*(r) + \left[\sum_{i=1}^{K} \begin{pmatrix} 1 \\ w_{i1} \\ w_{i2} \\ w_{i3} \end{pmatrix} \left[\pi_{(i)1}(1-\pi_{(i)}) \right] \begin{pmatrix} 1 \\ w_{i1} \\ w_{i2} \\ w_{i3} \end{pmatrix}' \right]^{-1}_{|\hat{\theta}^*(r)}$$

$$\times \sum_{i=1}^{K} \begin{pmatrix} 1 \\ w_{i1} \\ w_{i2} \\ w_{i3} \end{pmatrix} \left[y_i - \pi_{(i)1} \right]_{|\hat{\theta}^*(r)}, \tag{2.60}$$

and the variances of the estimator may be found from the covariance matrix

$$\text{var}[\hat{\theta}^*] = \left[\sum_{i=1}^{K} \begin{pmatrix} 1 \\ w_{i1} \\ w_{i2} \\ w_{i3} \end{pmatrix} \left[\pi_{(i)1}(1-\pi_{(i)1}) \right] \begin{pmatrix} 1 \\ w_{i1} \\ w_{i2} \\ w_{i3} \end{pmatrix}' \right]^{-1} \tag{2.61}$$

2.2.2 *Multinomial Likelihood Models Involving One Covariate with $L = p + 1$ Nominal Levels*

Suppose that the $L = p + 1$ levels of a covariate for an individual i may be represented by p dummy covariates as

$$(w_{i1}, \cdots, w_{ip}) \equiv \begin{cases} (1, 0, \cdots, 0) \longrightarrow \text{Level 1} \\ (0, 1, \cdots, 0) \longrightarrow \text{Level 2} \\ (\cdots\cdots\cdots\cdots) \\ (0, 0, \cdots, 1) \longrightarrow \text{Level p} \\ (0, 0, \cdots, 0) \longrightarrow \text{Level p+1} \end{cases} \tag{2.62}$$

Table 2.4 A notational display for cell counts and probabilities for J categories under each covariate level ℓ

		J categories of the response variable					
Covariate level	**Quantity**	1	...	j	...	J	**Total**
1	Cell count	$K_{[1]1}$	...	$K_{[1]j}$	...	$K_{[1]J}$	$K_{[1]}$
	Cell probability	$\pi_{[1]1}$	...	$\pi_{[1]j}$	...	$\pi_{[1]J}$	1
.	.	.	...	.	...	.	.
	.	.	...	.	...	.	.
ℓ	Cell count	$K_{[\ell]1}$	...	$K_{[\ell]j}$	...	$K_{[\ell]J}$	$K_{[\ell]}$
	Cell probability	$\pi_{[\ell]1}$	...	$\pi_{[\ell]j}$	...	$\pi_{[\ell]J}$	1
.	.	.	...	.	...	.	.
	.	.	...	.	...	.	.
$L=p+1$	Cell count	$K_{[p+1]1}$	...	$K_{[p+1]j}$	...	$K_{[p+1]J}$	$K_{[p+1]}$
	Cell probability	$\pi_{[p+1]1}$	...	$\pi_{[p+1]j}$	...	$\pi_{[p+1]J}$	1
	Total count	K_1	...	K_j	...	K_J	K

By (2.45), one may then write the probability for an individual i with covariate at level $\ell(\ell = 1,\ldots,p)$ to be in the jth category as

$$\pi_{[\ell]j} = \pi_{(i\in\ell)j} = \begin{cases} \frac{\exp(\beta_{j0}+\beta_{j\ell})}{1+\sum_{g=1}^{J-1}\exp(\beta_{g0}+\beta_{g\ell})} & \text{for } j = 1,\ldots,J-1 \\ \frac{1}{1+\sum_{g=1}^{J-1}\exp(\beta_{g0}+\beta_{g\ell})} & \text{for } j = J, \end{cases} \tag{2.63}$$

whereas for $\ell = p+1$, these probabilities are written as

$$\pi_{[p+1]j} = \pi_{(i\in(p+1))j} = \begin{cases} \frac{\exp(\beta_{j0})}{1+\sum_{g=1}^{J-1}\exp(\beta_{g0})} & \text{for } j = 1,\ldots,J-1 \\ \frac{1}{1+\sum_{g=1}^{J-1}\exp(\beta_{g0})} & \text{for } j = J. \end{cases} \tag{2.64}$$

Using the level based probability notation from (2.63)–(2.64) into (2.46), one may write the likelihood function as

$$\begin{aligned} L(\theta^*) &= L[(\beta_1^*,\ldots,\beta_j^*,\ldots,\beta_{(J-1)}^*)|y] \\ &= \Pi_{\ell=1}^{p+1}\Pi_{i\in\ell}^{K_{[\ell]}} \frac{1!}{y_{i1}!y_{i2}!\ldots y_{iJ}!}\pi_{[i\in(\ell)]1}^{y_{i1}}\pi_{[i\in(\ell)]2}^{y_{i2}}\cdots,\pi_{[i\in(\ell)]J}^{y_{iJ}}, \end{aligned} \tag{2.65}$$

where $\beta_j^* = (\beta_{j0},\beta_{j1},\ldots,\beta_{jp})'$, and $K_{[\ell]}$ denotes the number of individuals with covariate level ℓ so that $\sum_{\ell=1}^{p+1} K_{[\ell]} = K$. Further suppose that $K_{[\ell]j}$ denote the number of individuals those belong to the jth response category with covariate level ℓ so that $\sum_{j=1}^{J} K_{[\ell]j} = K_{[\ell]}$. For convenience of writing the likelihood estimating equations, we have displayed these notations for cell counts and cell probabilities as in the $L \times J$ contingency Table 2.4.

Note that in our notation, the row dimension L refers to the combined L levels for the categorical covariates under consideration, and J refers to the number of categories of a response variable. By this token, in Chap. 4, a contingency table for a bivariate multinomial problem with L level categorical covariates will be referred to as the $L \times R \times J$ contingency table, where J refers to the number of categories of the multinomial response variable Y as in this chapter, and R refers to the number of categories of the other multinomial response variable Z, say. When this notational scheme is used, the contingency Table 2.2 with four categories for Y (physician visit status) but no covariates, has the dimension 1×4. Thus, for a model involving no covariates, $p = 0$, i.e., $L = 1$. Further, when there are, for example, two categorical covariates in the model one with $p_1 + 1$ levels and the other with $p_2 + 1$ levels, one uses $p_1 + p_2$ dummy covariates to represent these $L = (p_1 + 1)(p_2 + 1)$ levels.

Turning back to the likelihood function (2.65), because $y_{ij} = 1$ or 0, with $\sum_{j=1}^{J} y_{ij} = 1$, by using the cell counts from Table 2.4, one may re-express this likelihood function as

$$L(\theta^*) = L[(\beta_1^*, \ldots, \beta_j^*, \ldots, \beta_{(J-1)}^*|y] = \Pi_{\ell=1}^{p+1} (\pi_{[\ell]1})^{K_{[\ell]1}} \ldots (\pi_{[\ell]J})^{K_{[\ell]J}}. \tag{2.66}$$

which one will maximize to estimate the desired parameters in θ^*.

2.2.2.1 Product Multinomial Likelihood Based Estimating Equations with a Global Regression form Using all Parameters

In some situations, it may be appropriate to assume that the cell counts for a given level in Table 2.3 follow a multinomial distribution and the distributions corresponding to any two levels are independent. For example, in a gender related study, male and females may be interviewed separately and hence $K_{[\ell]}$ at ℓth level may be assumed to be known, and they may be distributed in J cells, i.e., J categories, following the multinomial distribution. Note that in this approach K is not needed to be known in advance, rather all values for $K_{[\ell]}$ together yield $\sum_{\ell=1}^{L} K_{[\ell]} = K$. Following Table 2.4, we write this multinomial probability function at level ℓ as

$$f(K_{[\ell]1}, \ldots, K_{[\ell](J-1)}) = \frac{K_{[\ell]}!}{K_{[\ell]1}! \ldots K_{[\ell]J}!} \Pi_{j=1}^{J} [\pi_{[\ell]j}]^{K_{[\ell]j}} = L_\ell, \tag{2.67}$$

yielding the product multinomial function as

$$L(\theta^*) = \Pi_{\ell=1}^{p+1} f(K_{[\ell]1}, \ldots, K_{[\ell](J-1)}) = \Pi_{\ell=1}^{p+1} L_\ell. \tag{2.68}$$

At a given level $\ell (\ell = 1, \ldots, p+1)$, one may then write the probabilities in (2.63)–(2.64) for all $j = 1, \ldots, J$, as

$$\pi_{[\ell]j} = \frac{\exp(x'_{[\ell]j}\theta^*)}{\sum_{g=1}^{J}\exp(x'_{[\ell]g}\theta^*)}, \tag{2.69}$$

where

$$\theta^* = [\beta_1^{*\prime}, \ldots, \beta_j^{*\prime}, \ldots, \beta_{J-1}^{*}{}']', \text{ with } \beta_j^* = [\beta_{j0}, \beta_j']',$$

and $x'_{[\ell]j}$ is the jth ($j = 1, \ldots, J$) row of the $J \times (J-1)(p+1)$ matrix X_ℓ, defined for ℓth level as follows:

$$X_\ell = \begin{pmatrix} x'_{[\ell]1} \\ x'_{[\ell]2} \\ \cdot \\ x'_{[\ell](J-1)} \\ x'_{[\ell]J} \end{pmatrix}$$

$$= \begin{pmatrix} 1\ 01'_{\ell-1}, 1, 01'_{p-\ell} & 0 & 01'_p & \cdot\ 0 & 01'_p \\ 0 & 01'_p & 1\ 01'_{\ell-1}, 1, 01'_{p-\ell} & \cdot\ 0 & 01'_p \\ \cdot & \cdot & \cdot & \cdot\ \cdot & \cdot \\ 0 & 01'_p & 0 & 01'_p & \cdot\ 1\ 01'_{\ell-1}, 1, 01'_{p-\ell} \\ 0 & 01'_p & 0 & 01'_p & \cdot\ 0 \quad 01'_p \end{pmatrix} \text{ for } \ell = 1, \ldots, p$$

$$X_{p+1} = \begin{pmatrix} x'_{[p+1]1} \\ x'_{[p+1]2} \\ \cdot \\ x'_{[p+1](J-1)} \\ x'_{[p+1]J} \end{pmatrix} = \begin{pmatrix} 1\ 01'_p\ 0\ 01'_p \cdot 0\ 01'_p \\ 0\ 01'_p\ 1\ 01'_p \cdot 0\ 01'_p \\ \cdot\ \cdot\ \cdot\ \cdot\ \cdot\ \cdot\ \cdot \\ 0\ 01'_p\ 0\ 01'_p \cdot 1\ 01'_p \\ 0\ 01'_p\ 0\ 01'_p \cdot 0\ 01'_p \end{pmatrix}. \tag{2.70}$$

Following (2.35), the likelihood function (2.68) yields the likelihood equations

$$\frac{\partial \log L(\theta^*)}{\partial \theta^*} = \sum_{\ell=1}^{p+1} X'_\ell \left[y_{[\ell]} - K_{[\ell]}\pi_{[\ell]}\right] = 0, \tag{2.71}$$

where

$$y_{[\ell]} = [K_{[\ell]1}, \ldots, K_{[\ell]j}, \ldots, K_{[\ell]J}]' \text{ and } \pi_{[\ell]} = [\pi_{[\ell]1}, \ldots, \pi_{[\ell]j}, \ldots, \pi_{[\ell]J}]',$$

and X_ℓ matrices for $\ell = 1, \ldots, p+1$ are given as in (2.70).

2.2.2.1.1 Likelihood Estimates and their Asymptotic Variances

Note that the likelihood estimating equation (2.35) was developed for the covariates free cases, that is, for the cases with $p = 0$, whereas the likelihood estimating equation (2.71) is developed for one covariate with $p+1$ levels, represented by p dummy covariates. Thus, the estimating equation (2.71) may be treated as a generalization of the estimating equation (2.35) to the p covariates case. Let $\hat{\theta}^*$ be the solution of $f(\theta^*)=0$ in (2.71). Assuming that $\hat{\theta}_0^*$ is not a solution for $f(\theta^*)=0$, but a trial estimate and hence $f(\hat{\theta}_0^*) \neq 0$, by similar calculations as in (2.36), the iterative equation for $\hat{\theta}^*$ is obtained as

$$\hat{\theta}^* = \hat{\theta}_0^* - \left[\{f'(\theta^*)\}^{-1} f(\theta^*)\right]|_{\theta^*=\hat{\theta}_0^*}. \tag{2.72}$$

Further, by similar calculations as in (2.38), one obtains from (2.71) that

$$K_{[\ell]}\frac{\partial \pi_{[\ell]j}}{\partial \theta^{*\prime}} = K_{[\ell]}\left[\pi_{[\ell]j}x'_{[\ell]j} - \pi_{[\ell]j}\pi'_{[\ell]}X_\ell\right]. \tag{2.73}$$

Consequently, it follows from (2.71) that

$$\begin{aligned} f'(\theta^*) = -\sum_{\ell=1}^{p+1} K_{[\ell]}X'_\ell \frac{\partial \pi_{[\ell]}}{\partial \theta^{*\prime}} &= -\sum_{\ell=1}^{p+1} K_{[\ell]}X'_\ell\left[\mathrm{diag}(\pi_{[\ell]1},\ldots,\pi_{[\ell]J}) - \pi_{[\ell]}\pi'_{[\ell]}\right]X_\ell \\ &= -\sum_{\ell=1}^{p+1} K_{[\ell]}X'_\ell\left[D_{\pi_{[\ell]}} - \pi_{[\ell]}\pi'_{[\ell]}\right]X_\ell, \end{aligned} \tag{2.74}$$

and the iterative equation (2.72) takes the form

$$\begin{aligned} \widehat{\theta^*}(r+1) = \widehat{\theta^*}(r) &+ \left[\sum_{\ell=1}^{p+1} K_{[\ell]}X'_\ell\left[D_{\pi_{[\ell]}} - \pi_{[\ell]}\pi'_{[\ell]}\right]X_\ell\right]^{-1} \\ &\times \left[\sum_{\ell=1}^{p+1} X'_\ell\left(y_{[\ell]} - K_{[\ell]}\pi_{[\ell]}\right)\right]_{\theta^*=\widehat{\theta^*}(r)}, \end{aligned} \tag{2.75}$$

yielding the final estimate $\widehat{\theta^*}$. The covariance matrix of $\widehat{\theta^*}$ has the formula

$$\mathrm{var}(\widehat{\theta^*}) = \left[\sum_{\ell=1}^{p+1} K_{[\ell]}X'_\ell\{D_{\pi_{[\ell]}} - \pi_{[\ell]}\pi'_{[\ell]}\}X_\ell\right]^{-1}. \tag{2.76}$$

2.2.2.2 Product Multinomial Likelihood Based Estimating Equations with Local (Level Specified) Regression form Using Level Based Parameters

Note that in the last two sections, regression parameters were grouped category wise, that is, $\theta^* = [\beta_1^{*'}, \ldots, \beta_j^{*'}, \ldots, \beta_{J-1}^{*'}]'$, where $\beta_j^* = [\beta_{j0}, \beta_{j1}, \ldots, \beta_{jp}]'$ is formed corresponding to the covariates from all $p+1$ levels under the jth category response. Under product multinomial approach, it however makes more sense to group the parameters for all categories together under a given level $\ell(\ell = 1, \ldots, p+1)$, and write the estimating equations for these parameters of the multinomial distribution corresponding to the level ℓ, and then combine all estimating equations for overall parameters. Thus, we first use

$$\theta_\ell == \begin{cases} (\beta_{10}, \cdots, \beta_{J-1,0}, \beta_{1\ell}, \cdots, \beta_{J-1,\ell})' = (\beta_0', \beta_\ell')' : 2(J-1) \times 1, & \text{for } \ell = 1, \ldots, p \\ (\beta_{10}, \cdots, \beta_{J-1,0})' = \beta_0 : (J-1) \times 1 & \text{for } \ell = p+1, \end{cases}$$

and define

$$log\ m_{\ell j} = \tilde{x}'_{[\ell]j} \theta_\ell$$

satisfying the probability formulas

$$\pi_{[\ell]j} = \frac{m_{\ell j}}{\sum_{j=1}^J m_{\ell j}} = \frac{\exp(\tilde{x}'_{[\ell]j} \theta_\ell)}{\sum_{j=1}^J \exp(\tilde{x}'_{[\ell]j} \theta_\ell)}$$

in (2.63)–(2.64) for all $j = 1, \ldots, J$ at a given level ℓ. In regression form, it is equivalent to construct the $J \times 2(J-1)$ dummy covariate matrix $\tilde{X}_\ell$ for $\ell = 1, p$, and $J \times (J-1)$ dummy covariate matrix $\tilde{X}_{p+1}$, so that

$$\log \tilde{m}_\ell = [\log m_{\ell 1}, \cdots, \log m_{\ell j}, \cdots, \log m_{\ell J}]' = \tilde{X}_\ell \theta_\ell.$$

It follows that $\tilde{X}_\ell$ must have the form

$$\tilde{X}_\ell = \begin{pmatrix} 1\,0\,0 \cdot 0\,1\,0 \cdot 0 \\ 0\,1\,0 \cdot 0\,0\,1 \cdot 0 \\ \cdot\ \cdot\ \cdot\ \cdot\ \cdot\ \cdot\ \cdot\ \cdot\ \cdot \\ 0\,0\,0 \cdot 1\,0\,0 \cdot 1 \\ 0\,0\,0 \cdot 0\,0\,0 \cdot 0 \end{pmatrix} : J \times 2(J-1), \text{ for } \ell = 1, \ldots, p \tag{2.77}$$

$$\tilde{X}_\ell = \begin{pmatrix} 1\,0\,0 \cdot 0 \\ 0\,1\,0 \cdot 0 \\ \cdot\ \cdot\ \cdot\ \cdot\ \cdot \\ 0\,0\,0 \cdot 1 \\ 0\,0\,0 \cdot 0 \end{pmatrix} : J \times (J-1), \text{ for } \ell = p+1. \tag{2.78}$$

By similar calculations as in (2.35) (no covariate case), it follows from (2.67) (for covariate level ℓ) that the likelihood equation for θ_ℓ has the form

$$f(\theta_\ell) = \tilde{X}'_\ell(y_{[\ell]} - K_{[\ell]}\pi_{[\ell]}) = 0 \tag{2.79}$$

where $\tilde{X}_\ell$ have the forms as in (2.77) and (2.78), and

$$y_{[\ell]} = [K_{[\ell]1}, \ldots, K_{[\ell]j}, \ldots, K_{[\ell]J}]' \text{ and } \pi_{[\ell]} = [\pi_{[\ell]1}, \ldots, \pi_{[\ell]j}, \ldots, \pi_{[\ell]J}]'.$$

We then write a vector of distinct parameters, say θ, collecting them from all levels and append the estimating equation (2.79) for θ_ℓ to the final estimating equation for θ simply by using the chain rule of derivatives. In the present case for a single categorical covariate with $p+1$ levels, the θ vector can be written as

$$\theta = [\beta'_0, \beta'_1, \ldots, \beta'_\ell, \ldots, \beta'_p]' : (J-1)(p+1) \times 1,$$

with

$$\beta_0 = (\beta_{10}, \ldots, \beta_{j0}, \ldots, \beta_{(J-1)0})' \text{ and } \beta_\ell = (\beta_{1\ell}, \ldots, \beta_{j\ell}, \ldots, \beta_{(J-1)\ell})' \text{ for } \ell = 1, \ldots, p,$$

and by appending (2.79), the likelihood estimating equation for θ has the form

$$\begin{aligned} f(\theta) &= \sum_{\ell=1}^{p+1} [\frac{\partial \theta'_\ell}{\partial \theta} \tilde{X}'_\ell (y_{[\ell]} - K_{[\ell]}\pi_{[\ell]}) \\ &= \sum_{\ell=1}^{p+1} Q_\ell \tilde{X}'_\ell (y_{[\ell]} - K_{[\ell]}\pi_{[\ell]}) = 0, \end{aligned} \tag{2.80}$$

where Q_ℓ, for $\ell = 1, \ldots, p$, is the $(p+1)(J-1) \times 2(J-1)$ matrix and of dimension $(p+1)(J-1) \times (J-1)$ for $\ell = p+1$. These coefficient matrices are given by

$$Q_\ell = \begin{pmatrix} I_{J-1} & 0_{(J-1)\times(J-1)} \\ 0_{(\ell-1)(J-1)\times(J-1)} & 0_{(\ell-1)(J-1)\times(J-1)} \\ 0_{(J-1)\times(J-1)} & I_{J-1} \\ 0_{(p-\ell)(J-1)\times(J-1)} & 0_{(p-\ell)(J-1)\times(J-1)} \end{pmatrix} \text{ for } \ell = 1, \ldots, p$$

$$Q_{p+1} = \begin{pmatrix} I_{J-1} \\ 0_{(p)(J-1)\times(J-1)} \end{pmatrix}.$$

2.2.2.3 Illustration 2.3 (Continuation of Illustration 2.2): Partitioning the Product Binary ($J = 2$) Likelihood into Four Groups Corresponding to Four Nominal Levels of the Snoring Covariate

Note that Table 2.3 shows that the data were collected from 2,484 independent individuals. Because the individual status was recorded with regard to both snoring and heart disease problems, it is reasonable to consider the snoring status and heart disease status as two response variables. One would then analyze this data set by using a bivariate multinomial model to be constructed by accommodating the correlation between two multinomial response variables. This will be discussed in Chap. 5.

2.2.2.3.1 Product Binomial Approach

If one is, however, interested to examine the effect of snoring levels on the heart disease status, then the same data set may be analyzed by conditioning on the snoring levels and fitting a binary distribution at a given snoring level. This leads to a product binomial model that we use in this section to fit this snoring and heart disease data. To be specific, following the notations from Sect. 2.2.1.1(b), let $K_{[\ell]}$ be the number of individuals at ℓth snoring level. The responses of these individuals are distributed into two categories with regard to the heart disease problem. Thus the two cell counts at level ℓ will follow a binomial distribution. More specifically, because the $L = p+1 = 4$ levels are non-overlapping, one may first rewrite the product binary likelihood function (2.65) as

$$L^*[(\beta_{10}, \beta_{11}, \beta_{12}, \beta_{13})|y] = \Pi_{\ell=1}^{p+1} \Pi_{i=1}^{K_{[\ell]}} \frac{1!}{y_{i1}!y_{i2}!} \pi_{[i\in(\ell)]1}^{y_{i1}} \pi_{[i\in(\ell)]2}^{y_{i2}}, \tag{2.81}$$

where

$$y_{i2} = 1 - y_{i1} \text{ and } \pi_{[i\in(\ell)]2} = 1 - \pi_{[i\in(\ell)]1}.$$

Further note that because $\pi_{[i\in(\ell)]j}$ is not a function of i any more, without any loss of generality we denote this by $\pi_{[\ell]j}$, for $j = 1, 2$. Also suppose that $\pi_{[\ell]2} = 1 - \pi_{[\ell]1}$, and $K_{[\ell]1} + K_{[\ell]2} = K_{[\ell]}$, where $\Sigma_{i=1}^{K_\ell} y_{i1} = K_{[\ell]1}$. When these notations are used, the binary likelihood function from (2.81) at a given level ℓ reduces to the binomial distribution

$$f(K_{[\ell]1}) = \frac{K_{[\ell]}!}{K_{[\ell]1}!K_{[\ell]2}!} (\pi_{[\ell]1})^{K_{[\ell]1}} (\pi_{[\ell]2})^{K_{[\ell]2}}, \tag{2.82}$$

for all $\ell = 1, \ldots, p+1$, yielding the product binomial likelihood as

$$L[(\beta_{10},\beta_{11},\beta_{12},\beta_{13})|K] = \Pi_{\ell=1}^{p+1} \frac{K_{[\ell]}!}{K_{[\ell]1}!K_{[\ell]2}!}(\pi_{[\ell]1})^{K_{[\ell]1}}(\pi_{[\ell]2})^{K_{[\ell]2}}. \quad (2.83)$$

This product binomial (2.83) likelihood function may be maximized to obtain the likelihood estimates for the parameters involved, i.e., for $\beta_{10},\beta_{11},\beta_{12}$, and β_{13}.

2.2.2.3.1 (a) Estimating Equations: Global Regression Approach

Because in this example $J = 2$ and $p+1 = 4$, it follows from (2.69) that

$$\theta^* = (\beta_{10},\beta_{11},\beta_{12},\beta_{13})',$$

and by following (2.70), one writes

$$X_1 = \begin{pmatrix} 1 & 1 & 0 & 0 \\ 0 & 0 & 0 & 0 \end{pmatrix}$$

$$X_2 = \begin{pmatrix} 1 & 0 & 1 & 0 \\ 0 & 0 & 0 & 0 \end{pmatrix}$$

$$X_3 = \begin{pmatrix} 1 & 0 & 0 & 1 \\ 0 & 0 & 0 & 0 \end{pmatrix}$$

$$X_4 = \begin{pmatrix} 1 & 0 & 0 & 0 \\ 0 & 0 & 0 & 0 \end{pmatrix}.$$

Thus, by (2.71), the estimating equation for θ^* has the form

$$\sum_{\ell=1}^{p+1} X_\ell' \left[y_{[\ell]} - K_{[\ell]}\pi_{[\ell]}\right] = 0, \quad (2.84)$$

where

$$y_{[\ell]} = \begin{pmatrix} K_{[\ell]1} \\ K_{[\ell]2} \end{pmatrix} \text{ and } \pi_{[\ell]} = \begin{pmatrix} \pi_{[\ell]1} \\ \pi_{[\ell]2} \end{pmatrix}.$$

Note that for this heart disease and snoring relationship problem, the data and probabilities in terms of global parameters $\theta^* = (\beta_{10},\beta_{11},\beta_{12},\beta_{13})'$ are given by
Level 1 (Occasional snoring):
Response count: $K_{[1]1} = 35,\ K_{[1]2} = 603,\ K_{[1]} = 638.$
Probabilities: $\pi_{[1]1} = \frac{\exp(\beta_{10}+\beta_{11})}{1+\exp(\beta_{10}+\beta_{11})}$, and $\pi_{[1]2} = \frac{1}{1+\exp(\beta_{10}+\beta_{11})}$.

Global regression form: $\pi_{[1]1} = \frac{\exp(x'_{[1]1}\theta^*)}{\sum_{g=1}^{2}\exp(x'_{[1]g}\theta^*)}$, and $\pi_{[1]2} = \frac{\exp(x'_{[1]2}\theta^*)}{\sum_{g=1}^{2}\exp(x'_{[1]g}\theta^*)}$, where $x'_{[1]1}$, for example, is the first row vector of the above written $X_1 : 2 \times 4$ matrix.
Level 2 (Nearly every night snoring):
Response count: $K_{[2]1} = 21,\ K_{[2]2} = 192,\ K_{[2]} = 213.$
Probabilities: $\pi_{[2]1} = \frac{\exp(\beta_{10}+\beta_{12})}{1+\exp(\beta_{10}+\beta_{12})}$, and $\pi_{[2]2} = \frac{1}{1+\exp(\beta_{10}+\beta_{12})}$.
Global regression form: $\pi_{[2]1} = \frac{\exp(x'_{[2]1}\theta^*)}{\sum_{g=1}^{2}\exp(x'_{[2]g}\theta^*)}$, and $\pi_{[2]2} = \frac{\exp(x'_{[2]2}\theta^*)}{\sum_{g=1}^{2}\exp(x'_{[2]g}\theta^*)}$.
Level 3 (Every night snoring):
Response count: $K_{[3]1} = 30,\ K_{[3]2} = 224,\ K_{[3]} = 254.$
Probabilities: $\pi_{[3]1} = \frac{\exp(\beta_{10}+\beta_{13})}{1+\exp(\beta_{10}+\beta_{13})}$, and $\pi_{[3]2} = \frac{1}{1+\exp(\beta_{10}+\beta_{13})}$.
Global regression form: $\pi_{[3]1} = \frac{\exp(x'_{[3]1}\theta^*)}{\sum_{g=1}^{2}\exp(x'_{[3]g}\theta^*)}$, and $\pi_{[3]2} = \frac{\exp(x'_{[3]2}\theta^*)}{\sum_{g=1}^{2}\exp(x'_{[3]g}\theta^*)}$.
Level 4 (Never snoring):
Response count: $K_{[4]1} = 24,\ K_{[4]2} = 1355,\ K_{[4]} = 1379.$
Probabilities: $\pi_{[4]1} = \frac{\exp(\beta_{10})}{1+\exp(\beta_{10})}$, and $\pi_{[4]2} = \frac{1}{1+\exp(\beta_{10})}$.
Global regression form: $\pi_{[4]1} = \frac{\exp(x'_{[4]1}\theta^*)}{\sum_{g=1}^{2}\exp(x'_{[4]g}\theta^*)}$, and $\pi_{[4]2} = \frac{\exp(x'_{[4]2}\theta^*)}{\sum_{g=1}^{2}\exp(x'_{[4]g}\theta^*)}$.

2.2.2.3.1 (b) Estimating Equations: Local Regression Approach

For convenience we rewrite the binary probabilities under all four levels as
Level 1 (Occasional snoring):
Probabilities: $\pi_{[1]1} = \frac{\exp(\beta_{10}+\beta_{11})}{1+\exp(\beta_{10}+\beta_{11})}$, and $\pi_{[1]2} = \frac{1}{1+\exp(\beta_{10}+\beta_{11})}$.
Local regression parameters: $\theta_1 = (\beta_{10}, \beta_{11})'$.
Local regression form: $\pi_{[1]1} = \frac{\exp(\tilde{x}'_{[1]1}\theta_1)}{\sum_{g=1}^{2}\exp(\tilde{x}'_{[1]g}\theta_1)}$, and $\pi_{[1]2} = \frac{\exp(\tilde{x}'_{[1]2}\theta_1)}{\sum_{g=1}^{2}\exp(\tilde{x}'_{[1]g}\theta_1)}$, yielding the $\tilde{X}_1 : J \times 2(J-1)$ matrix (see (2.78)) as

$$\tilde{X}_1 = \begin{pmatrix} 1 & 1 \\ 0 & 0 \end{pmatrix}.$$

Level 2 (Nearly every night snoring):
Probabilities: $\pi_{[2]1} = \frac{\exp(\beta_{10}+\beta_{12})}{1+\exp(\beta_{10}+\beta_{12})}$, and $\pi_{[2]2} = \frac{1}{1+\exp(\beta_{10}+\beta_{12})}$.
Local regression parameters: $\theta_2 = (\beta_{10}, \beta_{12})'$.
Local regression form: $\pi_{[2]1} = \frac{\exp(\tilde{x}'_{[2]1}\theta_2)}{\sum_{g=1}^{2}\exp(\tilde{x}'_{[2]g}\theta_2)}$, and $\pi_{[2]2} = \frac{\exp(\tilde{x}'_{[2]2}\theta_2)}{\sum_{g=1}^{2}\exp(\tilde{x}'_{[2]g}\theta_2)}$, yielding the $\tilde{X}_2 : J \times 2(J-1)$ matrix (see (2.78)) as

$$\tilde{X}_2 = \begin{pmatrix} 1 & 1 \\ 0 & 0 \end{pmatrix}.$$

Level 3 (Every night snoring):
Probabilities: $\pi_{[3]1} = \frac{\exp(\beta_{10}+\beta_{13})}{1+\exp(\beta_{10}+\beta_{13})}$, and $\pi_{[3]2} = \frac{1}{1+\exp(\beta_{10}+\beta_{13})}$.
Local regression parameters: $\theta_3 = (\beta_{10}, \beta_{13})'$.
Local regression form: $\pi_{[3]1} = \frac{\exp(\tilde{x}'_{[3]1}\theta_3)}{\sum_{g=1}^{2}\exp(\tilde{x}'_{[3]g}\theta_3)}$, and $\pi_{[3]2} = \frac{\exp(\tilde{x}'_{[3]2}\theta_3)}{\sum_{g=1}^{2}\exp(\tilde{x}'_{[3]g}\theta_3)}$, yielding the $\tilde{X}_3 : J \times 2(J-1)$ matrix (see (2.78)) as

$$\tilde{X}_3 = \begin{pmatrix} 1 & 1 \\ 0 & 0 \end{pmatrix}.$$

Level 4 (Never snoring):
Probabilities: $\pi_{[4]1} = \frac{\exp(\beta_{10})}{1+\exp(\beta_{10})}$, and $\pi_{[4]2} = \frac{1}{1+\exp(\beta_{10})}$.
Local regression parameters: $\theta_4 = (\beta_{10})$.
Local regression form: $\pi_{[4]1} = \frac{\exp(\tilde{x}'_{[4]1}\theta_4)}{\sum_{g=1}^{2}\exp(\tilde{x}'_{[4]g}\theta_4)}$, and $\pi_{[4]2} = \frac{\exp(\tilde{x}'_{[4]2}\theta_4)}{\sum_{g=1}^{2}\exp(\tilde{x}'_{[4]g}\theta_4)}$, yielding the $\tilde{X}_4 : J \times (J-1)$ matrix (see (2.79)) as

$$\tilde{X}_4 = \begin{pmatrix} 1 \\ 0 \end{pmatrix}.$$

The likelihood estimating equation for

$$\theta_\ell = \begin{cases} (\beta'_0, \beta'_\ell)' = (\beta_{10}, \beta_{1\ell})' : 2(J-1) \times 1; & \text{for } \ell = 1, \ldots, p, \\ \beta_{10} & \text{for } \ell = p+1 = 4, \end{cases}$$

by (2.79), has the form

$$\tilde{X}'_\ell(y_{[\ell]} - K_{[\ell]}\pi_{[\ell]}) = 0,$$

for $\ell = 1, \ldots, 4$. Next in this special case with

$$\theta = (\beta'_0, \beta'_1, \ldots, \beta'_p)' = (\beta_{10}, \beta_{11}, \beta_{12}, \beta_{13})'$$

the estimating equation for this parameter θ, by (2.80), has the form

$$\sum_{\ell=1}^{4} Q_\ell \tilde{X}'_\ell(y_{[\ell]} - K_{[\ell]}\pi_{[\ell]}) = 0, \tag{2.85}$$

where

$$Q_\ell = \frac{\partial \theta'_\ell}{\partial \theta},$$

for all $\ell = 1, \ldots, 4$, have the forms

$$Q_1 = \begin{pmatrix} 1 & 0 \\ 0 & 1 \\ 0 & 0 \\ 0 & 0 \end{pmatrix}, Q_2 = \begin{pmatrix} 1 & 0 \\ 0 & 0 \\ 0 & 1 \\ 0 & 0 \end{pmatrix}, Q_3 = \begin{pmatrix} 1 & 0 \\ 0 & 0 \\ 0 & 0 \\ 0 & 1 \end{pmatrix}, Q_4 = \begin{pmatrix} 1 \\ 0 \\ 0 \\ 0 \end{pmatrix}.$$

2.2.2.3.1 (c) Equivalence of the Likelihood Equations (2.59)(i), (2.84)(ii), and (2.85)(iii)

(i) The estimating equation (2.59) has the form

$$\sum_{i=1}^{K} \begin{pmatrix} 1 \\ w_{i1} \\ w_{i2} \\ w_{i3} \end{pmatrix} [y_{i1} - \pi_i] = 0,$$

which, by using

$$\begin{aligned}
&\sum_{i=1}^{K} y_{i1} = K_{[\cdot]1}, \sum_{i=1}^{K} \pi_{(i)1} = \sum_{\ell=1}^{4} K_{[\ell]}\pi_{[\ell]1} \\
&\sum_{i=1}^{K} y_{i1}z_{i1} = K_{[1]1}, \sum_{i=1}^{K} w_{i1}\pi_{(i)1} = K_{[1]}\pi_{[1]1} \\
&\sum_{i=1}^{K} y_{i1}w_{i2} = K_{[2]1}, \sum_{i=1}^{K} w_{i2}\pi_{(i)1} = K_{[2]}\pi_{[2]1} \\
&\sum_{i=1}^{K} y_{i1}w_{i3} = K_{[3]1}, \sum_{i=1}^{K} w_{i3}\pi_{(i)1} = K_{[3]}\pi_{[3]1},
\end{aligned} \tag{2.86}$$

reduces to

$$\begin{pmatrix} K_{[\cdot]1} - \sum_{\ell=1}^{4} K_{[\ell]}\pi_{[\ell]1} \\ K_{[1]1} - K_{[1]}\pi_{[1]1} \\ K_{[2]1} - K_{[2]}\pi_{[2]1} \\ K_{[3]1} - K_{[3]}\pi_{[3]1} \end{pmatrix} = 0. \tag{2.87}$$

(ii) Next, the estimating equation in (2.84) has the form

$$\sum_{\ell=1}^{p+1} X'_\ell \left[y_{[\ell]} - K_{[\ell]}\pi_{[\ell]}\right] = 0,$$

which, for convenience, we re-express as

$$\begin{pmatrix}1&0\\1&0\\0&0\\0&0\end{pmatrix}\begin{pmatrix}K_{[1]1}-K_{[1]}\pi_{[1]1}\\K_{[1]2}-K_{[1]}\pi_{[1]2}\end{pmatrix}+\begin{pmatrix}1&0\\0&0\\1&0\\0&0\end{pmatrix}\begin{pmatrix}K_{[2]1}-K_{[2]}\pi_{[2]1}\\K_{[2]2}-K_{[2]}\pi_{[2]2}\end{pmatrix}$$

$$+\begin{pmatrix}1&0\\0&0\\0&0\\1&0\end{pmatrix}\begin{pmatrix}K_{[3]1}-K_{[3]}\pi_{[3]1}\\K_{[3]2}-K_{[3]}\pi_{[3]2}\end{pmatrix}+\begin{pmatrix}1&0\\0&0\\0&0\\0&0\end{pmatrix}\begin{pmatrix}K_{[4]1}-K_{[4]}\pi_{[4]1}\\K_{[4]2}-K_{[4]}\pi_{[4]2}\end{pmatrix}=0. \quad (2.88)$$

After a simple algebra, (2.88) reduces to (2.87).

(iii) Further, the estimating equation (2.85) has the form

$$\sum_{\ell=1}^{p+1} Q_\ell \tilde{X}'_\ell (y_{[\ell]} - K_{[\ell]}\pi_{[\ell]}) = 0.$$

Now to see that this estimating equation is the same as (2.88), one has to simply verify that $Q_\ell \tilde{X}'_\ell = X'_\ell$ for $\ell = 1,\ldots,p+1$. As the algebra below shows, this equality holds. Here

$$Q_1\tilde{X}'_1=\begin{pmatrix}1&0\\0&1\\0&0\\0&0\end{pmatrix}\begin{pmatrix}1&0\\1&0\end{pmatrix}=\begin{pmatrix}1&0\\1&0\\0&0\\0&0\end{pmatrix}=X'_1,$$

$$Q_2\tilde{X}'_2=\begin{pmatrix}1&0\\0&0\\0&1\\0&0\end{pmatrix}\begin{pmatrix}1&0\\1&0\end{pmatrix}=\begin{pmatrix}1&0\\0&0\\1&0\\0&0\end{pmatrix}=X'_2,$$

$$Q_3\tilde{X}'_3=\begin{pmatrix}1&0\\0&0\\0&0\\0&1\end{pmatrix}\begin{pmatrix}1&0\\1&0\end{pmatrix}=\begin{pmatrix}1&0\\0&0\\0&0\\1&0\end{pmatrix}=X'_3,$$

$$Q_4\tilde{X}'_4=\begin{pmatrix}1\\0\\0\\0\end{pmatrix}(1\ 0)=\begin{pmatrix}1&0\\0&0\\0&0\\0&0\end{pmatrix}=X'_4.$$

Hence, as expected, all three estimating equations are same. Note that the estimating equation (2.59) requires individual level information, whereas the estimating equations (2.84) and (2.85) are based on grouped or contingency type data. Between

(2.84) and (2.85), it is easier to construct the $\tilde{X}_\ell$ matrices in (2.85) as coefficients of the local level parameters than constructing similar matrices X_ℓ for (2.84) corresponding to global parameters. However, unlike in (2.85), there is no need of constructing the chain derivative matrices Q_ℓ, in (2.84). Thus, it is up to the users to choose between (2.84) and (2.85). In this book we will mostly follow the global parameters based estimating equation (2.84).

2.2.2.3.1 (d) Illustration 2.3 Continued: Application of the Product Binomial Model to the Snoring and Heart Disease Problem

Forming the $X_\ell(\ell = 1,\ldots,4)$ matrices and writing the probabilities in global regression form as in Sect. 2.2.2.3.1(a), and using the 4×2 cross-table data from Table 2.3, we now solve the likelihood estimating equation (2.85) (see also (2.71)) using the iterative equation (2.75). To be specific, because the observed probabilities under category one (having heart disease) are relatively much smaller as compared to those under category two, starting with an initial value of $\beta_{10,0} = -3.0$ and small positive initial values for other parameters ($\beta_{11,0} = \beta_{12,0} = \beta_{13,0} = 0.10$), the iterative equation (2.75) yielded converged estimates for these four parameters in five iterations. These estimates were then used in (2.76) to compute the estimated variances and pair-wise covariances of the estimators. The estimates and their corresponding estimated standard errors are given in Table 2.5 below.

Note that as the snoring status is considered to be a fixed covariate (as opposed to a response variable) with four levels, the heart disease status of an individual follow a binary distribution at a given level. For example, it is clear from Sect. 2.2.2.3.1(a) that an individual belonging to level 4, i.e., who snores every night (see Table 2.3), has the probability $\pi_{[4]1} = \frac{\exp(\beta_{10})}{1+\exp(\beta_{10})}$ for having a heart disease.

Table 2.5 Parameter estimates for the snoring and heart disease data of Table 2.3

	Regression parameters			
Quantity	β_{10}	β_{20}	β_{30}	β_{40}
Estimate	−4.034	1.187	1.821	2.023
Standard error	0.206	0.269	0.309	0.283

Table 2.6 Observed and estimated probabilities for the snoring and heart disease data

	Heart disease			
	Yes		No	
Snoring level	**Observed**	**Estimated**	**Observed**	**Estimated**
Occasionally	0.055	0.055	0.945	0.945
Nearly every night	0.099	0.099	0.901	0.901
Every night	0.118	0.118	0.882	0.882
Never	0.017	0.017	0.983	0.983

These probabilities at all four levels may now be estimated by using the parameter estimates from Table 2.5. These estimated probabilities along with their respective observed probabilities are shown in Table 2.6.

Notice from the results in Table 2.6 that there is no difference between the observed and estimated probabilities at any snoring level. This result is expected because of the fact that the product binomial model is constructed with four independent regression parameters to fit data in four independent cells. This type of models are known as saturated models. In summary, the product binomial model and the estimation of its parameters by using the likelihood approach appear to be perfect for both fitting and interpretation of the data. Note that the observed and estimated probabilities appear to support that as the snoring level increases the probability for an individual to have a heart disease gets larger.

Remark that when the same snoring data is analyzed by using the snoring as a covariate with arbitrary codes, as it was done in Sect. 2.2.1.1(a) following Agresti (2002, Section 4.2.3, p. 121–123), one obtains the estimated probabilities for an individual to have a heart disease as

$$0.049,\ 0.094,\ 0.134,\ 0.020$$

based on individual's corresponding snoring level: occasional; nearly every night; every night; or never. Agresti (2002, Table 4.2) reported these probabilities as

$$0.044,\ 0.093,\ 0.132,\ 0.021,$$

which are slightly different. In any case, these estimated probabilities, as opposed to the estimated probabilities shown in Table 2.6, appear to be far apart from the corresponding observed probabilities under the 'yes' heart disease category. Thus, it is recommended not to use any modeling approach based on arbitrary coding for the fixed categorical covariates.

2.2.2.4 Illustrations Using Multinomial Regression Models Involving Responses with $J > 2$ Categories Along with One Two Levels Categorical Covariate

2.2.2.4.1 Illustration 2.4: Analysis of $2 \times J(= 3)$ Aspirin and Heart Attacks Data Using Product Multinomial Approach

To illustrate the application of product multinomial model (2.68)–(2.69) we revisit here the aspirin use and heart attack data set earlier described by Agresti (2002, Section 2.1.1), for example, using a full multinomial (or log linear model) approach. We reproduce the data set below in Table 2.7. We describe and analyze this data using product multinomial approach.

This data set was originally recorded from a report on the relationship between aspirin use and heart attacks by the Physicians Health Study Research Group at

Table 2.7
Cross-classification of aspirin use and myocardial infarction

	Myocardial infarction			
	Fatal Attack	Non-Fatal Attack	No Attack	Total
Aspirin	5	99	10,933	11,037
Placebo	18	171	10,845	11,034
Total	23	270	21,778	22,071

Harvard Medical School. The Physicians Health Study was a 5 year randomized study of whether regular aspirin intake reduces mortality from cardiovascular disease. A physician participating in the study took either one aspirin tablet or a placebo, every other day, over the 5 year study period. This was a blind study for the participants as they did not know whether they were taking aspirin or a placebo for all these 5 years. By considering the heart attack status as one multinomial response variable with three categories (fatal, non-fatal, and no attacks) and the treatment as another multinomial response variable with two categories (placebo and aspirin use), Agresti (2002) used a full multinomial approach and described the association (correlation equivalent) between the two variables through computing certain odds ratios. In notation, let $z_i = (z_{i1}, \ldots, z_{ir}, \ldots, z_{i,R-1})'$ be the second multinomial response, but, with R categories, so that when z_i is realized at the rth category, one writes

$$z_i^{(r)} = (01'_{r-1}, 1, 01'_{R-1-r})', \text{ for } r = 1, \ldots, R-1; \text{ and } z_i^{(R)} = 01'_{R-1}.$$

Then many existing approaches write the joint probabilities, for example, for the aspirin use and heart attack data, as

$$\begin{aligned}\pi_{rj} &= P[z_i = z_i^{(r)}, y_i = y_i^{(j)}], \text{for all } i = 1, \ldots, 22071,\ r = 1, 2,\ j = 1, \ldots, 3 \\ &= \frac{\exp(\alpha_r + \beta_j + \phi_{rj})}{\sum_{r=1}^{2}\sum_{j=1}^{3}\exp(\alpha_r + \beta_j + \phi_{rj})} \\ &= \frac{m_{rj}}{\sum_{r=1}^{2}\sum_{j=1}^{3} m_{rj}} = \frac{m_{rj}}{m},\end{aligned} \tag{2.89}$$

where α_r is the rth category effect of the z variable, β_j is the jth category effect of the y variable, and ϕ_{rj} is the corresponding interaction effect of y and z variables, on any individual. These parameters are restricted by the dependence of the last category of each variable on their remaining independent categories. Thus, in this example, one may use

$$\alpha_2 = \beta_3 = \phi_{13} = \phi_{21} = \phi_{22} = \phi_{23} = 0,$$

and fit the full multinomial model to the data in Table 2.7 by estimating the parameters

$$\alpha_1, \beta_1, \beta_2, \phi_{11}, \text{ and } \phi_{12}.$$

The estimation is achieved by maximizing the full multinomial likelihood

$$L(\theta^*) = \Pi_{r=1}^{2} \Pi_{j=1}^{3} \pi_{rj}^{K_{rj}}, \tag{2.90}$$

with respect to $\theta^* = (\alpha_1, \beta_1, \beta_2, \phi_{11}, \phi_{12})'$, where K_{rj} is the number of individuals in the (r, j)th cell in Table 2.7, for example, $K_{12} = 99$.

This full multinomial approach, that is, considering the treatment as a response variable, lacks justification. This can be understood simply by considering a question that, under the study condition, can the response of one randomly chosen individual out of 22,071 participants belong to one of the six cells in the Table 2.7. This is not possible, because, even though, the placebo pill or aspirin was chosen by some one for a participant with a prior probability, the treatment was made fixed for an individual participant for the whole study period. Thus, treatment variable here must be considered as a fixed regression covariate with two levels. This prompted one to reanalyze this data set by using the product multinomial model (2.68)–(2.69) by treating heart attack status as the multinomial response variable only and the treatment as a categorical covariate with two levels. By this token, for both cross-sectional and longitudinal analysis, this book emphasizes on appropriate modeling for the categorical data by distinguishing categorical covariates from categorical responses.

Product multinomial global regression approach:

Turning back to the analysis of the categorical data in Table 2.7, following (2.69) we first write the multinomial probabilities at two levels of the treatment covariate as follows. Note that in notation of the model (2.69), for this heart attack and aspirin use data, we write $J = 3$ and $p + 1 = 2$, and

$$\theta^* = (\beta_{10}, \beta_{11}, \beta_{20}, \beta_{21})'.$$

When the model (2.68)–(2.69) is compared with (2.90)–(2.91), α_1 from the latter model is not needed. Also, even though

$$\beta_{10}, \beta_{20}, \beta_{11}, \beta_{21}$$

in the model (2.69) are, respectively, equivalent to the notations

$$\beta_1, \beta_2, \phi_{11}, \phi_{12}$$

of the model (2.90), they do not have, however, the same interpretation. This is because, β_{11} and β_{21} in (2.69) are simply regression effects of the covariate level 1 on first two categories, whereas ϕ_{11} and ϕ_{12} in (2.90) are treated to be association or odds ratio parameters. But, there is a definition problem with these odds ratio parameters in this situation, because treatment here cannot represent a response variable.

Now for the product multinomial model (2.68)–(2.69), one writes the level based $\{J \times (J-1)(p+1)\} \equiv \{3 \times 4\}$ covariate matrices as

$$X_1 = \begin{pmatrix} 1 & 1 & 0 & 0 \\ 0 & 0 & 1 & 1 \\ 0 & 0 & 0 & 0 \end{pmatrix}$$

$$X_2 = \begin{pmatrix} 1 & 0 & 0 & 0 \\ 0 & 0 & 1 & 0 \\ 0 & 0 & 0 & 0 \end{pmatrix}.$$

Then the cell probabilities and their forms in terms of the global parameters $\theta^* = (\beta_{10}, \beta_{11}, \beta_{20}, \beta_{21})'$ are given by

Level 1 (Aspirin user):

Response count: $K_{[1]1} = 5,\ K_{[1]2} = 99,\ K_{[1]3} = 10{,}933,\ K_{[1]} = 11{,}037.$

Probabilities:

$$\pi_{[1]1} = \frac{\exp(\beta_{10} + \beta_{11})}{1 + \sum_{g=1}^{2} \exp(\beta_{g0} + \beta_{g1})},\ \pi_{[1]2} = \frac{\exp(\beta_{20} + \beta_{21})}{1 + \sum_{g=1}^{2} \exp(\beta_{g0} + \beta_{g1})},$$
$$\pi_{[1]3} = \frac{1}{1 + \sum_{g=1}^{2} \exp(\beta_{g0} + \beta_{g1})}. \tag{2.91}$$

Global regression form:

$$\pi_{[1]1} = \frac{\exp(x'_{[1]1}\theta^*)}{\sum_{j=1}^{3} \exp(x'_{[1]j}\theta^*)},\ \pi_{[1]2} = \frac{\exp(x'_{[1]2}\theta^*)}{\sum_{j=1}^{3} \exp(x'_{[1]j}\theta^*)},$$
$$\pi_{[1]3} = \frac{\exp(x'_{[1]3}\theta^*)}{\sum_{j=1}^{3} \exp(x'_{[1]j}\theta^*)},$$

where $x'_{[1]2}$, for example, is the second row vector of the above written $X_1 : 3 \times 4$ matrix.

Level 2 (Placebo user):

Response count: $K_{[2]1} = 18,\ K_{[2]2} = 171,\ K_{[2]3} = 10{,}845,\ K_{[2]} = 11{,}034.$

Probabilities:

$$\pi_{[2]1} = \frac{\exp(\beta_{10})}{1 + \sum_{g=1}^{2} \exp(\beta_{g0})},\ \pi_{[2]2} = \frac{\exp(\beta_{20})}{1 + \sum_{g=1}^{2} \exp(\beta_{g0})},$$
$$\pi_{[2]3} = \frac{1}{1 + \sum_{g=1}^{2} \exp(\beta_{g0})}. \tag{2.92}$$

Table 2.8 Parameter estimates for the treatment and heart attack status data of Table 2.7

	Regression parameters			
Quantity	β_{10}	β_{11}	β_{20}	β_{21}
Estimate	−6.401	−1.289	−4.150	−0.555
Standard error	0.2360	0.5057	0.0771	0.1270

Global regression form:

$$\pi_{[2]1} = \frac{\exp(x'_{[2]1}\theta^*)}{\sum_{j=1}^{3}\exp(x'_{[2]j}\theta^*)}, \; \pi_{[2]2} = \frac{\exp(x'_{[2]2}\theta^*)}{\sum_{j=1}^{3}\exp(x'_{[2]j}\theta^*)},$$

$$\pi_{[2]3} = \frac{\exp(x'_{[2]3}\theta^*)}{\sum_{j=1}^{3}\exp(x'_{[2]j}\theta^*)}.$$

Now following (2.71) and using the iterative equation (2.75), we solve the product multinomial based likelihood estimating equation

$$\sum_{\ell=1}^{2} X'_\ell \left[y_{[\ell]} - K_{[\ell]}\pi_{[\ell]}\right] = 0, \tag{2.93}$$

where

$$y_{[\ell]} = \begin{pmatrix} K_{[\ell]1} \\ K_{[\ell]2} \\ K_{[\ell]3} \end{pmatrix} \text{ and } \pi_{[\ell]} = \begin{pmatrix} \pi_{[\ell]1} \\ \pi_{[\ell]2} \\ \pi_{[\ell]3} \end{pmatrix}.$$

These estimates and their corresponding standard errors computed by using (2.76) are reported in Table 2.8.

In order to interpret these parameter estimates, notice from the formulas from the probabilities under level 2 (placebo group) that the values of β_{10} and β_{20} would determine the probabilities of a placebo user individual to be in the 'fatal attack' or 'non-fatal attack' group, as compared to $\beta_{30} = 0$ used for probability for the same individual to be in the reference group, that is, in the 'no attack' group. To be specific, when the large negative values of $\beta_{10}(= -6.401)$ and $\beta_{20}(= -4.150)$ are compared to $\beta_{30} = 0$, it becomes clear by (2.92) that the probability of a placebo user to be in the 'no attack' group is very large, as expected, followed by the probabilities for the individual to be in the 'non-fatal' and fatal groups, respectively. Further because the value of $\beta_{10} + \beta_{11}$ would determine the probability of an aspirin user in the 'fatal attack' group, the negative value of $\beta_{11}(= -1.289)$ shows that an aspirin user has smaller probability than a placebo user to be in the 'fatal attack' group. Other estimates can be interpreted similarly. Now by using these estimates from Table 2.8, the estimates for all three categorized multinomial probabilities in (2.91) under aspirin user treatment level, and in (2.92) under placebo user treatment level, may be computed. These estimated probabilities along

Table 2.9 Observed and estimated multinomial probabilities for the treatment versus heart attack status data of Table 2.7

		Myocardial Infarction			
	Proportion/ Probability	Fatal Attack	Non-Fatal Attack	No Attack	Total
Aspirin	Observed	0.00045	0.00897	0.99058	1.00
	Estimated	0.00045	0.00897	0.99058	1.00
Placebo	Observed	0.00163	0.01550	0.98287	1.00
	Estimated	0.00163	0.01550	0.98287	1.00

with their counterpart (observed proportions) are displayed in Table 2.9. Similar to Table 2.6 for the snoring and heart disease problem data, it is clear from Table 2.9 that the observed and estimated probabilities are same. This happens because the four independent parameters, namely β_{10}, β_{11}, β_{20}, and β_{21} are used to define the probabilities in (2.91)–(2.92) (see also (2.68)–(2.69)) to fit four independent observations, two under aspirin user treatment level and another two under the placebo user treatment level. Thus a saturated model is fitted through solving the corresponding optimal likelihood estimating equations (2.93), and the parameter estimates shown in Table 2.8 are consistent and highly efficient (details are not discussed here).

Remark that the estimates of the regression parameters under two (independent) categories shown in Table 2.8 were obtained by applying the product multinomial estimating equation (2.93) to the observed data given in the contingency Table 2.7. However, because the data in this table are clearly laid out under each of the two treatment levels, one may easily reconstruct the individual level response and covariate information without any identity of the individual. Suppose that the treatment covariate is defined as

$$w_i = \begin{cases} 1 \text{ for aspirin taken by the } i\text{th individual} \\ 0 \text{ otherwise,} \end{cases}$$

and the multinomial response of this individual is given by

$$y_i = \begin{cases} (1,0)' \text{ if this ith individual had fatal attack} \\ (0,1)' \text{ if this ith individual had non fatal attack} \\ (0,0)' \text{ otherwise, i.e., if this ith individual had no attack.} \end{cases}$$

Consequently, one may directly solve the individual history based multinomial likelihood estimating equation (2.48) to obtain the same estimates (as in Table 2.8) of the regression parameters involved in the probability model (2.45).

Turning back to the results shown in Table 2.9, it is clear that the estimated proportion of individuals whose heart attack was either fatal or non-fatal is shown to

Table 2.10 Cross-classification of gender and physician visit

	Physician visit status				
Gender	None	Few	Not so few	High	Total
Male	28	40	16	12	96
Female	11	20	21	32	84
Total	38	62	36	44	180

be $(0.00045+0.00897)=0.00942$ for the aspirin group, and $(0.00164+0.01562)=0.01726$ for the placebo group, indicating the advantage of using aspirin as opposed to using none. This type of comparison is also available in Agresti (1990, Section 2.2.4, page 17), but by using only observed data. Later on it was emphasized in Agresti (2002, Section 2.1.1) for the comparison of the distribution of responses under each treatment level, but unlike in this section, no model was fitted.

2.2.2.4.2 Analysis of Physician Visits Data with $J=4$ Categories

We continue to illustrate the application of the product multinomial likelihood models now by considering the physician visits data described in Table 2.1. We consider the physician visits in four categories: none, few, not so few, and high visits, as indicated in Table 2.2, whereas there were three categories for heart attack status in the treatment versus heart attack data considered in the last section. To be specific, for the physician visits data, we will fit the product multinomial models to examine the marginal effects of (1) gender; (2) chronic disease; and (3) education levels, on the physician visits, in the following Sects. 2.2.2.4.2(a), (b), and (c), respectively.

2.2.2.4.2 (a) Illustration 2.5: Analysis for Gender Effects on Physician Visits

To examine the gender effects on the physician visits we use the data from Table 2.1 and display them in the 2×4 contingency Table 2.10. For convenience of fitting the product multinomial model (2.67)–(2.69) to this data, for each gender level we write the multinomial observation, probabilities under each of four categories, and the global regression form along with corresponding covariate matrix, as follows:
Level 1 (Male):
Response count: $K_{[1]1}=27,\ K_{[1]2}=42,\ K_{[1]3}=15,\ K_{[1]4}=12,\ K_{[1]}=96.$
Probabilities:

$$\pi_{[1]1}=\frac{\exp(\beta_{10}+\beta_{11})}{1+\sum_{g=1}^{3}\exp(\beta_{g0}+\beta_{g1})},\ \pi_{[1]2}=\frac{\exp(\beta_{20}+\beta_{21})}{1+\sum_{g=1}^{3}\exp(\beta_{g0}+\beta_{g1})},$$
$$\pi_{[1]3}=\frac{\exp(\beta_{30}+\beta_{31})}{1+\sum_{g=1}^{3}\exp(\beta_{g0}+\beta_{g1})},\ \pi_{[1]4}=\frac{1}{1+\sum_{g=1}^{3}\exp(\beta_{g0}+\beta_{g1})}. \quad (2.94)$$

Global regression form:

$$\pi_{[1]1} = \frac{\exp(x'_{[1]1}\theta^*)}{\sum_{j=1}^4 \exp(x'_{[1]j}\theta^*)},\ \pi_{[1]2} = \frac{\exp(x'_{[1]2}\theta^*)}{\sum_{j=1}^4 \exp(x'_{[1]j}\theta^*)},$$

$$\pi_{[1]3} = \frac{\exp(x'_{[1]3}\theta^*)}{\sum_{j=1}^4 \exp(x'_{[1]j}\theta^*)},\ \pi_{[1]4} = \frac{\exp(x'_{[1]4}\theta^*)}{\sum_{j=1}^4 \exp(x'_{[1]j}\theta^*)},$$

where

$$\theta^* = (\beta_{10}, \beta_{11}, \beta_{20}, \beta_{21}, \beta_{30}, \beta_{31})',$$

and $x'_{[1]3}$, for example, is the third row vector of the $X_1 : 4 \times 6$ matrix given by

$$X_1 = \begin{pmatrix} 1\ 1\ 0\ 0\ 0\ 0 \\ 0\ 0\ 1\ 1\ 0\ 0 \\ 0\ 0\ 0\ 0\ 1\ 1 \\ 0\ 0\ 0\ 0\ 0\ 0 \end{pmatrix}. \tag{2.95}$$

Level 2 (Female):
Response count: $K_{[2]1} = 11,\ K_{[2]2} = 20,\ K_{[2]3} = 21,\ K_{[2]4} = 32,\ K_{[2]} = 84.$
Probabilities:

$$\pi_{[2]1} = \frac{\exp(\beta_{10})}{1 + \sum_{g=1}^3 \exp(\beta_{g0})},\ \pi_{[2]2} = \frac{\exp(\beta_{20})}{1 + \sum_{g=1}^3 \exp(\beta_{g0})},$$

$$\pi_{[2]3} = \frac{\exp(\beta_{30})}{1 + \sum_{g=1}^3 \exp(\beta_{g0})},\ \pi_{[2]4} = \frac{1}{1 + \sum_{g=1}^3 \exp(\beta_{g0})}. \tag{2.96}$$

Global regression form:

$$\pi_{[2]1} = \frac{\exp(x'_{[2]1}\theta^*)}{\sum_{j=1}^4 \exp(x'_{[2]j}\theta^*)},\ \pi_{[2]2} = \frac{\exp(x'_{[2]2}\theta^*)}{\sum_{j=1}^4 \exp(x'_{[2]j}\theta^*)},$$

$$\pi_{[2]3} = \frac{\exp(x'_{[2]3}\theta^*)}{\sum_{j=1}^4 \exp(x'_{[2]j}\theta^*)},\ \pi_{[2]4} = \frac{\exp(x'_{[2]4}\theta^*)}{\sum_{j=1}^4 \exp(x'_{[2]j}\theta^*)},$$

where θ^* remains the same as

$$\theta^* = (\beta_{10}, \beta_{11}, \beta_{20}, \beta_{21}, \beta_{30}, \beta_{31})',$$

and $x'_{[2]3}$, for example, is the third row vector of the $X_2 : 4 \times 6$ matrix given by

Table 2.11 Parameter estimates for the gender and physician visit status data of Table 2.10

	Regression parameters					
Quantity	β_{10}	β_{11}	β_{20}	β_{21}	β_{30}	β_{31}
Estimate	−1.068	1.915	−0.470	1.674	−0.421	0.709
Standard error	0.3495	0.4911	0.2850	0.4354	0.2808	0.4740

$$X_2 = \begin{pmatrix} 1 & 0 & 0 & 0 & 0 & 0 \\ 0 & 0 & 1 & 0 & 0 & 0 \\ 0 & 0 & 0 & 0 & 1 & 0 \\ 0 & 0 & 0 & 0 & 0 & 0 \end{pmatrix}. \tag{2.97}$$

Now following (2.71) and using the iterative equation (2.75), we solve the product multinomial based likelihood estimating equation

$$\sum_{\ell=1}^{2} X'_\ell \left[y_{[\ell]} - K_{[\ell]} \pi_{[\ell]} \right] = 0, \tag{2.98}$$

where

$$y_{[\ell]} = \begin{pmatrix} K_{[\ell]1} \\ K_{[\ell]2} \\ K_{[\ell]3} \\ K_{[\ell]4} \end{pmatrix} \text{ and } \pi_{[\ell]} = \begin{pmatrix} \pi_{[\ell]1} \\ \pi_{[\ell]2} \\ \pi_{[\ell]3} \\ \pi_{[\ell]3} \end{pmatrix}.$$

These estimates and their corresponding standard errors computed by using (2.76) are reported in Table 2.11.

Notice from (2.96) that the estimates of β_{10}, β_{20}, and β_{30} indicate the relative probability for a female to be in none, few, and not so few categories, respectively, as compared to the probability for high category determined by $\beta_{40} = 0$ (by assumption).

Because all three estimates are negative, the estimate for β_{10} being large negative, it follows that a female has the highest probability to be in 'high visit' group and smallest probability to be in the 'none' (never visited) group. By the same token, it follows from (2.94) that the largest value for $\beta_{20} + \beta_{21} = 1.204$ estimate as compared to its reference value 0.0 indicates that a male has the highest probability to be in the 'few visits' group. These probabilities can be verified from Table 2.12 where we have displayed the estimated as well as observed probabilities. In summary, the estimated probabilities in Table 2.12 show that a female visits the physician for more number of times as compared to a male. These results are in agreement with those of health care utilization study reported in Sutradhar (2011, Section 4.2.8) where

Table 2.12 Observed and estimated multinomial probabilities for the gender versus physician visits data of Table 2.10

		Physician visit status				
Gender	Probability	None	Few	Not so few	High	Total
Male	Observed	0.2917	0.4166	0.1667	0.1250	1.0
	Estimated	0.2917	0.4166	0.1667	0.1250	1.0
Female	Observed	0.1309	0.2381	0.2500	0.3810	1.0
	Estimated	0.1309	0.2381	0.2500	0.3810	1.0

Table 2.13 Cross-classification of chronic condition and physician visit

	Physician visit status				
Chronic condition	None	Few	Not so few	High	Total
Yes	13	25	21	33	92
No	26	35	16	11	88
Total	39	60	37	44	180

the actual number of visits (as opposed to visit category) were analyzed by fitting a familial/clustered model using the so-called generalized quasi-likelihood (GQL) estimation approach.

2.2.2.4.2 (b) Illustration 2.6: Analysis for Chronic Condition Effects on Physician Visits

To examine the chronic condition effects on the number of visits, we first display the physician visit data in the form a contingency (cross-classified) table. More specifically, the 2×4 cross-classified Table 2.13 shows the distribution of the number of the respondents under four visit categories at a given chronic condition level. The chronic condition covariate has two levels. One of the levels represents the individuals with no chronic disease, and the individuals with one or more chronic disease have been assigned to the other group (level). Note that because both Tables 2.10 and 2.13 contain one categorical covariate with two levels, the probability models for the data in Table 2.13 would be the same as that of Table 2.10. The only difference is in the names of the levels. For this reason we do not reproduce the probability formulas and the form of X_ℓ matrices. However because the data are naturally different we write them in notation as follows:
Chronic condition level 1 (Yes):
Response count: $K_{[1]1} = 13,\ K_{[1]2} = 25,\ K_{[1]3} = 21,\ K_{[1]4} = 33,\ K_{[1]} = 92.$
Chronic condition level 2 (No):
Response count: $K_{[2]1} = 25,\ K_{[2]2} = 37,\ K_{[2]3} = 15,\ K_{[2]4} = 11,\ K_{[2]} = 88.$
We then solve the product multinomial likelihood estimating equation (2.98). The estimates of the regression parameters involved in the probability formulas (2.94) and (2.96) for the cross-classified data in Table 2.13 are given in Table 2.14. The estimates probabilities are shown in Table 2.15.

Table 2.14 Parameter estimates for the chronic condition and physician visit status data of Table 2.13

	Regression parameters					
Quantity	β_{10}	β_{11}	β_{20}	β_{21}	β_{30}	β_{31}
Estimate	0.860	−1.792	1.157	−1.435	0.375	−0.827
Standard error	0.3597	0.4864	0.3457	0.4356	0.3917	0.4810

Table 2.15 Observed and estimated multinomial probabilities for the chronic condition versus physician visits data of Table 2.13

		Physician visit status				
Chronic condition	Probability	None	Few	Not so few	High	Total
Yes	Observed	0.1413	0.2717	0.2283	0.3587	1.0
	Estimated	0.1413	0.2717	0.2283	0.3587	1.0
No	Observed	0.2955	0.3977	0.1818	0.1250	1.0
	Estimated	0.2955	0.3977	0.1818	0.1250	1.0

Notice from (2.96) that the estimates of β_{10}, β_{20}, and β_{30}, would indicate the relative probability for an individual with no chronic disease to be in none, few, and not so few categories, respectively, as compared to the probability for being in high category determined by $\beta_{40} = 0$ (by assumption). Consequently,

$$\hat{\beta}_{20} = 1.157 > \hat{\beta}_{10} > \hat{\beta}_{30} > \beta_{40} = 0$$

indicates that an individual with no chronic disease has higher probability of paying no visits or a few visits, as compared to paying higher number of visits, which is expected. By the same token,

$$[\hat{\beta}_{10} + \hat{\beta}_{11} = 0.860 - 1.792 = -0.932] < [\hat{\beta}_{30} + \hat{\beta}_{31}] < [\hat{\beta}_{20} + \hat{\beta}_{21}] < 0,$$

indicates that an individual with chronic disease has higher probability of paying larger number of visits. Note however that these estimates also indicate that irrespective of chronic condition a considerably large number of individuals pay at least a few visits, which may be natural or due to other covariate conditions.

2.2.2.4.2 (c) Illustration 2.7: Analysis for Education Level Effects on Physician Visits

We continue to illustrate the application of product multinomial approach now by examining the marginal effects of education status of an individual on the physician visit. Three levels of education are considered, namely low (less than high school education), medium (high school education), and high (more than high school education). The cross-classified data for education level versus physician visits, obtained from Table 2.1, are shown in Table 2.16.

Table 2.16 Cross-classification of education level and physician visit

	Physician visit status				
Education level	None	Few	Not so few	High	Total
Low (< High School)	17	16	10	15	58
Medium (High School)	6	8	8	11	33
High (> High School)	16	36	19	18	89
Total	39	60	37	44	180

Notice that it is appropriate to consider the education level at a given year (1985) as a fixed covariate. Here this covariate has three levels and two dummy covariates can be used to represent these three levels of education. Now to construct the likelihood estimating equation (2.71), following (2.69), we, for convenience, present the probabilities and their regression form as follows.

Level 1 (Low education):

Response count: $K_{[1]1} = 17,\ K_{[1]2} = 16,\ K_{[1]3} = 10,\ K_{[1]4} = 15,\ K_{[1]} = 58.$

Probabilities:

$$\pi_{[1]1} = \frac{\exp(\beta_{10}+\beta_{11})}{1+\sum_{g=1}^{3}\exp(\beta_{g0}+\beta_{g1})},\ \pi_{[1]2} = \frac{\exp(\beta_{20}+\beta_{21})}{1+\sum_{g=1}^{3}\exp(\beta_{g0}+\beta_{g1})},$$
$$\pi_{[1]3} = \frac{\exp(\beta_{30}+\beta_{31})}{1+\sum_{g=1}^{3}\exp(\beta_{g0}+\beta_{g1})},\ \pi_{[1]4} = \frac{1}{1+\sum_{g=1}^{3}\exp(\beta_{g0}+\beta_{g1})}. \quad (2.99)$$

Global regression form: For

$$\theta^* = (\beta_{10},\beta_{11},\beta_{12},\beta_{20},\beta_{21},\beta_{22},\beta_{30},\beta_{31},\beta_{32})',$$

the above probabilities may be re-expressed as

$$\pi_{[1]1} = \frac{\exp(x'_{[1]1}\theta^*)}{\sum_{j=1}^{4}\exp(x'_{[1]j}\theta^*)},\ \pi_{[1]2} = \frac{\exp(x'_{[1]2}\theta^*)}{\sum_{j=1}^{4}\exp(x'_{[1]j}\theta^*)},$$
$$\pi_{[1]3} = \frac{\exp(x'_{[1]3}\theta^*)}{\sum_{j=1}^{4}\exp(x'_{[1]j}\theta^*)},\ \pi_{[1]4} = \frac{\exp(x'_{[1]4}\theta^*)}{\sum_{j=1}^{4}\exp(x'_{[1]j}\theta^*)},$$

where $x'_{[1]3}$, for example, is the third row vector of the $X_1 : 4 \times 9$ matrix given by

$$X_1 = \begin{pmatrix} 1\,1\,0\,0\,0\,0\,0\,0\,0 \\ 0\,0\,0\,1\,1\,0\,0\,0\,0 \\ 0\,0\,0\,0\,0\,0\,1\,1\,0 \\ 0\,0\,0\,0\,0\,0\,0\,0\,0 \end{pmatrix}. \quad (2.100)$$

Level 2 (Medium education):
Response count: $K_{[2]1} = 6,\ K_{[2]2} = 8,\ K_{[2]3} = 8,\ K_{[2]4} = 11,\ K_{[2]} = 33.$
Probabilities:

$$\pi_{[2]1} = \frac{\exp(\beta_{10}+\beta_{12})}{1+\sum_{g=1}^{3}\exp(\beta_{g0}+\beta_{g2})},\ \pi_{[2]2} = \frac{\exp(\beta_{20}+\beta_{22})}{1+\sum_{g=1}^{3}\exp(\beta_{g0}+\beta_{g2})},$$
$$\pi_{[2]3} = \frac{\exp(\beta_{30}+\beta_{32})}{1+\sum_{g=1}^{3}\exp(\beta_{g0}+\beta_{g2})},\ \pi_{[2]4} = \frac{1}{1+\sum_{g=1}^{3}\exp(\beta_{g0}+\beta_{g2})}. \quad (2.101)$$

Global regression form:

$$\pi_{[2]1} = \frac{\exp(x'_{[2]1}\theta^*)}{\sum_{j=1}^{4}\exp(x'_{[2]j}\theta^*)},\ \pi_{[2]2} = \frac{\exp(x'_{[2]2}\theta^*)}{\sum_{j=1}^{4}\exp(x'_{[2]j}\theta^*)},$$
$$\pi_{[2]3} = \frac{\exp(x'_{[2]3}\theta^*)}{\sum_{j=1}^{4}\exp(x'_{[2]j}\theta^*)},\ \pi_{[2]4} = \frac{\exp(x'_{[2]4}\theta^*)}{\sum_{j=1}^{4}\exp(x'_{[2]j}\theta^*)},$$

where θ^* remains the same, but the covariate matrix X_2 is given by

$$X_2 = \begin{pmatrix} 1\ 0\ 1\ 0\ 0\ 0\ 0\ 0\ 0 \\ 0\ 0\ 0\ 1\ 0\ 1\ 0\ 0\ 0 \\ 0\ 0\ 0\ 0\ 0\ 0\ 1\ 0\ 1 \\ 0\ 0\ 0\ 0\ 0\ 0\ 0\ 0\ 0 \end{pmatrix}. \quad (2.102)$$

Level 3 (High education):
Response count: $K_{[3]1} = 16,\ K_{[2]2} = 36,\ K_{[3]3} = 19,\ K_{[3]4} = 18,\ K_{[3]} = 89.$
Probabilities:

$$\pi_{[3]1} = \frac{\exp(\beta_{10})}{1+\sum_{g=1}^{3}\exp(\beta_{g0})},\ \pi_{[3]2} = \frac{\exp(\beta_{20})}{1+\sum_{g=1}^{3}\exp(\beta_{g0})},$$
$$\pi_{[3]3} = \frac{\exp(\beta_{30})}{1+\sum_{g=1}^{3}\exp(\beta_{g0})},\ \pi_{[3]4} = \frac{1}{1+\sum_{g=1}^{3}\exp(\beta_{g0})}. \quad (2.103)$$

Global regression form:

$$\pi_{[3]1} = \frac{\exp(x'_{[3]1}\theta^*)}{\sum_{j=1}^{4}\exp(x'_{[3]j}\theta^*)},\ \pi_{[3]2} = \frac{\exp(x'_{[3]2}\theta^*)}{\sum_{j=1}^{4}\exp(x'_{[3]j}\theta^*)},$$
$$\pi_{[3]3} = \frac{\exp(x'_{[3]3}\theta^*)}{\sum_{j=1}^{4}\exp(x'_{[3]j}\theta^*)},\ \pi_{[3]4} = \frac{\exp(x'_{[3]4}\theta^*)}{\sum_{j=1}^{4}\exp(x'_{[3]j}\theta^*)},$$

Table 2.17 Parameter estimates for the education level and physician visit status data of Table 2.16

	Regression parameters								
Quantity	β_{10}	β_{11}	β_{12}	β_{20}	β_{21}	β_{22}	β_{30}	β_{31}	β_{32}
Estimate	−0.118	0.243	−0.488	0.693	−0.629	−1.012	0.054	−0.460	−0.373
Standard error	0.3436	0.4935	0.6129	0.2887	0.4610	0.5470	0.3289	0.5243	0.5693

where θ^* remains the same, but the covariate matrix X_3 is given by

$$X_3 = \begin{pmatrix} 1 & 0 & 0 & 0 & 0 & 0 & 0 & 0 & 0 \\ 0 & 0 & 0 & 1 & 0 & 0 & 0 & 0 & 0 \\ 0 & 0 & 0 & 0 & 0 & 0 & 1 & 0 & 0 \\ 0 & 0 & 0 & 0 & 0 & 0 & 0 & 0 & 0 \end{pmatrix}. \tag{2.104}$$

Now following (2.71) and using the iterative equation (2.75), we solve the product multinomial based likelihood estimating equation

$$\sum_{\ell=1}^{2} X'_\ell \left[y_{[\ell]} - K_{[\ell]}\pi_{[\ell]}\right] = 0, \tag{2.105}$$

where

$$y_{[\ell]} = \begin{pmatrix} K_{[\ell]1} \\ K_{[\ell]2} \\ K_{[\ell]3} \\ K_{[\ell]4} \end{pmatrix} \text{ and } \pi_{[\ell]} = \begin{pmatrix} \pi_{[\ell]1} \\ \pi_{[\ell]2} \\ \pi_{[\ell]3} \\ \pi_{[\ell]4} \end{pmatrix}.$$

These estimates and their corresponding standard errors computed by using (2.76) are reported in Table 2.17. Further by using these estimates in the probability formulas in (2.99), (2.101), and (2.103), we compute the estimated probabilities, which are same as the corresponding observed probabilities. For the sake of completeness, these probabilities are displayed in Table 2.18.

Notice from (2.103) that the estimates of β_{10}, β_{20}, and β_{30} indicate the relative probability for an individual with high education to be in none, few, and not so few categories, respectively, as compared to the probability for high category determined by $\beta_{40} = 0$ (by assumption). A large positive value of $\hat{\beta}_{20} = 0.693$ as compared to $\beta_{40} = 0$ shows that a large proportion of individuals belonging to the high education group paid a few visits to the physician. Similarly, for the individuals with medium level education, the negative values of $\hat{\beta}_{j0} + \hat{\beta}_{j2}$ for $j = 1,2,3$, such as $\hat{\beta}_{20} + \hat{\beta}_{22} = (0.693 - 1.012) = -0.319$, as compared to 0 show that a large proportion of individuals in this group paid high visits to the physician. On the contrary, by using (2.99), the largest positive value of $\hat{\beta}_{10} + \hat{\beta}_{11} = (-0.118 + 0.243) = 0.125$ indicates that a large proportion of individuals in the low education group did not pay any

Table 2.18 Observed and estimated multinomial probabilities for the education level versus physician visits data of Table 2.16

		Physician visit status				
Education level	Probability	None	Few	Not so few	High	Total
Low	Observed	0.2931	0.2759	0.1724	0.2586	1.0
	Estimated	0.2931	0.2759	0.1724	0.2586	1.0
Medium	Observed	0.1819	0.2424	0.2424	0.3333	1.0
	Estimated	0.1819	0.2424	0.2424	0.3333	1.0
High	Observed	0.1798	0.4045	0.2135	0.2022	1.0
	Estimated	0.1798	0.4045	0.2135	0.2022	1.0

visits. Thus, in general, most of the individuals in the low education group paid no visits to the physician, whereas most of the individuals with higher education paid a moderate number of visits (few visits). These categorical data based results agree, in general, with those reported in Sutradhar (2011, Section 4.2.8) based on original counts. However, the present categorical data based analysis naturally reveals more detailed pattern of visits.

2.2.3 Multinomial Likelihood Models with L= $(p+1)(q+1)$ Nominal Levels for Two Covariates with Interactions

Let there be two categorical covariates, one with $p+1$ levels and the other with $q+1$ levels. Following (2.45), for an individual i, we use the p-dimensional vector $w_i = [w_{i1},\ldots,w_{is},\ldots,w_{ip}]'$ containing p dummy covariates to represent $p+1$ levels of the first categorical covariate, and the q-dimensional vector $v_i = [v_{i1},\ldots,v_{im},\ldots,v_{iq}]'$ containing q dummy covariates to represent the $q+1$ levels of the second categorical covariate. Further, let $w_i(v_i)$ be a pq-dimensional nested covariate vector with v_i nested within w_i. That is,

$$w_i(v_i) = [w_{i1}v_{i1},\ldots,w_{i1}v_{iq},w_{i2}v_{11},\ldots,w_{is}v_{im},\ldots,w_{ip}v_{iq}]'.$$

Similar to (2.45), one may then write the probability for the response of the ith individual to be in the jth $(j=1,\ldots,J)$ category as

$$P[y_i = y_i^{(j)} = \delta_{ij}] = \pi_{(i)j} = \begin{cases} \frac{\exp(\beta_{j0}+\beta_j' w_i+\xi_j' v_i+\phi_j^{*\prime} w_i(v_i))}{1+\sum_{g=1}^{J-1}\exp(\beta_{g0}+\beta_g' w_i+\xi_g' v_i+\phi_g^{*\prime} w_i(v_i))} & \text{for } j=1,\ldots,J-1 \\ \frac{1}{1+\sum_{g=1}^{J-1}\exp(\beta_{g0}+\beta_g' w_i+\xi_g' v_i+\phi_g^{*\prime} w_i(v_i))} & \text{for } j=J, \end{cases} \tag{2.106}$$

where $\beta_j = [\beta_{j1},\ldots,\beta_{js},\ldots,\beta_{jp}]'$, $\xi_j = [\xi_{j1},\ldots,\xi_{jm},\ldots,\xi_{jq}]'$, and ϕ_j^* be the pq-dimensional vector of interaction effects of the covariates defined as

$$\phi_j^* = [\phi_{j11}^*,\ldots,\phi_{j1q}^*,\phi_{j21}^*,\ldots,\phi_{jsm}^*,\ldots,\phi_{jpq}^*]'.$$

Note that in (2.89), the interaction effects of two response variables are denoted by $\{\phi_{rj}\}$ whereas in (2.106), $\{\phi^*_{jum}\}$ represent the interaction effects of two covariates on the response $y_i = y_i^{(j)}$. Thus, a clear difference is laid out so that one does not use the same model to deal with contingency tables between two responses, and the contingency tables between one response and one or two or more categorical covariates. To be more explicit, one must use the probabilities in (2.89) to construct a full multinomial model, whereas the probabilities in (2.106) should be used to construct the product multinomial model.

Note that the $p+1$ levels corresponding to the covariate vector w_i may be formed as

$$(w_{i1},\cdots,w_{ip}) \equiv \begin{cases} (\,1,\,01'_{p-1}) & \longrightarrow \text{Level 1} \\ (\,01'_1,\,1,\,01'_{p-2}) & \longrightarrow \text{Level 2} \\ (\cdots\cdots\cdots\cdots) & \\ (\,01'_{\ell_1-1},\,1,\,01'_{p-\ell_1}) & \longrightarrow \text{Level } \ell_1 \\ (\cdots\cdots\cdots\cdots) & \\ (\,01'_{p-1},\,1\,) & \longrightarrow \text{Level p} \\ (\,01'_p) & \longrightarrow \text{Level p+1} \end{cases} \tag{2.107}$$

Similarly, the $q+1$ levels corresponding to the covariate vector v_i may be formed as

$$(v_{i1},\cdots,v_{iq}) \equiv \begin{cases} (\,1,\,01'_{q-1}) & \longrightarrow \text{Level 1} \\ (\,01'_1,\,1,\,01'_{q-2}) & \longrightarrow \text{Level 2} \\ (\cdots\cdots\cdots\cdots) & \\ (\,01'_{\ell_2-1},\,1,\,01'_{q-\ell_2}) & \longrightarrow \text{Level } \ell_2 \\ (\cdots\cdots\cdots\cdots) & \\ (\,01'_{q-1},\,1\,) & \longrightarrow \text{Level q} \\ (\,01'_q) & \longrightarrow \text{Level q+1} \end{cases} \tag{2.108}$$

Consequently, by (2.106), we may write the level based probabilities for an individual i, with covariates at level (ℓ_1,ℓ_2), to be in the jth category as

$$\pi_{[\ell_1,\ell_2]j} = \pi_{(i\in\{\ell_1,\ell_2\})j}$$
$$= \begin{cases} \frac{\exp(\beta_{j0}+\beta_{j\ell_1}+\xi_{j\ell_2}+\phi^*_{j,\ell_1\ell_2})}{1+\sum_{g=1}^{J-1}\exp(\beta_{g0}+\beta_{g\ell_1}+\xi_{g\ell_2}+\phi^*_{g,\ell_1\ell_2})} & \text{for } j=1,\ldots,J-1;\ell_1=1,\ldots,p;\ell_2=1,\ldots,q \\ \frac{1}{1+\sum_{g=1}^{J-1}\exp(\beta_{g0}+\beta_{g\ell_1}+\xi_{g\ell_2}+\phi^*_{g,\ell_1\ell_2})} & \text{for } j=J;\ \ell_1=1,\ldots,p;\ell_2=1,\ldots,q, \end{cases} \tag{2.109}$$

$$\pi_{[\ell_1,q+1]j} = \pi_{(i\in\{\ell_1,q+1\})j}$$
$$= \begin{cases} \frac{\exp(\beta_{j0}+\beta_{j\ell_1})}{1+\sum_{g=1}^{J-1}\exp(\beta_{g0}+\beta_{g\ell_1})} & \text{for } j=1,\ldots,J-1; \ell_1=1,\ldots,p \\ \frac{1}{1+\sum_{g=1}^{J-1}\exp(\beta_{g0}+\beta_{g\ell_1})} & \text{for } j=J;\ \ell_1=1,\ldots,p, \end{cases} \tag{2.110}$$

$$\pi_{[p+1,\ell_2]j} = \pi_{(i\in\{p+1,\ell_2\})j}$$
$$= \begin{cases} \frac{\exp(\beta_{j0}+\xi_{j\ell_2})}{1+\sum_{g=1}^{J-1}\exp(\beta_{g0}+\xi_{g\ell_2})} & \text{for } j=1,\ldots,J-1; \ell_2=1,\ldots,q \\ \frac{1}{1+\sum_{g=1}^{J-1}\exp(\beta_{g0}+\xi_{g\ell_2})} & \text{for } j=J;\ \ell_2=1,\ldots,q, \end{cases} \tag{2.111}$$

and

$$\pi_{[p+1,q+1]j} = \pi_{(i\in\{p+1,q+1\})j}$$
$$= \begin{cases} \frac{\exp(\beta_{j0})}{1+\sum_{g=1}^{J-1}\exp(\beta_{g0})} & \text{for } j=1,\ldots,J-1 \\ \frac{1}{1+\sum_{g=1}^{J-1}\exp(\beta_{g0})} & \text{for } j=J. \end{cases} \tag{2.112}$$

Next we display the observed cell counts in notation under all J categories and covariates level (ℓ_1,ℓ_2). Note that by transforming the rectangular levels to a real valued level, that is, using the relabeling formula $\{\ell \equiv [(\ell_1-1)(q+1)+\ell_2], \ell_1=1,\ldots,p+1; \ell_2=1,\ldots,q+1\}$, one may still use the Table 2.4 after a slight adjustment to display the cell counts in the present setup with two covariates. The cell counts with level adjustment are shown in Table 2.19.

Note that even though the cell probabilities in Tables 2.4 and 2.19 are denoted by the same notation $\pi_{[\ell]j}$, they are however different. The difference lies in the form of global regression parameter θ^*. To be more specific, the probabilities in Table 2.4 follow the formulas in (2.63)–(2.64), which were further re-expressed by (2.69) as

$$\pi_{[\ell]j} = \frac{\exp(x'_{[\ell]j}\theta^*)}{\sum_{g=1}^{J}\exp(x'_{[\ell]g}\theta^*)},$$

with

$$\theta^* = [\beta_1^{*\prime},\ldots,\beta_j^{*\prime},\ldots,\beta_{J-1}^{*}{}']', \text{ where } \beta_j^* = [\beta_{j0},\beta_j']'.$$

Note that once θ^* is written, the row vector $x'_{[\ell]j}$ becomes specified from the probability formulas. Now because $\pi_{[\ell]j}$ in Table 2.19 represent the two covariates level based probabilities defined in (2.109)–(2.112), the global regression parameters are different than θ^* in (2.69).

Table 2.19 A notational display for cell counts and probabilities for J categories under covariates level $(\ell_1, \ell_2) \longrightarrow$ Newlevel $\ell = (\ell_1 - 1)(\mathrm{q}+1) + \ell_2$

			***J* response categories**			
Covariates level	**New level**	**Quantity**	**1**	...	***J***	**Total**
$(1,1)$	1	Count	$K_{[1]1}$	...	$K_{[1]J}$	$K_{[1]}$
		Probability	$\pi_{[1]1}$	...	$\pi_{[1]J}$	1
.	.	.	.	...	.	.
		.	.	...	.	.
$(1,q+1)$	$q+1$	Count	$K_{[q+1]1}$	...	$K_{[q+1]J}$	$K_{[q+1]}$
		Probability	$\pi_{[q+1]1}$	...	$\pi_{[q+1]J}$	1
$(2,1)$	$q+2$	Count	$K_{[q+2]1}$	...	$K_{[q+2]J}$	$K_{[q+2]}$
		Probability	$\pi_{[q+2]1}$	...	$\pi_{[q+2]J}$	1
.	.	.	.	...	.	.
		.	.	...	.	.
(ℓ_1,ℓ_2)	ℓ	Count	$K_{[\ell]1}$	...	$K_{[\ell]J}$	$K_{[\ell]}$
		Probability	$\pi_{[\ell]1}$	...	$\pi_{[\ell]J}$	1
.	.	.	.	...	.	.
		.	.	...	.	.
$(p+1,q+1)$	$(p+1)(q+1)$	Count	$K_{[(p+1)(q+1)]1}$	...	$K_{[(p+1)(q+1)]J}$	$K_{[(p+1)(q+1)]}$
		Probability	$\pi_{[(p+1)(q+1)]1}$	...	$\pi_{[(p+1)(q+1)]J}$	1

Let θ^{**} denote the regression parameters used in two covariates level based probabilities in (2.109)–(2.112). To be specific, we write

$$\theta^{**} = [\beta_1^{**\prime}, \ldots, \beta_j^{**\prime}, \ldots, \beta_{J-1}^{**\prime}]' : \{(J-1)(p+1)(q+1)\} \times 1, \tag{2.113}$$

where

$$\beta_j^{**} = [\beta_{j0},\ \beta_j',\ \xi_j',\ \phi^{*\prime}_j]' : \{(p+1)(q+1)\} \times 1,$$

with

$$\begin{aligned}\beta_j' &= [\beta_{j1}, \ldots, \beta_{js}, \ldots, \beta_{jp}] \\ \xi_j' &= [\xi_{j1}, \ldots, \xi_{jm}, \ldots, \xi_{jq}] \\ \phi^{*\prime}_j &= [\phi^*_{j,11}, \ldots, \phi^*_{j,1q}, \phi^*_{j,21}, \ldots, \phi^*_{j,sm}, \ldots, \phi^*_{j,pq}],\end{aligned}$$

by (2.106).

Consequently, at level

$$\ell = (\ell_1 - 1)(q+1) + \ell_2,\ \ell_1 = 1,\ldots,p+1;\ \ell_2 = 1,\ldots,q+1,$$

all probabilities defined in (2.109)–(2.112) may be expressed as

$$\pi_{[\ell]j} = \frac{\exp(x'_{[\ell]j}\theta^{**})}{\sum_{g=1}^{J}\exp(x'_{[\ell]g}\theta^{**})}, \tag{2.114}$$

where $x'_{[\ell]j}: 1\times(J-1)(p+1)(q+1)$ is the jth $(j=1,\ldots,J)$ row vector of the $X_\ell : J\times(J-1)(p+1)(q+1)$ matrix at the ℓth level $(\ell = 1,\ldots,(p+1)(q+1))$. We construct this jth row vector of the X_ℓ matrix in four groups as follows.

Group 1: $\ell = \{(\ell_1-1)q+\ell_2\}$ for $\ell_1 = 1,\ldots,p;\ \ell_2 = 1,\ldots,q$

$$\begin{aligned} x'_{[\ell]j} &= x'_{[(\ell_1-1)q+\ell_2]j} \\ &= \begin{cases} \Big[01'_{(j-1)(p+1)(q+1)}, \\ \{1, 01'_{\ell_1-1}, 1, 01'_{p-\ell_1}, 01'_{\ell_2-1}, 1, 01'_{q-\ell_2}, 01'_{(\ell_1-1)q+\ell_2-1}, 1, 01'_{pq-[(\ell_1-1)q+\ell_2]}\}, \\ 01'_{(J-1-j)(p+1)(q+1)}\Big], \text{ for } j = 1,\ldots,J-1 \\ 01'_{(J-1)(p+1)(q+1)}, \text{ for } j = J. \end{cases} \end{aligned} \tag{2.115}$$

Group 2: $\ell = \{(\ell_1-1)(q+1)+(q+1)\}$ for $\ell_1 = 1,\ldots,p$

$$\begin{aligned} x'_{[\ell]j} &= x'_{[(\ell_1-1)(q+1)+(q+1)]j} \\ &= \begin{cases} \Big[01'_{(j-1)(p+1)(q+1)}, \\ \{1, 01'_{\ell_1-1}, 1, 01'_{p-\ell_1}, 01'_{q}, 01'_{pq}, \}, \\ 01'_{(J-1-j)(p+1)(q+1)}\Big], \text{ for } j = 1,\ldots,J-1 \\ 01'_{(J-1)(p+1)(q+1)}, \text{ for } j = J. \end{cases} \end{aligned} \tag{2.116}$$

Group 3: $\ell = \{p(q+1)+\ell_2\}$ for $\ell_2 = 1,\ldots,q$

$$\begin{aligned} x'_{[\ell]j} &= x'_{[p(q+1)+\ell_2]j} \\ &= \begin{cases} \Big[01'_{(j-1)(p+1)(q+1)}, \\ \{1, 01'_{p}, 01'_{\ell_2-1}, 1, 01'_{q-\ell_2}, 01'_{pq}, \}, \\ 01'_{(J-1-j)(p+1)(q+1)}\Big], \text{ for } j = 1,\ldots,J-1 \\ 01'_{(J-1)(p+1)(q+1)}, \text{ for } j = J. \end{cases} \end{aligned} \tag{2.117}$$

Group 4: $\ell = \{(p+1)(q+1)\}$

$$x'_{[\ell]j} = x'_{[(p+1)(q+1)]j}$$

$$= \begin{cases} \Big[01'_{(j-1)(p+1)(q+1)}, \\ \{1, 01'_p, 01'_q, 01'_{pq}, \}, \\ 01'_{(J-1-j)(p+1)(q+1)}\Big], \quad \text{for } j = 1, \ldots, J-1 \\ 01'_{(J-1)(p+1)(q+1)}, \quad \text{for } j = J. \end{cases} \tag{2.118}$$

Now by replacing θ^* with θ^{**} in (2.67)–(2.68), by similar calculations as in (2.71), one obtains the likelihood equations for θ^{**} as

$$\frac{\partial \log L(\theta^{**})}{\partial \theta^{**}} = \sum_{\ell=1}^{(p+1)(q+1)} X'_\ell \left[y_{[\ell]} - K_{[\ell]}\pi_{[\ell]}\right] = 0, \tag{2.119}$$

where

$$y_{[\ell]} = [K_{[\ell]1}, \ldots, K_{[\ell]j}, \ldots, K_{[\ell]J}]' \text{ and } \pi_{[\ell]} = [\pi_{[\ell]1}, \ldots, \pi_{[\ell]j}, \ldots, \pi_{[\ell]J}]',$$

with probabilities are being given by (2.114) or equivalently by (2.109)–(2.112), and furthermore X_ℓ matrices for $\ell = 1, \ldots, (p+1)(q+1)$ are given as in (2.115)–(2.118).

Note that after slight adjustment in notation, one may use the iterative equation (2.75) to solve this likelihood equation in (2.119). To be specific, the iterative equation to solve (2.119) for the final estimate for θ^{**} is given by

$$\widehat{\theta^{**}}(r+1) = \widehat{\theta^{**}}(r) + \left[\sum_{\ell=1}^{(p+1)(q+1)} K_{[\ell]} X'_\ell \left[D_{\pi_{[\ell]}} - \pi_{[\ell]}\pi'_{[\ell]}\right] X_\ell\right]^{-1}$$
$$\times \left[\sum_{\ell=1}^{(p+1)(q+1)} X'_\ell \left(y_{[\ell]} - K_{[\ell]}\pi_{[\ell]}\right)\right]_{\theta^{**} = \widehat{\theta^{**}}(r)}, \tag{2.120}$$

where $D_{\pi_{[\ell]}} = \text{diag}[\pi_{[\ell]1}, \ldots, \pi_{[\ell]j}, \ldots, \pi_{[\ell]J}]$. Furthermore, the covariance matrix of $\widehat{\theta^{**}}$ has the formula

$$\text{var}(\widehat{\theta^{**}}) = \left[\sum_{\ell=1}^{(p+1)(q+1)} K_{[\ell]} X'_\ell \{D_{\pi_{[\ell]}} - \pi_{[\ell]}\pi'_{[\ell]}\} X_\ell\right]^{-1}. \tag{2.121}$$

2.2.3.1 Illustration 2.8: Analysis for the Effects of Both Gender and Chronic Condition on the Physician Visits

The marginal effects of gender and chronic condition on the physician visits were discussed in Sects. 2.2.2.4.2(a) and (b), respectively. To illustrate the product multinomial model for a response variable (physician visit) based on two categorical covariates, discussed in the last section, we now consider gender and chronic

Table 2.20 $2 \times 2 \times 4$ contingency table for the physician visit data corresponding to gender and chronic condition of the individuals

		Physician visit status				
Gender	Chronic condition	None	Few	Not so few	High	Level total (K_ℓ)
Male	One or more	8	13	9	10	40
	None	20	27	7	2	56
Female	One or more	5	12	12	23	52
	None	6	8	9	9	32

Table 2.21 Cell counts and probabilities for $J = 4$ physician visit categories under covariates level (ℓ_1, ℓ_2) for $\ell_1 = 1, 2$; and $\ell_2 = 1, 2$

			Physician visit status				
Covariates level	New level (ℓ)	Quantity	None	Few	Not so few	High	Level total ($K_{[\ell]}$)
(1,1)	1	Count	8	13	9	10	40
		Probability	$\pi_{[1]1}$	$\pi_{[1]2}$	$\pi_{[1]3}$	$\pi_{[1]4}$	1.0
(1,2)	2	Count	20	27	7	2	56
		Probability	$\pi_{[2]1}$	$\pi_{[2]2}$	$\pi_{[2]3}$	$\pi_{[2]4}$	1.0
(2,1)	3	Count	5	12	12	23	52
		Probability	$\pi_{[3]1}$	$\pi_{[3]2}$	$\pi_{[3]3}$	$\pi_{[3]4}$	1.0
(2,2)	4	Count	6	8	9	9	32
		Probability	$\pi_{[4]1}$	$\pi_{[4]2}$	$\pi_{[4]3}$	$\pi_{[4]4}$	1.0

condition as two covariates and examine their marginal as well as joint (interaction between the two covariates) effects on the physician visit. For the purpose, following the Table 2.19, we first present the observed counts as in the $2 \times 2 \times 4$ contingency Table 2.20. Note that this contingency table is not showing the distribution for three response variables, rather, it shows the distribution of one response variable at different marginal and joint levels for the two covariates. Consequently, it is appropriate to use the product multinomial approach to analyze the data of this Table 2.20.

Further to make the cell probability formulas clear and precise, we use the data from Table 2.20 and put them in Table 2.21 along with probabilities following the format of Table 2.19.

Next, we write the formulas for the probabilities in Table 2.21 in the form of (2.109)–(2.112), and also in global regression form as follows:

Level 1 (Group 1) (based on $\ell_1 = 1, \ell_2 = 1$):

Probabilities:

$$\pi_{[1]1} = \frac{\exp(\beta_{10} + \beta_{11} + \xi_{11} + \phi^*_{1,11})}{1 + \sum_{g=1}^{3} \exp(\beta_{g0} + \beta_{g1} + \xi_{g1} + \phi^*_{g,11})}, \quad \pi_{[1]2} = \frac{\exp(\beta_{20} + \beta_{21} + \xi_{21} + \phi^*_{2,11})}{1 + \sum_{g=1}^{3} \exp(\beta_{g0} + \beta_{g1} + \xi_{g1} + \phi^*_{g,11})},$$

$$\pi_{[1]3} = \frac{\exp(\beta_{30} + \beta_{31} + \xi_{31} + \phi^*_{3,11})}{1 + \sum_{g=1}^{3} \exp(\beta_{g0} + \beta_{g1} + \xi_{g1} + \phi^*_{g,11})}, \; \pi_{[1]4} = \frac{1}{1 + \sum_{g=1}^{3} \exp(\beta_{g0} + \beta_{g1} + \xi_{g1} + \phi^*_{g,11})}. \tag{2.122}$$

Global regression form:

$$\pi_{[1]1} = \frac{\exp(x'_{[1]1}\theta^{**})}{\sum_{j=1}^{4} \exp(x'_{[1]j}\theta^{**})}, \; \pi_{[1]2} = \frac{\exp(x'_{[1]2}\theta^{**})}{\sum_{j=1}^{4} \exp(x'_{[1]j}\theta^{**})},$$

$$\pi_{[1]3} = \frac{\exp(x'_{[1]3}\theta^{**})}{\sum_{j=1}^{4} \exp(x'_{[1]j}\theta^{**})}, \; \pi_{[1]4} = \frac{\exp(x'_{[1]4}\theta^{**})}{\sum_{j=1}^{4} \exp(x'_{[1]j}\theta^{**})},$$

where

$$\theta^{**} = (\beta_{10}, \beta_{11}, \xi_{11}, \phi^*_{1,11}, \beta_{20}, \beta_{21}, \xi_{21}, \phi^*_{2,11}, \beta_{30}, \beta_{31}, \xi_{31}, \phi^*_{3,11},)',$$

and $x'_{[1]3}$, for example, is the third row vector of the $X_1 : 4 \times 12$ matrix given by

$$X_1 = \begin{pmatrix} 1'_4 & 01'_4 & 01'_4 \\ 01'_4 & 1'_4 & 01'_4 \\ 01'_4 & 01'_4 & 1'_4 \\ 01'_4 & 01'_4 & 01'_4 \end{pmatrix}. \tag{2.123}$$

Level 2 (Group 2) (based on $\ell_1 = 1$):
Probabilities:

$$\pi_{[2]1} = \frac{\exp(\beta_{10} + \beta_{11})}{1 + \sum_{g=1}^{3} \exp(\beta_{g0} + \beta_{g1})}, \; \pi_{[2]2} = \frac{\exp(\beta_{20} + \beta_{21})}{1 + \sum_{g=1}^{3} \exp(\beta_{g0} + \beta_{g1})},$$

$$\pi_{[2]3} = \frac{\exp(\beta_{30} + \beta_{31})}{1 + \sum_{g=1}^{3} \exp(\beta_{g0} + \beta_{g1})}, \; \pi_{[2]4} = \frac{1}{1 + \sum_{g=1}^{3} \exp(\beta_{g0} + \beta_{g1})}. \tag{2.124}$$

Global regression form:

$$\pi_{[2]1} = \frac{\exp(x'_{[2]1}\theta^{**})}{\sum_{j=1}^{4} \exp(x'_{[2]j}\theta^{**})}, \; \pi_{[2]2} = \frac{\exp(x'_{[2]2}\theta^{**})}{\sum_{j=1}^{4} \exp(x'_{[2]j}\theta^{**})},$$

$$\pi_{[2]3} = \frac{\exp(x'_{[2]3}\theta^{**})}{\sum_{j=1}^{4} \exp(x'_{[2]j}\theta^{**})}, \; \pi_{[2]4} = \frac{\exp(x'_{[2]4}\theta^{**})}{\sum_{j=1}^{4} \exp(x'_{[2]j}\theta^{**})},$$

where θ^{**} is the same as above, that is,

$$\theta^{**} = (\beta_{10}, \beta_{11}, \xi_{11}, \phi^*_{1,11}, \beta_{20}, \beta_{21}, \xi_{21}, \phi^*_{2,11}, \beta_{30}, \beta_{31}, \xi_{31}, \phi^*_{3,11},)',$$

and $x'_{[2]3}$, for example, is the third row vector of the $X_2 : 4 \times 12$ matrix given by

$$X_2 = \begin{pmatrix} 1'_2 & 01'_2 & 01'_4 & 01'_4 \\ 01'_4 & 1'_2 & 01'_2 & 01'_4 \\ 01'_4 & 01'_4 & 1'_2 & 01'_2 \\ 01'_2 & 01'_2 & 01'_4 & 01'_4 \end{pmatrix}. \tag{2.125}$$

Level 3 (Group 3) (based on $\ell_2 = 1$):
Probabilities:

$$\pi_{[3]1} = \frac{\exp(\beta_{10} + \xi_{11})}{1 + \sum_{g=1}^{3} \exp(\beta_{g0} + \xi_{g1})}, \ \pi_{[3]2} = \frac{\exp(\beta_{20} + \xi_{21})}{1 + \sum_{g=1}^{3} \exp(\beta_{g0} + \xi_{g1})},$$
$$\pi_{[3]3} = \frac{\exp(\beta_{30} + \xi_{31})}{1 + \sum_{g=1}^{3} \exp(\beta_{g0} + \xi_{g1})}, \ \pi_{[3]4} = \frac{1}{1 + \sum_{g=1}^{3} \exp(\beta_{g0} + \xi_{g1})}. \tag{2.126}$$

Global regression form:

$$\pi_{[3]1} = \frac{\exp(x'_{[3]1}\theta^{**})}{\sum_{j=1}^{4} \exp(x'_{[3]j}\theta^{**})}, \ \pi_{[3]2} = \frac{\exp(x'_{[3]2}\theta^{**})}{\sum_{j=1}^{4} \exp(x'_{[3]j}\theta^{**})},$$
$$\pi_{[3]3} = \frac{\exp(x'_{[3]3}\theta^{**})}{\sum_{j=1}^{4} \exp(x'_{[3]j}\theta^{**})}, \pi_{[3]4} = \frac{\exp(x'_{[3]4}\theta^{**})}{\sum_{j=1}^{4} \exp(x'_{[3]j}\theta^{**})},$$

where $x'_{[3]3}$, for example, is the third row vector of the $X_3 : 4 \times 12$ matrix given by

$$X_3 = \begin{pmatrix} 1 & 0 & 1 & 0 & 01'_4 & 01'_4 \\ 01'_4 & 1 & 0 & 1 & 0 & 01'_4 \\ 01'_4 & 01'_4 & 1 & 0 & 1 & 0 \\ 01'_4 & 01'_4 & 0 & 0 & 0 & 0 \end{pmatrix}. \tag{2.127}$$

Level 4 (Group 4)
Probabilities:

$$\pi_{[4]1} = \frac{\exp(\beta_{10})}{1 + \sum_{g=1}^{3} \exp(\beta_{g0})}, \ \pi_{[4]2} = \frac{\exp(\beta_{20})}{1 + \sum_{g=1}^{3} \exp(\beta_{g0})},$$
$$\pi_{[4]3} = \frac{\exp(\beta_{30})}{1 + \sum_{g=1}^{3} \exp(\beta_{g0})}, \ \pi_{[4]4} = \frac{1}{1 + \sum_{g=1}^{3} \exp(\beta_{g0})}. \tag{2.128}$$

Global regression form:

$$\pi_{[4]1} = \frac{\exp(x'_{[4]1}\theta^{**})}{\sum_{j=1}^{4} \exp(x'_{[4]j}\theta^{**})}, \ \pi_{[4]2} = \frac{\exp(x'_{[4]2}\theta^{**})}{\sum_{j=1}^{4} \exp(x'_{[4]j}\theta^{**})},$$

Table 2.22 Parameter estimates for the gender and chronic condition versus physician visit status data of Table 2.21

	Regression parameters							
Quantity	β_{10}	β_{11}	ξ_{11}	$\phi^*_{1,11}$	β_{20}	β_{21}	ξ_{21}	$\phi^*_{2,11}$
Estimate	−0.405	2.708	−1.121	−1.405	−0.118	2.720	−.533	−1.808
Standard error	0.5270	0.9100	0.7220	1.1385	0.4859	0.8793	0.6024	1.0377
Quantity	β_{30}	β_{31}	ξ_{31}	$\phi^*_{3,11}$				
Estimate	0.000	1.253	−0.651	−0.708				
Standard error	0.4714	0.9301	0.5908	1.0968				

Table 2.23 Estimated/observed probabilities corresponding to the data given in $2 \times 2 \times 4$ contingency Table 2.20

		Physician visit status			
Gender	Chronic condition	None	Few	Not so few	High
Male	One or more	0.2000	0.3250	0.2250	0.2500
	None	0.3572	0.4821	0.1250	0.0357
Female	One or more	0.0962	0.2308	0.2308	0.4422
	None	0.1874	0.2500	0.2813	0.2813

$$\pi_{[4]3} = \frac{\exp(x'_{[4]3}\theta^{**})}{\sum_{j=1}^{4}\exp(x'_{[4]j}\theta^{**})}, \pi_{[4]4} = \frac{\exp(x'_{[4]4}\theta^{**})}{\sum_{j=1}^{4}\exp(x'_{[4]j}\theta^{**})},$$

where $x'_{[4]3}$, for example, is the third row vector of the $X_4 : 4 \times 12$ matrix given by

$$X_4 = \begin{pmatrix} 1 & 01'_3 & 01'_4 & 01'_4 \\ 01'_4 & 1 & 01'_3 & 01'_4 \\ 01'_4 & 01'_4 & 1 & 01'_3 \\ 01'_4 & 01'_4 & 01'_3 & 0 \end{pmatrix}. \tag{2.129}$$

Using the gender and chronic condition versus physician visits data from Table 2.21, we now solve the likelihood estimating equation (2.119), i.e.,

$$\frac{\partial \log L(\theta^{**})}{\partial \theta^{**}} = \sum_{\ell=1}^{(p+1)(q+1)} X'_\ell \left[y_{[\ell]} - K_{[\ell]}\pi_{[\ell]}\right] = 0,$$

for θ^{**}. The estimates for all components in θ^{**} along with their standard errors are given in Table 2.22.

Now by using the regression estimates from Table 2.22 into the probability formulas (2.112), (2.124), (2.126), and (2.128), one obtains the estimated probabilities as in Table 2.23. The estimated and observed probabilities are the same.

We now interpret the estimates of the parameters from Table 2.22. Because at level 4, i.e., for a female with no chronic disease, the category probabilities for the first three categories are determined by the respective estimates of β_{10}, β_{20}, and β_{30}, as compared to the conventional value $\beta_{40} = 0$, it is easier to interpret their role first. For example, $\hat{\beta}_{30} = 0.0$ shows that an individual in this group has the same probability to be in the third (not so few) or fourth (high) physician visits category. Further, smaller negative value for $\hat{\beta}_{20} = -0.118$ as compared to $\hat{\beta}_{10} = -0.405$ shows that the individual in this group has a much higher probability to pay a few visits to the physician as opposed to paying no visits at all.

Next the values of $(\hat{\beta}_{j0} + \hat{\xi}_{j1})$ for $j = 1,2,3$, as compared to $\beta_{40} + \xi_{41} = 0.0$ would determine relative probability of an individual at level 3 (group 3) to be in the jth category. Note that group 3 individuals are female with one or more chronic disease. For example, the small negative and equal values of $\hat{\beta}_{20} + \hat{\xi}_{21} = -0.651 = \hat{\beta}_{30} + \hat{\xi}_{31}$ as compared to large negative value of $\hat{\beta}_{10} + \hat{\xi}_{11} = -1.526$ indicate that a female with chronic disease has increasing probabilities to pay more visit to the physicians. But a male with chronic disease, i.e., an individual belonging to group 1 (level 1), has smaller probability to pay a high physician visit. This follows from relatively large positive value of $\hat{\beta}_{20} + \hat{\beta}_{21} + \hat{\xi}_{21} + \hat{\phi}^*{}_{2,11} = 0.261$ as compared to small negative value of $\hat{\beta}_{30} + \hat{\beta}_{31} + \hat{\xi}_{31} + \hat{\phi}^*{}_{3,11} = -0.106$, and $\beta_{40} + \beta_{41} + \xi_{41} + \phi^*{}_{4,11} = 0.0$.

2.3 Cumulative Logits Model for Univariate Ordinal Categorical Data

There are situations where the categories for a response may also be ordinal by nature. For example, when the individuals in a study are categorized to examine their agreement or disagreement on a policy issue with, say, three political groups A, B, and C, these three categories are clearly nominal. However, in the treatment versus heart attack status data analyzed in Sect. 2.2.2.4.1, the three categories accommodating the heart attack status, namely no attack, non-fatal, and fatal attacks, can also be treated as ordinal categories. Similarly, in the physician visit study in Sect. 2.2.2.4.2, four physician visit status, namely none, few, not so few, and high visits, can be treated as ordinal categories. Now because of this additional ordinal property of the categorical responses, one may collapse the $J > 2$ categories in a cumulative fashion into two $(J' = 2)$ categories and use simpler binary model to fit such collapsed data. Note however that there will be various binary groups depending on which category in the middle is used as a cut point. This approach is referred to as the cumulative logits model approach and we discuss this alternative modeling of the categorical data in this section provided the categories also exhibit order in them.

2.3.1 Cumulative Logits Model Involving One Covariate with $L = p+1$ Levels

Suppose that similar to Sect. 2.2.2, $\pi_{[\ell]j}$ denotes the probability for an individual i with covariate at level $\ell(\ell = 1,\ldots,p+1)$ to be in the jth category, but because categories are ordered, one may collapse the J categories based multinomial model to a binary model with

$$F_{[\ell]j} = \sum_{c=1}^{j} \pi_{[\ell]c}$$

representing the probability for the binary response to be in any categories between 1 and j, and

$$1 - F_{[\ell]j} = \sum_{c=j+1}^{J} \pi_{[\ell]c}$$

representing the probability for the binary response to be in any categories beyond j. Consequently, unlike in Sect. 2.2.2, instead of modeling individual category based probabilities $\pi_{[\ell]j}$, one may model the binary probability $F_{[\ell]j}$ by using the linear logits relationship

$$L_{[\ell]j} = log\left[\frac{1-F_{[\ell]j}}{F_{[\ell]j}}\right] = \begin{cases} \alpha_{j0}+\alpha_{j\ell} & \text{for } j=1,\ldots,J-1;\ \ell=1,\ldots,p \\ \alpha_{j0} & \text{for } j=1,\ldots,J-1;\ \ell=p+1. \end{cases} \quad (2.130)$$

We refer to this model (2.130) as the logit model 1 (LM1). Also, three other logit models are considered in the next section with relation to a real life data example.

Note that for $j = 1,\ldots,J-1$, the logit relationship in (2.130) is equivalent to write

$$1 - F_{[\ell]j} = \begin{cases} \frac{\exp(\alpha_{j0}+\alpha_{j\ell})}{1+\exp(\alpha_{j0}+\alpha_{j\ell})} & \text{for } \ell = 1,\ldots,p \\ \frac{\exp(\alpha_{j0})}{1+\exp(\alpha_{j0})} & \text{for } \ell = p+1. \end{cases} \quad (2.131)$$

Remark that the logits in (2.130) satisfy the monotonic constraint given in the following lemma.

Lemma 2.3.1. *The logits in (2.130) satisfy the monotonic property*

$$L_{[\ell]1} \geq L_{[\ell]2} \geq \ldots \geq L_{[\ell](J-1)}. \quad (2.132)$$

Proof. Since

$$F_{[\ell]1} \leq F_{[\ell]2} \leq \ldots \leq F_{[\ell](J-1)},$$

and

$$(1 - F_{[\ell]1}) \geq (1 - F_{[\ell]2}) \geq \ldots \geq (1 - F_{[\ell](J-1)}),$$

one obtains

$$\frac{F_{[\ell]1}}{1 - F_{[\ell]1}} \leq \frac{F_{[\ell]2}}{1 - F_{[\ell]2}} \leq \cdots \leq \frac{F_{[\ell](J-1)}}{1 - F_{[\ell](J-1)}}.$$

Hence the lemma follows because $L_{[\ell]j} = log\left[\frac{1-F_{[\ell]j}}{F_{[\ell]j}}\right]$ for all $j = 1, \ldots, J-1$.

2.3.1.1 Weighted Least Square Estimation for the Parameters of the Cumulative Logits Model (2.130)

We describe this estimation technique in the following steps.

Step 1. Writing the logits in linear regression form

Let $F(\pi)$ be a vector consisting of all possible logits, where π represents all $J(p+1)$ individual cell probabilities. That is,

$$F = F(\pi) = \left[L'_1, \ldots, L'_\ell, \ldots, L'_{p+1}\right]' : (J-1)(p+1) \times 1, \tag{2.133}$$

where L_ℓ is the vector of $J-1$ logits given by

$$L_\ell = \left[L_{[\ell]1}, \ldots, L_{[\ell]j}, \ldots, L_{[\ell](J-1)}\right]', \tag{2.134}$$

with $L_{[\ell]j}$ defined as in (2.130). Note that these logits for $j = 1, \ldots, J-1$ are functions of all J individual probabilities $\pi_{[\ell]1}, \ldots, \pi_{[\ell]J}$ at the covariate level ℓ.

Now define the regression parameters vector α as

$$\alpha = \left[\alpha'_0, \alpha'_1, \ldots, \alpha'_\ell, \ldots, \alpha'_p\right]', \tag{2.135}$$

where

$$\alpha_0 = [\alpha_{10}, \ldots, \alpha_{(J-1)0}]' \text{ and } \alpha_\ell = [\alpha_{1\ell}, \ldots, \alpha_{(J-1)\ell}]',$$

for $\ell = 1, \ldots, p$. Next by using (2.135) and (2.130), one may then express the logits vector (2.133) in the linear regression form as

$$F = X\alpha, \tag{2.136}$$

where

$$X = \begin{bmatrix} I_{J-1} \; X_1 \\ I_{J-1} \; X_2 \\ \cdot \quad \cdot \\ I_{J-1} \; X_p \\ I_{J-1} \; X_{p+1} \end{bmatrix} : (J-1)(p+1) \times (J-1)(p+1), \tag{2.137}$$

with

$$X_\ell = \begin{pmatrix} x'_{[\ell]1} \\ x'_{[\ell]2} \\ \cdot \\ x'_{[\ell](J-1)} \end{pmatrix} : (J-1) \times (J-1)p, \text{ for } \ell = 1, \ldots, p+1 \tag{2.138}$$

where, for $j = 1, \ldots, J-1$,

$$\begin{aligned} x'_{[\ell]j} &= \left(01'_{(\ell-1)(J-1)} \; 01'_{j-1} \; 1 \; 01'_{J-1-j} \; 01'_{(p-\ell)(J-1)} \right) \text{ for } \ell = 1, \ldots, p \\ x'_{[p+1]j} &= 01'_{p(J-1)}. \end{aligned} \tag{2.139}$$

Step 2. Formulation of $F(\pi)$ in terms of π

Write

$$\pi = [\pi'_{[1]}, \ldots, \pi'_{[\ell]}, \ldots, \pi'_{[p+1]}]' : J(p+1) \times 1, \tag{2.140}$$

where at covariate level ℓ, as in Sect. 2.2.2, all J cell probabilities are denoted by $\pi_{[\ell]}$, that is,

$$\pi_{[\ell]} = [\pi_{[\ell]1}, \ldots, \pi_{[\ell]j}, \ldots, \pi_{[\ell]J}]',$$

$\pi_{[\ell]j}$ being the probability for the response of an individual with ℓth level covariate information to be in the jth category.

Notice from (2.130) that $L_{[\ell]j}$ has the form

$$\begin{aligned} L_{[\ell]j} &= log \left[\frac{1 - F_{[\ell]j}}{F_{[\ell]j}} \right] \\ &= log \left[\frac{\sum_{c=j+1}^{J} \pi_{[\ell]c}}{\sum_{c=1}^{j} \pi_{[\ell]c}} \right] \end{aligned}$$

$$= \left[log\{ \sum_{c=j+1}^{J} \pi_{[\ell]c}\} - log\{\sum_{c=1}^{j} \pi_{[\ell]c}\} \right]. \tag{2.141}$$

Consequently, L_ℓ defined in (2.134) can be expressed as

$$\begin{aligned} L_\ell &= [L_{[\ell]1}, \ldots, L_{[\ell](J-1)}]' \\ &= [\left(log\{\sum_{c=2}^{J} \pi_{[\ell]c}\} - log\{\sum_{c=1}^{1} \pi_{[\ell]c}\} \right), \ldots, \left(log\{\sum_{c=J}^{J} \pi_{[\ell]c}\} - log\{\sum_{c=1}^{J-1} \pi_{[\ell]c}\} \right)]' \\ &= M^* log\,(A^* \pi_{[\ell]}), \end{aligned} \tag{2.142}$$

where $\pi_{[\ell]}$ is defined by (2.140), and A^* and K^* have the forms:

$$A^* = \begin{bmatrix} 1'_1 & 01'_{J-1} \\ 01'_1 & 1'_{J-1} \\ 1'_2 & 01'_{J-2} \\ 01'_2 & 1'_{J-2} \\ \cdot & \cdot \\ \cdot & \cdot \\ 1'_{J-1} & 01'_1 \\ 01'_{J-1} & 1'_1 \end{bmatrix} : 2(J-1) \times J, \tag{2.143}$$

and

$$M^* = \begin{bmatrix} -1 & 1 & 01'_2 & 01'_{2(J-3)} \\ 01'_2 & -1 & 1 & 01'_{2(J-3)} \\ \cdot & \cdot & \cdot & \cdot \\ 01'_{2(J-3)} & 01'_2 & -1 & 1 \end{bmatrix} : (J-1) \times 2(J-1), \tag{2.144}$$

respectively. Now by using (2.142), it follows from (2.133) that

$$
\begin{aligned}
F = F(\pi) = \begin{pmatrix} L_1 \\ L_2 \\ \cdot \\ \cdot \\ L_\ell \\ \cdot \\ \cdot \\ L_{p+1} \end{pmatrix} &= \begin{pmatrix} M^* log\,(A^* \pi_{[1]}) \\ M^* log\,(A^* \pi_{[2]}) \\ \cdot \\ \cdot \\ M^* log\,(A^* \pi_{[\ell]}) \\ \cdot \\ \cdot \\ M^* log\,(A^* \pi_{[p+1]}) \end{pmatrix} \\
&= [I_{p+1} \otimes M^*]\, log\, [(I_{p+1} \otimes A^*)\, \pi] \\
&= M log\,(A\pi),
\end{aligned} \tag{2.145}
$$

where $\pi = [\pi'_{[1]}, \ldots, \pi'_{[\ell]}, \ldots, \pi'_{[p+1]}]'$, and '$\otimes$' denotes the direct or Kronecker product.

Step 3. Forming a 'working' linear model

Using notations from Step 2 (2.145) in (2.136) under Step 1, one consequently solves α satisfying

$$
F = F(\pi) = M log\,(A\pi) = X\alpha. \tag{2.146}
$$

Note that this (2.146) is not an estimating equation yet as π is unknown in practice. This means the model (population average) Eq. (2.146) does not involve any data. However, by using the observed proportion p for π, one may write an approximate (working) linear regression model with correlated errors as follows:

$$
F(p) \approx F(\pi) + \frac{\partial F(\pi)}{\partial \pi'} [p - \pi] = F(\pi) + \varepsilon,\ (J-1)(p+1) \times 1 \tag{2.147}
$$

where ε may be treated as an error vector. Next, because for a given ℓ, the cell counts $\{K_{[\ell]j},\ j = 1, \ldots, J\}$ follow the multinomial probability distribution (2.67) [see also Table 2.4 for data display], it follows that

$$
E[p_{[\ell]j}] = E[\frac{K_{[\ell]j}}{K_{[\ell]}}] = \pi_{[\ell]j}, \text{ for all j and } \ell,
$$

that is $E[p] = \pi$, where π is defined by (2.140), and p is the corresponding observed proportion vector, with $p_{[\ell]} = [p_{[\ell]j}, \ldots, p_{[\ell]j}, \ldots, p_{[\ell]J}]'$. It then follows that

$$
\begin{aligned}
E[\varepsilon] &= 0, \\
\text{cov}[\varepsilon] &= \left[\frac{\partial F(\pi)}{\partial \pi'}\right] \text{cov}(p) \left[\frac{\partial F'(\pi)}{\partial \pi}\right]
\end{aligned}
$$

$$= \left[\frac{\partial F(\pi)}{\partial \pi'}\right] V \left[\frac{\partial F'(\pi)}{\partial \pi}\right] = \Sigma_\varepsilon \text{ (say)}, \; (J-1)(p+1) \times (J-1)(p+1). \tag{2.148}$$

Note that the approximation in (2.147) follows from the so-called Taylor's series expansion for $F(p)$. To be specific, for $u = 1, \ldots, (J-1)(p+1)$, the uth component of $F(p)$ may be expanded in Taylor's series form as

$$\begin{aligned} F_u(p) &= F_u(\pi) + (p-\pi)' \frac{\partial F_u(\pi)}{\partial \pi} \\ &\quad + \varepsilon^*_{u,K}(||p_{[1]} - \pi_{[1]}||, \ldots, ||p_{[\ell]} - \pi_{[\ell]}||, \ldots, ||p_{[p+1]} - \pi_{[p+1]}||), \end{aligned} \tag{2.149}$$

where for $K = \sum_{\ell=1}^{p+1} K_{[\ell]}$, $\varepsilon^*_{u,K}(\cdot)$ is a higher order remainder term in the Taylor's expansion, and it is a function of Euclidian distances

$$||p_{[\ell]} - \pi_{[\ell]}|| = \sqrt{\sum_{j=1}^{J} [p_{[\ell]j} - \pi_{[\ell]j}]^2}, \text{ for all } \ell = 1, \ldots, p+1.$$

Further note that when $\min_\ell\{K_{[\ell]}\} \to \infty$ it can be shown that

$$\varepsilon^*_{u,K}(\cdot) \to 0 \text{ in probability} \tag{2.150}$$

(see, for example, Rao (1973, p. 387); Bishop et al. (1975, Sec. 14.6) for details on this convergence property). Thus, for all $u = 1, \ldots, (J-1)(p+1)$, and using (2.150), one obtains the approximate linear relationship (2.147) from (2.149). Finally by using (2.146), one may fit the linear model

$$\begin{aligned} F(p) &= F(\pi) + \varepsilon \\ &= X\alpha + \varepsilon, \end{aligned} \tag{2.151}$$

(see also Grizzle et al. (1969), Haberman (1978, pp. 64–77)) where $F(p) = M\log\,(Ap)$ with M and A as given by (2.145), and the error vector ε has the zero mean vector and covariance matrix Σ_ε as given by (2.148).

Step 4. WLS (weighted least square) estimating equation

Consequently, one may write the WLS estimating equation for α as

$$X'\Sigma_\varepsilon^{-1}[F(p) - X\alpha] = 0, \tag{2.152}$$

and obtain the WLS estimator of α as

$$\hat{\alpha}_{WLS} = [X'\Sigma_\varepsilon^{-1}X]^{-1}X'\Sigma_\varepsilon^{-1}F(p). \tag{2.153}$$

For similar use of the WLS approach in fitting models to ordinal data, one may be referred to Semenya and Koch (1980) and Semenya et al. (1983) (see also Agresti (1984, Section 7.2, Appendix A.2); Koch et al. (1992)). For computation convenience, one may further simplify Σ_ε from (2.148) as

$$\begin{aligned}\Sigma_\varepsilon = \text{cov}[F(p)] &= \left[\frac{\partial F(\pi)}{\partial \pi'}\right] V \left[\frac{\partial F'(\pi)}{\partial \pi}\right] \\ &= \left[\frac{\partial M log\, A\pi}{\partial \pi'}\right] V \left[\frac{\partial M log\, A\pi}{\partial \pi'}\right]' \\ &= MD^{-1}AVA'D^{-1}M' = QVQ', \text{ (say)}, \end{aligned} \quad (2.154)$$

where $D = \text{diag}[A\pi] : 2(J-1)(p+1) \times 2(J-1)(p+1)$, $A\pi : 2(J-1)(p+1) \times 1$ being given by (2.145). Hence, using Σ_ε from (2.154) into (2.153), one may re-express $\hat{\alpha}_{WLS}$ as

$$\hat{\alpha}_{WLS} = \left[X'(QVQ')^{-1}X\right]^{-1} X'(QVQ')^{-1}F(p), \quad (2.155)$$

with $F(p) = Mlog\, Ap$. Note that to compute $\hat{\alpha}_{WLS}$ by (2.155), one requires to replace the D matrix by its unbiased estimate $\hat{D} = \text{diag}[Ap]$. Next, because, $\text{cov}[F(p)] = QVQ'$ by (2.154), by treating D as a known matrix, one may compute the covariance of the WLS estimator of α as

$$\text{cov}[\hat{\alpha}_{WLS}] = \left[X'(QVQ')^{-1}X\right]^{-1}, \quad (2.156)$$

which can be estimated by replacing π with p, that is,

$$\hat{\text{cov}}[\hat{\alpha}_{WLS}] = \left[X'(QVQ')^{-1}X\right]^{-1}_{|\pi=p}. \quad (2.157)$$

Further note that the V matrix in (2.154)–(2.157) has the block diagonal form given by

$$V = \bigoplus_{\ell=1}^{p+1} [\text{cov}(p_{[\ell]})] : (p+1)J \times (p+1)J, \quad (2.158)$$

where

$$\text{cov}(p_{[\ell]}) = \frac{1}{K_{[\ell]}} \left[\text{diag}[\pi_{[\ell]1}, \ldots, \pi_{[\ell]j}, \ldots, \pi_{[\ell]J}] - \pi_{[\ell]}\pi'_{[\ell]}\right]. \quad (2.159)$$

Table 2.24 Cross-classification of gender and physician visit along with observed proportions

	Physician visit status				
Gender	None	Few	Not so few	High	Total
Male	28	40	16	12	96
Cell proportion	0.2917	0.4166	0.1667	0.1250	1.0
Female	11	20	21	32	84
Cell proportion	0.1309	0.2381	0.2500	0.3810	1.0

2.3.1.1.1 Illustration 2.9: Weighted Least Square Fitting of the Cumulative Logits Model to the Gender Versus Physician Visit Data

Recall the physician visit status data for male and female from Table 2.10. For convenience, we redisplay these data along with observed proportions as in the following Table 2.24. Note that the physician visit status can be treated as ordinal categorical. However, among others, this data set was analyzed in Sect. 2.2.2.4 by applying the product multinomial likelihood approach discussed in Sects. 2.2.2.1 and 2.2.2.2, where categories were treated to be nominal. As discussed in last section, when categories are treated to be ordinal, one may fit the cumulative probability ratios based logits model to analyze such data. The logit models are different than standard multinomial models used for the analysis of nominal categorical data. We now follow the logit model and inferences discussed in the last section to reanalyze the gender versus physician visit status data shown in Table 2.24.

We first write the observed proportion vector p as

$$p = [p'_{[1]}, p'_{[2]}]', \tag{2.160}$$

with

$$\begin{aligned} p_{[1]} &= [p_{[1]1}, p_{[1]2}, p_{[1]3}, p_{[1]4}]' = [0.2917,\ 0.4166,\ 0.1667,\ 0.1250]' \\ p_{[2]} &= [p_{[2]1}, p_{[2]2}, p_{[2]3}, p_{[2]4}]' = [0.1309,\ 0.2381,\ 0.2500,\ 0.3810]'. \end{aligned}$$

Next we follow the steps from the previous section and formulate the matrices and vectors to compute $\hat{\alpha}$ by (2.155).

Step 1. Constructing $F(\pi) = X\alpha$ under LM 1

To define X and α, we write the vector of logits by (2.133) as

$$F(\pi) = [L'_1, L'_2]' : 6 \times 1, \tag{2.161}$$

with

$$L_1 = [L_{[1]1}, L_{[1]2}, L_{[1]3}]'$$
$$L_2 = [L_{[2]1}, L_{[2]2}, L_{[2]3}]',$$

where by (2.130)

$$L_{[1]1} = \alpha_{10} + \alpha_{11}$$
$$L_{[1]2} = \alpha_{20} + \alpha_{21}$$
$$L_{[1]3} = \alpha_{30} + \alpha_{31},$$

and

$$L_{[2]1} = \alpha_{10}$$
$$L_{[2]2} = \alpha_{20}$$
$$L_{[2]3} = \alpha_{30},$$

producing α by (2.135) as

$$\begin{aligned}\alpha &= [\alpha_0', \alpha_1']' \\ &= [\alpha_{10}, \alpha_{20}, \alpha_{30}, \alpha_{11}, \alpha_{21}, \alpha_{31}]'.\end{aligned} \quad (2.162)$$

Now to express $F(\pi)$ in (2.161) as $F(\pi) = X\alpha$ with α as in (2.162), one must write the 6×6 matrix X as

$$X = \begin{bmatrix} 1\,0\,0\,1\,0\,0 \\ 0\,1\,0\,0\,1\,0 \\ 0\,0\,1\,0\,0\,1 \\ 1\,0\,0\,0\,0\,0 \\ 0\,1\,0\,0\,0\,0 \\ 0\,0\,1\,0\,0\,0 \end{bmatrix} \quad (2.163)$$

This matrix satisfies the notations from (2.137) to (2.139).

Note that as indicated in the last section, we also consider three other logit models as follows:

LM2. Instead of using the model (2.130), one may use different restriction on the level effect parameters and write the logit model as

$$L_{[\ell]j} = log\left[\frac{1-F_{[\ell]j}}{F_{[\ell]j}}\right] = \begin{cases} \alpha_{j0}+\alpha_{j\ell} & \text{for } j=1,\ldots,J-1;\ \ell=1,\ldots,p \\ \alpha_{j0}-\Sigma_{\ell=1}^{p}\alpha_{j\ell} & \text{for } j=1,\ldots,J-1;\ \ell=p+1. \end{cases} \quad (2.164)$$

yielding six logits for the gender versus physician visit data as

$$\begin{aligned} L_{[1]1} &= \alpha_{10}+\alpha_{11} \\ L_{[1]2} &= \alpha_{20}+\alpha_{21} \\ L_{[1]3} &= \alpha_{30}+\alpha_{31}, \end{aligned}$$

and

$$\begin{aligned} L_{[2]1} &= \alpha_{10}-\alpha_{11} \\ L_{[2]2} &= \alpha_{20}-\alpha_{21} \\ L_{[2]3} &= \alpha_{30}-\alpha_{31}. \end{aligned}$$

For

$$\begin{aligned} \alpha &= [\alpha_0', \alpha_1']' \\ &= [\alpha_{10},\alpha_{20},\alpha_{30},\alpha_{11},\alpha_{21},\alpha_{31}]', \end{aligned}$$

the aforementioned six logits produce the X matrix as

$$X = \begin{bmatrix} 1 & 0 & 0 & 1 & 0 & 0 \\ 0 & 1 & 0 & 0 & 1 & 0 \\ 0 & 0 & 1 & 0 & 0 & 1 \\ 1 & 0 & 0 & -1 & 0 & 0 \\ 0 & 1 & 0 & 0 & -1 & 0 \\ 0 & 0 & 1 & 0 & 0 & -1 \end{bmatrix}. \quad (2.165)$$

LM3. Now suppose that unlike the models (2.130) and (2.164), one uses the same level effect parameter, say $\alpha_{1\ell}$, under all response categories. Then, similar to LM1, the logits can be expressed as

$$L_{[\ell]j} = log\left[\frac{1-F_{[\ell]j}}{F_{[\ell]j}}\right] = \begin{cases} \alpha_{j0}+\alpha_{1\ell} & \text{for } j=1,\ldots,J-1;\ \ell=1,\ldots,p \\ \alpha_{j0} & \text{for } j=1,\ldots,J-1;\ \ell=p+1. \end{cases} \quad (2.166)$$

yielding six logits for the gender versus physician visit data as

$$\begin{aligned} L_{[1]1} &= \alpha_{10} + \alpha_{11} \\ L_{[1]2} &= \alpha_{20} + \alpha_{11} \\ L_{[1]3} &= \alpha_{30} + \alpha_{11}, \end{aligned}$$

and

$$\begin{aligned} L_{[2]1} &= \alpha_{10} \\ L_{[2]2} &= \alpha_{20} \\ L_{[2]3} &= \alpha_{30}. \end{aligned}$$

For

$$\begin{aligned} \alpha &= [\alpha_0', \alpha_1']' \\ &= [\alpha_{10}, \alpha_{20}, \alpha_{30}, \alpha_{11}]', \end{aligned}$$

the aforementioned six logits produce the $X : 6 \times 4$ matrix as

$$X = \begin{bmatrix} 1\,0\,0\,1 \\ 0\,1\,0\,1 \\ 0\,0\,1\,1 \\ 1\,0\,0\,0 \\ 0\,1\,0\,0 \\ 0\,0\,1\,0 \end{bmatrix}. \tag{2.167}$$

LM4. Suppose that we use the same regression parameters as in the model (2.166), but use the restriction on the level effect parameters as in (2.164). One may then express the logits as

$$L_{[\ell]j} = log\left[\frac{1 - F_{[\ell]j}}{F_{[\ell]j}}\right] = \begin{cases} \alpha_{j0} + \alpha_{1\ell} & \text{for } j = 1, \ldots, J-1;\ \ell = 1, \ldots, p \\ \alpha_{j0} - \Sigma_{\ell=1}^{p} \alpha_{1\ell} & \text{for } j = 1, \ldots, J-1;\ \ell = p+1. \end{cases} \tag{2.168}$$

yielding six logits for the gender versus physician visit data as

$$\begin{aligned} L_{[1]1} &= \alpha_{10} + \alpha_{11} \\ L_{[1]2} &= \alpha_{20} + \alpha_{11} \\ L_{[1]3} &= \alpha_{30} + \alpha_{11}, \end{aligned}$$

and

$$L_{[2]1} = \alpha_{10} - \alpha_{11}$$
$$L_{[2]2} = \alpha_{20} - \alpha_{11}$$
$$L_{[2]3} = \alpha_{30} - \alpha_{11}.$$

For

$$\begin{aligned}\alpha &= [\alpha_0', \alpha_1']' \\ &= [\alpha_{10}, \alpha_{20}, \alpha_{30}, \alpha_{11}]',\end{aligned}$$

the aforementioned six logits produce the $X : 6 \times 4$ matrix as

$$X = \begin{bmatrix} 1\,0\,0\,1 \\ 0\,1\,0\,1 \\ 0\,0\,1\,1 \\ 1\,0\,0\,-1 \\ 0\,1\,0\,-1 \\ 0\,0\,1\,-1 \end{bmatrix}. \tag{2.169}$$

Step 2. Developing notations to write $F(\pi) = Mlog\,(A\pi)$ satisfying (2.145)

Now because $J = 4$, for a given $\ell(\ell = 1, 2)$, A^* and M^* matrices by (2.143) and (2.144), are written as

$$A^* = \begin{bmatrix} 1\,0\,0\,0 \\ 0\,1\,1\,1 \\ 1\,1\,0\,0 \\ 0\,0\,1\,1 \\ 1\,1\,1\,0 \\ 0\,0\,0\,1 \end{bmatrix} : 6 \times 4, \tag{2.170}$$

and

$$M^* = \begin{bmatrix} -1\,1\,0 & 0\,0 & 0 \\ 0 & 0\,-1\,1\,0 & 0 \\ 0 & 0\,0 & 0\,-1\,1 \end{bmatrix} : 3 \times 6, \tag{2.171}$$

respectively. Note that these matrices are constructed following the definition of the logits, that is, satisfying

$$L_\ell = [L_{[\ell]1}, L_{[\ell]2}, L_{[\ell]3}]' = M^* log\,(A^* \pi_{[\ell]}),$$

as shown by (2.141)–(2.142). Thus, for the present gender versus physician visit status data, by (2.145), we write

$$M = \begin{pmatrix} M^* & 0U_{3\times 6} \\ 0U_{3\times 6} & M^* \end{pmatrix} : 6 \times 12,\; A = \begin{pmatrix} A^* & 0U_{6\times 4} \\ 0U_{6\times 4} & A^* \end{pmatrix} : 12 \times 8, \tag{2.172}$$

with $U_{3\times 6}$, for example, as the 3×6 unit matrix, satisfying $F(\pi) = Mlog\,(A\pi)$, where

$$\begin{aligned} \pi &= [\pi'_{[1]}, \pi'_{[2]}]' \\ &= [\pi_{[1]1}, \pi_{[1]2}, \pi_{[1]3}, \pi_{[1]4}, \pi_{[2]1}, \pi_{[2]2}, \pi_{[2]3}, \pi_{[2]4}]'. \end{aligned}$$

We now directly go to Step 4 and use (2.155) to compute the WLS estimate for the regression parameter vector α.

Step 4. Computation of $\hat{\alpha}_{WLS}$ by (2.155)

Notice that V matrix in (2.155) is computed by (2.158), that is,

$$\begin{aligned} V = \text{var}[p] &= \text{var}[p'_{[1]}, p'_{[2]}]' \\ &= \begin{pmatrix} \text{var}[p_{[1]}] & \text{cov}[p_{[1]}, p'_{[2]}] \\ \text{cov}[p_{[2]}, p'_{[1]}] & \text{var}[p_{[2]}] \end{pmatrix} \\ &= \begin{pmatrix} V_1 & 0 \\ 0 & V_2 \end{pmatrix}, \end{aligned} \tag{2.173}$$

where

$$\begin{aligned} K_{[1]}V_1 &= \text{diag}[\pi_{[1]1}, \pi_{[1]2}, \pi_{[1]3}, \pi_{[1]4}] - \pi_{[1]}\pi'_{[1]} \\ K_{[2]}V_2 &= \text{diag}[\pi_{[2]1}, \pi_{[2]2}, \pi_{[2]3}, \pi_{[2]4}] - \pi_{[2]}\pi'_{[2]}. \end{aligned}$$

Table 2.25 Parameter estimates and their standard errors under selected cumulative logit models for gender versus physician visit status data

	Logit model parameters based on gender and 4 visit categories						
Logit model	Quantity	$\hat{\alpha}_{10}$	$\hat{\alpha}_{20}$	$\hat{\alpha}_{30}$	$\hat{\alpha}_{11}$	$\hat{\alpha}_{21}$	$\hat{\alpha}_{31}$
LM1	Estimate	1.893	0.537	−0.485	−1.006	−1.424	−1.461
	Standard error	0.324	0.226	0.225	0.394	0.319	0.382
LM2	Estimate	1.390	−0.175	−1.216	−0.503	−0.712	−0.750
	Standard error	0.197	0.159	0.190	0.197	0.159	0.191
LM3	Estimate	2.107	0.508	−0.524	−1.312	-	-
	Standard error	0.261	0.215	0.214	0.285	-	-
LM4	Estimate	1.451	−0.148	−1.180	−0.656	-	-
	Standard error	0.189	0.157	0.181	0.142	-	-

One however needs to use an estimate of this V matrix to compute $\hat{\alpha}_{WLS}$ by (2.155). Now because $p_{[1]}$ and $p_{[2]}$ are unbiased estimates for $\pi_{[1]}$ and $\pi_{[2]}$, respectively, V matrix may be estimated as

$$\hat{V} = \begin{pmatrix} \hat{V}_1 & 0 \\ 0 & \hat{V}_2 \end{pmatrix}, \tag{2.174}$$

where

$$K_{[1]}\hat{V}_1 = \text{diag}[p_{[1]1}, p_{[1]2}, p_{[1]3}, p_{[1]4}] - p_{[1]}p'_{[1]}$$
$$K_{[2]}\hat{V}_2 = \text{diag}[p_{[2]1}, p_{[2]2}, p_{[2]3}, p_{[2]4}] - p_{[2]}p'_{[2]},$$

with $p[1]$ and $p_{[2]}$ as given by (2.160).

Next we compute $\hat{D} = \text{diag}[Ap]$, where A is given in (2.172). Further compute $\hat{Q} = M\hat{D}^{-1}A$. Finally by using these estimates $\hat{V}, \hat{Q}$, and $F(p) = Mlog\ (Ap)$ into (2.155), we obtain $\hat{\alpha}_{WLS}$ by using X matrix from (2.163), (2.165), (2.167), and (2.169), under the models LM1, LM2, LM3, and LM4, respectively. These estimates along with their standard errors computed by (2.157) are reported in Table 2.25.

We now use the estimates from Table 2.25 and compute the logits under all four models. The observed logits are also computed using the observed proportions from Table 2.24. For interpretation convenience we display the exponent of the logits, i.e., $\exp(L_{[\ell]j})$ under all four models in Table 2.26. Notice that LM1 and LM2 produce the same logits, similarly LM3 and LM4 also produce the same logits. Thus, proper restriction on level based parameters is important but restrictions can vary. Next, it is clear from the table that LM1 (or LM2) fits the observed logits exactly, whereas the logits produced by LM3 (or LM4) are slightly different than the observed logits. This shows that level (gender) based covariates do not play the same role under all four response categories. Thus, using three different regression parameters, namely α_{1j} for $j = 1, \ldots, 3$, is more appropriate than using only one parameter, namely α_{11}.

Table 2.26 Observed and estimated logits under selected cumulative logit models for gender versus physician visit status data

		Logit estimates				
Gender	Logits	Observed	LM1	LM2	LM3	LM4
Male	$\exp(L_{[1]1})$	2.428	2.428	2.428	2.214	2.214
	$\exp(L_{[1]2})$	0.411	0.411	0.411	0.447	0.447
	$\exp(L_{[1]3})$	0.143	0.143	0.143	0.159	0.159
Female	$\exp(L_{[2]1})$	6.639	6.639	6.639	8.225	8.225
	$\exp(L_{[2]2})$	1.710	1.710	1.710	1.662	1.662
	$\exp(L_{[2]3})$	0.616	0.616	0.616	0.592	0.592

Furthermore, when logits of males are compared to those of the females, all three logits for the male group appear to be smaller than the corresponding logits for the female group, i.e.,

$$L_{[1]j} \leq L_{[2]j}, \text{ for all } j = 1,2,3,$$

showing that more females pay large number of visits to their physician as compared to males. These results agree with the analysis discussed in Sect. 2.2.2.4.2(a) and the results reported in Table 2.12, where it was found through direct multinomial regression fitting that females paid relatively more visits as compared to males.

2.3.1.2 Binary Mapping Based Pseudo-Likelihood Estimation Approach

Based on the form of the cumulative logits from (2.130)–(2.131), in this approach we utilize the binary information at every cut point for an individual and write a likelihood function. For the purpose, for an individual i with covariate level ℓ and responding in category $h (h = 1,\ldots,J)$ [this identifies the ith individual as $i \in (\ell,h)$], we define a cut point j $(j = 1,\ldots,J-1)$ based 'working' or 'pseudo' binary variable

$$b^{(j)}_{i\in(\ell,h)} = \begin{cases} 1 \text{ for given response category } h > j \\ 0 \text{ for given response category } h \leq j, \end{cases} \tag{2.175}$$

with probabilities following (2.130)–(2.131) as

$$\begin{aligned} Pr[b^{(j)}_{i\in(\ell,h)} = 1] &= \sum_{c=j+1}^{J} \pi_{[\ell]c} = 1 - F_{[\ell]j} \\ &= \begin{cases} \frac{\exp(\alpha_{j0}+\alpha_{j\ell})}{1+\exp(\alpha_{j0}+\alpha_{j\ell})} & \text{for } \ell = 1,\ldots,p \\ \frac{\exp(\alpha_{j0})}{1+\exp(\alpha_{j0})} & \text{for } \ell = p+1. \end{cases} \end{aligned} \tag{2.176}$$

Table 2.27 Cumulative counts as responses at cut points $j = 1,\ldots,J-1$, reflecting the cumulative probabilities (2.176), under covariate level ℓ

	Binomial response		
Cut point	**Low group ($g^* = 1$)**	**High group ($g^* = 2$)**	**Total**
1	$K^*_{[\ell]1} = \sum_{c=1}^{1} K_{[\ell]c}$	$K_{[\ell]} - K^*_{[\ell]1}$	$K_{[\ell]}$
.	.	.	.
j	$K^*_{[\ell]j} = \sum_{c=1}^{j} K_{[\ell]c}$	$K_{[\ell]} - K^*_{[\ell]j}$	$K_{[\ell]}$
.	.	.	.
$J-1$	$K^*_{[\ell](J-1)} = \sum_{c=1}^{J-1} K_{[\ell]c}$	$K_{[\ell]} - K^*_{[\ell](J-1)}$	$K_{[\ell]}$

representing the probability for the binary response to be in category h beyond j; and

$$Pr[b^{(j)}_{i\in(\ell,h)} = 0] = \sum_{c=1}^{j} \pi_{[\ell]c} = F_{[\ell]j}$$
$$= = \begin{cases} \frac{1}{1+\exp(\alpha_{j0}+\alpha_{j\ell})} & \text{for } \ell = 1,\ldots,p \\ \frac{1}{1+\exp(\alpha_{j0})} & \text{for } \ell = p+1. \end{cases} \quad (2.177)$$

representing the probability for the binary response to be in a category h between 1 and j inclusive.

Now as a reflection of the cut points based cumulative probabilities (2.176)–(2.177), for convenience, we display the response counts computed from Table 2.4, at every cut points, as in Table 2.27. We use the notation $K^*_{[\ell]j} = \sum_{c=1}^{j} K_{[\ell]c}$, whereas in Table 2.4, $K_{[\ell]c}$ is the number of individuals with covariate at level ℓ those belong to category c for their responses.

Note that $K_{[\ell]} - K^*_{[\ell]j}$ follows the binomial distribution $\text{Bin}(K_{[\ell]}, 1-F_{[\ell]j})$, where $[1-F_{[\ell]j}] = \sum_{c=j+1}^{J} \pi_{[\ell]c} = \pi^*_{[\ell]j}$ by (2.176). Furthermore, the regression parameters in (2.176)–(2.177) may be expressed by a vector α as in (2.135), that is,

$$\alpha = \left[\alpha_0', \alpha_1', \ldots, \alpha_\ell', \ldots, \alpha_p'\right]',$$

where

$$\alpha_0 = [\alpha_{10}, \ldots, \alpha_{(J-1)0}]' \text{ and } \alpha_\ell = [\alpha_{1\ell}, \ldots, \alpha_{(J-1)\ell}]',$$

for $\ell = 1,\ldots,p$. Alternatively, similar to (2.69), these parameters may be represented by

$$\alpha = [\alpha_1^{*\prime}, \ldots, \alpha_j^{*\prime}, \ldots, \alpha_{J-1}^{*}{}'\,]', \text{ with } \alpha_j^* = [\alpha_{j0}, \alpha_{j1}, \ldots, \alpha_{j\ell}, \ldots, \alpha_{jp}]'. \quad (2.178)$$

Now for a given form of α, we first write a pseudo-likelihood function by using the pseudo binary probabilities from (2.175)–(2.177), as

$$\begin{aligned} L(\alpha) &= \Pi_{\ell=1}^{p+1}\Pi_{j=1}^{J-1}\Pi_{[i\in(\ell,h)|j,\ell]}^{K_{[\ell]}}\left[\{F_{[\ell]j}\}^{1-b_{i\in(\ell,h)}^{(j)}}\right]\left[\{1-F_{[\ell]j}\}^{b_{i\in(\ell,h)}^{(j)}}\right] \\ &= \Pi_{\ell=1}^{p+1}\Pi_{j=1}^{J-1}\left[\{F_{[\ell]j}\}^{\Sigma_{c=1}^{j}K_{[\ell]c}}\right]\left[\{1-F_{[\ell]j}\}^{\Sigma_{c=j+1}^{J}K_{[\ell]c}}\right] \\ &= \Pi_{\ell=1}^{p+1}\Pi_{j=1}^{J-1}\left[\{F_{[\ell]j}\}^{\Sigma_{c=1}^{j}K_{[\ell]c}}\right]\left[\{1-F_{[\ell]j}\}^{K_{[\ell]}-\Sigma_{c=1}^{j}K_{[\ell]c}}\right] \qquad (2.179) \\ &= \Pi_{j=1}^{J-1}\left[\Pi_{\ell=1}^{p}\frac{\exp\{(K_{[\ell]}-K_{[\ell]j}^{*})(\alpha_{j0}+\alpha_{j\ell})\}}{[1+\exp(\alpha_{j0}+\alpha_{j\ell})]^{K_{[\ell]}}}\right] \\ &\times\left[\frac{\exp\{(K_{[p+1]}-K_{[p+1]j}^{*})(\alpha_{j0})\}}{[1+\exp(\alpha_{j0})]^{K_{[p+1]}}}\right], \qquad (2.180) \end{aligned}$$

where $K_{[\ell]j}^{*}=\Sigma_{c=1}^{j}K_{[\ell]c}$ for $j=1,\ldots,J-1$, and for all $\ell=1,\ldots,p+1$.

Next, in order to write the log likelihood estimating equation in an algebraic convenient form, we use the α in the form of (2.178) and first re-express $1-F_{[\ell]j}$ and $F_{[\ell]j}$ from (2.176)–(2.177) as

$$\begin{aligned} 1-F_{[\ell]j} &= \frac{\exp(x_{[\ell]j}'\alpha)}{1+\exp(x_{[\ell]j}'\alpha)} \\ F_{[\ell]j} &= \frac{1}{1+\exp(x_{[\ell]j}'\alpha)}, \qquad (2.181) \end{aligned}$$

where $x_{[\ell]j}'$ is the jth $(j=1,\ldots,J-1)$ row of the $(J-1)\times(J-1)(p+1)$ matrix X_ℓ, defined for ℓth level as follows:

$$\begin{aligned} X_\ell &= \begin{pmatrix} x_{[\ell]1}' \\ x_{[\ell]2}' \\ \cdot \\ x_{[\ell](J-1)}' \end{pmatrix} \\ &= \begin{pmatrix} 1\ 01_{\ell-1}',1,01_{p-\ell}' & 0 & 01_p' & \cdot\ 0 & 01_p' \\ 0 & 01_p' & 1\ 01_{\ell-1}',1,01_{p-\ell}' & \cdot\ 0 & 01_p' \\ \cdot & \cdot & \cdot & \cdot & \cdot\ \cdot & \cdot \\ 0 & 01_p' & 0 & 01_p' & \cdot\ 1\ 01_{\ell-1}',1,01_{p-\ell}' \end{pmatrix} \text{ for } \ell=1,\ldots,p \end{aligned}$$

$$X_{p+1} = \begin{pmatrix} x'_{[p+1]1} \\ x'_{[p+1]2} \\ \cdot \\ x'_{[p+1](J-1)} \end{pmatrix} = \begin{pmatrix} 1\ 01'_p\ 0\ 01'_p\ \cdot\ 0\ 01'_p \\ 0\ 01'_p\ 1\ 01'_p\ \cdot\ 0\ 01'_p \\ \cdot\ \cdot\ \cdot\ \cdot\ \cdot\ \cdot\ \cdot\ \cdot \\ 0\ 01'_p\ 0\ 01'_p\ \cdot\ 1\ 01'_p \end{pmatrix}. \tag{2.182}$$

The log likelihood equation for α may then be written from (2.179) as

$$\begin{aligned}
\frac{\partial Log\, L(\alpha)}{\partial \alpha} &= \sum_{\ell=1}^{p+1}\sum_{j=1}^{J-1}\left[(K_{[\ell]} - K^*_{[\ell]j})\frac{\partial}{\partial \alpha}\{log\,(1-F_{[\ell]j})\}\right. \\
&+ \left. K^*_{[\ell]j}\frac{\partial}{\partial \alpha}\{log\, F_{[\ell]j}\}\right] \\
&= \sum_{\ell=1}^{p+1}\sum_{j=1}^{J-1}\left[(K_{[\ell]} - K^*_{[\ell]j})\frac{\partial}{\partial \alpha}\{log\,(\frac{\exp(x'_{[\ell]j}\alpha)}{1+\exp(x'_{[\ell]j}\alpha)})\}\right. \\
&+ \left. K^*_{[\ell]j}\frac{\partial}{\partial \alpha}\{log\,\frac{1}{1+\exp(x'_{[\ell]j}\alpha)}\}\right] \\
&= \sum_{\ell=1}^{p+1}\sum_{j=1}^{J-1}\left[(K_{[\ell]} - K^*_{[\ell]j})\{F_{[\ell]j}x_{[\ell]j}\}\right. \\
&- \left. K^*_{[\ell]j}\{(1-F_{[\ell]j})x_{[\ell]j}\}\}\right] \\
&= \sum_{\ell=1}^{p+1}\sum_{j=1}^{J-1} x_{[\ell]j}\left[K_{[\ell]}F_{[\ell]j} - K^*_{[\ell]j}\right] \\
&= -\sum_{\ell=1}^{p+1}\sum_{j=1}^{J-1} x_{[\ell]j}\left[K^*_{[\ell]j} - K_{[\ell]}F_{[\ell]j}\right] \\
&= \sum_{\ell=1}^{p+1}\sum_{j=1}^{J-1} x_{[\ell]j}\left[(K_{[\ell]} - K^*_{[\ell]j}) - K_{[\ell]}(1-F_{[\ell]j})\right] \qquad (2.183) \\
&= \sum_{\ell=1}^{p+1} X'_\ell\left[y^*_{[\ell]} - K_{[\ell]}\pi^*_{[\ell]}\right] = f(\alpha) = 0, \qquad (2.184)
\end{aligned}$$

where

$$y^*_{[\ell]} = [K_{[\ell]} - K^*_{[\ell]1}, \ldots, K_{[\ell]} - K^*_{[\ell]j}, \ldots, K_{[\ell]} - K^*_{[\ell](J-1)}]' \text{ and}$$

$$\pi^*_{[\ell]} \equiv [\pi^*_{[\ell]1}, \ldots, \pi^*_{[\ell]j}, \ldots, \pi^*_{[\ell](J-1)}]' = [1-F_{[\ell]1}, \ldots, 1-F_{[\ell]j}, \ldots, 1-F_{[\ell](J-1)}]',$$

with X_ℓ matrices for $\ell = 1,\ldots,p+1$ as given in (2.182). Note that this estimating equation form in (2.184) is similar to (2.71), but they are quite different estimating equations.

2.3.1.2.1 Pseudo-Likelihood Estimates and their Asymptotic Variances

Let $\hat{\alpha}$ be the solution of $f(\alpha) = 0$ in (2.184). Assuming that $\hat{\alpha}_0$ is not a solution for $f(\alpha) = 0$ but a trial estimate, and hence $f(\hat{\alpha}_0) \neq 0$, by similar calculations as in (2.36), the iterative equation for $\hat{\alpha}*$ is obtained as

$$\hat{\alpha} = \hat{\alpha}_0 - \left[\{f'(\alpha)\}^{-1} f(\alpha)\right] |_{\alpha=\hat{\alpha}_0}. \tag{2.185}$$

Next, by similar calculations as in (2.183), one writes

$$\begin{aligned}\frac{\partial \pi^*_{[\ell]j}}{\partial \alpha'} &= \frac{\partial(1-F_{[\ell]j})}{\partial \alpha'} \\ &= F_{[\ell]j}(1-F_{[\ell]j})x'_{[\ell]j} = \pi^*_{[\ell]j}(1-\pi^*_{[\ell]j})x'_{[\ell]j},\end{aligned} \tag{2.186}$$

yielding

$$\begin{aligned}\frac{\partial \pi^*_{[\ell]}}{\partial \alpha'} &= \text{diag}[\pi^*_{[\ell]1}(1-\pi^*_{[\ell]1}),\ldots,\pi^*_{[\ell](J-1)}(1-\pi^*_{[\ell](J-1)})]X_\ell \\ &= D_{\pi^*_{[\ell]}} X_\ell.\end{aligned} \tag{2.187}$$

By (2.187), it then follows from (2.184) that

$$\begin{aligned}f'(\alpha) &= \frac{\partial^2 Log\, L(\alpha)}{\partial \alpha \partial \alpha'} \\ &= -\sum_{\ell=1}^{p+1} K_{[\ell]} X'_\ell D_{\pi^*_{[\ell]}} X_\ell.\end{aligned} \tag{2.188}$$

Thus, by (2.188), the iterative equation (2.185) takes the form

$$\begin{aligned}\hat{\alpha}(r+1) = \hat{\alpha}(r) &+ \left[\sum_{\ell=1}^{p+1} K_{[\ell]} X'_\ell D_{\pi^*_{[\ell]}} X_\ell\right]^{-1} \\ &\times \left[\sum_{\ell=1}^{p+1} X'_\ell \left(y^*_{[\ell]} - K_{[\ell]}\pi^*_{[\ell]}\right)\right]_{\alpha=\hat{\alpha}(r)},\end{aligned} \tag{2.189}$$

yielding the final estimate $\hat{\alpha}$.

Next because

$$\text{var}[y^*_{[\ell]j} - K_{[\ell]}\pi^*_{[\ell]j}] = \text{var}[K^*_{[\ell]j} - K_{[\ell]}F_{[\ell]j}]$$
$$= \text{var}[\sum_{c=1}^{j} K_{[\ell]c}], \quad (2.190)$$

and $K^*_{[\ell]j}$ follows the binomial distribution with parameters $K_{[\ell]}$ and $\pi^*_{[\ell]j} = [1 - F_{[\ell]j}]$, one writes

$$\text{var}[y^*_{[\ell]j} - K_{[\ell]}\pi^*_{[\ell]j}] = K_{[\ell]}F_{[\ell]j}[1 - F_{[\ell]j}] = K_{[\ell]}\pi^*_{[\ell]j}[1 - \pi^*_{[\ell]j}]. \quad (2.191)$$

It then follows from (2.189) that $\text{var}(\hat{\alpha})$ has the formula given by

$$\text{var}(\hat{\alpha}) = \left[\sum_{\ell=1}^{p+1} K_{[\ell]}X'_\ell D_{\pi^*_{[\ell]}} X_\ell\right]^{-1}. \quad (2.192)$$

2.3.1.3 Binary Mapping Based GQL Estimation Approach

By Table 2.27, consider the response vector

$$y^*_{[\ell]} = [K_{[\ell]} - K^*_{[\ell]1}, \ldots, K_{[\ell]} - K^*_{[\ell]j}, \ldots, K_{[\ell]} - K^*_{[\ell](J-1)}]'$$

[see also (2.184)], where

$$y^*[\ell]j = [K_{[\ell]} - K^*_{[\ell]j}] \sim \text{Bin}(K_{[\ell]}, \pi^*_{[\ell]j}),$$

with

$$\pi^*_{[\ell]j} = 1 - F_{[\ell]j} = \frac{\exp(x'_{[\ell]j}\alpha)}{1 + \exp(x'_{[\ell]j}\alpha)}$$

by (2.181). By following Sutradhar (2003, Section 3), one may then write a GQL estimating equation for α as

$$\sum_{\ell=1}^{p+1} \frac{\partial [K_{[\ell]}\pi^{*\prime}_{[\ell]}]}{\partial \alpha} \left[\text{cov}(Y^*_{[\ell]})\right]^{-1} [y^*_{[\ell]} - K_{[\ell]}\pi^*_{[\ell]}] = 0, \quad (2.193)$$

where

$$\frac{\partial \pi^{*\prime}_{[\ell]}}{\partial \alpha} = X'_\ell D_{\pi^*_{[\ell]}}$$

by (2.187), and

$$\text{cov}[Y^*_{[\ell]}] = K_{[\ell]} D_{\pi^*_{[\ell]}}$$

by (2.191). The GQL estimating equation (2.193) then reduces to

$$\sum_{\ell=1}^{p+1} X'_\ell [y^*_{[\ell]} - K_{[\ell]} \pi^*_{[\ell]}] = 0,$$

which is the same as the pseudo-likelihood estimating equation given by (2.184). Hence the GQL estimate of α is the same as the likelihood estimate found by (2.189), and its asymptotic covariance matrix is the same as that of the likelihood estimates given by (2.192).

2.3.1.4 Some Remarks on GQL Estimation for Fitting the Multinomial Model (3.63) Subject to Category Order Restriction

Notice from (2.184) that

$$\begin{aligned} y^*_{[\ell]} &= [K_{[\ell]} - K^*_{[\ell]1}, \ldots, K_{[\ell]} - K^*_{[\ell]j}, \ldots, K_{[\ell]} - K^*_{[\ell](J-1)}]' \\ &= [y^*_{[\ell]1}, \ldots, y^*_{[\ell]j}, \ldots, y^*_{[\ell](J-1)}]', \end{aligned} \tag{2.194}$$

is a cumulative response vector with its expectation

$$\begin{aligned} E[y^*_{[\ell]}] &= K_{[\ell]} \pi^*_{[\ell]} \\ &\equiv K_{[\ell]} [\pi^*_{[\ell]1}, \ldots, \pi^*_{[\ell]j}, \ldots, \pi^*_{[\ell](J-1)}]' \\ &= K_{[\ell]} [1 - F_{[\ell]1}, \ldots, 1 - F_{[\ell]j}, \ldots, 1 - F_{[\ell](J-1)}]', \end{aligned} \tag{2.195}$$

with

$$\pi^*_{[\ell]j} = 1 - F_{[\ell]j} = \sum_{c=j+1}^{J} \pi_{[\ell]c}, \tag{2.196}$$

where, by (2.63) and (2.64), the multinomial probabilities are defined as

$$\pi_{[\ell]c} = \begin{cases} \frac{\exp(\beta_{c0}+\beta_{c\ell})}{1+\sum_{g=1}^{J-1}\exp(\beta_{g0}+\beta_{g\ell})} & \text{for } c = 1, \ldots, J-1 \\ \frac{1}{1+\sum_{g=1}^{J-1}\exp(\beta_{g0}+\beta_{g\ell})} & \text{for } c = J, \end{cases} \tag{2.197}$$

for $\ell = 1, \ldots, p$, whereas for $\ell = p+1$, these probabilities are given as

$$\pi_{[p+1]c} = \begin{cases} \frac{\exp(\beta_{c0})}{1+\sum_{g=1}^{J-1}\exp(\beta_{g0})} & \text{for } c = 1,\ldots,J-1 \\ \frac{1}{1+\sum_{g=1}^{J-1}\exp(\beta_{g0})} & \text{for } c = J. \end{cases} \tag{2.198}$$

Use $x_{[\ell]J} = 01_{(J-1)(p+1)}$ for all $\ell = 1,\ldots,p+1$, along with $x_{[\ell]c}$ from (2.182) for $c = 1,\ldots,J-1$; and $\ell = 1,\ldots,p+1$, and re-express all $\pi_{[\ell]c}$ in (2.196)–(2.197) as

$$\pi_{[\ell]c} = \frac{\exp(x'_{[\ell]c}\beta)}{\sum_{g=1}^{J}\exp(x'_{[\ell]g}\beta)}, \tag{2.199}$$

where, similar to (2.178),

$$\beta = [\beta_1^{*\prime},\ldots,\beta_j^{*\prime},\ldots,\beta_{J-1}^{*\prime}]', \text{ with } \beta_j^* = [\beta_{j0},\beta_{j1},\ldots,\beta_{j\ell},\ldots,\beta_{jp}]'. \tag{2.200}$$

Note that α parameters in (2.178) and β parameters in (2.198) are different, even though they have some implicit connection. Here, one is interested to estimate β for the purpose of comparing $\pi^*_{[\ell]j} = \sum_{c=1}^{J}\pi_{[\ell]c}$ with $1-\pi^*_{[\ell]j} = \sum_{c=1}^{j}\pi_{[\ell]c}$. We construct a GQL estimating equation (Sutradhar 2004, 2011) for β as follows.

2.3.1.4.1 GQL Estimating Equation for β

2.3.1.4.1 (a) Computation of $\mathrm{cov}(y^*_{[\ell]}) = \Gamma_{[\ell]} = (\gamma_{[\ell]jh}) : (J-1)\times(J-1)$

The elements of the Γ matrix are computed as follows.

$$\begin{aligned} \gamma_{[\ell]jj} &= \mathrm{var}[y^*_{[\ell]j} - K_{[\ell]}\pi^*_{[\ell]j}] \\ &= \mathrm{var}[K^*_{[\ell]j} - K_{[\ell]}F_{[\ell]j}] \\ &= \mathrm{var}[\sum_{c=1}^{j} K_{[\ell]c}] \\ &= K_{[\ell]}\left[\sum_{c=1}^{j}\pi_{[\ell]c}(1-\pi_{[\ell]c}) - \sum_{c\neq c'}^{j}\pi_{[\ell]c}\pi_{[\ell]c'}\right], \text{ for } j = 1,\ldots,J-1. \end{aligned} \tag{2.201}$$

Next, for $j < h, j,h = 1,\ldots,J-1$,

$$\begin{aligned} \gamma_{[\ell]jh} &= \mathrm{cov}[y^*_{[\ell]j} - K_{[\ell]}\pi^*_{[\ell]j}, y^*_{[\ell]h} - K_{[\ell]}\pi^*_{[\ell]h}] \\ &= \mathrm{cov}[\sum_{c=1}^{j} K_{[\ell]c}, \sum_{c=1}^{h} K_{[\ell]c}] \end{aligned}$$

$$= K_{[\ell]}\left[\sum_{c=1}^{j}\pi_{[\ell]c}(1-\pi_{[\ell]c}) - \sum_{c\neq c'}^{j}\pi_{[\ell]c}\pi_{[\ell]c'} - \sum_{c=1}^{j}\sum_{c'=j+1}^{h}\pi_{[\ell]c}\pi_{[\ell]c'}\right] \quad (2.202)$$

Also it follows that $\gamma_{[\ell]jh} = \gamma_{[\ell]hj}$.

2.3.1.4.1 (b) Computation of $\frac{\partial \pi^{*\prime}_{[\ell]}}{\partial \beta} : (J-1)(p+1) \times (J-1)$

It is sufficient to compute the derivative of a general element, say $\pi^{*}_{[\ell]j}$ with respect to β. That is,

$$\begin{aligned}
\frac{\partial \pi^{*}_{[\ell]j}}{\partial \beta} &= \sum_{c=j+1}^{J}\frac{\partial \pi_{[\ell]c}}{\partial \beta} \\
&= \sum_{c=j+1}^{J}\left[\pi_{[\ell]c}\left\{x_{[\ell]c} - \sum_{u=1}^{J}\pi_{[\ell]u}x_{[\ell]u}\right\}\right] \\
&= \sum_{c=j+1}^{J}\left[\pi_{[\ell]c}\left\{x_{[\ell]c} - X'_{\ell}\pi_{[\ell]}\right\}\right] \\
&= A^{*}_{[\ell]j}(x,\beta) : \ (J-1)(p+1)\times 1, \text{ (say)},
\end{aligned} \quad (2.203)$$

yielding

$$\begin{aligned}
\frac{\partial \pi^{*\prime}_{[\ell]}}{\partial \beta} &= \left(A^{*}_{[\ell]1}(x,\beta) \ \ldots \ A^{*}_{[\ell]j}(x,\beta) \ \ldots \ A^{*}_{[\ell](J-1)}(x,\beta)\right) \ (J-1)(p+1)\times(J-1) \\
&= A^{*}_{[\ell]}(x,\beta), \text{ (say)}.
\end{aligned} \quad (2.204)$$

Next, by following Sutradhar (2004), and using (2.200)–(2.201), and (2.203), we can write a GQL estimating equation for β as

$$\begin{aligned}
&\sum_{\ell=1}^{p+1} K_{[\ell]}\frac{\partial \pi^{*\prime}_{[\ell]}}{\partial \beta}\Gamma^{-1}_{[\ell]}\left(y^{*}_{[\ell]} - K_{[\ell]}\pi^{*}_{[\ell]}\right) \\
&= \sum_{\ell=1}^{p+1} K_{[\ell]}A^{*}_{[\ell]}(x,\beta)\Gamma^{-1}_{[\ell]}\left(y^{*}_{[\ell]} - K_{[\ell]}\pi^{*}_{[\ell]}\right) = 0
\end{aligned} \quad (2.205)$$

The solution of this GQL estimating equation (2.204) for β may be obtained iteratively by using the iterative formula

$$\hat{\beta}(r+1) = \hat{\beta}(r) + \left[\left\{ \sum_{\ell=1}^{p+1} K_{[\ell]}^2 A_{[\ell]}^*(x,\beta) \Gamma_{[\ell]}^{-1} A_{[\ell]}^{*\prime}(x,\beta) \right\}^{-1} \times \sum_{\ell=1}^{p+1} K_{[\ell]} A_{[\ell]}^*(x,\beta) \Gamma_{[\ell]}^{-1} \left(y_{[\ell]}^* - K_{[\ell]} \pi_{[\ell]}^* \right) \right]_{\beta=\hat{\beta}(r)}, \quad (2.206)$$

yielding the final GQL estimate $\hat{\beta}_{GQL}$, along with its asymptotic (as $\min_{1\leq \ell \leq p+1} K_{[\ell]} \rightarrow \infty$) covariance matrix

$$\text{cov}[\hat{\beta}_{GQL}] = \left[\sum_{\ell=1}^{p+1} K_{[\ell]}^2 A_{[\ell]}^*(x,\beta) \Gamma_{[\ell]}^{-1} A_{[\ell]}^{*\prime}(x,\beta) \right]^{-1}. \quad (2.207)$$

References

Agresti, A. (1984). *Analysis of ordinal categorical data.* New York: Wiley.

Agresti, A. (1990). *Categorical data analysis* (1st ed.). New York: Wiley.

Agresti, A. (2002). *Categorical data analysis* (2nd ed.). New York: Wiley.

Bishop, Y. M. M., Fienberg, S. E., & Holland, P. W. (1975). *Discrete multivariate analysis: Theory and practice*. Cambridge: MIT Press.

Grizzle, J. E., Starmer, C. F., & Koch, G. G. (1969). Analysis of categorical data by linear models. *Biometrics, 25*, 489–504.

Haberman, S. J. (1978). *Analysis of qualitative data. Introductory topics* (Vol. 1). New York: Academic Press.

Koch, G. G., Singer, J. M., & Stokes, M. E. (1992). Some aspects of weighted least squares analysis for longitudinal categorical data. In J. H. Dwyer, M. Feinleib, P. Lippert, & H. Hoffmeister (Eds.), *Statistical Models for Longitudinal Studies of Health, Monographs in Epidemiology and Biostatistics* (Vol. 16, pp. 215–258). New York: Oxford University Press. ISBN: 0-19-505473-3

Rao, C. R. (1973). *Linear statistical inference and its applications.* New York: Wiley.

Semenya, K., & Koch, G. G. (1980). *Compound function and linear model methods for the multivariate analysis of ordinal categorical data. Mimeo Series* (Vol. 1323). Chapel Hill: University of North Carolina Institute of Statistics.

Semenya, K., Koch, G. G., Stokes, M. E., & Forthofer, R. N. (1983). Linear models methods for some rank function analyses of ordinal categorical data. *Communication in Statistics Series A, 12*, 1277–1298.

Sutradhar, B. C. (2003). An overview on regression models for discrete longitudinal responses. *Statistical Science, 18*, 377–393.

Sutradhar, B. C. (2004). On exact quasilikelihood inference in generalized linear mixed models. *Sankhya B: The Indian Journal of Statistics, 66*, 261–289.

Sutradhar, B. C. (2011). *Dynamic mixed models for familial longitudinal data.* New York: Springer.

Chapter 3
Regression Models For Univariate Longitudinal Stationary Categorical Data

3.1 Model Background

Note that the multinomial model discussed in Chap. 2 and the inferences therein for this model are described for a cross-sectional study, where the multinomial responses with corresponding covariates are collected from a large number of independent individuals at a single point of time. There are, however, situations in practice where this type of multinomial responses are collected over a small period of time. Here the repeated multinomial responses are likely to be correlated. But, the modeling and inferences for such repeated multinomial data are not addressed adequately in the literature. One of the main reasons for this is the difficulty of modeling the correlations among the repeated categorical responses. This is not surprising as the modeling for repeated binary data has also been a challenging problem over the last few decades (e.g., Park et al. 1996; Prentice 1988; Oman and Zucker 2001; Qaqish 2003; Farrell and Sutradhar 2006; Sutradhar 2010a, 2011, Chapter 7), indicating that the modeling for correlations for repeated multinomial responses would naturally be more complex.

Let $y_{it} = (y_{it1}, \ldots, y_{itj}, \ldots, y_{it,J-1})'$ be the $(J-1)$-dimensional multinomial response variable and for $j = 1, \ldots, J-1$,

$$y_{it}^{(j)} = (y_{it1}^{(j)}, \ldots, y_{itj}^{(j)}, \ldots, y_{it,J-1}^{(j)})' = (01'_{j-1}, 1, 01'_{J-1-j})' \equiv \delta_{itj} \tag{3.1}$$

indicates that the multinomial response of ith individual belongs to jth category at time t. For $j = J$, one writes $y_{it}^{(J)} = \delta_{itJ} = 01_{J-1}$. Here 1_m, for example, denotes the m-dimensional unit vector. Also, let

$$w_{it} = [w_{it1}, \ldots, w_{its}, \ldots, w_{itp}]' \tag{3.2}$$

B.C. Sutradhar, *Longitudinal Categorical Data Analysis*, Springer Series in Statistics, DOI 10.1007/978-1-4939-2137-9_3

be the $p \times 1$ vector of fixed and known covariates corresponding to y_{it}, and β_j denote its effect on y_{it} belonging to the jth category. For example, in a longitudinal obesity study, w_{it} may represent the epidemiological/socio-economic variables such as

$$w_{it} \equiv [\text{age, gender, education level, marital status, geographical region,} \\ \text{chronic conditions and lifestyle including smoking and food habits}]' \quad (3.3)$$

at a given year (t) for the ith individual. This w_{it} will have β_j influence to put the response y_{it} in the jth obesity level, where for $J = 5$, for example, standard obesity levels are normal, overweight, obese class 1, 2, and 3.

3.1.1 Non-stationary Multinomial Models

Next, as a generalization to the longitudinal setup, one may follow (2.45) from Chap. 2, and write the marginal probability for y_{it} to belong to the jth category as

$$P[y_{it} = y_{it}^{(j)} = \delta_{itj}] = \pi_{(it)j} = \begin{cases} \frac{\exp(\beta_{j0}+\beta_j' w_{it})}{1+\sum_{g=1}^{J-1}\exp(\beta_{g0}+\beta_g' w_{it})} & \text{for } j = 1,\ldots,J-1 \\ \frac{1}{1+\sum_{g=1}^{J-1}\exp(\beta_{g0}+\beta_g' w_{it})} & \text{for } j = J, \end{cases} \quad (3.4)$$

where $\beta_j = [\beta_{j1},\ldots,\beta_{js},\ldots,\beta_{jp}]'$ for $j = 1,\ldots,J-1$, is the same as in (2.45) indicating that the regression effects remain the same for all $t = 1,\ldots,T$, even though we now have time dependent covariates w_{it}, whereas in the cross-sectional setup, i.e., in (2.45), w_i is expressed as $w_i = [w_{i1},\ldots,w_{is},\ldots,w_{ip}]'$. Note that except for gender, all other covariates used to illustrate w_{it} through (3.3) can be time dependent. Thus, w_{it} in (3.3) may be referred to as a time dependent (non-stationary) covariate vector, which makes the marginal multinomial probabilities (3.4) non-stationary over time. For example, to understand the time effect on longitudinal multinomial responses, some authors such as Agresti (2002, Chapter 11, Eqs. (11.3)–(11.6)) (see also Agresti 1989, 1990) have modeled the marginal multinomial probabilities at a given time $t (t = 1,\ldots,T)$ by adding a deterministic time effect to the category effect of the response variable. To be specific, for

$$w_{it} = [\text{time, gender, time} \times \text{gender}]' = [t, G, tG]'$$

the marginal probability in (3.4) reduces to

$$P[y_{it} = y_{it}^{(j)} = \delta_{itj}] = \pi_{(it)j} = \begin{cases} \frac{\exp(\beta_{j0}+\beta_{j1}t+\beta_{j2}G+\beta_{j3}Gt)}{1+\sum_{g=1}^{J-1}\exp(\beta_{g0}+\beta_{g1}t+\beta_{g2}G+\beta_{g3}Gt)} & \text{for } j = 1,\ldots,J-1 \\ \frac{1}{1+\sum_{g=1}^{J-1}\exp(\beta_{g0}+\beta_{g1}t+\beta_{g2}G+\beta_{g3}Gt)} & \text{for } j = J, \end{cases} \quad (3.5)$$

which is similar to the marginal probability model (11.6) in Agresti (2002). Note that when w_{it} is properly constructed using associated time dependent covariates such as in (3.3), it is unlikely that time (t) will directly influence the probability as in (3.5). Thus, any model similar to (3.5) will have little practical values. To understand the time effect, it is however important to exploit the possible correlation structure for the repeated multinomial responses $y_{i1}, \ldots, y_{it}, \ldots, y_{iT}$, when marginal probabilities are modeled by (3.4). Here y_{it} is the $(J-1) \times 1$ response vector defined as $y_{it} = [y_{it1}, \ldots, y_{itj}, \ldots, y_{it,J-1}]'$. As far as the correlation structure is concerned, Agresti (2002, Section 11.4) made an attempt to use the so-called working correlation structure for the repeated multinomial responses, and the regression effects were suggested to be computed by solving the so-called generalized estimating equations (GEE) (Liang and Zeger 1986). But, as discussed in detail by Sutradhar (2011, Chapter 7), for example in the context of longitudinal binary data, this type of GEE approach can produce less efficient estimates than the 'independence' assumption based moment or QL (quasi-likelihood) approaches, which makes the GEE approach useless. Further as a remedy, Sutradhar (2010a, 2011) suggested to use an auto-correlation structure based GQL (generalized quasi-likelihood) (see also Sutradhar 2010b, www.statprob.com) estimation approach that always produces more efficient estimates than the aforementioned 'independence' assumption based estimates. However, in this book, instead of using the whole auto-correlation class, we will exploit the most likely auto-regressive type model but in both linear and non-linear forms. These linear and non-linear non-stationary multinomial models and parameter estimation are discussed in detail in Chap. 4. The so-called odds ratio based existing correlation models will also be discussed.

3.1.2 Stationary Multinomial Models

In some situations, covariates of an individual can be time independent. In such cases, it is sufficient to use the notation

$$w_i = [w_{i1}, \ldots, w_{is}, \ldots, w_{ip}]'$$

in place of w_{it} (3.2) for all $t = 1, \ldots, T$, to represent p covariates of the ith individual. For example, suppose that one is interested to study the effects of gender and race on the repeated multinomial responses $y_{it} : (J-1) \times 1$ collected over T time periods. For this problem, for the ith $(i = 1, \ldots, K)$, one writes

$$w_i = [\text{gender}_i,\ \text{race}_i]' = [w_{i1}, w_{i2}]',$$

and consequently, the marginal multinomial probability, similar to (3.4), may be written as

$$P[y_{it} = y_{it}^{(j)}] = \pi_{(i)j} = \begin{cases} \frac{\exp(\beta_{j0}+\beta_j' w_i)}{1+\sum_{g=1}^{J-1}\exp(\beta_{g0}+\beta_g' w_i)} & \text{for } j = 1,\ldots,J-1;\ t = 1,\ldots,T \\ \frac{1}{1+\sum_{g=1}^{J-1}\exp(\beta_{g0}+\beta_g' w_i)} & \text{for } j = J;\ t = 1,\ldots,T, \end{cases} \tag{3.6}$$

where β_j for $j = 1,\ldots,J-1$, has the same notation as in (3.4), that is, $\beta_j = [\beta_{j1},\ldots,\beta_{js},\ldots,\beta_{jp}]'$. Notice that these marginal multinomial probabilities in (3.6) are the same as the multinomial probability (2.45) used in the cross-sectional case, that is, for the $t = 1$ case. However, unlike the probability formula in (2.45), the marginal probability in (3.6) cannot represent the complete model in the longitudinal setup. More specifically, a complete model involving (3.6) also must accommodate, at least, the correlation structure for the repeated multinomial responses $y_{i1},\ldots,y_{it},\ldots,y_{iT}$. We deal with the inferences for this type of complete longitudinal stationary multinomial models in Sect. 3.3 for the binary case ($J = 2$) for simplicity and in Sect. 3.5 for general case with more than two categories ($J > 2$). To be specific, in these Sects. 3.3 and 3.5 we will generalize the cross-sectional level inferences discussed in Sect. 2.2 (of Chap. 2) to the longitudinal setup.

3.1.3 More Simpler Stationary Multinomial Models: Covariates Free (Non-regression) Case

Similar to Sect. 2.1 (Chap. 2), it may happen in some situations that the multinomial (categorical) data are collected from a group of individuals with similar covariates background. For example, suppose that a treatment is applied to 500 males and a multinomial response with three categories such as 'highly effective,' 'somewhat effective,' and 'not effective at all' is collected from every individual. Further suppose that this survey is repeated for $T = 3$ times with the same 500 individuals. To model this type of data, it is appropriate to use the marginal probability as

$$P[y_{it} = y_{it}^{(j)}] = \pi_j = \begin{cases} \frac{\exp(\beta_{j0})}{1+\sum_{g=1}^{J-1}\exp(\beta_{g0})} & \text{for } j = 1,\ldots,J-1;\ t = 1,\ldots,T \\ \frac{1}{1+\sum_{g=1}^{J-1}\exp(\beta_{g0})} & \text{for } j = J;\ t = 1,\ldots,T, \end{cases} \tag{3.7}$$

which is a covariates free and hence a simpler version of the marginal probability relationship in (3.6). This marginal probability is the same as (2.2) which was defined under a cross-sectional setup. In the present case, the repeated multinomial responses $y_{i1},\ldots,y_{it},\ldots,y_{iT}$ are likely to be correlated. In Sects. 3.2–3.5, we accommodate the correlations of the repeated responses and develop the inference procedure for efficient estimation of the parameters $\beta_{10},\ldots,\beta_{j0},\ldots,\beta_{J-1,0}$. For simplicity, the binary case ($J = 2$) is discussed in Sect. 3.2 with no covariates involved in the model, and in Sect. 3.4 we deal with the general longitudinal multinomial ($J > 2$) cases without covariates in the model. To be specific, in these sections, we generalize the cross-sectional level inference discussed in Sect. 2.1.3 (of Chap. 2) to the longitudinal setup. Both likelihood and GQL estimating equation approaches will be discussed.

3.2 Covariate Free Basic Univariate Longitudinal Binary Models

For simplicity, in this section, we discuss various longitudinal binary models ($J=2$) and inferences, and turn back to the general longitudinal multinomial case with $J>2$ categories in Sect. 3.3.

3.2.1 *Auto-correlation Class Based Stationary Binary Model and Estimation of Parameters*

In the stationary longitudinal setup for binary ($J=2$) data, for $i=1,\ldots,K$, the marginal probabilities by (3.7) have the forms:

$$P[y_{it}=y_{it}^{(j)}]=\pi_j=\begin{cases}\frac{\exp(\beta_{10})}{1+\exp(\beta_{10})} & \text{for } j=1\\ \frac{1}{1+\exp(\beta_{10})} & \text{for } j=J=2,\end{cases} \tag{3.8}$$

for all $t=1,\ldots,T$, where

$$y_{it}^{(j)}=\begin{cases}1 \text{ for } j=1;\ t=1,\ldots,T\\ 0 \text{ for } j=J=2;\ t=1,\ldots,T.\end{cases}$$

For this stationary case, one may summarize the response frequencies over T time periods through following initial contingency Table 3.1 and $T-1$ lag ($h^*=1,\ldots,T-1$) contingency tables (Tables 3.2(1)–3.2(1)($T-1$)):

Table 3.1 Contingency table at initial time $t=1$

t ($t=1$)		
Category		
1	2	Total
$K_1(1)$	$K_2(1)$	K

Table 3.2 Lag h^* ($h^*=1,\ldots,T-1$) based $[h^*(T-h^*)]$ contingency tables

		t ($t=h^*+1,\ldots,T$)		
Time		Category		
Time	Category	1	2	Total
t-h^*	1	$K_{11}(t-h^*,t)$	$K_{12}(t-h^*,t)$	$K_1(t-h^*)$
	2	$K_{21}(t-h^*,t)$	$K_{22}(t-h^*,t)$	$K_2(t-h^*)$
	Total	$K_1(t)$	$K_2(t)$	K

As far as the correlation structure for the repeated binary responses is concerned, following Sutradhar (2010a, 2011), it is quite reasonable to assume that they follow an ARMA (auto-regressive moving average) type auto-correlation class which accommodates simpler AR(1), MA(1) and equi-correlations (EQC) correlation models. Note that the correlation structure of any correlation model within this auto-correlation class can be understood simply by consistently estimating all possible lag correlations, namely ρ_{h^*} for $h^* = 1,\ldots,T-1$. These auto-correlations for the stationary binary data form the common stationary $T \times T$ auto-correlation matrix, say $C_i(\rho) = \mathrm{Corr}(Y_i) = \mathrm{Corr}(Y_{i1},\ldots,Y_{it},\ldots,Y_{iT})'$ given by

$$C_i(\rho) = \begin{bmatrix} 1 & \rho_1 & \rho_2 & \cdots & \rho_{T-1} \\ \rho_1 & 1 & \rho_1 & \cdots & \rho_{T-2} \\ \vdots & \vdots & \vdots & & \vdots \\ \rho_{T-1} & \rho_{T-2} & \rho_{T-3} & \cdots & 1 \end{bmatrix} = C(\rho), \quad (3.9)$$

which is same for all $i = 1,\ldots,K$.

3.2.1.1 GQL Estimation of β_{10}

To develop the GQL estimating equation for β_{10}, we first provide a moment estimating equation for ρ_{h^*} by assuming that β_{10} is known. Following Sutradhar (2011, Eq. 7.67), for example, this moment equation is given by

$$\hat{\rho}_{h^*} = \frac{\sum_{i=1}^{K}\sum_{t=h^*+1}^{T} \tilde{y}_{i,t-h^*}\tilde{y}_{it}/K(T-h^*)}{\sum_{i=1}^{K}\sum_{t=1}^{T}\tilde{y}_{it}^2/KT}, \quad (3.10)$$

where $\tilde{y}_{it}$ is the standardized deviance, defined as

$$\tilde{y}_{it} = \frac{y_{it}-\pi_1}{\{\pi_1(1-\pi_1)\}^{1/2}},$$

where π_1 is defined by (3.8). Now by using the frequencies from the contingency Tables 3.1 and 3.2, one writes

$$\sum_{i=1}^{K}\sum_{t=1}^{T} y_{it} = \sum_{t=1}^{T}\sum_{i=1}^{K} y_{it} = \sum_{t=1}^{T} K_1(t), \text{ or}$$

$$\sum_{i=1}^{K}\sum_{t=h^*+1}^{T} y_{it} = \sum_{t=h^*+1}^{T}\sum_{i=1}^{K} y_{it} = \sum_{t=h^*+1}^{T} K_1(t); \text{ and}$$

$$\sum_{i=1}^{K}\sum_{t=h^*+1}^{T} y_{i,t-h^*} = \sum_{t=h^*+1}^{T}\sum_{i=1}^{K} y_{i,t-h^*} = \sum_{t=h^*+1}^{T} K_1(t-h^*)$$

$$\sum_{i=1}^{K}\sum_{t=h^*+1}^{T} y_{i,t-h^*}y_{it} = \sum_{t=h^*+1}^{T}\sum_{i=1}^{K} y_{i,t-h^*}y_{it} = \sum_{t=h^*+1}^{T} K_{11}(t-h^*,\, t). \tag{3.11}$$

By using (3.11), it then follows from (3.10) that

$$\hat{\rho}_{h^*} = \frac{\frac{1}{T-h^*}\sum_{t=h^*+1}^{T}\left[K_{11}(t-h^*,\, t) - \pi_1\{K_1(t) + K_1(t-h^*)\} + \pi_1^2 K\right]}{\frac{1}{T}\sum_{t=1}^{T}\left[(1-2\pi_1)K_1(t) + \pi_1^2 K\right]}. \tag{3.12}$$

For the GQL estimation of β_{10} we follow the steps below.

Step 1. Use $\rho_{h^*} = 0$, that is, $C_i(\rho) = C(\rho) = I_T$, the $T \times T$ identity matrix, and construct the covariance matrix $\Sigma_i(\beta_{10}, \rho)$ as

$$\Sigma_i(\beta_{10}, \rho) = A_i^{1/2} C(\rho) A_i^{1/2}, \tag{3.13}$$

where

$$A_i = \text{diag}[\sigma_{(i)11}, \ldots, \sigma_{(i)tt}, \ldots, \sigma_{(i)TT}], \tag{3.14}$$

with $\sigma_{(i)tt} = \text{var}[Y_{it}]$. Now because, in the present stationary case $\sigma_{(i),tt} = \pi_1(1-\pi_1)$, that is $A_i = \pi_1(1-\pi_1)I_T$, the covariance matrix in (3.13) has the simpler form given by

$$\Sigma_i(\beta_{10}, \rho) = \pi_1(1-\pi_1)C(\rho). \tag{3.15}$$

Step 2. Then for

$$\pi_{(i)} = E[Y_i] = E[Y_{i1}, \ldots, Y_{it}, \ldots, Y_{iT}]' = \pi_1 1_T,$$

solve the GQL estimating equation

$$\begin{aligned}
&\sum_{i=1}^{K} \frac{\partial \pi'_{(i)}}{\partial \beta_{10}} \Sigma_i^{-1}(\rho)(y_i - \pi_{(i)}) \\
&= \sum_{i=1}^{K} 1'_T C^{-1}(\rho)(y_i - \pi_1 1_T) \\
&= \sum_{i=1}^{K} (\omega_1, \ldots, \omega_t, \ldots, \omega_T)(y_i - \pi_1 1_T) \\
&= \sum_{t=1}^{T} \omega_t K_1(t) - K\pi_1 \sum_{t=1}^{T} \omega_t = 0,
\end{aligned} \tag{3.16}$$

(Sutradhar 2011, Section 7.3.5) for β_{10}, by using the iterative equation

$$\hat{\beta}_{10}(r+1) = \hat{\beta}_{10}(r) + \left[\left\{\sum_{i=1}^{K} \frac{\partial \pi'_{(i)}}{\partial \beta_{10}} \Sigma_i^{-1}(\rho) \frac{\partial \pi'_{(i)}}{\partial \beta_{10}}\right\}^{-1} \sum_{i=1}^{K} \frac{\partial \pi'_{(i)}}{\partial \beta_{10}} \Sigma_i^{-1}(\rho)(y_i - \pi_{(i)})\right]_{|\beta_{10}=\hat{\beta}_{10}(r)}$$

$$= \hat{\beta}_{10}(r) + \frac{1}{K\{\pi_1(1-\pi_1)\}\sum_{t=1}^{T}\omega_t}\left[\sum_{t=1}^{T}\omega_t K_1(t) - K\pi_1\sum_{t=1}^{T}\omega_t\right] \quad (3.17)$$

Step 3. Use this estimate of β_{10} from (3.17) into π_1 and compute $\hat{\rho}_{h^*}$ by (3.12), and then compute the $C_i(\rho)$ by (3.9). Next, use this $C_i(\rho)$ in Step 1 to construct the covariance matrix Σ_i by (3.15), and then obtain improved estimate of β_{10} by using (3.17) from Step 2.

These three steps continue until convergence for β_{10} yielding the converged value as the estimate.

Note that one can conveniently use the above iterative formula (3.17) to obtain the standard error of the GQL estimate for β_{10}. To be specific, because the variance of the estimator depends on the variance of second term in the right-hand side of (3.17), and because K individuals are independent, for known ρ, it follows that the variance of the estimator $\hat{\beta}_{10}$ has the formula

$$\mathrm{var}[\hat{\beta}_{10}] = \left[\sum_{i=1}^{K} \frac{\partial \pi'_{(i)}}{\partial \beta_{10}} \Sigma_i^{-1}(\rho) \frac{\partial \pi'_{(i)}}{\partial \beta_{10}}\right]^{-1} \sum_{i=1}^{K} \frac{\partial \pi'_{(i)}}{\partial \beta_{10}} \Sigma_i^{-1}(\rho)\mathrm{var}[y_i - \pi_{(i)}]\Sigma_i^{-1}(\rho)\frac{\partial \pi_{(i)}}{\partial \beta_{10}}$$

$$\times \left[\sum_{i=1}^{K} \frac{\partial \pi'_{(i)}}{\partial \beta_{10}} \Sigma_i^{-1}(\rho) \frac{\partial \pi'_{(i)}}{\partial \beta_{10}}\right]^{-1}$$

$$= \left[\sum_{i=1}^{K} \frac{\partial \pi'_{(i)}}{\partial \beta_{10}} \Sigma_i^{-1}(\rho) \frac{\partial \pi'_{(i)}}{\partial \beta_{10}}\right]^{-1} = \frac{1}{K\{\pi_1(1-\pi_1)\}\sum_{t=1}^{T}\omega_t}, \quad (3.18)$$

because $\mathrm{var}[y_i - \pi_{(i)}] = \Sigma_i(\rho)$.

3.2.1.2 A Simpler Alternative Estimation Formula for β_{10}

Note that in the present covariate free stationary case, one can first write a closed formula for the estimate of π_1 and then solve for β_{10} from the formula for $\pi_1 = \frac{\exp(\beta_{10})}{1+\exp(\beta_{10})}$. To be specific, the estimating equation (3.16) provides

$$\hat{\pi}_1 = \frac{\sum_{t=1}^{T}\omega_t K_1(t)}{K\sum_{t=1}^{T}\omega_t}, \quad (3.19)$$

where $K_1(t)$ is the number of individuals those belong to category 1 (yes group) at time t, and ω_t is the t-th element of the row vector

$$\omega' = [\omega_1, \ldots, \omega_t, \ldots, \omega_T] \equiv 1'_T C^{-1}(\rho).$$

Next, by equating $\hat{\pi}_1$ from (3.19) to $\frac{\exp(\beta_{10})}{1+\exp(\beta_{10})}$, one writes

$$\exp(\hat{\beta}_{10}) = \frac{\sum_{t=1}^{T} \omega_t K_1(t)}{K\sum_{t=1}^{T} \omega_t - \sum_{t=1}^{T} \omega_t K_1(t)},$$

and obtains the estimate of β_{10} as

$$\hat{\beta}_{10} = log\left[\frac{\sum_{t=1}^{T} \omega_t K_1(t)}{K\sum_{t=1}^{T} \omega_t - \sum_{t=1}^{T} \omega_t K_1(t)}\right]. \tag{3.20}$$

which is easy to compute. However, finding the standard error of this estimate is somewhat complex but can be done by using the so-called delta method, whereas it is relatively much easier to use the variance formula (3.18) to obtain this standard error.

3.2.1.3 Illustration 3.1: Analysis of Longitudinal Asthma Data Using Auto-correlations Class Based GQL Approach

Consider the asthma data for 537 children from Ohio collected over a period of 4 years. This data set containing yearly asthma status for these children along with their mother's smoking habits was earlier analyzed by Zeger et al. (1988), Sutradhar (2003), and Sutradhar and Farrell (2007), among others. The data set is available in Appendix 7F in Sutradhar (2011, p. 320) (see also Zeger et al. 1988). Children with asthma problem are coded as 1 and no asthma attack is coded as 0. However to match with the notation of Table 3.2, we rename them (coded response) as category 1 and 2, respectively. Note that it is assumed in this study that mother's smoking habit remains unchanged over the study period. Thus, there is no time dependent covariate. Consequently, it is reasonable to assume that probability of an asthma attack to a child is not time dependent, but the repeated responses over 4 time periods will be auto-correlated. It is, therefore, of interest to compute this probability after taking the correlations into account. Further note that to compute this probability, in this section, we even ignore the mother's smoking habits as a covariate. In Sect. 3.3, we reanalyze this data set again by including the smoking habits of the mother as a binary covariate.

To be clear and precise, we first display all transitional contingency tables corresponding to Tables 3.1 and 3.2, as follows:

Now to compute the probability (3.8) of having an asthma attack for a child, we need to compute β_{10}, taking into account that the asthma status of a child over two different times is correlated. For the purpose, we however compute this parameter first by treating the repeated responses as independent. Thus, by putting $\rho_{h^*} = 0$ as guided by Step 1, we compute an initial estimate of β_{10} by solving (3.16). More

Table 3.3 *Contingency table for the asthma data at initial time* $t = 1$ for 537 children

t ($t = 1$)		
Category		
1 (Asthma attack)	2 (No attack)	Total
$K_1(1) = 87$	$K_2(1) = 450$	K=537

Table 3.4 (1): Lag $h^* = 1$ based transitional table from time $t - h^* = 1$ to $t = 2$ for the asthma data

		2		
Time		Category		
Time	Category	1	2	Total
1	1	$K_{11}(1,2) = 41$	$K_{12}(1,2) = 46$	$K_1(1) = 87$
	2	$K_{21}(1,2) = 50$	$K_{22}(1,2) = 400$	$K_2(1) = 450$
	Total	$K_1(2) = 91$	$K_2(2) = 446$	537

Table 3.4 (2): Lag $h^* = 1$ based transitional table from time $t - h^* = 2$ to $t = 3$ for the asthma data

		3		
Time		Category		
Time	Category	1	2	Total
2	1	$K_{11}(2,3) = 47$	$K_{12}(2,3) = 44$	$K_1(2) = 91$
	2	$K_{21}(2,3) = 38$	$K_{22}(2,3) = 408$	$K_2(2) = 446$
	Total	$K_1(3) = 85$	$K_2(3) = 452$	537

Table 3.4 (3): Lag $h^* = 1$ based transitional table from time $t - h^* = 3$ to $t = 4$ for the asthma data

		4		
Time		Category		
Time	Category	1	2	Total
3	1	$K_{11}(3,4) = 34$	$K_{12}(3,4) = 51$	$K_1(3) = 85$
	2	$K_{21}(3,4) = 29$	$K_{22}(3,4) = 423$	$K_2(1) = 452$
	Total	$K_1(4) = 63$	$K_2(4) = 474$	537

specifically we do this by using the iterative equation (3.17) under the assumption that all $\rho_{h^*} = 0$ $(h^* = 1, 2, 3)$. This initial estimate of β_{10} is found to be

$$\hat{\beta}_{10}(\text{initial}) = -1.7208.$$

Next we use this initial estimate of β_{10} and follow Step 3 to compute the auto-correlations by using the formula (3.12). These auto-correlation values are then used in (3.15) and (3.17) to obtain the improved estimate for β_{10}. In three cycles of iterations, the final estimates for 3 lag correlations were found to be

$$\hat{\rho}_1 = 0.40,\ \hat{\rho}_2 = 0.3129,\ \hat{\rho}_3 = 0.2979, \tag{3.21}$$

Table 3.4 (4): Lag $h^* = 2$ based transitional table from time $t - h^* = 1$ to $t = 3$ for the asthma data

		3		
Time		Category		
Time	Category	1	2	Total
1	1	$K_{11}(1,3) = 36$	$K_{12}(1,3) = 51$	$K_1(1) = 87$
	2	$K_{21}(1,3) = 49$	$K_{22}(1,3) = 401$	$K_2(1,3) = 450$
	Total	$K_1(3) = 85$	$K_2(3) = 452$	537

Table 3.4 (5): Lag $h^* = 2$ based transitional table from time $t - h^* = 2$ to $t = 4$ for the asthma data

		4		
Time		Category		
Time	Category	1	2	Total
2	1	$K_{11}(2,4) = 32$	$K_{12}(2,4) = 59$	$K_1(2) = 91$
	2	$K_{21}(2,4) = 31$	$K_{22}(2,4) = 415$	$K_2(2) = 446$
	Total	$K_1(4) = 63$	$K_2(4) = 474$	537

Table 3.4 (6): Lag $h^* = 3$ based transitional table from time $t - h^* = 1$ to $t = 4$ for the asthma data

		4		
Time		Category		
Time	Category	1	2	Total
1	1	$K_{11}(1,4) = 31$	$K_{12}(1,4) = 56$	$K_1(1) = 87$
	2	$K_{21}(1,4) = 32$	$K_{22}(1,4) = 418$	$K_2(1) = 450$
	Total	$K_1(4) = 63$	$K_2(4) = 474$	537

yielding the final binary category effect (regression effect) as

$$\hat{\beta}_{10} = -1.7284, \tag{3.22}$$

with its standard error, computed by (3.18) as

$$\text{s.e.}(\hat{\beta}_{10}) = \sqrt{0.00748} = 0.0865.$$

Note that the above correlation values are in agreement with those found in Sutradhar (2003, Section 5.2) but this regression estimate in (3.22) is computed by using a simpler regression model involving only binary category effect, whereas Sutradhar (2003) (see also Zeger et al. 1988) has used a slightly different regression model involving covariate (mother's smoking habits) specific category effects. This latter model but based on contingency (transitional) tables is discussed in the next section. Turning back to the marginal model (3.8), by using the final regression estimate from (3.22) into (3.8), one obtains the probability of having an asthma attack for a child as $\hat{\pi}_1 = 0.1508$, which appears to be a large probability and can be a matter of practical concern. Note that the direct estimating formula (3.19) also produces the same estimate 0.1508 for this probability and (3.20) consequently yields the same estimate for β_{10} as in (3.22).

3.2.2 *Stationary Binary AR(1) Type Model and Estimation of Parameters*

In the last section, the repeated categorical (binary) responses were assumed to follow a general class of auto-correlation structures, and the inferences were made by using the so-called GQL approach. Now suppose that one is interested to fit a specific such as lag 1 dynamic (AR(1)) model to the same repeated binary data. It is demonstrated below that one may use the likelihood approach in such cases for the estimation of the parameters. Also, one may alternatively use the specific correlation structure based GQL approach for the estimation.

3.2.2.1 LDCP Model and Likelihood Estimation

Refer to the repeated binary data for K individuals with transitional counts displayed through the contingency Tables 3.1 and 3.2. For example, $K_{11}(1,3)$ denotes the number of individuals with responses who were in category 1 at time $t = 1$ and also belong to category 1 at time $t = 3$. We now assume that the repeated binary responses of these individuals follow the so-called LDCP model (also known as Markovian or AR(1) type LDCP model (Zeger et al. 1985; Sutradhar 2011, Section 7.2.3.1)) given by

$$P[y_{i1} = y_{i1}^{(j)}] = \pi_j = \begin{cases} \frac{\exp(\beta_{10})}{1+\exp(\beta_{10})} & \text{for } j = 1 \\ \frac{1}{1+\exp(\beta_{10})} & \text{for } j = J = 2; \end{cases} \tag{3.23}$$

$$\begin{aligned} P[y_{it} = y_{it}^{(1)} | y_{i,t-1} = y_{i,t-1}^{(g)}] &= \pi_1 + \rho(y_{i,t-1}^{(g)} - \pi_1) \\ &= \lambda_{it|t-1}^{(1)}(g) \text{ (say)}, g = 1,2;\ t = 2,\ldots,T; \end{aligned} \tag{3.24}$$

and

$$\lambda_{it|t-1}^{(2)}(g) = 1 - \lambda_{it|t-1}^{(1)}(g), \text{ for } g = 1,2;\ t = 2,\ldots,T. \tag{3.25}$$

This LDCP model presented by (3.23)–(3.25) produces the marginal mean and variance of y_{it} for $t = 1,\ldots,T$, as

$$E[Y_{it}] = E_{Y_{i1}} E_{Y_{i2}} \cdots E_{Y_{it}} [Y_{it} | y_{i,t-1}] = \pi_1$$
$$\text{var}[Y_{it}] = E[Y_{it}] - [E[Y_{it}]]^2 = \pi_1(1 - \pi_1), \tag{3.26}$$

and for $u < t$, the Gaussian type lag $t - u$ auto-covariances as

$$\begin{aligned}\text{Cov}[Y_{iu}, Y_{it}] &= E[Y_{iu}Y_{it}] - E[Y_{iu}]E[Y_{it}] \\ &= E_{Y_{iu}}\left[Y_{iu}E_{Y_{i,t-(t-u-1)}} \cdots E_{Y_{i,t-1}} E_{Y_{it}}[Y_{it}|y_{i,t-1}]\right] - \pi_1^2 \\ &= \rho^{t-u}\text{var}[Y_{iu}],\end{aligned}$$

yielding the auto-correlations as

$$\text{Corr}[Y_{iu}, Y_{it}] = \rho^{t-u}. \tag{3.27}$$

3.2.2.1.1 Likelihood Function

In the LDCP model (3.23)–(3.25), there are 2 parameters, namely the intercept parameter β_{10} (categorical regression parameter) and correlation index parameter ρ. To construct the likelihood function, let $f_1(y_{i1})$ denote the binary density of the initial response variable y_{i1}, and $f_t(y_{it}|y_{i,t-1})$ denote the conditional binary distribution of response variable at time t given the response at previous time $t-1$. Because K individuals are independent, the likelihood function based on lag 1 dynamic dependent observations has the form

$$L(\beta_{10}, \rho) = \Pi_{i=1}^{K} L_i, \tag{3.28}$$

where

$$L_i = f_1(y_{i1}) f_2(y_{i2}|y_{i1}) \cdots f_T(y_{iT}|y_{i,T-1}),$$

with

$$f_1(y_{i1}) = [\pi_1]^{y_{i1}} [\pi_2]^{1-y_{i1}} = \frac{\exp[y_{i1}\beta_{10}]}{1+\exp(\beta_{10})}, \text{ and}$$
$$f_t(y_{it}|y_{i,t-1}) = [\lambda^{(1)}_{it|t-1}(y_{i,t-1})]^{y_{it}} [\lambda^{(2)}_{it|t-1}(y_{i,t-1})]^{1-y_{it}}, \text{ for } t = 2, \ldots, T, \tag{3.29}$$

yielding the log likelihood function as

$$\begin{aligned}\text{Log}L(\beta_{10}, \rho) &= \sum_{i=1}^{K} [y_{i1} \log \pi_1 + (1 - y_{i1}) \log \pi_2] \\ &+ \sum_{g=1}^{2} \sum_{i \in g}^{K} \sum_{t=2}^{T} [y_{it} \log \lambda^{(1)}_{it|t-1}(g) + (1 - y_{it}) \log \lambda^{(2)}_{it|t-1}(g)].\end{aligned} \tag{3.30}$$

Note that under the present stationary model, it follows from (3.24) that $\lambda^{(1)}_{it|t-1}(1)$ and $\lambda^{(1)}_{it|t-1}(2)$ are free from i and t. Consequently, for convenience, we suppress the subscripts from these conditional probabilities and use $\lambda^{(1)}(2)$ for $\lambda^{(1)}_{it|t-1}(2)$, for example. Next by using the cell frequencies from the contingency Table 3.2, we express the log likelihood function (3.30) as

$$\begin{aligned}\text{Log}\, L(\beta_{10},\rho) &= [K_1(1)\log \pi_1 + K_2(1)\log \pi_2] \\ &\quad + \log \lambda^{(1)}(1)\sum_{t=2}^{T} K_{11}(t-1,t) + \log \lambda^{(2)}(1)\sum_{t=2}^{T} K_{12}(t-1,t) \\ &\quad + \log \lambda^{(1)}(2)\sum_{t=2}^{T} K_{21}(t-1,t) + \log \lambda^{(2)}(2)\sum_{t=2}^{T} K_{22}(t-1,t), \quad (3.31)\end{aligned}$$

where by (3.24)–(3.25),

$$\begin{aligned}&\lambda^{(1)}(1) = \pi_1 + \rho(1-\pi_1),\ \lambda^{(2)}(1) = 1-\lambda^{(1)}(1) = (1-\rho)(1-\pi_1) \\ &\lambda^{(1)}(2) = (1-\rho)\pi_1,\ \lambda^{(2)}(2) = 1-\lambda^{(1)}(2) = 1-(1-\rho)\pi_1. \quad (3.32)\end{aligned}$$

This log likelihood function is maximized in the next section to estimate the parameters β_{10} and ρ. We remark that unlike the computation of the likelihood function under the present AR(1) type model (3.24), the likelihood computation under other linear dynamic models such as MA(1) and EQC, however, would be impossible or extremely complicated (see Sutradhar 2011, Section 7.3.4).

3.2.2.1.2 Likelihood Estimating Equations

The following derivatives, first, with respect to β_{10} and then with respect to ρ will be helpful to write the likelihood estimating equations for β_{10} and ρ, respectively.

Derivatives with Respect to β_{10} and ρ

It follows from (3.24)–(3.25) and (3.32) that

$$\begin{aligned}\frac{\partial \pi_1}{\partial \beta_{10}} &= \pi_1(1-\pi_1);\ \frac{\partial \pi_2}{\partial \beta_{10}} = -\pi_1(1-\pi_1), \\ \frac{\partial \lambda^{(1)}(1)}{\partial \beta_{10}} &= (1-\rho)\pi_1(1-\pi_1) = \frac{\partial \lambda^{(1)}(2)}{\partial \beta_{10}}, \\ \frac{\partial \lambda^{(2)}(1)}{\partial \beta_{10}} &= -(1-\rho)\pi_1(1-\pi_1) = \frac{\partial \lambda^{(2)}(2)}{\partial \beta_{10}}, \quad (3.33)\end{aligned}$$

and

$$
\begin{aligned}
\frac{\partial \pi_1}{\partial \rho} &= 0;\ \frac{\partial \pi_2}{\partial \rho} = 0,\\
\frac{\partial \lambda^{(1)}(1)}{\partial \rho} &= (1-\pi_1);\ \frac{\partial \lambda^{(2)}(1)}{\partial \rho} = -(1-\pi_1),\\
\frac{\partial \lambda^{(1)}(2)}{\partial \rho} &= -\pi_1;\ \frac{\partial \lambda^{(2)}(2)}{\partial \rho} = \pi_1.
\end{aligned}
\tag{3.34}
$$

By (3.33), it then follows from (3.31) that the likelihood estimating equation for β_{10} has the form

$$
\begin{aligned}
\frac{\partial \mathrm{Log}\, L(\beta_{10},\rho)}{\partial \beta_{10}} &= [\pi_1(1-\pi_1)]\left[\frac{K_1(1)}{\pi_1} - \frac{K_2(1)}{\pi_2}\right]\\
&+ [(1-\rho)\pi_1(1-\pi_1)]\left[\frac{\sum_{t=2}^{T} K_{11}(t-1,t)}{\lambda^{(1)}(1)} - \frac{\sum_{t=2}^{T} K_{12}(t-1,t)}{\lambda^{(2)}(1)}\right]\\
&+ [(1-\rho)\pi_1(1-\pi_1)]\left[\frac{\sum_{t=2}^{T} K_{21}(t-1,t)}{\lambda^{(1)}(2)} - \frac{\sum_{t=2}^{T} K_{22}(t-1,t)}{\lambda^{(2)}(2)}\right]\\
&= [\pi_2 K_1(1) - \pi_1 K_2(1)]\\
&+ [(1-\rho)\pi_1(1-\pi_1)]\left[\frac{\sum_{t=2}^{T} K_{11}(t-1,t)}{\lambda^{(1)}(1)} - \frac{\sum_{t=2}^{T} K_{12}(t-1,t)}{\lambda^{(2)}(1)}\right.\\
&+ \left.\frac{\sum_{t=2}^{T} K_{21}(t-1,t)}{\lambda^{(1)}(2)} - \frac{\sum_{t=2}^{T} K_{22}(t-1,t)}{\lambda^{(2)}(2)}\right] = 0.
\end{aligned}
\tag{3.35}
$$

Similarly, the likelihood estimating equation for ρ has the form

$$
\begin{aligned}
\frac{\partial \mathrm{Log}\, L(\beta_{10},\rho)}{\partial \rho} &= [1-\pi_1]\left[\frac{\sum_{t=2}^{T} K_{11}(t-1,t)}{\lambda^{(1)}(1)} - \frac{\sum_{t=2}^{T} K_{12}(t-1,t)}{\lambda^{(2)}(1)}\right]\\
&- [\pi_1]\left[\frac{\sum_{t=2}^{T} K_{21}(t-1,t)}{\lambda^{(1)}(2)} - \frac{\sum_{t=2}^{T} K_{22}(t-1,t)}{\lambda^{(2)}(2)}\right] = 0.
\end{aligned}
\tag{3.36}
$$

Note that it is relatively easier to solve these score equations (3.35) for β_{10} and (3.36) for ρ, marginally, as opposed to their joint estimation. To be specific, for known ρ, the marginal likelihood estimate for β_{10} may be obtained by using the iterative equation

$$
\hat{\beta}_{10}(r+1) = \hat{\beta}_{10}(r) - \left[\left\{\frac{\partial^2 \mathrm{Log}\, L(\beta_{10},\rho)}{\partial \beta_{10}^2}\right\}^{-1} \frac{\partial \mathrm{Log}\, L(\beta_{10},\rho)}{\partial \beta_{10}}\right]_{|\beta_{10}=\hat{\beta}_{10}(r)},
\tag{3.37}
$$

where the second derivative by (3.35) has the formula

$$\begin{aligned}\frac{\partial^2 \text{Log } L(\beta_{10},\rho)}{\partial \beta_{10}^2} &= -K\pi_1(1-\pi_1) \\ &+ [(1-\rho)\pi_1(1-\pi_1)(1-2\pi_1)]\left[\frac{\sum_{t=2}^{T} K_{11}(t-1,t)}{\lambda^{(1)}(1)} - \frac{\sum_{t=2}^{T} K_{12}(t-1,t)}{\lambda^{(2)}(1)}\right. \\ &+ \left.\frac{\sum_{t=2}^{T} K_{21}(t-1,t)}{\lambda^{(1)}(2)} - \frac{\sum_{t=2}^{T} K_{22}(t-1,t)}{\lambda^{(2)}(2)}\right] \\ &- [(1-\rho)\pi_1(1-\pi_1)]^2\left[\frac{\sum_{t=2}^{T} K_{11}(t-1,t)}{\{\lambda^{(1)}(1)\}^2} + \frac{\sum_{t=2}^{T} K_{12}(t-1,t)}{\{\lambda^{(2)}(1)\}^2}\right. \\ &+ \left.\frac{\sum_{t=2}^{T} K_{21}(t-1,t)}{\{\lambda^{(1)}(2)\}^2} + \frac{\sum_{t=2}^{T} K_{22}(t-1,t)}{\{\lambda^{(2)}(2)\}^2}\right]. \end{aligned} \tag{3.38}$$

Similarly, for known β_{10}, the marginal likelihood estimate for ρ may be obtained by using the iterative equation

$$\hat{\rho}(r+1) = \hat{\rho}(r) - \left[\left\{\frac{\partial^2 \text{Log } L(\beta_{10},\rho)}{\partial \rho^2}\right\}^{-1} \frac{\partial \text{Log } L(\beta_{10},\rho)}{\partial \rho}\right]_{|\rho=\hat{\rho}(r)}, \tag{3.39}$$

where the second derivative by (3.36) has the formula

$$\begin{aligned}\frac{\partial^2 \text{Log } L(\beta_{10},\rho)}{\partial \rho^2} &= -[1-\pi_1]^2\left[\frac{\sum_{t=2}^{T} K_{11}(t-1,t)}{\{\lambda^{(1)}(1)\}^2} + \frac{\sum_{t=2}^{T} K_{12}(t-1,t)}{\{\lambda^{(2)}(1)\}^2}\right] \\ &- [\pi_1^2]\left[\frac{\sum_{t=2}^{T} K_{21}(t-1,t)}{\{\lambda^{(1)}(2)\}^2} + \frac{\sum_{t=2}^{T} K_{22}(t-1,t)}{\{\lambda^{(2)}(2)\}^2}\right]. \end{aligned} \tag{3.40}$$

3.2.2.1.3 Illustration 3.2 (Continuation of Illustration 3.1 for Longitudinal Asthma Data Analysis): AR(1) Correlation Model Based Likelihood Estimates

To use the iterative equations (3.37) and (3.39) for maximum likelihood estimates for β_{10} and ρ, we follow the cyclical iterations as follows. Starting with initial values $\hat{\beta}_{10}(0) = 0$ and $\rho = \hat{\rho}(0) = 0$, the iterative equation (3.37) is used to obtain an improved estimate for β_{10}. This improved estimate for β_{10}, along with initial value $\hat{\rho}(0) = 0$, is then used in (3.39) to obtain an improved estimate for ρ. Next, the β_{10} estimate is further improved by (3.37) using this new estimate for ρ. This cycle of computations continues until convergence. The resulting likelihood (L) estimates were

$$\hat{\beta}_{10,L} = -1.7306, \text{ and } \hat{\rho}_L = 0.5258.$$

Note that the likelihood estimate of ρ is much larger than lag 1 correlation estimate $\hat{\rho}_1 = 0.40$ found in Sect. 3.2.1.3, by using the method of moments based on a general auto-correlation structure. This is not surprising as the lag correlations found in (3.21) indicate an equi-correlation structure for the data whereas we have fitted the likelihood method to the data assuming that they follow AR(1) structure. Nevertheless, the estimates of β_{10} ($\hat{\beta}_{10,L} = -1.7306$) and the resulting probability of an asthma attack ($\hat{\pi}_1 = 0.1505$) were found to be almost the same as those ($\hat{\beta}_{10} = -1.7284$, $\hat{\pi}_1 = 0.1508$) under the general auto-correlation model.

3.2.2.2 LDCP Model and GQL Estimation

Note that under the lag 1 based LDCP model (3.23)–(3.25), the stationary correlation structure specified by (3.27) has the form

$$C_i(\rho) = \begin{bmatrix} 1 & \rho & \rho^2 & \cdots \rho^{T-1} \\ \rho^1 & 1 & \rho^1 & \cdots \rho^{T-2} \\ \vdots & \vdots & \vdots & \vdots \\ \rho^{T-1} & \rho^{T-2} & \rho^{T-3} \cdots & 1 \end{bmatrix} = \tilde{C}(\rho), \tag{3.41}$$

for all $i = 1, \ldots, K$. Consequently, similar to (3.16), one may use this known correlation matrix $\tilde{C}(\rho)$ and construct the GQL estimating equation as

$$\begin{aligned} &\sum_{i=1}^{K} \frac{\partial \pi'_{(i)}}{\partial \beta_{10}} \Sigma_i^{-1}(\rho)(y_i - \pi_{(i)}) \\ &= \sum_{i=1}^{K} 1'_T \tilde{C}^{-1}(\rho)(y_i - \pi_1 1_T) \\ &= \sum_{i=1}^{K} (\tilde{\omega}_1, \ldots, \tilde{\omega}_t, \ldots, \tilde{\omega}_T)(y_i - \pi_1 1_T) \\ &= \sum_{t=1}^{T} \tilde{\omega}_t K_1(t) - K\pi_1 \sum_{t=1}^{T} \tilde{\omega}_t = 0, \end{aligned} \tag{3.42}$$

and solve it iteratively by using

$$\hat{\beta}_{10}(r+1) = \hat{\beta}_{10}(r) + \frac{1}{K\{\pi_1(1-\pi_1)\}\sum_{t=1}^{T} \tilde{\omega}_t} \left[\sum_{t=1}^{T} \tilde{\omega}_t K_1(t) - K\pi_1 \sum_{t=1}^{T} \tilde{\omega}_t \right]. \tag{3.43}$$

Note that this GQL estimation by (3.42) and (3.43) is much simpler than obtaining the estimate of β_{10} by using the likelihood based iterative equation (3.37). Furthermore, the moment estimate of ρ parameter may be obtained easily either by (a) an approximation, or (b) exact moment matching, as follows.

(a) **Approximate moment estimate**
To estimate the correlation matrix (3.41) one may argue that once ρ is estimated by using the lag 1 sample correlations, the other elements can be computed. Note that this would however yield an approximate moment estimate as higher order sample moments, in relation to lag 1 moment, may not satisfy the pattern in (3.41). Nevertheless, it would be simpler to use such an approximation which may not affect adversely the regression, that is, β_{10} estimation. This simpler estimate can be computed by (3.12) using $h^* = 1$. Thus,

$$\hat{\rho} \equiv \hat{\rho}_1 = \frac{\frac{1}{T-1}\sum_{t=2}^{T}\left[K_{11}(t-1,\,t) - \pi_1\{K_1(t) + K_1(t-1)\} + \pi_1^2 K\right]}{\frac{1}{T}\sum_{t=1}^{T}\left[(1-2\pi_1)K_1(t) + \pi_1^2 K\right]}. \tag{3.44}$$

(b) **Exact moment estimate**
When sample moments of all possible lags are used, a moment equation for ρ is constructed by matching the decaying correlation pattern in (3.41). To be specific, ρ may be computed by solving the polynomial moment equation

$$\sum_{h^*=1}^{T-1}(T-h^*)\rho^{h^*} = \sum_{h^*=1}^{T-1}(T-h^*)\hat{\rho}_{h^*}, \tag{3.45}$$

where $\hat{\rho}_{h^*}$ is computed by (3.12) for all $h^* = 1,\ldots,T-1$.

3.2.2.2.1 Illustration 3.3 (Continuation of Illustration 3.1 for Longitudinal Asthma Data Analysis): AR(1) Correlation Model Based GQL Estimates

(a) **Using approximate correlation estimate:**
For the asthma data considered in illustrations 3.1 and 3.2, the GQL estimating equation (3.43) for β_{10} and the approximate moment equation (3.41) for ρ, produce by iteration, their estimates as

$$\hat{\beta}_{10} = -1.7445 \text{ and } \hat{\rho} = 0.40,$$

with standard error of $\hat{\beta}_{10}$, by (3.43) and (3.18), as s.e.$(\hat{\beta}_{10}) = 0.0802$. Notice that the approximate moment estimate $\hat{\rho} = 0.40$ under AR(1) model is different than the likelihood estimate $\hat{\rho}_L = 0.5258$ under the same AR(1) model. However, the β_{10} QL estimate under the AR(1) model, that is, $\hat{\beta}_{10} = -1.7445$

produces similar but slightly different probability of asthma attack, namely $\hat{\pi}_1 = 0.1487$, whereas under the general auto-correlation model (illustration 3.1), the probability was found to be 0.1508.

(b) **Using exact correlation estimate:**
In this approach, β_{10} is estimated by (3.43), but the moment estimate of ρ is obtained by solving the polynomial equation (3.45). To be specific, for $T = 4$, by (3.45), we write the moment estimating equation as

$$f(\rho) = 3\rho + 2\rho^2 + \rho^3 - (3\hat{\rho}_1 + 2\hat{\rho}_2 + \hat{\rho}_3) = 0, \tag{3.46}$$

where $\hat{\rho}_{h^*}$ for $h^* = 1,2,3$ are computed by using the formula (3.12) with adjusted value of π_1 using β_{10} estimate from (3.43). This moment equation may be solved by using the iterative equation

$$\hat{\rho}(r+1) = \hat{\rho}(r) - \left[\{\frac{\partial f(\rho)}{\partial \rho}\}^{-1} f(\rho)\right]_{\rho=\hat{\rho}(r)}. \tag{3.47}$$

After five iterations, (3.43) and (3.47) yielded

$$\hat{\beta}_{10} = -1.7525, \text{ and } \hat{\rho} = 0.4998.$$

These estimates are very close to the likelihood estimates computed for illustration 3.2. This is expected as both likelihood and the present GQL approach use the exact correlation estimate for the AR(1) model. The GQL estimate $\hat{\beta}_{10} = -1.7525$ has the s.e.$(\hat{\beta}_{10}) = \sqrt{0.007393} = 0.0860$, and this yields the probability estimate as $\hat{\pi}_1 = 0.1477$.

3.2.3 *Stationary Binary EQC Model and Estimation of Parameters*

In Sect. 3.2.1.3, the lag correlations for the longitudinal asthma data were found to indicate equal correlations (3.21) among binary responses. For this and other similar data, one may like to consider an EQC model as opposed to AR(1) type linear dynamic conditional probability (LDCP) model discussed in Sect. 3.2.2.1.

3.2.3.1 EQC Model and Likelihood Estimation

Unlike the AR(1) model, the EQC model for binary responses may be modeled as follows (Sutradhar 2011, Section 7.3.3). Let y_{i0} be an unobservable initial binary response with its mean $\pi_1 = \frac{\exp(\beta_{10})}{1+\exp(\beta_{10})}$. That is

$$P[y_{i1} = y_{i0}^{(j)}] = \pi_j = \begin{cases} \frac{\exp(\beta_{10})}{1+\exp(\beta_{10})} & \text{for } j = 1 \\ \frac{1}{1+\exp(\beta_{10})} & \text{for } j = J = 2; \end{cases} \tag{3.48}$$

$$\begin{aligned} P[y_{it} = y_{it}^{(1)} | y_{i0} = y_{i0}^{(g)}] &= \pi_1 + \rho(y_{i0}^{(g)} - \pi_1) \\ &= \lambda_{it|0}^{(1)}(g) \text{ (say)}, g = 1,2;\ t = 1,\ldots,T; \end{aligned} \tag{3.49}$$

and

$$\lambda_{it|0}^{(2)}(g) = 1 - \lambda_{it|0}^{(1)}(g), \text{ for } g = 1,2;\ t = 1,2,\ldots,T. \tag{3.50}$$

This model (3.48)–(3.50) has the following basic properties:

$$\begin{aligned} E[Y_{it}] &= \pi_1, \text{ and } \mathrm{var}[Y_{it}] = \pi_1(1-\pi_1), \text{ for all } t = 1,\ldots,T \\ \mathrm{cov}[Y_{iu}, Y_{it}] &= \rho^2\pi_1(1-\pi_1), \text{ for } u \neq t, \end{aligned} \tag{3.51}$$

yielding

$$\mathrm{Corr}[Y_{iu}, Y_{it}] = \rho^2, \text{ for all } u \neq t.$$

3.2.3.1.1 Likelihood Function and Estimation Complexity

Refer to the conditional probability model (3.49). It is clear that given y_{i0}, all repeated responses are independent, whereas the latent binary response y_{i0} follows the binary distribution with parameter π_1 given in (3.48). Also, conditional on y_{i0}, each of the responses $y_{i1},\ldots,y_{iT}$ follows the binary distribution with proportion parameter $0 < \lambda_{it|0}^{(1)}(g) < 1$. Thus, one writes the likelihood function as

$$\begin{aligned} L(\beta_{10},\rho) &= \Pi_{i=1}^{K} \sum_{y_{i0}=0}^{1} \Pi_{t=1}^{T} [f(y_{it}|y_{i0}) f(y_{i0})] \\ &= \Pi_{i=1}^{K} \sum_{g=1}^{2} \Pi_{t=1}^{T} \left[\{\lambda_{it|0}^{(1)}(g)\}^{y_{it}} \{1-\lambda_{it|0}^{(1)}(g)\}^{1-y_{it}} \pi_g^{y_{i0}^{(g)}} \right] \\ &= \Pi_{i=1}^{K} \left[\left(\pi_1^T \Pi_{t=1}^{T} \{\lambda_{it|0}^{(1)}(1)\}^{y_{it}} \{1-\lambda_{it|0}^{(1)}(1)\}^{1-y_{it}} \right) \right. \\ &\quad \left. + \left(\Pi_{t=1}^{T} \{\lambda_{it|0}^{(1)}(2)\}^{y_{it}} \{1-\lambda_{it|0}^{(1)}(2)\}^{1-y_{it}} \right) \right], \end{aligned} \tag{3.52}$$

where

$$\lambda^{(1)}_{it|0}(1) = \pi_1 + \rho(1-\pi_1) \equiv \lambda^{(1)}(1), \text{ and } \lambda^{(1)}_{it|0}(2) = \pi_1(1-\rho) \equiv \lambda^{(1)}(2).$$

The log likelihood function may then be written as

$$Log\, L(\beta_{10},\rho) = \sum_{i=1}^{K} \log\, [a_i(\beta_{10},\rho) + b_i(\beta_{10},\rho)], \quad (3.53)$$

where

$$a_i(\beta_{10},\rho) = \pi_1^T \Pi_{t=1}^T \{\lambda^{(1)}(1)\}^{y_{it}} \{1-\lambda^{(1)}(1)\}^{1-y_{it}}$$
$$b_i(\beta_{10},\rho) = \Pi_{t=1}^T \{\lambda^{(1)}(2)\}^{y_{it}} \{1-\lambda^{(1)}(2)\}^{1-y_{it}}.$$

Notice that the log likelihood function became complicated for the purpose of writing likelihood estimating equations for β_{10} and ρ, which happened mainly because of the summation over the binary distribution of the latent response y_{i0} to derive the likelihood function as in (3.52). Nevertheless, interested readers may go through some algebras as in the next section and derive the desired likelihood estimating equations.

3.2.3.1.2 Likelihood Estimating Equation

The likelihood equations have the forms

$$\frac{\partial LogL(\beta_{10},\rho)}{\partial \beta_{10}} = \sum_{i=1}^{K} \frac{\frac{\partial a_i(\beta_{10},\rho)}{\partial \beta_{10}} + \frac{\partial b_i(\beta_{10},\rho)}{\partial \beta_{10}}}{a_i(\beta_{10},\rho) + b_i(\beta_{10},\rho)} = 0, \text{ and}$$
$$\frac{\partial LogL(\beta_{10},\rho)}{\partial \rho} = \sum_{i=1}^{K} \frac{\frac{\partial a_i(\beta_{10},\rho)}{\partial \rho} + \frac{\partial b_i(\beta_{10},\rho)}{\partial \rho}}{a_i(\beta_{10},\rho) + b_i(\beta_{10},\rho)} = 0, \quad (3.54)$$

for β_{10} and ρ, respectively. Now write

$$a_i(\beta_{10},\rho) = \exp\left[T \log \pi_1 + \log\lambda^{(1)}(1) \sum_{t=1}^{T} y_{it} + \log \lambda^{(2)}(1) \sum_{t=1}^{T}(1-y_{it})\right]$$
$$b_i(\beta_{10},\rho) = \exp\left[\log \lambda^{(1)}(2) \sum_{t=1}^{T} y_{it} + \log \lambda^{(2)}(2) \sum_{t=1}^{T}(1-y_{it})\right]. \quad (3.55)$$

Notice that the forms $a_i(\beta_{10},\rho)$ and $b_i(\beta_{10},\rho)$ are determined by the categorical status of the ith individual collectively over all T time period. Thus, if an individual belongs to category 1 in any d time points, say, and in category two

Table 3.5 Contingency table with overall status for the whole period

Distribution of individuals based on number of times (d) in category 1							
0	1	2	...	d	...	T	Total
$K_1^*(0)$	$K_1^*(1)$	$K_1^*(2)$	...	$K_1^*(d)$	...	$K_1^*(T)$	K

in remaining times $T-d$, then $\sum_{t=2}^{T} y_{it} = d$. Note that this d ranges from 0 to T. Now for convenience of taking summation over all i to compute the likelihood equations (3.54), one can form the contingency Table 3.5.

Using the frequency Table 3.5, one may then simplify the likelihood equations in (3.54) as

$$\frac{\partial LogL(\beta_{10},\rho)}{\partial \beta_{10}} = \sum_{d=0}^{T} \frac{\frac{\partial a_d^*(\beta_{10},\rho)}{\partial \beta_{10}} + \frac{\partial b_d^*(\beta_{10},\rho)}{\partial \beta_{10}}}{a_d^*(\beta_{10},\rho)+b_d^*(\beta_{10},\rho)} = 0, \text{ and}$$

$$\frac{\partial LogL(\beta_{10},\rho)}{\partial \rho} = \sum_{d=0}^{T} \frac{\frac{\partial a_d^*(\beta_{10},\rho)}{\partial \rho} + \frac{\partial b_d^*(\beta_{10},\rho)}{\partial \rho}}{a_d^*(\beta_{10},\rho)+b_d^*(\beta_{10},\rho)} = 0, \tag{3.56}$$

for β_{10} and ρ, respectively, with

$$a_d^*(\beta_{10},\rho) = \exp\left[K_1^*(d)\left\{T\log \pi_1 + d\log \lambda^{(1)}(1) + (T-d)\log \lambda^{(2)}(1)\right\}\right]$$
$$b_d^*(\beta_{10},\rho) = \exp\left[K_1^*(d)\left\{d\log \lambda^{(1)}(2) + (T-d)\log \lambda^{(2)}(2)\right\}\right]. \tag{3.57}$$

Next by using the derivatives from (3.33) one writes

$$\frac{\partial a_d^*(\beta_{10},\rho)}{\partial \beta_{10}} = a_d^*(\beta_{10},\rho)\left[K_1^*(d)(1-\pi_1)\left\{T+(1-\rho)\pi_1\left(\frac{d}{\lambda^{(1)}(1)} - \frac{T-d}{\lambda^{(2)}(1)}\right)\right\}\right]$$
$$\frac{\partial b_d^*(\beta_{10},\rho)}{\partial \beta_{10}} = b_d^*(\beta_{10},\rho)\left[K_1^*(d)(1-\rho)\pi_1(1-\pi_1)\left(\frac{d}{\lambda^{(1)}(2)} - \frac{T-d}{\lambda^{(2)}(2)}\right)\right], \tag{3.58}$$

yielding, by (3.56), the likelihood estimating equation for β_{10} as

$$\frac{\partial LogL(\beta_{10},\rho)}{\partial \beta_{10}} = \sum_{d=0}^{T} K_1^*(d)(1-\pi_1)$$
$$\times \left[\frac{a_d^*(\beta_{10},\rho)}{a_d^*(\beta_{10},\rho)+b_d^*(\beta_{10},\rho)}\left\{T+(1-\rho)\pi_1\left(\frac{d}{\lambda^{(1)}(1)} - \frac{T-d}{\lambda^{(2)}(1)}\right)\right\}\right.$$
$$\left. + \frac{b_d^*(\beta_{10},\rho)}{a_d^*(\beta_{10},\rho)+b_d^*(\beta_{10},\rho)}\left\{\pi_1(1-\rho)\left(\frac{d}{\lambda^{(1)}(2)} - \frac{T-d}{\lambda^{(2)}(2)}\right)\right\}\right] = 0. \tag{3.59}$$

Similarly, by using the basic derivatives from (3.34) into (3.56), one obtains the likelihood estimating equation for ρ as

$$\frac{\partial LogL(\beta_{10},\rho)}{\partial\rho} = \sum_{d=0}^{T} K_1^*(d) \times \left[\frac{a_d^*(\beta_{10},\rho)}{a_d^*(\beta_{10},\rho)+b_d^*(\beta_{10},\rho)}\left\{(1-\pi_1)\left(\frac{d}{\lambda^{(1)}(1)}-\frac{T-d}{\lambda^{(2)}(1)}\right)\right\} - \frac{b_d^*(\beta_{10},\rho)}{a_d^*(\beta_{10},\rho)+b_d^*(\beta_{10},\rho)}\left\{\pi_1\left(\frac{d}{\lambda^{(1)}(2)}-\frac{T-d}{\lambda^{(2)}(2)}\right)\right\}\right] = 0. \quad (3.60)$$

These equations (3.59) and (3.60) are then solved iteratively to obtain the likelihood estimates for β_{10} and ρ under the EQC model, ρ^2 being the common correlations between any two binary responses. Note that writing the iterative equations, similar to (3.37) and (3.39) under the AR(1) model, requires to compute the second order derivatives

$$\frac{\partial^2 LogL(\beta_{10},\rho)}{\partial\beta_{10}^2}, \text{ and } \frac{\partial^2 LogL(\beta_{10},\rho)}{\partial\rho^2},$$

respectively. However the calculus is straightforward but lengthy and hence not given here.

Remark that the computation for the likelihood estimates obtained in Sect. 3.2.2.1 for the AR(1) model (3.23)–(3.27) was much more involved than that of the GQL estimation in Sect. 3.2.2.2. Under the equi-correlation model (3.48)–(3.51), the likelihood estimation became more cumbersome. In the next section, it is demonstrated that obtaining the GQL estimates for the parameters of the EQC model is rather straightforward, and hence much easier than obtaining the likelihood estimates.

3.2.3.2 EQC Model and GQL Estimation

Note that the marginal means and variances produced by the EQC model (3.48)–(3.50) are the same as those of the AR(1) model (3.23)–(3.25). The difference between the two models lies in the correlation structure, with decaying correlations (as lag increases) as given by (3.41) under the AR(1) model, whereas the equi-correlation model (3.48)–(3.50) yields the equi-correlation matrix as

$$C_i(\rho) = \begin{bmatrix} 1 & \rho^2 & \rho^2 & \cdots & \rho^2 \\ \rho^2 & 1 & \rho^2 & \cdots & \rho^2 \\ \vdots & \vdots & \vdots & & \vdots \\ \rho^2 & \rho^2 & \rho^2 & \cdots & 1 \end{bmatrix} = C^*(\rho), \text{ (say)}, \quad (3.61)$$

for all $i = 1,\ldots,K$. Thus, similar to the AR(1) case (Eqs. (3.42)–(3.43)), the GQL estimating equation for β_{10} under the EQC model may be written as

$$\sum_{i=1}^{K} \frac{\partial \pi'_{(i)}}{\partial \beta_{10}} \Sigma_i^{-1}(\rho)(y_i - \pi_{(i)})$$
$$= \sum_{i=1}^{K} 1'_T C^{*-1}(\rho)(y_i - \pi_1 1_T)$$
$$= \sum_{i=1}^{K} (\omega^*{}_1,\ldots,\omega^*{}_t,\ldots,\omega^*{}_T)(y_i - \pi_1 1_T)$$
$$= \sum_{t=1}^{T} \omega^*{}_t K_1(t) - K\pi_1 \sum_{t=1}^{T} \omega^*{}_t = 0, \quad (3.62)$$

and solve it iteratively by using

$$\hat{\beta}_{10}(r+1) = \hat{\beta}_{10}(r) + \frac{1}{K\{\pi_1(1-\pi_1)\}\sum_{t=1}^{T} \omega^*{}_t} \left[\sum_{t=1}^{T} \omega^*{}_t K_1(t) - K\pi_1 \sum_{t=1}^{T} \omega^*{}_t \right]. \quad (3.63)$$

As far as the estimation of the common correlation ρ^2 is concerned in this EQC setup, similar to the exact moment estimating equation (3.46) under the AR(1) case, one may equate the data based auto-correlation matrix (3.9)–(3.10) with the model based correlation matrix $C^*(\rho)$ (3.61), and obtain the moment estimating equation for ρ^2 as

$$\{T(T-1)/2\}\rho^2 = \sum_{h^*=1}^{T-1} (T-h^*)\hat{\rho}_{h^*}, \quad (3.64)$$

(see (3.45)) where $\hat{\rho}_{h^*}$ is computed by (3.12), that is,

$$\hat{\rho}_{h^*} = \frac{\frac{1}{T-h^*}\sum_{t=h^*+1}^{T}\left[K_{11}(t-h^*,\,t) - \pi_1\{K_1(t) + K_1(t-h^*)\} + \pi_1^2 K\right]}{\frac{1}{T}\sum_{t=1}^{T}\left[(1-2\pi_1)K_1(t) + \pi_1^2 K\right]},$$

where $K_1(t)$ and $K_{11}(t-h,t)$ are counts from the contingency Tables 3.1 and 3.2.

Note that when correlations are known to be common for all individuals at any two time points u and t, $(u < t)$, instead of the weighted sum of the lag correlations as shown in (3.64), similar to (3.10), one may compute, say ρ_{ut} by

$$\hat{\rho}_{ut} = \frac{\sum_{i=1}^{K} \tilde{y}_{iu}\tilde{y}_{it}/K}{\sqrt{[\sum_{i=1}^{K}\tilde{y}_{iu}^2/K][\sum_{i=1}^{K}\tilde{y}_{it}^2/K]}}, \quad (3.65)$$

where $\tilde{y}_{it}$, for example, is the standardized deviance, defined as

$$\tilde{y}_{it} = \frac{y_{it} - \pi_1}{\{\pi_1(1-\pi_1)\}^{1/2}},$$

with π_1 as in (3.48) (also same as (3.8)). Note that in terms of cell counts, this estimate in (3.65) is equivalent to

$$\hat{\rho}_{ut} = \frac{[K_{11}(u,t) - \pi_1(K_1(u) + K_1(t)) + K\pi_1^2]/K}{\sqrt{[\{(1-2\pi_1)K_1(u) + K\pi_1^2\}/K][\{(1-2\pi_1)K_1(t) + K\pi_1^2\}/K]}}, \tag{3.66}$$

Next, because $\rho_{ut} \equiv \rho^2$ for all u,t, under the EQC structure (3.61), one may estimate this parameter as

$$\hat{\rho}^2 = \frac{2}{T(T-1)} \sum_{t=u+1}^{T} \sum_{u=1}^{T-1} \hat{\rho}_{ut}. \tag{3.67}$$

In summary, once ρ^2 is computed by (3.64) or (3.67), we use this estimate in (3.63) to compute $\hat{\beta}_{10}$, and the iterations continue until convergence.

3.2.3.2.1 Illustration 3.4 (Continuation of Illustration 3.1 for Longitudinal Asthma Data Analysis): EQC Correlation Model Based GQL Estimates

Recall from Sect. 3.2.1.3 that the lag correlations for the asthma data were found to be

$$\hat{\rho}_1 = 0.40,\ \hat{\rho}_2 = 0.3129,\ \hat{\rho}_3 = 0.2979,$$

(Eq. (3.21)) indicating EQC perhaps would be a better model to fit the data as compared to the AR(1) model. Now to illustrate the application of the EQC model (3.48)–(3.50), we have estimated the correlations by using both the lag correlations (3.64) and pair-wise correlations (3.67) based moment equations, and in each case β_{10} was estimated by solving the GQL estimating equation (3.62). To be specific, the moment formula (3.64) for correlation ρ^2 and the GQL equation (3.62) yielded

$$\hat{\rho}^2 = 0.3538,\ \hat{\beta}_{10} = -1.7208, \tag{3.68}$$

with s.e.$(\hat{\beta}_{10}) = 0.0863$. Furthermore, this estimate of β_{10} from (3.68) yielded the estimated probability as $\hat{\pi}_1 = 0.1518$. Similarly, the pair-wise correlations based moment formula (3.67) and the GQL estimating equation (3.62) produced the estimates as

$$\hat{\rho}^2 = 0.3470,\ \hat{\beta}_{10} = -1.7208, \tag{3.69}$$

with s.e.$(\hat{\beta}_{10}) = 0.0859$, further yielding the same probability estimate as $\hat{\pi}_1 = 0.1518$. Thus two approaches using slightly different moment formulas for correlations produce almost the same results. For the sake of completeness, one may note the pair-wise correlation values as

$$\hat{\rho}_{12} = 0.3545,\ \hat{\rho}_{23} = 0.4435,\ \hat{\rho}_{34} = 0.3768,$$
$$\hat{\rho}_{13} = 0.3081,\ \hat{\rho}_{24} = 0.2772,$$
$$\hat{\rho}_{14} = 0.3216,$$

which again tend to support the EQC model for the data. By the same token, the correlation estimate from (3.47) under the AR(1) model assumption was found to be $\hat{\rho} = 0.4998$, which is much larger than $\hat{\rho}^2 = 0.3545$. Furthermore, as expected, the EQC model based estimate $\hat{\rho}^2 = 0.3545$ is close to the aforementioned lag correlations (see also Eq. (3.21)).

3.2.4 Binary Dynamic Logit Model and Estimation of Parameters

As opposed to the LDCP model discussed in Sect. 3.2.2.1, there exists a non-linear (in logit form) dynamic conditional probability model for the analysis of binary and multinomial panel data. See, for example, Amemiya (1985, p. 422), Farrell and Sutradhar (2006), Sutradhar and Farrell (2007) for such models in the regression setup with fixed covariates (resulting to fixed effects model); and Fienberg et al. (1985), Manski (1987), Conaway (1989), Honore and Kyriazidou (2000), Sutradhar et al. (2008) and Sutradhar et al. (2010) for similar models in the regression setup with random effects (resulting to mixed effects model). This type of non-linear dynamic models is useful when the mean response level at a given time appears to maintain a recursive relationship with other past mean levels. In this section, we consider the binary dynamic logit (BDL) models in the most simple stationary setup with no covariates. The multinomial dynamic logit (MDL) models involving no covariates will be discussed in Sect. 3.4, whereas similar models with time independent (stationary) covariates will be discussed in Sect. 3.3 for the binary data and in Sect. 3.5 for general categorical data.

3.2.4.1 BDL Model and Basic Properties

For the BDL model, the marginal probability function for the initial binary response y_{i1} has the form

$$P[y_{i1} = y_{i1}^{(j)}] = \pi_{([\cdot]1)j} = \begin{cases} \frac{\exp(\beta_{10})}{1+\exp(\beta_{10})} & \text{for } j = 1 \\ \frac{1}{1+\exp(\beta_{10})} & \text{for } j = J = 2, \end{cases} \tag{3.70}$$

which is same as in the LDCP model (3.23). However, for $t = 2, \ldots, T$, the conditional probability, unlike the LDCP model (3.24), has the dynamic logit form given by

$$\eta_{it|t-1}^{(j)}(g) = P\left(Y_{it} = y_{it}^{(j)} \,\middle|\, Y_{i,t-1} = y_{i,t-1}^{(g)}\right)$$
$$= \begin{cases} \frac{\exp\left[\beta_{10}+\gamma_1 y_{i,t-1}^{(g)}\right]}{1+\exp\left[\beta_{10}+\gamma_1 y_{i,t-1}^{(g)}\right]}, & \text{for } j = 1; g = 1,2; t = 2,\ldots,T \\ \frac{1}{1+\exp\left[\beta_{10}+\gamma_1 y_{i,t-1}^{(g)}\right]}, & \text{for } j = J = 2; g = 1,2; t = 2,\ldots,T, \end{cases} \tag{3.71}$$

where γ_1 denotes the dynamic dependence parameter, which is neither a correlation nor an odds ratio parameter. But it is clear that the correlations of the repeated multinomial responses will be function of this γ_1 parameter. Furthermore, the marginal probabilities (3.70) at time $t = 1$ and conditional probabilities (3.71) for $t = 2, \ldots, T$, yield the marginal probabilities at time $t(t = 2, \ldots)$ as functions of β_{10} and they are also influenced by γ_1 parameter. For example, in the binary case $(J = 1)$ the unconditional (marginal) probabilities have the forms

$$E[Y_{it}] = \pi_{([\cdot]t)1} == Pr[Y_{it} = y_{it}^{(1)}]$$
$$= \begin{cases} \frac{\exp(\beta_{10})}{1+\exp(\beta_{10})}, & \text{for } t = 1 \\ \eta_1^* + \pi_{([\cdot](t-1))1}[\tilde{\eta}_1 - \eta_1^*], & \text{for } t = 2, \ldots, T, \end{cases} \tag{3.72}$$

(Sutradhar and Farrell 2007) for all $i = 1, \ldots, K$, with

$$\tilde{\eta}_1 = \frac{\exp(\beta_{10}+\gamma_1)}{1+\exp(\beta_{10}+\gamma_1)} \text{ and } \eta_1^* = \frac{\exp(\beta_{10})}{1+\exp(\beta_{10})}.$$

Note that in (3.72), $\pi_{([\cdot]1)1} = \eta_1^*$. Now, to see the role of γ_1 parameter on the correlations of the repeated responses, one may, for example, compute the correlations for the repeated binary responses y_{iu} and y_{it} $(u < t)$ as

$$\text{corr}(Y_{iu}, Y_{it}) = \sqrt{\frac{\pi_{([\cdot]u)1}(1-\pi_{([\cdot]u)1})}{\pi_{([\cdot]t)1}(1-\pi_{([\cdot]t)1})}} \Pi_{k=u+1}^{t}(\tilde{\eta}_1 - \eta_1^*)$$
$$= \sqrt{\frac{\pi_{([\cdot]u)1}(1-\pi_{([\cdot]u)1})}{\pi_{([\cdot]t)1}(1-\pi_{([\cdot]t)1})}} (\tilde{\eta}_1 - \eta_1^*)^{t-u}, \text{ for all } i, \text{ and } u < t, \tag{3.73}$$

where the marginal probability $\pi_{([\cdot]t)1}$ at time t is given by (3.72).

3.2.4.2 Likelihood Estimation of Parameters

For the BDL model (3.70)–(3.71), the likelihood function for the parameters β_{10} and γ_1 has the formula

$$L(\beta_{10},\gamma_1) = \Pi_{i=1}^{K} L_i, \tag{3.74}$$

where

$$L_i = f_1(y_{i1}) f_2(y_{i2}|y_{i1}) \cdots f_T(y_{iT}|y_{i,T-1}),$$

with

$$f_1(y_{i1}) = [\pi_{([\cdot]1)1}]^{y_{i1}} [\pi_{([\cdot]t)2}]^{1-y_{i1}} = \frac{\exp[y_{i1}\beta_{10}]}{1+\exp(\beta_{10})}, \text{ and}$$

$$f_t(y_{it}|y_{i,t-1}) = [\eta^{(1)}_{it|t-1}(g)]^{y_{it}} [\eta^{(2)}_{it|t-1}(g)]^{1-y_{it}}, \text{ for } t = 2,\ldots,T, \tag{3.75}$$

yielding the log likelihood function as

$$\begin{aligned}\text{Log } L(\beta_{10},\gamma_1) &= \sum_{i=1}^{K} [y_{i1}\log \pi_{([\cdot]1)1} + (1-y_{i1})\log \pi_{([\cdot]1)2}] \\ &+ \sum_{g=1}^{2}\sum_{i\in g}^{K}\sum_{t=2}^{T} [y_{it}\log \eta^{(1)}_{it|t-1}(g) + (1-y_{it})\log \eta^{(2)}_{it|t-1}(g)]. \end{aligned}\tag{3.76}$$

Note that under the present stationary model, similar to (3.30), it follows from (3.71) that $\eta^{(1)}_{it|t-1}(1)$ and $\eta^{(1)}_{it|t-1}(2)$ are free from i and t. Thus, for convenience, suppressing the subscripts from these conditional probabilities and using $\eta^{(1)}(1)$ for $\eta^{(1)}_{it|t-1}(1)$, for example, and by using the cell frequencies from the contingency Table 3.2, one can express the log likelihood function (3.76) as

$$\begin{aligned}\text{Log } L(\beta_{10},\gamma_1) &= [K_1(1)\log \pi_{([\cdot]1)1} + K_2(1)\log \pi_{([\cdot]1)2}] \\ &+ \log \eta^{(1)}(1)\sum_{t=2}^{T} K_{11}(t-1,t) + \log \eta^{(2)}(1)\sum_{t=2}^{T} K_{12}(t-1,t) \\ &+ \log \eta^{(1)}(2)\sum_{t=2}^{T} K_{21}(t-1,t) + \log \eta^{(2)}(2)\sum_{t=2}^{T} K_{22}(t-1,t), \end{aligned}\tag{3.77}$$

where by (3.71)–(3.72)

$$\pi_{([\cdot]1)1} = \eta_1^*, \; \pi_{([\cdot]1)2} = 1-\eta_1^*$$

$$\eta^{(1)}(1) = \tilde{\eta}_1,\ \eta^{(2)}(1) = 1 - \eta^{(1)}(1) = 1 - \tilde{\eta}_1$$
$$\eta^{(1)}(2) = \eta_1^*,\ \eta^{(2)}(2) = 1 - \eta^{(1)}(2) = 1 - \eta_1^*. \quad (3.78)$$

Also it follows from the formulas for η_1^* and $\tilde{\eta}_1$ in (3.72) that

$$\frac{\partial \pi_{([\cdot]1)1}}{\partial \beta_{10}} = \frac{\partial \eta^{(1)}(2)}{\partial \beta_{10}} = \eta_1^*(1-\eta_1^*)$$
$$\frac{\partial \pi_{([\cdot]1)2}}{\partial \beta_{10}} = \frac{\partial \eta^{(2)}(2)}{\partial \beta_{10}} = -\eta_1^*(1-\eta_1^*)$$
$$\frac{\partial \eta^{(1)}(1)}{\partial \beta_{10}} = \tilde{\eta}_1(1-\tilde{\eta}_1),\ \frac{\partial \eta^{(2)}(1)}{\partial \beta_{10}} = -\tilde{\eta}_1(1-\tilde{\eta}_1); \quad (3.79)$$

and

$$\frac{\partial \pi_{([\cdot]1)1}}{\partial \gamma_1} = \frac{\partial \eta^{(1)}(2)}{\partial \gamma_1} = \frac{\partial \pi_{([\cdot]1)2}}{\partial \gamma_1} = \frac{\partial \eta^{(2)}(2)}{\partial \gamma_1} = 0$$
$$\frac{\partial \eta^{(1)}(1)}{\partial \gamma_1} = \tilde{\eta}_1(1-\tilde{\eta}_1),\ \frac{\partial \eta^{(2)}(1)}{\partial \gamma_1} = -\tilde{\eta}_1(1-\tilde{\eta}_1). \quad (3.80)$$

3.2.4.2.1 Likelihood Estimating Equations

By using (3.79), it follows from (3.77) that the likelihood estimating equation for β_{10} has the form

$$\frac{\partial \mathrm{Log}\, L(\beta_{10},\gamma_1)}{\partial \beta_{10}} = [\eta_1^*(1-\eta_1^*)]\left[\frac{K_1(1)}{\eta_1^*} - \frac{K_2(1)}{\eta_2^*}\right]$$
$$+ [\tilde{\eta}_1(1-\tilde{\eta}_1)]\left[\frac{\sum_{t=2}^T K_{11}(t-1,t)}{\eta^{(1)}(1)} - \frac{\sum_{t=2}^T K_{12}(t-1,t)}{\eta^{(2)}(1)}\right]$$
$$+ [\eta_1^*(1-\eta_1^*)]\left[\frac{\sum_{t=2}^T K_{21}(t-1,t)}{\eta^{(1)}(2)} - \frac{\sum_{t=2}^T K_{22}(t-1,t)}{\eta^{(2)}(2)}\right] = 0. \quad (3.81)$$

Similarly, by using (3.80), the likelihood function (3.77) yields the likelihood estimating equation for γ_1 as

$$\frac{\partial \mathrm{Log}\, L(\beta_{10},\gamma_1)}{\partial \gamma_1} = [\tilde{\eta}_1(1-\tilde{\eta}_1)]\left[\frac{\sum_{t=2}^T K_{11}(t-1,t)}{\eta^{(1)}(1)} - \frac{\sum_{t=2}^T K_{12}(t-1,t)}{\eta^{(2)}(1)}\right] = 0. \quad (3.82)$$

As opposed to the joint estimation, the estimating equations (3.81) and (3.82) may be solved marginally through iterations. To be specific, for known γ_1, the marginal likelihood estimate for β_{10} may be obtained by using the iterative equation

$$\hat{\beta}_{10}(r+1) = \hat{\beta}_{10}(r) - \left[\left\{ \frac{\partial^2 \text{Log}\, L(\beta_{10}, \gamma_1)}{\partial \beta_{10}^2} \right\}^{-1} \frac{\partial \text{Log}\, L(\beta_{10}, \gamma_1)}{\partial \beta_{10}} \right]_{|\beta_{10}=\hat{\beta}_{10}(r)}, \tag{3.83}$$

and using this estimate, that is, for known β_{10}, the marginal likelihood estimate of γ_1 may be obtained as a solution of (3.82) by using the iterative equation

$$\hat{\gamma}_1(r+1) = \hat{\gamma}_1(r) - \left[\left\{ \frac{\partial^2 \text{Log}\, L(\beta_{10}, \gamma_1)}{\partial \gamma_1^2} \right\}^{-1} \frac{\partial \text{Log}\, L(\beta_{10}, \gamma_1)}{\partial \gamma_1} \right]_{|\rho=\hat{\rho}(r)}. \tag{3.84}$$

In (3.83), the second derivative of the likelihood function with respect to β_{10} has the formula

$$\begin{aligned} \frac{\partial^2 \text{Log}\, L(\beta_{10}, \gamma_1)}{\partial \beta_{10}^2} &= -K[\eta_1^*(1-\eta_1^*)] \\ &+ [\tilde{\eta}_1(1-\tilde{\eta}_1)(1-2\tilde{\eta}_1)] \left[\frac{\sum_{t=2}^T K_{11}(t-1,t)}{\eta^{(1)}(1)} - \frac{\sum_{t=2}^T K_{12}(t-1,t)}{\eta^{(2)}(1)} \right] \\ &+ [\eta_1^*(1-\eta_1^*)(1-2\eta_1^*)] \left[\frac{\sum_{t=2}^T K_{21}(t-1,t)}{\eta^{(1)}(2)} - \frac{\sum_{t=2}^T K_{22}(t-1,t)}{\eta^{(2)}(2)} \right] \\ &- [\tilde{\eta}_1(1-\tilde{\eta}_1)]^2 \left[\frac{\sum_{t=2}^T K_{11}(t-1,t)}{\{\eta^{(1)}(1)\}^2} + \frac{\sum_{t=2}^T K_{12}(t-1,t)}{\{\eta^{(2)}(1)\}^2} \right] \\ &- [\eta_1^*(1-\eta_1^*)] \left[\frac{\sum_{t=2}^T K_{21}(t-1,t)}{\{\eta^{(1)}(2)\}^2} + \frac{\sum_{t=2}^T K_{22}(t-1,t)}{\{\eta^{(2)}(2)\}^2} \right], \end{aligned} \tag{3.85}$$

and in (3.84), the second derivative of the likelihood function with respect to γ_1 has the formula given by

$$\begin{aligned} \frac{\partial^2 \text{Log}\, L(\beta_{10}, \gamma_1)}{\partial \gamma_1^2} &= [\tilde{\eta}_1(1-\tilde{\eta}_1)(1-2\tilde{\eta}_1)] \left[\frac{\sum_{t=2}^T K_{11}(t-1,t)}{\eta^{(1)}(1)} - \frac{\sum_{t=2}^T K_{12}(t-1,t)}{\eta^{(2)}(1)} \right] \\ &- [\tilde{\eta}_1(1-\tilde{\eta}_1)]^2 \left[\frac{\sum_{t=2}^T K_{11}(t-1,t)}{\{\eta^{(1)}(1)\}^2} + \frac{\sum_{t=2}^T K_{12}(t-1,t)}{\{\eta^{(2)}(1)\}^2} \right]. \end{aligned} \tag{3.86}$$

3.2.4.2.2 Illustration 3.5 (Continuation of Illustration 3.1 for Longitudinal Asthma Data Analysis): BDL Model Based Likelihood Estimates

Notice that the longitudinal asthma status data described through contingency type Tables 3.3 and 3.4(1)–3.4(6) were analyzed in Sect. 3.2.1.3 by fitting a general auto-correlation structure for repeated binary (asthma status) data. A LDCP model was fitted to the same data set using likelihood approach in Sect. 3.2.2.1.3, and the GQL approach in Sect. 3.2.2.2.1. Also an EQC model was fitted by using the GQL estimation approach and the results were discussed in Sect. 3.2.3.2.1. We now illustrate the fitting of a completely different, namely non-linear dynamic model, to be more specific the BDL model, to the same asthma status data, by using the likelihood approach.

The estimation was carried out as follows.

Step 1. Using initial values $\beta_{10} = 0$ and $\gamma_1 = 0$, and applying the iterative equation (3.83), β_{10} was estimated as -1.6394, in a few iterations.

Step 2. Using the initial value $\gamma_1 = 0.0$ and β_{10} value from Step 1, the iterative equation (3.84) was applied only once to obtain the value for γ_1 as 2.2137.

Step 3. The γ_1 value from Step 2 was used in Step 1 to obtain an improved estimate for β_{10} by (3.83), and this improved β_{10} estimate was applied in (3.84) as in Step 2 to obtain an improved estimate for γ_1.

Step 4. The above three steps constitute a cycle of iterations. This cycle was repeated a few times (5 times to be precise) to obtain the final estimates as

$$\hat{\beta}_{10} = -2.1184, \text{ and } \hat{\gamma}_1 = 1.9737.$$

Next, to understand the model parameters such as recursive means $(\pi_{([\cdot]t)1})$ and variances $(\pi_{([\cdot]t)1}\{1-\pi_{([\cdot]t)1}\})$ over time, we have applied the final estimates from Step 4 to (3.72), which were found to be as in the following Table 3.6. Note that the means reported in Table 3.6, found by using the recursive relation (3.72), appear to reflect well the observed proportions calculated by $K_1(t)/K$ at a time point t. Further to understand the longitudinal correlations of the data, we have computed them by using the BDL model based correlation formula given by (3.73). These correlations are given in Table 3.7. It is interesting to observe that these lag correlations appear to satisfy a Gaussian AR(1) type structure. Note that if the marginal variances over time are almost equal, then following (3.73), one would have computed the correlations by

Table 3.6 Marginal means and variances for the asthma data over time based on BDL model (3.70)–(3.71)

	Time			
Quantity	Year 1	Year 2	Year 3	Year 4
Mean	0.1073	0.1456	0.1592	0.1641
Variance	0.0958	0.1244	0.1339	0.1372
Observed Proportion	0.1620	0.1694	0.1583	0.1173

Table 3.7 BDL model based pair-wise correlations (3.73) for the asthma data

	Time			
Time	Year 1	Year 2	Year 3	Year 4
Year 1	1.0	0.3129	0.1075	0.0.0379
Year 2	0.3129	1.0	0.3437	0.1210
Year 3	0.1075	0.3437	1.0	0.3522
Year 4	0.0379	0.1210	0.3522	1.0

$$\text{corr}(Y_{iu}, Y_{it}) = [\tilde{\pi}_1 - \pi_1^*]^{t-u},$$

indicating AR(1) type correlations. Further note that these results are not directly comparable with likelihood estimates under the LDCP model found in Sect. 3.2.2.1(b). This is because, even though the same likelihood approach is used for the estimation of the model parameters, models are, however, quite different, one being linear and the present model in this section is non-linear. Nevertheless, the probability of having an asthma attack under the LDCP model was found to be 0.1447, for any time points, which is close to the probabilities (means) at time points 2, 3, and 4, shown in Table 3.6.

3.3 Univariate Longitudinal Stationary Binary Fixed Effect Regression Models

In Sect. 3.2, individuals were categorized into one of the two ($J = 2$) categories at a given time t, without considering their covariates. But in many practical situations, information about some of their possibly influential covariates are also collected.

Recall from Chap. 2, specifically from Sect. 2.2.2 that at a cross-sectional setup as opposed to the longitudinal setup, the probability for an individual i with a single covariate, say, at level $\ell(\ell = 1,\ldots,p)$ to be in the jth category (see Eqs. (2.63)–(2.64)) has the form

$$\pi_{[\ell]j} = \pi_{(i\in\ell)j} = \begin{cases} \frac{\exp(\beta_{10}+\beta_{1\ell})}{1+\exp(\beta_{10}+\beta_{1\ell})} & \text{for } j = 1 \\ \frac{1}{1+\exp(\beta_{10}+\beta_{1\ell})} & \text{for } j = J = 2, \end{cases}$$

and for $\ell = p+1$, these probabilities have the formulas

$$\pi_{[p+1]j} = \pi_{(i\in(p+1))j} = \begin{cases} \frac{\exp(\beta_{10})}{1+\exp(\beta_{10})} & \text{for } j = 1 \\ \frac{1}{1+\exp(\beta_{10})} & \text{for } j = J = 2. \end{cases}$$

Now using the notation from (3.6), in the stationary binary ($J = 2$) longitudinal setup, for all time points $t = 1,\ldots,T$, these probabilities may be written as

Table 3.8 *Contingency table at initial time* $t = 1$ for binary category versus covariate level data

	t ($t=1$)		
	Category		
Covariate level	1	2	Total
1	$K_{[1]1}(1)$	$K_{[1]2}(1)$	$K_{[1]}$
2	$K_{[2]1}(1)$	$K_{[2]2}(1)$	$K_{[2]}$
·	...	...	·
ℓ	$K_{[\ell]1}(1)$	$K_{[\ell]2}(1)$	$K_{[\ell]}$
·	...	...	·
$p+1$	$K_{[p+1]1}(1)$	$K_{[p+1]2}(1)$	$K_{[p+1]}$
Total	$K_1(1)$	$K_2(1)$	K

Table 3.9 Lag h^* ($h^* = 1,\ldots,T-1$) based $[h^*(T-h^*)]$ transitional counts for binary responses for individuals belonging to ℓ-th ($\ell = 1,\ldots,p+1$) level of a covariate

			t ($t = h^*+1,\ldots,T$)		
	Time		Category		
Covariate level	Time	Category	1	2	Total
ℓ	t-h^*	1	$K_{[\ell]11}(t-h^*,t)$	$K_{[\ell]12}(t-h^*,t)$	$K_{[\ell]1}(t-h^*)$
		2	$K_{[\ell]21}(t-h^*,t)$	$K_{[\ell]22}(t-h^*,t)$	$K_{[\ell]2}(t-h^*)$
		Total	$K_{[\ell]1}(t)$	$K_{[\ell]2}(t)$	$K_{[\ell]}$

$$P[y_{it} = y_{it}^{(j)}|i \in \ell] = \pi_{([i\in\ell]t)j} \equiv \pi_{[\ell]j}$$
$$= \begin{cases} \frac{\exp(\beta_{10}+\beta_{1\ell})}{1+\exp(\beta_{10}+\beta_{1\ell})} & \text{for } j=1;\ \ell=1,\ldots,p \\ \frac{1}{1+\exp(\beta_{10}+\beta_{1\ell})} & \text{for } j=J=2;\ \ell=1,\ldots,p, \end{cases} \tag{3.87}$$

and for $\ell = p+1$, these probabilities have the formulas

$$P[y_{it} = y_{it}^{(j)}|i \in (p+1)] = = \pi_{(i\in(p+1)t)j} \equiv \pi_{[p+1]j}$$
$$= \begin{cases} \frac{\exp(\beta_{10})}{1+\exp(\beta_{10})} & \text{for } j=1;\ \ell=p+1 \\ \frac{1}{1+\exp(\beta_{10})} & \text{for } j=J=2;\ \ell=p+1. \end{cases} \tag{3.88}$$

For this stationary case, as an extension of the contingency Tables 3.1 and 3.2, one may accommodate the covariates or a covariate with $p+1$ levels, and summarize the response frequencies over T time periods, through following the contingency Table 3.8 at the initial time point, and $T-1$ lag ($h^* = 1,\ldots,T-1$) contingency tables (Tables 3.9(1)–3.9($T-1$)):

3.3.1 LDCP Model Involving Covariates and Estimation of Parameters

Similar to the covariate free LDCP model given in (3.23)–(3.25), we first write the probabilities at initial time point $t = 1$ as

$$P[y_{i1} = y_{i1}^{(j)} | i \in \ell] = \pi_{[(i\in\ell]1)j} \equiv \pi_{[\ell]j}$$
$$= \begin{cases} \frac{\exp(\beta_{10}+\beta_{1\ell})}{1+\exp(\beta_{10}+\beta_{1\ell})} & \text{for } j = 1;\ \ell = 1,\ldots,p \\ \frac{1}{1+\exp(\beta_{10}+\beta_{1\ell})} & \text{for } j = J = 2;\ \ell = 1,\ldots,p, \end{cases} \tag{3.89}$$

and for $\ell = p+1$, these probabilities have the formulas

$$P[y_{i1} = y_{i1}^{(j)} | i \in (p+1)] = = \pi_{(i\in(p+1)1)j} \equiv \pi_{[p+1]j}$$
$$= \begin{cases} \frac{\exp(\beta_{10})}{1+\exp(\beta_{10})} & \text{for } j = 1 \\ \frac{1}{1+\exp(\beta_{10})} & \text{for } j = J = 2. \end{cases} \tag{3.90}$$

Next, for $\ell = 1,\ldots,p+1$, and $t = 2,\ldots,T$, the lag 1 based LDC probabilities may be written as

$$P[y_{it} = y_{it}^{(1)} | y_{i,t-1} = y_{i,t-1}^{(g)}, i \in \ell] = \pi_{[\ell]1} + \rho(y_{i,t-1}^{(g)} - \pi_{[\ell]1})$$
$$= \lambda_{it|t-1}^{(1)}(g,\ell) \text{ (say)}, g = 1,2;\ t = 2,\ldots,T; \tag{3.91}$$

and

$$\lambda_{it|t-1}^{(2)}(g,\ell) = 1 - \lambda_{it|t-1}^{(1)}(g,\ell), \text{ for } g = 1,2;\ t = 2,\ldots,T. \tag{3.92}$$

3.3.1.1 GQL Estimation

It follows from (3.90)–(3.92) that the repeated binary observations for the ith individual follow the stationary auto-correlation model with correlation matrix $C_i(\rho) = \tilde{C}(\rho)$ as given by (3.41). That is,

$$\tilde{C}(\rho) = \begin{bmatrix} 1 & \rho & \rho^2 & \cdots & \rho^{T-1} \\ \rho^1 & 1 & \rho^1 & \cdots & \rho^{T-2} \\ \vdots & \vdots & \vdots & & \vdots \\ \rho^{T-1} & \rho^{T-2} & \rho^{T-3} & \cdots & 1 \end{bmatrix},$$

for all $i = 1,\ldots,K$. Thus, the LDCP model contains $p+1$ regression parameters, namely

$$\beta_{10};\ \beta_{11},\ldots,\beta_{1\ell},\ldots,\beta_{1p},$$

and one correlation parameter, namely ρ.

3.3.1.1.1 Estimation of Correlation Parameter

Now to develop the GQL estimating equations for these regression parameters, we first provide a moment estimating equation for ρ_{h^*} by assuming that these regression parameters are known, and then similar to (3.45), ρ may be estimated by solving the polynomial moment equation

$$\sum_{h^*=1}^{T-1}(T-h^*)\rho^{h^*} = \sum_{h^*=1}^{T-1}(T-h^*)\hat{\rho}_{h^*}, \tag{3.93}$$

where $\hat{\rho}_{h^*}$ is computed as follows.

$$\hat{\rho}_{h^*} = \frac{\sum_{\ell=1}^{p+1}\left[\sum_{i\in\ell}^{K}\sum_{t=h^*+1}^{T}\tilde{y}_{i\in\ell,t-h^*}\tilde{y}_{i\in\ell,t}/\{K_{[\ell]}(T-h^*)\}\right]}{\sum_{\ell=1}^{p+1}\left[\sum_{i\in\ell}^{K}\sum_{t=1}^{T}\tilde{y}^2_{i\in\ell,t}/\{K_{[\ell]}T\}\right]}, \tag{3.94}$$

where $\tilde{y}_{i\in\ell,t}$ is the standardized deviance, defined as

$$\tilde{y}_{i\in\ell,t} = \frac{y_{i\in\ell,t}-\pi_{[\ell]1}}{\{\pi_{[\ell]1}(1-\pi_{[\ell]1})\}^{1/2}},$$

where $\pi_{[\ell]1}$ is defined by (3.89)–(3.90). Note that this formula for $\hat{\rho}_h$ in (3.94) is written by modifying (3.10) in order to reflect the data and model involving the ℓ-th specified level ($\ell = 1,\ldots,p+1$) of the covariate. Further note that this pooling of quantities from all $p+1$ levels is appropriate because of the fact that one individual belongs to one level only and hence at a given level, the responses at a time point have a binomial or multinomial distribution. This is similar to product binomial approach used in Chap. 2 (see, for example, Sect. 2.2.2.3). The difference lies in the fact that in the present longitudinal setup, at each level of the covariate, binary responses are correlated over time, whereas in Chap. 2, models were developed at the cross-sectional level, that is, for $T = 1$ only.

Now by using the frequencies from the contingency Tables 3.8 and 3.9, one may modify the formulas in (3.11) as

$$\sum_{i\in\ell}^{K}\sum_{t=1}^{T} y_{i\in\ell,t} = \sum_{t=1}^{T}\sum_{i\in\ell}^{K} y_{i\in\ell,t} = \sum_{t=1}^{T} K_{[\ell]1}(t), \text{ or}$$

$$\sum_{i\in\ell}^{K}\sum_{t=h^*+1}^{T} y_{i\in\ell,t} = \sum_{t=h^*+1}^{T}\sum_{i\in\ell}^{K} y_{i\in\ell,t} = \sum_{t=h^*+1}^{T} K_{[\ell]1}(t); \text{ and}$$

$$\sum_{i\in\ell}^{K}\sum_{t=h^*+1}^{T} y_{i\in\ell,t-h^*} = \sum_{t=h^*+1}^{T}\sum_{i\in\ell}^{K} y_{i\in\ell,t-h^*} = \sum_{t=h^*+1}^{T} K_{[\ell]1}(t-h^*)$$

$$\sum_{i\in\ell}^{K}\sum_{t=h^*+1}^{T} y_{i\in\ell,t-h^*}y_{i\in\ell,t} = \sum_{t=h^*+1}^{T}\sum_{i\in\ell}^{K} y_{i\in\ell,t-h^*}y_{i\in\ell,t} = \sum_{t=h^*+1}^{T} K_{[\ell]11}(t-h^*,\, t). \quad (3.95)$$

By using (3.95), it then follows from (3.94) that

$$\hat{\rho}_{h^*} = \frac{\frac{1}{T-h^*}\sum_{t=h^*+1}^{T}\left[\sum_{\ell=1}^{p+1}\frac{1}{K_{[\ell]}}\left\{K_{[\ell]11}(t-h^*,\, t) - \pi_{[\ell]1}\{K_{[\ell]1}(t)+K_{[\ell]1}(t-h^*)\} + \pi_{[\ell]1}^2 K_{[\ell]}\right\}\right]}{\frac{1}{T}\sum_{t=1}^{T}\left[\sum_{\ell=1}^{p+1}\frac{1}{K_{[\ell]}}\left\{(1-2\pi_{[\ell]1})K_{[\ell]1}(t) + \pi_{[\ell]1}^2 K_{[\ell]}\right\}\right]}, \quad (3.96)$$

where, for all $\ell = 1,\ldots,p+1$, the marginal probabilities $\pi_{[\ell]1}$ are given by (3.87) and (3.88).

3.3.1.1.2 Estimation of Regression Parameters

Next, once the correlation parameter ρ is estimated by (3.93), one computes the $\tilde{C}(\rho)$ matrix (see also (3.41)) and then computes the covariance matrix for the ith individual having covariate level ℓ as

$$\Sigma_{i\in\ell}(\rho) = A_{i\in\ell}^{\frac{1}{2}}\tilde{C}(\rho)A_{i\in\ell}^{\frac{1}{2}}, \quad (3.97)$$

where

$$A_{i\in\ell} = \pi_{[\ell]1}(1-\pi_{[\ell]1})I_T,$$

I_T being the $T\times T$ identity matrix. Consequently, to reflect the covariate levels, one may modify the GQL estimating equation (3.42) for regression parameters as follows. By using the notation $\theta^* = [\beta_{10},\beta_{11},\ldots,\beta_{1p}]'$ as in Sect. 2.2.2.1 (from Chap. 2), first write

$$\pi_{[\ell]1} = \begin{cases} \frac{\exp(\beta_{10}+\beta_{1\ell})}{1+\exp(\beta_{10}+\beta_{1\ell})} & \text{for } \ell = 1,\ldots,p \\ \frac{\exp(\beta_{10})}{1+\exp(\beta_{10})} & \text{for } \ell = p+1 \end{cases}$$

$$= \frac{\exp(x'_{[\ell]1}\theta^*)}{1+\exp(x'_{[\ell]1}\theta^*)},$$

where

$$x'_{[\ell]1} = \begin{cases} \left(1\ 01'_{\ell-1}\ 1\ 01'_{p-\ell}\right) & \text{for } \ell = 1,\ldots,p \\ \left(1\ 01'_{p}\right) & \text{for } \ell = p+1, \end{cases}$$

and use

$$\begin{aligned} \pi_{(i\in\ell)} &= E\left\{[Y_{i1},\ldots,Y_{it},\ldots,Y_{iT}]'|i\in\ell\right\} \\ &= [\pi_{[\ell]1},\ldots,\pi_{[\ell]1},\ldots,\pi_{[\ell]1}]' \\ &= \pi_{[\ell]1}1_T \\ &= \bar{\pi}_{[\ell]}, \end{aligned}$$

and then construct the GQL estimating equation for θ^* as

$$\begin{aligned} &\sum_{\ell=1}^{p+1}\sum_{i\in\ell}^{K}\frac{\partial\pi'_{(i\in\ell)}}{\partial\theta^*}\Sigma^{-1}_{i\in\ell}(\rho)(y_i-\pi_{(i\in\ell)}) \\ &= \sum_{\ell=1}^{p+1}\sum_{i\in\ell}^{K}\frac{\partial\bar{\pi}'_{[\ell]}}{\partial\theta^*}\Sigma^{-1}_{i\in\ell}(\rho)(y_i-\bar{\pi}_{[\ell]}) = 0, \end{aligned} \tag{3.98}$$

where $y_i = (y_{i1},\ldots,y_{it},\ldots,y_{iT})'$. Note that the derivative matrix in (3.98) may be computed as

$$\begin{aligned} \frac{\partial\pi'_{(i\in\ell)}}{\partial\theta^*} &= X'_\ell A_{i\in\ell} \\ &= X'_\ell[\pi_{[\ell]1}(1-\pi_{[\ell]1})I_T, \end{aligned} \tag{3.99}$$

where X_ℓ is the $T\times(p+1)$ coefficient matrix defined as

$$\begin{aligned} X_\ell &= 1_T\otimes x'_{[\ell]1} \\ &= \begin{cases} 1_T\otimes\left(1\ 01'_{\ell-1}\ 1\ 01'_{p-\ell}\right) & \text{for } \ell=1,\ldots,p \\ 1_T\otimes\left(1\ 01'_{p}\right) & \text{for } \ell=p+1. \end{cases} \end{aligned} \tag{3.100}$$

Now by using (3.99) in (3.98), the GQL estimating equation for θ^* reduces to

$$\begin{aligned}
f(\theta^*) &= \sum_{\ell=1}^{p+1}\sum_{i\in\ell}^{K} X'_\ell \tilde{C}^{-1}(\rho)(y_i - \pi_{[\ell]1}1_T) \\
&= \sum_{\ell=1}^{p+1}\sum_{i\in\ell}^{K} \begin{pmatrix} \tilde{\omega}_{[\ell]11} & \cdots & \tilde{\omega}_{[\ell]1t} & \cdots & \tilde{\omega}_{[\ell]1T} \\ \vdots & \vdots & \vdots & \vdots & \vdots \\ \tilde{\omega}_{[\ell]s1} & \cdots & \tilde{\omega}_{[\ell]st} & \cdots & \tilde{\omega}_{[\ell]sT} \\ \vdots & \vdots & \vdots & \vdots & \vdots \\ \tilde{\omega}_{[\ell](p+1,1)} & \cdots & \tilde{\omega}_{[\ell](p+1,t)} & \cdots & \tilde{\omega}_{[\ell](p+1,T)} \end{pmatrix} (y_i - \pi_{[\ell]1}1_T) \\
&= \sum_{\ell=1}^{p+1}\left[\sum_{t=1}^{T} \begin{pmatrix} \tilde{\omega}_{[\ell]1t} \\ \vdots \\ \tilde{\omega}_{[\ell]st} \\ \vdots \\ \tilde{\omega}_{[\ell](p+1)t} \end{pmatrix} K_{[\ell]1}(t) - \pi_{[\ell]1}K_{[\ell]}\sum_{t=1}^{T} \begin{pmatrix} \tilde{\omega}_{[\ell]1t} \\ \vdots \\ \tilde{\omega}_{[\ell]st} \\ \vdots \\ \tilde{\omega}_{[\ell](p+1)t} \end{pmatrix}\right] \\
&= \sum_{\ell=1}^{p+1}\left[\sum_{t=1}^{T} \tilde{\omega}_{[\ell]t}K_{[\ell]1}(t) - \pi_{[\ell]1}K_{[\ell]}\sum_{t=1}^{T}\tilde{\omega}_{[\ell]t}\right] = 0,
\end{aligned} \tag{3.101}$$

where $K_{[\ell]1}(t)$ for all $\ell = 1,\ldots,p+1$, and $t = 1,\ldots,T$, and the values of $K_{[\ell]}$ are available from the contingency Table 3.9. Now to solve the GQL estimating equation (3.98) or (3.101), we first compute

$$\begin{aligned}
f'(\theta^*) &= \frac{\partial f(\theta^*)}{\partial \theta^{*\prime}} \\
&= -\sum_{\ell=1}^{p+1}\sum_{i\in\ell}^{K} \frac{\partial \bar{\pi}'_{[\ell]}}{\partial \theta^*}\Sigma^{-1}_{i\in\ell}(\rho)\frac{\partial \bar{\pi}_{[\ell]}}{\partial \theta^{*\prime}} \\
&= -\sum_{\ell=1}^{p+1}\sum_{i\in\ell}^{K} X'_\ell \tilde{C}^{-1}(\rho)\frac{\partial \pi_{[\ell]1}1_T}{\partial \theta^{*\prime}} \\
&= -\sum_{\ell=1}^{p+1}\sum_{i\in\ell}^{K} X'_\ell \tilde{C}^{-1}(\rho)A_{i\in\ell}X_\ell \\
&= -\sum_{\ell=1}^{p+1}\sum_{i\in\ell}^{K} [\pi_{[\ell]1}(1-\pi_{[\ell]1})]X'_\ell \tilde{C}^{-1}(\rho)X_\ell \\
&= -\sum_{\ell=1}^{p+1} [\pi_{[\ell]1}(1-\pi_{[\ell]1})]K_{[\ell]}
\end{aligned}$$

$$\times \begin{pmatrix} \tilde{\omega}^*_{[\ell]11} & \cdots & \tilde{\omega}^*_{[\ell]1s} & \cdots & \tilde{\omega}^*_{[\ell]1,p+1} \\ \vdots & \vdots & \vdots & \vdots & \vdots \\ \tilde{\omega}^*_{[\ell]s1} & \cdots & \tilde{\omega}^*_{[\ell]ss} & \cdots & \tilde{\omega}^*_{[\ell]s,p+1} \\ \vdots & \vdots & \vdots & \vdots & \vdots \\ \tilde{\omega}^*_{[\ell](p+1,1)} & \cdots & \tilde{\omega}^*_{[\ell](p+1,s)} & \cdots & \tilde{\omega}^*_{[\ell](p+1,p+1)} \end{pmatrix}$$

$$= -\sum_{\ell=1}^{p+1} [\pi_{[\ell]1}(1-\pi_{[\ell]1})] K_{[\ell]} \tilde{\Omega}^*_{[\ell]}. \tag{3.102}$$

One may then obtain the GQL estimate for θ^* by using the iterative equation

$$\hat{\theta}^*(r+1) = \hat{\theta}^*(r) + \left[\left\{ \sum_{\ell=1}^{p+1} [\pi_{[\ell]1}(1-\pi_{[\ell]1})] K_{[\ell]} \tilde{\Omega}^*_{[\ell]} \right\}^{-1} \right.$$
$$\left. \times \sum_{\ell=1}^{p+1} \left[\sum_{t=1}^{T} \tilde{\omega}_{[\ell]t} K_{[\ell]1}(t) - \pi_{[\ell]1} K_{[\ell]} \sum_{t=1}^{T} \tilde{\omega}_{[\ell]t} \right] \right]_{|(r)}. \tag{3.103}$$

Note that in the present setup, at a given covariate level ℓ, the $K_{[\ell]}$ individuals are independent. Further because levels are mutually exclusive, responses from any two levels are independent. Consequently, similar to (3.18), one may obtain the covariance matrix of $\hat{\theta}^*$ obtained from (3.103) as

$$\text{var}[\hat{\theta}^*] = \left[\sum_{\ell=1}^{p+1} \sum_{i\in\ell}^{K} \frac{\partial \bar{\pi}'_{[\ell]}}{\partial \theta^*} \Sigma^{-1}_{i\in\ell}(\rho) \frac{\partial \bar{\pi}_{[\ell]}}{\partial \theta^{*\prime}} \right]^{-1} \sum_{\ell=1}^{p+1} \sum_{i\in\ell}^{K} \frac{\partial \bar{\pi}'_{[\ell]}}{\partial \theta^*} \Sigma^{-1}_{i\in\ell}(\rho) \text{var}(y_i - \pi_{[\ell]1} 1_T) \Sigma^{-1}_{i\in\ell}(\rho) \frac{\partial \bar{\pi}_{[\ell]}}{\partial \theta^{*\prime}}$$
$$\times \left[\sum_{\ell=1}^{p+1} \sum_{i\in\ell}^{K} \frac{\partial \bar{\pi}'_{[\ell]}}{\partial \theta^*} \Sigma^{-1}_{i\in\ell}(\rho) \frac{\partial \bar{\pi}_{[\ell]}}{\partial \theta^{*\prime}} \right]^{-1}$$
$$= \left[\sum_{\ell=1}^{p+1} \sum_{i\in\ell}^{K} \frac{\partial \bar{\pi}'_{[\ell]}}{\partial \theta^*} \Sigma^{-1}_{i\in\ell}(\rho) \frac{\partial \bar{\pi}_{[\ell]}}{\partial \theta^{*\prime}} \right]^{-1} = \left\{ \sum_{\ell=1}^{p+1} [\pi_{[\ell]1}(1-\pi_{[\ell]1})] K_{[\ell]} \tilde{\Omega}^*_{[\ell]} \right\}^{-1}, \tag{3.104}$$

by (3.102)–(3.103).

3.3.1.1.3 Illustration 3.6 : Mothers Smoking Effect on Longitudinal Asthma Status: An Application of the GQL Approach

In the illustration 3.3(b) under the Sect. 3.2.2.2.1, this longitudinal asthma data were analyzed by ignoring any covariates, which is the same to say that the covariate 'mother's smoking habit' did not play any role to determine the asthma status of a child. This produced the AR(1) lag correlation $\hat{\rho} = 0.4998$ based regression estimate $\hat{\beta}_{10} = -1.7525$, yielding the probability for a child at any time point to have asthma as $\hat{\pi}_1 = 0.1477$. In this section, we have analyzed the same response data collected over 4 years but with a major difference that in the present case these responses are analyzed conditional on the covariate level. For the first year, that is at $t = 1$, the covariate 'mother's smoking habit' specific response data are given in Table 3.10, and for other years the transitional data are given in Tables 3.11(1)–3.11(6). More specifically, by using the data from these tables and the initial estimate $\hat{\rho} = 0$, we have computed the first step estimate of β_{10} and β_{11} by using their iterative equation (103) with initial values $\hat{\beta}_{10} = 0$, $\hat{\beta}_{11} = 0$. These first step estimate of β's are then used in (3.96) to estimate lag correlations for the computation of $\hat{\rho}$ by (3.93). This cycle of iteration continues until convergence. The convergence was very quick. The final estimate of lag correlations from (3.96) were found to be

$$\hat{\rho}_1 = 0.4017,\ \hat{\rho}_2 = 0.3148,\ \hat{\rho}_3 = 0.3038$$

Table 3.10 Maternal smoking versus children asthma status contingency table at initial time $t = 1$

	t ($t = 1$)		
	Asthma category		
Covariate level	Yes (1)	No (2)	Total
Smoking mother (1)	$K_{[1]1}(1) = 31$	$K_{[1]2}(1) = 156$	$K_{[1]} = 187$
Non-smoking mother (2)	$K_{[2]1}(1) = 56$	$K_{[2]2}(1) = 294$	$K_{[2]} = 350$
Total	$K_1(1) = 87$	$K_2(1) = 450$	$K = 537$

Table 3.11 (1): Lag $h^* = 1$ based transitional table from time $t - h^* = 1$ to $t = 2$ for the maternal smoking versus children asthma status data

			2		
	Time		Category		
Covariate level	Time	Category	1	2	Total
1	1	1	$K_{[1]11}(1,2) = 17$	$K_{[1]12}(1,2) = 14$	$K_{[1]1}(1) = 31$
		2	$K_{[1]21}(1,2) = 22$	$K_{[1]22}(1,2) = 134$	$K_{[1]2}(1) = 156$
		Total	$K_{[1]1}(2) = 39$	$K_{[1]2}(2) = 148$	$K_{[1]} = 187$
2	1	1	$K_{[2]11}(1,2) = 24$	$K_{[2]12}(1,2) = 32$	$K_{[2]1}(1) = 56$
		2	$K_{[2]21}(1,2) = 28$	$K_{[2]22}(1,2) = 266$	$K_{[2]2}(1) = 294$
		Total	$K_{[2]1}(2) = 52$	$K_{[2]2}(2) = 298$	$K_{[2]} = 350$

Table 3.11 (2): Lag $h^* = 1$ based transitional table from time $t - h^* = 2$ to $t = 3$ for the maternal smoking versus children asthma status data

			3		
	Time		Category		
Covariate level	Time	Category	1	2	Total
1	2	1	$K_{[1]11}(2,3) = 21$	$K_{[1]12}(2,3) = 18$	$K_{[1]1}(2) = 39$
		2	$K_{[1]21}(2,3) = 14$	$K_{[1]22}(2,3) = 134$	$K_{[1]2}(2) = 148$
		Total	$K_{[1]1}(3) = 35$	$K_{[1]2}(3) = 152$	$K_{[1]} = 187$
2	2	1	$K_{[2]11}(2,3) = 26$	$K_{[2]12}(2,3) = 26$	$K_{[2]1}(2) = 52$
		2	$K_{[2]21}(2,3) = 24$	$K_{[2]22}(2,3) = 274$	$K_{[2]2}(2) = 298$
		Total	$K_{[2]1}(3) = 50$	$K_{[2]2}(3) = 300$	$K_{[2]} = 350$

Table 3.11 (3): Lag $h^* = 1$ based transitional table from time $t - h^* = 3$ to $t = 4$ for the maternal smoking versus children asthma status data

			4		
	Time		Category		
Covariate level	Time	Category	1	2	Total
1	3	1	$K_{[1]11}(3,4) = 14$	$K_{[1]12}(3,4) = 21$	$K_{[1]1}(3) = 35$
		2	$K_{[1]21}(3,4) = 12$	$K_{[1]22}(3,4) = 140$	$K_{[1]2}(3) = 152$
		Total	$K_{[1]1}(4) = 26$	$K_{[1]2}(4) = 161$	$K_{[1]} = 187$
2	3	1	$K_{[2]11}(3,4) = 20$	$K_{[2]12}(3,4) = 30$	$K_{[2]1}(3) = 50$
		2	$K_{[2]21}(3,4) = 17$	$K_{[2]22}(3,4) = 283$	$K_{[2]2}(3) = 300$
		Total	$K_{[2]1}(4) = 37$	$K_{[2]2}(4) = 313$	$K_{[2]} = 350$

Table 3.11 (4): Lag $h^* = 2$ based transitional table from time $t - h^* = 1$ to $t = 3$ for the maternal smoking versus children asthma status data

			3		
	Time		Category		
Covariate level	Time	Category	1	2	Total
1	1	1	$K_{[1]11}(1,3) = 15$	$K_{[1]12}(1,3) = 16$	$K_{[1]1}(1) = 31$
		2	$K_{[1]21}(1,3) = 20$	$K_{[1]22}(1,3) = 136$	$K_{[1]2}(1) = 156$
		Total	$K_{[1]1}(3) = 35$	$K_{[1]2}(3) = 152$	$K_{[1]} = 187$
2	1	1	$K_{[2]11}(1,3) = 21$	$K_{[2]12}(1,3) = 35$	$K_{[2]1}(1) = 56$
		2	$K_{[2]21}(1,3) = 29$	$K_{[2]22}(1,3) = 265$	$K_{[2]2}(1) = 294$
		Total	$K_{[2]1}(3) = 50$	$K_{[2]2}(3) = 300$	$K_{[2]} = 350$

Table 3.11 (5): Lag $h^* = 2$ based transitional table from time $t - h^* = 2$ to $t = 4$ for the maternal smoking versus children asthma status data

			4		
	Time		Category		
Covariate level	Time	Category	1	2	Total
1	2	1	$K_{[1]11}(2,4) = 14$	$K_{[1]12}(2,4) = 25$	$K_{[1]1}(2) = 39$
		2	$K_{[1]21}(2,4) = 12$	$K_{[1]22}(2,4) = 136$	$K_{[1]2}(2) = 148$
		Total	$K_{[1]1}(4) = 26$	$K_{[1]2}(4) = 161$	$K_{[1]} = 187$
2	2	1	$K_{[2]11}(2,4) = 18$	$K_{[2]12}(2,4) = 34$	$K_{[2]1}(2) = 52$
		2	$K_{[2]21}(2,4) = 19$	$K_{[2]22}(2,4) = 279$	$K_{[2]2}(2) = 298$
		Total	$K_{[2]1}(4) = 37$	$K_{[2]2}(4) = 313$	$K_{[2]} = 350$

Table 3.11 (6): Lag $h^* = 3$ based transitional table from time $t - h^* = 1$ to $t = 4$ for the maternal smoking versus children asthma status data

			4		
	Time		Category		
Covariate level	Time	Category	1	2	Total
1	1	1	$K_{[1]11}(1,4) = 13$	$K_{[1]12}(1,4) = 18$	$K_{[1]1}(1) = 31$
		2	$K_{[1]21}(1,4) = 13$	$K_{[1]22}(1,4) = 143$	$K_{[1]2}(1) = 156$
		Total	$K_{[1]1}(4) = 26$	$K_{[1]2}(4) = 161$	$K_{[1]} = 187$
2	1	1	$K_{[2]11}(1,4) = 18$	$K_{[2]12}(1,4) = 38$	$K_{[2]1}(1) = 56$
		2	$K_{[2]21}(1,4) = 19$	$K_{[2]22}(1,4) = 275$	$K_{[2]2}(1) = 294$
		Total	$K_{[2]1}(4) = 37$	$K_{[2]2}(4) = 313$	$K_{[2]} = 350$

yielding the AR(1) correlation parameter estimate by (3.93) as $\hat{\rho} = 0.5024$. This final estimate of AR(1) correlation parameter yielded the GQL estimates for β_{10} and β_{11} by (3.102)–(3.103) as

$$\hat{\beta}_{10} = -1.8393 \text{ and } \hat{\beta}_{11} = 0.2360,$$

along with their standard errors ($s.e.$) computed by (3.104) as

$$s.e.\hat{\beta}_{10} = 0.1100 \text{ and } s.e.\hat{\beta}_{11} = 0.1770,$$

respectively.

Notice from (3.87) and (3.88) that β_{10} determines the probability for a child with a non-smoking mother to have an asthma attack, whereas both β_{10} and β_{11} play a role to determine the probability of an asthma attack to a child with a smoking mother. By using the aforementioned estimate of β_{10} in (3.88), and the estimates of both β_{10} and β_{11} in (3.87), the probabilities for an asthma attack to these two groups of children were found to be as follows (Table 3.12):

Table 3.12 Observed over the years and fitted stationary probabilities using GQL approach

		Asthma status probability	
Observed/fitted	Covariate level	Yes	No
Fitted	Smoking mother	0.1675	0.8325
	Non-smoking mother	0.1371	0.8639
Observed at $t = 1$	Smoking mother	0.1658	0.8342
	Non-smoking mother	0.1600	0.8400
Observed at $t = 2$	Smoking mother	0.2085	0.7915
	Non-smoking mother	0.1486	0.8514
Observed at $t = 3$	Smoking mother	0.1872	0.8128
	Non-smoking mother	0.1429	0.8571
Observed at $t = 4$	Smoking mother	0.1390	0.8610
	Non-smoking mother	0.1057	0.8943

The fitted probabilities show that the mother's smoking habit has a detrimental effect on the asthma status, and they agree with those results discussed in Sutradhar (2003, Section 5.2).

3.3.1.2 Likelihood Estimation

Because the response of an individual i with covariate level ℓ follows the multinomial (binary in the present case) at any given time t, using the notation from the last section, one may modify the likelihood function for the covariate free case (3.28) to accommodate the covariates as follows. Altogether there are $p+1$ regression parameters which are denoted by $\theta^* = [\beta_{10}, \beta_{11}, \ldots, \beta_{1p}]'$, and ρ is the correlation index parameter involved in the conditional probability relating $y_{i,t-1}$ and y_{it} for all i. Following (3.28), the likelihood function for the present problem may be written as

$$L(\theta^*, \rho) = \Pi_{\ell=1}^{p+1} \Pi_{i\in\ell}^{K} L_{i\in\ell}, \tag{3.105}$$

where

$$L_{i\in\ell} = f_{\ell,1}(y_{i1}) f_{\ell,2}(y_{i2}|y_{i1}) \cdots f_{\ell,T}(y_{iT}|y_{i,T-1}),$$

with

$$\begin{aligned} f_{\ell,1}(y_{i1}) &= [\pi_{[\ell]1}]^{y_{i1}} [\pi_{[\ell]2}]^{1-y_{i1}} \\ &= \begin{cases} \frac{\exp[y_{i1}(\beta_{10}+\beta_{1\ell})]}{1+\exp(\beta_{10}+\beta_{1\ell})} & \text{for } \ell = 1, \ldots, p \\ \frac{\exp[y_{i1}\beta_{10}]}{1+\exp(\beta_{10})}, & \text{for } \ell = p+1, \end{cases} \end{aligned} \tag{3.106}$$

and

$$f_{\ell,t}(y_{it}|y_{i,t-1}) = [\lambda^{(1)}_{it|t-1}(g,\ell)]^{y_{it}}[\lambda^{(2)}_{it|t-1}(g,\ell)]^{1-y_{it}}, \text{ for } t = 2,\ldots,T, \tag{3.107}$$

where

$$\begin{aligned}\lambda^{(1)}_{it|t-1}(g,\ell) &= \pi_{[\ell]1} + \rho(y^{(g)}_{i,t-1} - \pi_{[\ell]1})\\ \lambda^{(2)}_{it|t-1}(g,\ell) &= 1 - \lambda^{(1)}_{it|t-1}(g,\ell).\end{aligned} \tag{3.108}$$

Hence, by (3.105), the log likelihood function is given by

$$\begin{aligned}\mathrm{Log}L(\theta^*,\rho) &= \sum_{\ell=1}^{p+1}\sum_{i\in\ell}^{K}[y_{i1}\log \pi_{[\ell]1} + (1-y_{i1})\log \pi_{[\ell]2}]\\ &+ \sum_{\ell=1}^{p+1}\sum_{g=1}^{2}\sum_{i\in(g,\ell)}^{K}\sum_{t=2}^{T}[y_{it}\log \lambda^{(1)}_{it|t-1}(g,\ell)\\ &+ (1-y_{it})\log \lambda^{(2)}_{it|t-1}(g,\ell)].\end{aligned} \tag{3.109}$$

Note that because by (3.108), $\lambda^{(1)}_{it|t-1}(1,\ell)$ and $\lambda^{(1)}_{it|t-1}(2,\ell)$ are free from i and t, for convenience, we suppress the subscripts from these conditional probabilities and use $\lambda^{(1)}(2,\ell)$ for $\lambda^{(1)}_{it|t-1}(2,\ell)$, for example. Next by using the cell frequencies from the contingency Table 3.9, we express the log likelihood function (3.109) as

$$\begin{aligned}\mathrm{Log}\, L(\theta^*,\rho) = \sum_{\ell=1}^{p+1}\Big[\{K_{[\ell]1}(1)\log \pi_{[\ell]1} + K_{[\ell]2}(1)\log(1-\pi_{[\ell]1})\}\\ + \log \lambda^{(1)}(1,\ell)\sum_{t=2}^{T}K_{[\ell]11}(t-1,t) + \log \lambda^{(2)}(1,\ell)\sum_{t=2}^{T}K_{[\ell]12}(t-1,t)\\ + \log \lambda^{(1)}(2,\ell)\sum_{t=2}^{T}K_{[\ell]21}(t-1,t) + \log \lambda^{(2)}(2,\ell)\sum_{t=2}^{T}K_{[\ell]22}(t-1,t)\Big],\end{aligned} \tag{3.110}$$

where by (3.108),

$$\begin{aligned}&\lambda^{(1)}(1,\ell) = \pi_{[\ell]1} + \rho(1-\pi_{[\ell]1}),\ \lambda^{(2)}(1,\ell) = 1-\lambda^{(1)}(1,\ell) = (1-\rho)(1-\pi_{[\ell]1})\\ &\lambda^{(1)}(2,\ell) = (1-\rho)\pi_{[\ell]1},\ \lambda^{(2)}(2,\ell) = 1-\lambda^{(1)}(2,\ell) = 1-(1-\rho)\pi_{[\ell]1}.\end{aligned} \tag{3.111}$$

This log likelihood function in (3.110) is maximized in the next section to estimate the parameters θ^* and ρ.

3.3.1.2.1 Likelihood Estimating Equations

Note that as opposed to the covariate free likelihood estimation discussed in Sect. 3.2.2.1.1, it is now convenient to use the notation

$$\pi_{[\ell]1} = \frac{\exp(x'_{[\ell]1}\theta^*)}{1+\exp(x'_{[\ell]1}\theta^*)}, \tag{3.112}$$

as in (3.99)–(3.100), where $\theta^* = (\beta_{10}, \beta_{11}, \ldots, \beta_{1p})'$, and

$$x'_{[\ell]1} = \left(1\ 01'_{\ell-1}\ 1\ 01'_{p-\ell}\right) \text{ for } \ell = 1, \ldots, p; \text{ and } x'_{[p+1]1} = \left(1\ 01'_{p}\right).$$

The following derivatives, first, with respect to θ^* and then with respect to ρ will be helpful to write the likelihood estimating equations for θ^* and ρ, respectively.

Derivatives with Respect to θ^* and ρ

It follows from (3.110)–(3.112) that

$$\begin{aligned}
\frac{\partial \pi_{[\ell]1}}{\partial \theta^*} &= \left[\pi_{[\ell]1}(1-\pi_{[\ell]1})\right] x_{[\ell]1}, \\
\frac{\partial \lambda^{(1)}(1,\ell)}{\partial \theta^*} &= \frac{\partial \lambda^{(1)}(2,\ell)}{\partial \theta^*} = (1-\rho)\left[\pi_{[\ell]1}(1-\pi_{[\ell]1})\right] x_{[\ell]1}, \\
\frac{\partial \lambda^{(2)}(1,\ell)}{\partial \theta^*} &= \frac{\partial \lambda^{(2)}(2,\ell)}{\partial \theta^*} = -(1-\rho)\left[\pi_{[\ell]1}(1-\pi_{[\ell]1})\right] x_{[\ell]1},
\end{aligned} \tag{3.113}$$

and

$$\begin{aligned}
\frac{\partial \pi_{[\ell]1}}{\partial \rho} &= 0, \\
\frac{\partial \lambda^{(1)}(1,\ell)}{\partial \rho} &= (1-\pi_{[\ell]1}); \quad \frac{\partial \lambda^{(2)}(1,\ell)}{\partial \rho} = -(1-\pi_{[\ell]1}), \\
\frac{\partial \lambda^{(1)}(2,\ell)}{\partial \rho} &= -\pi_{[\ell]1}; \quad \frac{\partial \lambda^{(2)}(2,\ell)}{\partial \rho} = \pi_{[\ell]1}.
\end{aligned} \tag{3.114}$$

By (3.113), it then follows from (3.110) that the likelihood estimating equation for θ^* has the form

$$\frac{\partial \text{Log}\, L(\theta^*,\rho)}{\partial \theta^*} = \sum_{\ell=1}^{p+1} \left[K_{[\ell]1}(1) - \pi_{[\ell]1}K_{[\ell]}\right] x_{[\ell]1}$$
$$+ (1-\rho)\sum_{\ell=1}^{p+1}\left[\pi_{[\ell]1}(1-\pi_{[\ell]1})\left\{\frac{\sum_{t=2}^{T} K_{[\ell]11}(t-1,t)}{\lambda^{(1)}(1,\ell)} - \frac{\sum_{t=2}^{T} K_{[\ell]12}(t-1,t)}{\lambda^{(2)}(1,\ell)}\right.\right.$$
$$\left.\left. + \frac{\sum_{t=2}^{T} K_{[\ell]21}(t-1,t)}{\lambda^{(1)}(2,\ell)} - \frac{\sum_{t=2}^{T} K_{[\ell]22}(t-1,t)}{\lambda^{(2)}(2,\ell)}\right\} x_{[\ell]1}\right] = 0. \quad (3.115)$$

Similarly, the likelihood estimating equation for ρ has the form

$$\frac{\partial \text{Log}\, L(\theta^*,\rho)}{\partial \rho} = \sum_{\ell=1}^{p+1}\left[\frac{\sum_{t=2}^{T} K_{[\ell]11}(t-1,t)}{\lambda^{(1)}(1,\ell)} - \frac{\sum_{t=2}^{T} K_{[\ell]12}(t-1,t)}{\lambda^{(2)}(1,\ell)}\right]$$
$$- \sum_{\ell=1}^{p+1}\left[\pi_{[\ell]1}\left\{\frac{\sum_{t=2}^{T} K_{[\ell]11}(t-1,t)}{\lambda^{(1)}(1,\ell)} - \frac{\sum_{t=2}^{T} K_{[\ell]12}(t-1,t)}{\lambda^{(2)}(1,\ell)}\right.\right.$$
$$\left.\left. + \frac{\sum_{t=2}^{T} K_{[\ell]21}(t-1,t)}{\lambda^{(1)}(2,\ell)} - \frac{\sum_{t=2}^{T} K_{[\ell]22}(t-1,t)}{\lambda^{(2)}(2,\ell)}\right\}\right] = 0. \quad (3.116)$$

These likelihood equations (3.115)–(3.116) may be solved iteratively by using the iterative equations for θ^* and ρ given by

$$\hat{\theta}^*(r+1) = \hat{\theta}^*(r) - \left[\left\{\frac{\partial^2 \text{Log}\, L(\theta^*,\rho)}{\partial \theta^{*\prime}\partial \theta^*}\right\}^{-1} \frac{\partial \text{Log}\, L(\theta^*,\rho)}{\partial \theta^*}\right]_{|\theta^*=\hat{\theta}^*(r)}; \ (p+1)\times 1, \quad (3.117)$$

and

$$\hat{\rho}(r+1) = \hat{\rho}(r) - \left[\left\{\frac{\partial^2 \text{Log}\, L(\theta^*,\rho)}{\partial \rho^2}\right\}^{-1} \frac{\partial \text{Log}\, L(\theta^*,\rho)}{\partial \rho}\right]_{|\rho=\hat{\rho}(r)}, \quad (3.118)$$

respectively. In (3.117), the $(p+1)\times(p+1)$ second derivative matrix has the formula given by

$$\frac{\partial^2 \text{Log}\, L(\theta^*,\rho)}{\partial \theta^{*\prime}\partial \theta^*} = -\sum_{\ell=1}^{p+1}\left[\pi_{[\ell]1}(1-\pi_{[\ell]1})K_{[\ell]}\right] x_{[\ell]1}x'_{[\ell]1}$$
$$+ (1-\rho)\sum_{\ell=1}^{p+1}\left[\pi_{[\ell]1}(1-\pi_{[\ell]1})(1-2\pi_{[\ell]1})\left\{\frac{\sum_{t=2}^{T} K_{[\ell]11}(t-1,t)}{\lambda^{(1)}(1,\ell)} - \frac{\sum_{t=2}^{T} K_{[\ell]12}(t-1,t)}{\lambda^{(2)}(1,\ell)}\right.\right.$$
$$\left.\left. + \frac{\sum_{t=2}^{T} K_{[\ell]21}(t-1,t)}{\lambda^{(1)}(2,\ell)} - \frac{\sum_{t=2}^{T} K_{[\ell]22}(t-1,t)}{\lambda^{(2)}(2,\ell)}\right\} x_{[\ell]1}x'_{[\ell]1}\right]$$

$$- (1-\rho)^2 \sum_{\ell=1}^{p+1} \left[\{\pi_{[\ell]1}(1-\pi_{[\ell]1})\}^2 \left\{ \frac{\sum_{t=2}^{T} K_{[\ell]11}(t-1,t)}{\{\lambda^{(1)}(1,\ell)\}^2} + \frac{\sum_{t=2}^{T} K_{[\ell]12}(t-1,t)}{\{\lambda^{(2)}(1,\ell)\}^2} \right.\right.$$
$$\left.\left. + \frac{\sum_{t=2}^{T} K_{[\ell]21}(t-1,t)}{\{\lambda^{(1)}(2,\ell)\}^2} + \frac{\sum_{t=2}^{T} K_{[\ell]22}(t-1,t)}{\{\lambda^{(2)}(2,\ell)\}^2} \right\} x_{[\ell]1} x'_{[\ell]1} \right] \tag{3.119}$$

Similarly, by using (3.111), it follows that the scalar second derivative in (3.118) has the formula

$$\frac{\partial^2 \text{Log}\, L(\theta^*,\rho)}{\partial \rho^2} = -\sum_{\ell=1}^{p+1} (1-\pi_{[\ell]1}) \left[\frac{\sum_{t=2}^{T} K_{[\ell]11}(t-1,t)}{\{\lambda^{(1)}(1,\ell)\}^2} + \frac{\sum_{t=2}^{T} K_{[\ell]12}(t-1,t)}{\{\lambda^{(2)}(1,\ell)\}^2} \right]$$
$$+ \sum_{\ell=1}^{p+1} \pi_{[\ell]1}(1-\pi_{[\ell]1}) \left[\frac{\sum_{t=2}^{T} K_{[\ell]11}(t-1,t)}{\{\lambda^{(1)}(1,\ell)\}^2} + \frac{\sum_{t=2}^{T} K_{[\ell]12}(t-1,t)}{\{\lambda^{(2)}(1,\ell)\}^2} \right]$$
$$- \sum_{\ell=1}^{p+1} \{\pi_{[\ell]1}\}^2 \left[\frac{\sum_{t=2}^{T} K_{[\ell]21}(t-1,t)}{\{\lambda^{(1)}(2,\ell)\}^2} + \frac{\sum_{t=2}^{T} K_{[\ell]22}(t-1,t)}{\{\lambda^{(2)}(2,\ell)\}^2} \right]. \tag{3.120}$$

3.3.1.2.2 Illustration 3.7 : Mothers Smoking Effect on Longitudinal Asthma Status: Likelihood Approach for LDCP Regression Model

The likelihood estimates for $\theta^* = (\beta_{10}, \beta_{11})'$ and ρ were obtained as follows. Using initial values

$$\hat{\theta}^*(0) = (\hat{\beta}_{10}(0) = 0.0, \hat{\beta}_{11}(0) = 0.0)' \text{ and } \hat{\rho}(0) = 0.0,$$

we first obtain the first step estimate $\hat{\theta}^*(1)$ by (3.117). This first step estimate of θ^* and initial value $\hat{\rho}(0) = 0.0$ were then used in (3.118) to obtain the first step estimate of ρ, that is $\hat{\rho}(1)$, which was in turn used in (3.117) to obtain improved estimate for θ^*. This whole operation constitutes a cycle. This cycle of iterations continued until convergence. Only 4 cycles of iterations provide the final marginal likelihood estimates (MMLE) as

$$\hat{\theta}^*_{MMLE} = (\hat{\beta}_{10,MMLE} = -1.8317, \hat{\beta}_{11,MMLE} = 0.2410)' \text{ and } \hat{\rho}_{MMLE} = 0.3836.$$

These regression estimates are similar but slightly different than those found by the GQL approach in Sect. 3.3.1.1.3. However the GQL approach produced $\hat{\rho} = 0.5024$, which is considerably different than $\hat{\rho}_{MMLE} = 0.3836$. Thus, the GQL and MLE approaches would produce different estimates for conditional probabilities, and hence for joint cell probabilities, yielding slightly different estimates for marginal probabilities. The aforementioned MLE estimates for regression effects produces the marginal probabilities as in Table 3.13, which are slightly different than those found in Table 3.12 by the GQL approach.

Table 3.13 Fitted stationary probabilities using MMLE and JMLE approaches

		Asthma status probability	
Fitting approach	Covariate level	Yes	No
MMLE	Smoking mother	0.1693	0.8307
	Non-smoking mother	0.1380	0.8620
JMLE	Smoking mother	0.1693	0.8307
	Non-smoking mother	0.1380	0.8620

To obtain the joint maximum likelihood estimates (JMLE) for the parameters (θ^*, ρ), instead of (3.117)–(3.118), one uses the iterative equation

$$\begin{pmatrix} \hat{\theta}^*(r+1) \\ \hat{\rho}(r+1) \end{pmatrix} = \begin{pmatrix} \hat{\theta}^*(r) \\ \hat{\rho}(r) \end{pmatrix}$$

$$- \left[\begin{pmatrix} \left\{ \frac{\partial^2 \text{Log}\, L(\theta^*,\rho)}{\partial \theta^{*\prime} \partial \theta^*} \right\} & \left\{ \frac{\partial^2 \text{Log}\, L(\theta^*,\rho)}{\partial \rho \partial \theta^*} \right\} \\ \cdot & \left\{ \frac{\partial^2 \text{Log}\, L(\theta^*,\rho)}{\partial \rho^2} \right\} \end{pmatrix}^{-1} \begin{pmatrix} \frac{\partial \text{Log}\, L(\theta^*,\rho)}{\partial \theta^*} \\ \frac{\partial \text{Log}\, L(\theta^*,\rho)}{\partial \rho} \end{pmatrix} \right]_{|\theta^* = \hat{\theta}^*(r), \rho = \hat{\rho}(r)},$$

where

$$\begin{aligned} \frac{\partial^2 \text{Log}\, L(\theta^*,\rho)}{\partial \theta^* \partial \rho} &= -\sum_{\ell=1}^{p+1} \left[\pi_{[\ell]1}(1-\pi_{[\ell]1}) \left\{ \frac{\sum_{t=2}^T K_{[\ell]11}(t-1,t)}{\lambda^{(1)}(1,\ell)} - \frac{\sum_{t=2}^T K_{[\ell]12}(t-1,t)}{\lambda^{(2)}(1,\ell)} \right. \right. \\ &\quad \left. \left. + \frac{\sum_{t=2}^T K_{[\ell]21}(t-1,t)}{\lambda^{(1)}(2,\ell)} - \frac{\sum_{t=2}^T K_{[\ell]22}(t-1,t)}{\lambda^{(2)}(2,\ell)} \right\} x_{[\ell]1} \right] \\ &\quad + (1-\rho) \sum_{\ell=1}^{p+1} \left[\pi_{[\ell]1}(1-\pi_{[\ell]1}) \left\{ \left(\frac{\sum_{t=2}^T K_{[\ell]11}(t-1,t)}{\{\lambda^{(1)}(1,\ell)\}^2} + \frac{\sum_{t=2}^T K_{[\ell]12}(t-1,t)}{\{\lambda^{(2)}(1,\ell)\}^2} \right. \right. \right. \\ &\quad \left. + \frac{\sum_{t=2}^T K_{[\ell]21}(t-1,t)}{\{\lambda^{(1)}(2,\ell)\}^2} + \frac{\sum_{t=2}^T K_{[\ell]22}(t-1,t)}{\{\lambda^{(2)}(2,\ell)\}^2} \right) \pi_{[\ell]1} \\ &\quad \left. \left. - \left(\frac{\sum_{t=2}^T K_{[\ell]11}(t-1,t)}{\{\lambda^{(1)}(1,\ell)\}^2} + \frac{\sum_{t=2}^T K_{[\ell]12}(t-1,t)}{\{\lambda^{(2)}(1,\ell)\}^2} \right) \right\} x_{[\ell]1} \right]. \end{aligned}$$

Using the initial values

$$\hat{\theta}^*(0) = (\hat{\beta}_{10}(0) = 0.0, \hat{\beta}_{11}(0) = 0.0)' \text{ and } \hat{\rho}(0) = 0.0,$$

the aforementioned iterative equations in 5 cycles of iterations produced the JMLE as

$$\hat{\theta}^*_{JMLE} = (\hat{\beta}_{10,JMLE} = -1.8317, \hat{\beta}_{11,JMLE} = 0.2410)' \text{ and } \hat{\rho}_{JMLE} = 0.3836,$$

which are the same as the MMLE Thus for this particular data set, the MMLE and JMLE produce the same probability estimates as shown in Table 3.13.

3.3.2 BDL Regression Model and Estimation of Parameters

The probabilities at initial time point $t = 1$ have the same formulas (3.89)–(3.90) under both LDCP and this BDL models involving covariates, that is,

$$P[y_{i1} = y_{i1}^{(j)} | i \in \ell] = \pi_{[(i \in \ell]1)j} \equiv \pi_{[\ell]j}$$
$$= \begin{cases} \frac{\exp(\beta_{10}+\beta_{1\ell})}{1+\exp(\beta_{10}+\beta_{1\ell})} & \text{for } j = 1;\ \ell = 1,\ldots,p \\ \frac{1}{1+\exp(\beta_{10}+\beta_{1\ell})} & \text{for } j = J = 2;\ \ell = 1,\ldots,p, \end{cases} \quad (3.121)$$

and for $\ell = p+1$, these probabilities have the formulas

$$P[y_{i1} = y_{i1}^{(j)} | i \in (p+1)] = = \pi_{(i \in (p+1))1)j} \equiv \pi_{[p+1]j}$$
$$= \begin{cases} \frac{\exp(\beta_{10})}{1+\exp(\beta_{10})} & \text{for } j = 1 \\ \frac{1}{1+\exp(\beta_{10})} & \text{for } j = J = 2. \end{cases} \quad (3.122)$$

However, for $t = 2,\ldots,T$, the conditional probability, unlike the LDCP model (3.90)–(3.91) (see also (3.24)), has the dynamic logit form given by

$$\eta_{it|t-1}^{(j)}(g,\ell) = P\left(Y_{it} = y_{it}^{(j)} \middle| Y_{i,t-1} = y_{i,t-1}^{(g)}, i \in \ell\right)$$
$$= \begin{cases} \frac{\exp\left[\beta_{10}+\beta_{1\ell}+\gamma_1 y_{i,t-1}^{(g)}\right]}{1+\exp\left[\beta_{10}+\beta_{1\ell}+\gamma_1 y_{i,t-1}^{(g)}\right]}, & \text{for } j = 1; g = 1,2; \ell = 1,\ldots,p \\ \frac{1}{1+\exp\left[\beta_{10}+\beta_{1\ell}+\gamma_1 y_{i,t-1}^{(g)}\right]}, & \text{for } j = J = 2; g = 1,2; \ell = 1,\ldots,p, \end{cases} \quad (3.123)$$

where γ_1 denotes the dynamic dependence parameter, which is neither a correlation nor an odds ratio parameter. But it is clear that the correlations of the repeated multinomial responses will be function of this γ_1 parameter. For $\ell = p+1$, these conditional probabilities have the formulas

$$\eta_{it|t-1}^{(j)}(g,p+1) = P\left(Y_{it} = y_{it}^{(j)} \middle| Y_{i,t-1} = y_{i,t-1}^{(g)}, i \in \ell\right)$$
$$= \begin{cases} \frac{\exp\left[\beta_{10}+\gamma_1 y_{i,t-1}^{(g)}\right]}{1+\exp\left[\beta_{10}+\gamma_1 y_{i,t-1}^{(g)}\right]}, & \text{for } j = 1; g = 1,2; \ell = p+1 \\ \frac{1}{1+\exp\left[\beta_{10}+\gamma_1 y_{i,t-1}^{(g)}\right]}, & \text{for } j = J = 2; g = 1,2; \ell = p+1. \end{cases} \quad (3.124)$$

Define

$$\tilde{\eta}_{[\ell]1} = \begin{cases} \frac{\exp(\beta_{10}+\beta_{1\ell}+\gamma_1)}{1+\exp(\beta_{10}+\beta_{1\ell}+\gamma_1)}, & \text{for } \ell = 1,\ldots,p \\ \frac{\exp(\beta_{10}+\gamma_1)}{1+\exp(\beta_{10}+\gamma_1)}, & \text{for } \ell = p+1, \end{cases} \tag{3.125}$$

and

$$\eta^*_{[\ell]1} = \begin{cases} \frac{\exp(\beta_{10}+\beta_{1\ell})}{1+\exp(\beta_{10}+\beta_{1\ell})}, & \text{for } \ell = 1,\ldots,p \\ \frac{\exp(\beta_{10})}{1+\exp(\beta_{10})}, & \text{for } \ell = p+1. \end{cases} \tag{3.126}$$

For the individuals with covariate level ℓ, it then follows that (see also (3.72)) the marginal probabilities at time $t = 1,\ldots,T$, are given by

$$\begin{aligned} E[Y_{it}|i \in \ell] &= \pi_{([\ell]t)1} = Pr[Y_{it} = y_{it}^{(1)}|i \in \ell] \\ &= \begin{cases} \eta^*_{[\ell]1}, & \text{for } t = 1 \\ \eta^*_{[\ell]1} + \pi_{([\ell](t-1))1}[\tilde{\eta}_{[\ell]1} - \eta^*_{[\ell]1}], & \text{for } t = 2,\ldots,T, \end{cases} \end{aligned} \tag{3.127}$$

(Sutradhar and Farrell 2007) for $i = 1,\ldots,K_{[\ell]}$.

Note that as the marginal probabilities in (3.127) are covariate level (ℓ) dependent, the lag correlations can be different for individuals belonging to different groups corresponding to their covariate levels. To be specific, for $u < t$, the $t-u$ lag correlations under the ℓ-th group (that is, for individuals $i \in \ell$) have the formulas

$$\begin{aligned} \rho_{\{[\ell],t-u\}} &= \text{corr}\{(Y_{iu}, Y_{it})|i \in \ell\} = \sqrt{\frac{\pi_{([\ell]u)1}(1-\pi_{([\ell]u)1})}{\pi_{([\ell]t)1}(1-\pi_{([\ell]t)1})}}\, \Pi_{k=u+1}^{t}(\tilde{\eta}_{[\ell]1} - \eta^*_{[\ell]1}) \\ &= \sqrt{\frac{\pi_{([\ell]u)1}(1-\pi_{([\ell]u)1})}{\pi_{([\ell]t)1}(1-\pi_{([\ell]t)1})}} \left(\tilde{\eta}_{[\ell]1} - \eta^*_{[\ell]1}\right)^{t-u}, \text{ for all } i \in \ell, \text{ and } u < t, \end{aligned} \tag{3.128}$$

where the marginal probability $\pi_{([\ell]t)1}$ at time t is given by (3.127).

3.3.2.1 Likelihood Estimation

Similar to the LDCP model, denote all regression parameters involved in the BDL regression model (3.121)–(3.124) by θ^*. That is, $\theta^* = [\beta_{10}, \beta_{11}, \ldots, \beta_{1p}]'$. Note however that γ_1 in the present model describes the dynamic dependence parameter in a logit function, whereas ρ was used in (3.91) as a dynamic dependence parameter in a linear conditional probability function. Thus, similar to (3.105), one writes the likelihood function in θ^* and γ_1 as

$$L(\theta^*, \gamma_1) = \Pi_{\ell=1}^{p+1} \Pi_{i\in\ell}^{K} L_{i\in\ell}, \tag{3.129}$$

where

$$L_{i\in\ell} = f_{\ell,1}(y_{i1}) f_{\ell,2}(y_{it}|y_{i1}) \cdots f_{\ell,T}(y_{iT}|y_{i,T-1}),$$

with

$$f_{\ell,1}(y_{i1}) = [\pi_{[\ell]1}]^{y_{i1}} [\pi_{[\ell]2}]^{1-y_{i1}} = \begin{cases} \frac{\exp[y_{i1}(\beta_{10}+\beta_{1\ell})]}{1+\exp(\beta_{10}+\beta_{1\ell})} \text{ for } \ell = 1,\ldots,p \\ \frac{\exp[y_{i1}\beta_{10}]}{1+\exp(\beta_{10})}, \text{ for } \ell = p+1, \end{cases} \quad (3.130)$$

and

$$f_{\ell,t}(y_{it}|y_{i,t-1}) = [\eta^{(1)}_{it|t-1}(g,\ell)]^{y_{it}} [\eta^{(2)}_{it|t-1}(g,\ell)]^{1-y_{it}}, \text{ for } t = 2,\ldots,T, \quad (3.131)$$

where $\eta^{(1)}_{it|t-1}(g,\ell)$ and $\eta^{(2)}_{it|t-1}(g,\ell) = 1 - \eta^{(1)}_{it|t-1}(g,\ell)$ are given by (3.123) for $\ell = 1,\ldots,p$, and by (3.124) for $\ell = p+1$.

Hence, by (3.129), the log likelihood function is given by

$$\text{Log}L(\theta^*,\gamma_1) = \sum_{\ell=1}^{p+1}\sum_{i\in\ell}^{K}[y_{i1}\log\pi_{[\ell]1} + (1-y_{i1})\log\pi_{[\ell]2}]$$
$$+\sum_{\ell=1}^{p+1}\sum_{g=1}^{2}\sum_{i\in(g,\ell)}^{K}\sum_{t=2}^{T}[y_{it}\log\eta^{(1)}_{it|t-1}(g,\ell) + (1-y_{it})\log\eta^{(2)}_{it|t-1}(g,\ell)]. \quad (3.132)$$

Next because $\eta^{(1)}_{it|t-1}(1,\ell)$ and $\eta^{(1)}_{it|t-1}(2,\ell)$ are free from i and t, by using the cell frequencies from the contingency Tables 3.8 and 3.9, the log likelihood function (3.132) may be expressed as

$$\text{Log }L(\theta^*,\gamma_1) = \sum_{\ell=1}^{p+1}\Big[\{K_{[\ell]1}(1)\log\pi_{[\ell]1} + K_{[\ell]2}(1)\log(1-\pi_{[\ell]1})\}$$
$$+\log\eta^{(1)}(1,\ell)\sum_{t=2}^{T}K_{[\ell]11}(t-1,t) + \log\eta^{(2)}(1,\ell)\sum_{t=2}^{T}K_{[\ell]12}(t-1,t)$$
$$+\log\eta^{(1)}(2,\ell)\sum_{t=2}^{T}K_{[\ell]21}(t-1,t) + \log\eta^{(2)}(2,\ell)\sum_{t=2}^{T}K_{[\ell]22}(t-1,t)\Big], \quad (3.133)$$

where by (3.121)–(3.122) and (3.125)–(3.126),

$$\pi_{[\ell]1} = \eta^{(1)}(2,\ell) = \eta^*_{[\ell]1} = \begin{cases} \frac{\exp(\beta_{10}+\beta_{1\ell})}{1+\exp(\beta_{10}+\beta_{1\ell})}, \text{ for } \ell = 1,\ldots,p \\ \frac{\exp(\beta_{10})}{1+\exp(\beta_{10})}, \quad \text{for } \ell = p+1, \end{cases} \quad (3.134)$$

and

$$\eta^{(1)}(1,\ell) = \tilde{\eta}_{[\ell]1} = \begin{cases} \frac{\exp(\beta_{10}+\beta_{1\ell}+\gamma_1)}{1+\exp(\beta_{10}+\beta_{1\ell}+\gamma_1)}, & \text{for } \ell = 1,\ldots,p \\ \frac{\exp(\beta_{10}+\gamma_1)}{1+\exp(\beta_{10}+\gamma_1)}, & \text{for } \ell = p+1. \end{cases} \tag{3.135}$$

3.3.2.1.1 Likelihood Estimating Equations

Note that unlike the parameters θ^* and ρ in the LDCP model (3.90)–(3.91), θ^* and γ_1 in the present BDL model (3.121)–(3.124) appear in the same exponent used to define the associated probabilities. Consequently, for computational convenience, one may treat the dynamic dependence parameter γ_1 as a regression parameter and estimate θ^* and γ_1 jointly. Furthermore, the exponents in the probabilities may be expressed in standard linear regression form in the manner similar to that of (3.112) used under the likelihood estimation approach. Remark that the likelihood estimation for the regression parameter β_{10} and dynamic dependence parameter γ_1 under the covariate free BDL model discussed in Sect. 3.2.4.2.1 could be done jointly using similar linear regression form for the exponents, but they were estimated marginally because of smaller (scalar) dimension for regression effects.

We now turn back to the probability functions (3.134)–(3.135) and re-express them as follows using the linear regression form in the exponents. Note however that there are two groups ($g = 1,2$) of probability functions and consequently we define two regression variables $x_{[\ell]1}(1)$ and $x_{[\ell]1}(2)$ to represent these groups. That is, for the joint estimation of the elements of parameter vector

$$\tilde{\theta} = [\beta_{10}, \beta_{11}, \ldots, \beta_{1\ell}, \ldots, \beta_{1p}, \gamma_1]',$$

we re-express the functions in (3.135) and (3.134), in terms of $\tilde{\theta}$ as

$$\eta^{(1)}(1,\ell) = \tilde{\eta}_{[\ell]1} = \frac{\exp(x'_{[\ell]1}(1)\tilde{\theta})}{1+\exp(x'_{[\ell]1}(1)\tilde{\theta})}, \tag{3.136}$$

and

$$\pi_{[\ell]1} = \eta^{(1)}(2,\ell) = \eta^*_{[\ell]1} = \frac{\exp(x'_{[\ell]1}(2)\tilde{\theta})}{1+\exp(x'_{[\ell]1}(2)\tilde{\theta})}, \tag{3.137}$$

respectively, where

$$x'_{[\ell]1}(1) = \begin{cases} \begin{pmatrix} 1 \; 01'_{\ell-1} \; 1 \; 01'_{p-\ell} \; 1 \end{pmatrix}, & \text{for } \ell = 1,\ldots,p \\ \begin{pmatrix} 1 \; 01'_p \; 1 \end{pmatrix}, & \text{for } \ell = p+1, \end{cases} \tag{3.138}$$

and

$$x'_{[\ell]1}(2) = \begin{cases} \left(1\ 01'_{\ell-1}\ 1\ 01'_{p-\ell}\ 0\right), & \text{for } \ell = 1,\ldots,p \\ \left(1\ 01'_{p}\ 0\right), & \text{for } \ell = p+1. \end{cases} \tag{3.139}$$

Notice that

$$\begin{aligned} \frac{\partial \pi_{[\ell]1}}{\partial \tilde{\theta}} = \frac{\partial \eta^{(1)}(2,\ell)}{\partial \tilde{\theta}} &= \frac{\partial \eta^*_{[\ell]1}}{\partial \tilde{\theta}} \\ &= \eta^*_{[\ell]1}[1-\eta^*_{[\ell]1}]x_{[\ell]1}(2), \end{aligned}$$

and

$$\begin{aligned} \frac{\partial \eta^{(1)}(1,\ell)}{\partial \tilde{\theta}} &= \frac{\partial \tilde{\eta}_{[\ell]1}}{\partial \tilde{\theta}} \\ &= \tilde{\eta}_{[\ell]1}[1-\tilde{\eta}_{[\ell]1}]x_{[\ell]1}(1). \end{aligned}$$

Consequently, it follows from (3.133) that the likelihood estimating equation for $\tilde{\theta}$ has the form

$$\begin{aligned} \frac{\partial \text{Log}\, L(\theta^*,\gamma_1)}{\partial \tilde{\theta}} &= \sum_{\ell=1}^{p+1} \left[K_{[\ell]1}(1) - \pi_{[\ell]1}K_{[\ell]}\right] x_{[\ell]1}(2) \\ &+ \sum_{\ell=1}^{p+1}\left[\tilde{\eta}_{[\ell]1}(1-\tilde{\eta}_{[\ell]1})\left\{\frac{\sum_{t=2}^{T} K_{[\ell]11}(t-1,t)}{\eta^{(1)}(1,\ell)} - \frac{\sum_{t=2}^{T} K_{[\ell]12}(t-1,t)}{\eta^{(2)}(1,\ell)}\right\} x_{[\ell]1}(1)\right] \\ &+ \sum_{\ell=1}^{p+1}\left[\eta^*_{[\ell]1}(1-\eta^*_{[\ell]1})\left\{\frac{\sum_{t=2}^{T} K_{[\ell]21}(t-1,t)}{\eta^{(1)}(2,\ell)}\right.\right. \\ &- \left.\left.\frac{\sum_{t=2}^{T} K_{[\ell]22}(t-1,t)}{\eta^{(2)}(2,\ell)}\right\} x_{[\ell]1}(2)\right] = 0. \end{aligned} \tag{3.140}$$

These likelihood equations in (3.140) may be solved iteratively by using the iterative equations for $\tilde{\theta}$ given by

$$\hat{\tilde{\theta}}(r+1) = \hat{\tilde{\theta}}(r) - \left[\left\{\frac{\partial^2 \text{Log}\, L(\theta^*,\gamma_1)}{\partial \tilde{\theta}' \partial \tilde{\theta}}\right\}^{-1} \frac{\partial \text{Log}\, L(\theta^*,\gamma_1)}{\partial \tilde{\theta}}\right]_{|\tilde{\theta}=\hat{\tilde{\theta}}(r)} ;\ (p+2)\times 1. \tag{3.141}$$

In (3.141), the $(p+2)\times(p+2)$ second derivative matrix has the formula given by

$$\frac{\partial^2 \text{Log}\, L(\theta^*,\gamma_1)}{\partial \tilde{\theta}' \partial \tilde{\theta}} = -\sum_{\ell=1}^{p+1}\left[\pi_{[\ell]1}(1-\pi_{[\ell]1})K_{[\ell]}\right] x_{[\ell]1}(2)x'_{[\ell]1}(2)$$

$$+\sum_{\ell=1}^{p+1}\left[\tilde{\eta}_{[\ell]1}(1-\tilde{\eta}_{[\ell]1})(1-2\tilde{\eta}_{[\ell]1})\left\{\frac{\sum_{t=2}^{T}K_{[\ell]11}(t-1,t)}{\eta^{(1)}(1,\ell)}-\frac{\sum_{t=2}^{T}K_{[\ell]12}(t-1,t)}{\eta^{(2)}(1,\ell)}\right\}x_{[\ell]1}(1)x'_{[\ell]1}(1)\right]$$
$$-\sum_{\ell=1}^{p+1}\left[\{\tilde{\eta}_{[\ell]1}(1-\tilde{\eta}_{[\ell]1})\}^2\left\{\frac{\sum_{t=2}^{T}K_{[\ell]11}(t-1,t)}{\{\eta^{(1)}(1,\ell)\}^2}+\frac{\sum_{t=2}^{T}K_{[\ell]12}(t-1,t)}{\{\eta^{(2)}(1,\ell)\}^2}\right\}x_{[\ell]1}(1)x'_{[\ell]1}(1)\right]$$
$$+\sum_{\ell=1}^{p+1}\left[\eta^*_{[\ell]1}(1-\eta^*_{[\ell]1})(1-2\eta^*_{[\ell]1})\left\{\frac{\sum_{t=2}^{T}K_{[\ell]21}(t-1,t)}{\eta^{(1)}(2,\ell)}-\frac{\sum_{t=2}^{T}K_{[\ell]22}(t-1,t)}{\eta^{(2)}(2,\ell)}\right\}x_{[\ell]1}(2)x'_{[\ell]1}(2)\right]$$
$$-\sum_{\ell=1}^{p+1}\left[\{\eta^*_{[\ell]1}(1-\eta^*_{[\ell]1})\}^2\left\{\frac{\sum_{t=2}^{T}K_{[\ell]21}(t-1,t)}{\{\eta^{(1)}(2,\ell)\}^2}+\frac{\sum_{t=2}^{T}K_{[\ell]22}(t-1,t)}{\{\eta^{(2)}(2,\ell)\}^2}\right\}x_{[\ell]1}(2)x'_{[\ell]1}(2)\right]. \tag{3.142}$$

3.3.2.1.2 Illustration 3.8 : Mothers Smoking Effect on Longitudinal Asthma Status: Likelihood Approach for BDL Regression Model

Under the LDCP regression model (3.89)–(3.92), the marginal probabilities at $p+1$ level of covariates are determined only by the regression parameters $\beta_{10};\ \beta_{11},\ldots,\beta_{1\ell},\ldots,\beta_{1p}$ which were however estimated in Sect. 3.3.1.2.1 by exploiting the AR(1) correlation parameter ρ under the likelihood approach. These marginal probabilities remain the same for all times $t=1,\ldots,T$. But the marginal probabilities under the present BDL regression model are determined by (3.127) and they change over time unless the dynamic dependence parameter is $\gamma_1=0$.

Now to fit the BDL model with 2 level of covariates to the asthma data, the model parameters, that is,

$$\tilde{\theta}=[\beta_{10},\beta_{11},\gamma_1]',$$

are estimated by solving the likelihood iterative equation (3.141) by using the initial values

$$\hat{\tilde{\theta}}(0)=[\hat{\beta}_{10}(0)=0.0,\hat{\beta}_{11}(0)=0.0\ \hat{\gamma}_1(0)=0.0].$$

After 5 iterations, we obtain the likelihood estimates as

$$\hat{\tilde{\theta}}_{MLE}=[\hat{\beta}_{10,MLE}=-2.1886,\hat{\beta}_{11,MLE}=0.2205\ \hat{\gamma}_{1,MLE}=1.9554]$$

which are the same as in Sutradhar and Farrell (2007) (see also lower half of Table 7.10 in Sutradhar 2011).

Notice from (3.127) that the marginal probabilities at a given level of the covariate maintain a recursive relationship over time. The above likelihood estimates for the parameters produce the asthma status probabilities for two groups of children (with smoking or non-smoking mother) as in Table 3.14.

Table 3.14 Asthma status probabilities over time by fitting BDL model with MLE (maximum likelihood estimation) approach

		Asthma status probability	
Time (t)	Covariate level	Yes	No
$t = 1$	Smoking mother	0.1226	0.8774
	Non-smoking mother	0.1008	0.8992
$t = 2$	Smoking mother	0.1685	0.8315
	Non-smoking mother	0.1352	0.8648
$t = 3$	Smoking mother	0.1856	0.8144
	Non-smoking mother	0.1469	0.8531
$t = 4$	Smoking mother	0.1921	0.8079
	Non-smoking mother	0.1506	0.8494

Table 3.15 Lag correlations for asthma responses for children belonging to ℓ-th ($\ell = 1,2$) level of the smoking mother covariate

		Time			
Covariate level	Time	1	2	3	4
Smoking mother	1	1.0	0.3279	0.1181	0.0436
	2		1.0	0.3603	0.1331
	3			1.0	0.3694
	4				1.0
Non-smoking mother	1	1.0	0.3004	0.0990	0.0340
	2		1.0	0.3295	0.1112
	3			1.0	.3374
	4				1.0

The results of this table show that while the probabilities having asthma for both groups of children are increasing over time, the children with smoking mother always have larger probability for having asthma as compared to their counterparts with non-smoking other. Note that the LDCP model produces constant probabilities over time for both groups as shown in Table 3.13 which appear to be very close for the case with $t = 2$ produced by the BDL model as seen from Table 3.14.

Furthermore, on top of marginal probabilities, the dynamic dependence parameter γ_1 of the BDL model naturally influences the lag correlations of the asthma status responses. For simplicity, the lag correlations among the responses of two groups of children computed by (3.128) are shown in Table 3.15.

The results of this Table 3.15 show that the lag 1 correlations are only large and positive, and they are slightly larger under the smoking mother group as compared to the non-smoking mother group.

3.4 Covariate Free Basic Univariate Longitudinal Multinomial Models

Recall from Sect. 3.1 that $y_{it} = (y_{it1}, \ldots, y_{itj}, \ldots, y_{it,J-1})'$ denotes the $(J-1)$-dimensional multinomial response variable and for $j = 1, \ldots, J-1$,

$$y_{it}^{(j)} = (y_{it1}^{(j)}, \ldots, y_{itj}^{(j)}, \ldots, y_{it,J-1}^{(j)})' = (01'_{j-1}, 1, 01'_{J-1-j})' \equiv \delta_{itj} \tag{3.143}$$

indicates that the multinomial response of ith individual belongs to jth category at time t. For $j = J$, one writes $y_{it}^{(J)} = \delta_{itJ} = 01_{J-1}$. Also recall from Sect. 3.1.3 that in the stationary case one uses the same marginal probability for all time points $t = 1, \ldots, T$. This becomes much more simpler when the data is covariate free for all individuals $i = 1, \ldots, K$. In such cases, the constant multinomial probability has the form (see Eq. (3.7))

$$P[y_{it} = y_{it}^{(j)}] = \pi_{(it)j} \equiv \pi_j = \begin{cases} \frac{\exp(\beta_{j0})}{1+\sum_{g=1}^{J-1}\exp(\beta_{g0})} & \text{for } j = 1, \ldots, J-1;\ t = 1, \ldots, T \\ \frac{1}{1+\sum_{g=1}^{J-1}\exp(\beta_{g0})} & \text{for } j = J;\ t = 1, \ldots, T, \end{cases} \tag{3.144}$$

and the elements of $y_{it} = (y_{it1}, \ldots, y_{itj}, \ldots, y_{it,J-1})'$ follow the multinomial probability distribution given by

$$P[y_{it1}, \ldots, y_{itj}, \ldots, y_{it,J-1}] = \frac{1!}{y_{it1}! \ldots y_{itj}! \ldots y_{it,J-1}! y_{itJ}!} \Pi_{j=1}^{J} \pi_j^{y_{itj}}, \tag{3.145}$$

for all $t = 1, \ldots, T$. In (3.145),

$$y_{itJ} = 1 - \sum_{j=1}^{J-1} y_{itj}, \text{ and } \pi_J = \sum_{j=1}^{J-1} \pi_j.$$

As far as the nature of the longitudinal multinomial data is concerned, in this covariate free case, they may be displayed as in the contingency Tables 3.16 and 3.17, as a generalization of the binary longitudinal contingency Tables 3.1 and 3.2, respectively.

Table 3.16 Contingency table for $J > 2$ categories at initial time $t = 1$

t ($t = 1$)					
Category					
1	…	j	…	J	Total
$K_1(1)$	…	$K_j(1)$	…	$K_J(1)$	K

Table 3.17 Lag h^* ($h^* = 1,\ldots,T-1$) based $[h^*(T-h^*)]$ contingency tables for $J > 2$ categories

		t ($t = h^*+1,\ldots,T$)					
Time		Category (j)					
Time	Category (g)	1	...	j	...	J	Total
t-h^*	1	$K_{11}(t-h^*,\, t)$	...	$K_{1j}(t-h^*,\, t)$	...	$K_{1J}(t-h^*,\, t)$	$K_1(t-h^*)$
	.	...	...	...	...	...	.
	g	$K_{g1}(t-h^*,\, t)$	...	$K_{gj}(t-h^*,\, t)$	...	$K_{gJ}(t-h^*,\, t)$	$K_g(t-h^*)$
	.	...	...	...	...	...	.
	J	$K_{J1}(t-h^*,\, t)$	...	$K_{Jj}(t-h^*,\, t)$	...	$K_{JJ}(t-h^*,\, t)$	$K_J(t-h^*)$
	Total	$K_1(t)$	...	$K_j(t)$	...	$K_J(t)$	K

3.4.1 Linear Dynamic Conditional Multinomial Probability Models

For the longitudinal binary data, an LDCP model was used in Sect. 3.2.2 to study the correlations among repeated binary data. There exist some studies, where this LDCP model has been generalized to the time series setup (Loredo-Osti and Sutradhar 2012, for example), as well as to the longitudinal setup (Chowdhury 2011, for example), to study the role of correlations among repeated multinomial data in the inferences for regression effects. In the present stationary longitudinal setup, this generalized LDCMP (linear dynamic conditional multinomial probability) model may be constructed as follows. For $t = 2,\ldots,T$, suppose that the response of the ith individual at time $t-1$ was in gth category. Because g can take a value from 1 to J, the conditional probability for y_{it} to be in jth category, given that the previous response was in gth category, may have the linear form

$$\begin{aligned} P[Y_{it} = y_{it}^{(j)} | Y_{i,t-1} = y_{i,t-1}^{(g)}] &= \pi_{(it)j} + \sum_{h=1}^{J-1} \rho_{jh} \left[y_{i,t-1,h}^{(g)} - \pi_{(i,t-1)h} \right] \\ &= \pi_j + \sum_{h=1}^{J-1} \rho_{jh} \left[y_{i,t-1,h}^{(g)} - \pi_h \right] \text{ by stationary property (3.144)} \\ &= \pi_j + \rho_j' \left(y_{i,t-1}^{(g)} - \pi \right) \\ &= \lambda_{it|t-1}^{(j)}(g), \text{ (say), for } g = 1,\ldots,J; j = 1,\ldots,J-1, \end{aligned} \quad (3.146)$$

and

$$P[Y_{it} = y_{it}^{(J)} | Y_{i,t-1} = y_{i,t-1}^{(g)}] = \lambda_{it|t-1}^{(J)}(g) = 1 - \sum_{j=1}^{J-1} \lambda_{it|t-1}^{(j)}(g), \quad (3.147)$$

where

$$\rho_j = (\rho_{j1},\ldots,\rho_{jc},\ldots,\rho_{j,J-1})' : (J-1)\times 1;\; \pi = [\pi_1,\ldots,\pi_j,\ldots,\pi_{J-1}]' : (J-1)\times 1.$$

3.4.1.1 Correlation Properties of the LDCMP Model

3.4.1.1.1 Marginal Mean Vector and Covariance Matrix at a Given Time t

By (3.143) and (3.144), the multinomial response $y_{it} = (y_{it1}, \ldots, y_{itj}, \ldots, y_{it,J-1})'$ has the stationary mean vector given by

$$E[Y_{it}] = \sum_{g=1}^{J-1} y_{it}^{(g)} P[Y_{it} = y_{it}^{(g)}] = \sum_{g=1}^{J-1} y_{it}^{(g)} \pi_g$$
$$= [\pi_1, \ldots, \pi_j, \ldots, \pi_{J-1}]' = \pi : (J-1) \times 1, \quad (3.148)$$

for all $t = 1, \ldots, T$, and the stationary covariance matrix $\Sigma(\pi)$ given by

$$\mathrm{var}[Y_{it}] = E[\{Y_{it} - \pi\}\{Y_{it} - \pi\}']$$
$$= E[Y_{it}Y_{it}'] - \pi\pi', \quad (3.149)$$

by (3.148).

Note that in general, $E[Y_{it}]$ in (3.148) is derived by using the formula

$$E[Y_{it}] = E_{Y_{i1}} E_{Y_{i2}} \cdots E_{Y_{i,t-1}} E_{Y_{it}}[Y_{it} | y_{i,t-1}],$$

where by (3.146), the conditional expectation vector may be written as

$$E_{Y_{it}}[Y_{it} | y_{i,t-1}] = \pi + \rho_M (y_{i,t-1} - \pi)$$

(see (3.154) below) with ρ_M as defined in (3.153). The above successive expectations in the end produces

$$E[Y_{it}] = \pi + E_{Y_{i1}}[\rho_M^{t-1}(Y_{i1} - \pi)] = \pi$$

as in (3.148). Here, for example, $\rho_M^2 = \rho_M \rho_M$.

Next because for $j \neq k$, the jth and kth categories are mutually exclusive, it follows that

$$E[Y_{itj} Y_{itk}] = P[Y_{itj} = 1, Y_{itk} = 1] = P[Y_{it} = y_{it}^{(j)}, Y_{it} = y_{it}^{(k)}] = 0.$$

Furthermore,

$$E[Y_{itj}^2] = E[Y_{itj}] = P[Y_{itj} = 1] = 1 P[Y_{it} = y_{it}^{(j)}] + 0 \sum_{g \neq j}^{J} P[Y_{it} = y_{it}^{(g)}] = \pi_{(it)j} = \pi_j.$$

Consequently, the covariance matrix in (3.149) has the form

$$\Sigma(\pi) = \text{var}[Y_{it}] = \text{diag}[\pi_1, \ldots, \pi_j, \ldots, \pi_{J-1}] - \pi\pi', \tag{3.150}$$

for all $t = 1, \ldots, T$; and $i = 1, \ldots, K$. For a similar formula for the covariance matrix at a cross-sectional level, see Lemma 2.1.1 in Chap. 2.

3.4.1.1.2 Auto-correlations Among Repeated Multinomial Responses

For the computations of any lag auto-correlations, it is convenient to compute the lag $h\,(h = 1, \ldots, T-1)$ auto-covariance matrix $\text{cov}[Y_{iu}, Y'_{it}]$ for $u < t$, which is defined as

$$\begin{aligned} \text{cov}[Y_{it}, Y'_{iu}] &= E[\{Y_{it} - \pi\}\{Y_{iu} - \pi\}'] \\ &= E[Y_{it}Y'_{iu}] - \pi\pi', \end{aligned} \tag{3.151}$$

where $\pi = E[Y_{it}]$ by (3.148) for all $t = 1, \ldots, T$. Next it follows from the model (3.147) that

$$\begin{aligned} E[Y_{it}|y^{(g)}_{i,t-1}] &= \begin{pmatrix} \pi_1 + \rho'_1(y^{(g)}_{i,t-1} - \pi) \\ \pi_2 + \rho'_2(y^{(g)}_{i,t-1} - \pi) \\ \cdots \\ \pi_j + \rho'_j(y^{(g)}_{i,t-1} - \pi) \\ \cdots \\ \pi_{J-1} + \rho'_{J-1}(y^{(g)}_{i,t-1} - \pi) \end{pmatrix} \\ &= \pi + \rho_M(y^{(g)}_{i,t-1} - \pi),\ g = 1, \ldots, J, \end{aligned} \tag{3.152}$$

where ρ_M is the $(J-1) \times (J-1)$ linear dependence parameters matrix given by

$$\rho_M = \begin{pmatrix} \rho'_1 \\ \vdots \\ \rho'_j \\ \vdots \\ \rho'_{J-1} \end{pmatrix} : (J-1) \times (J-1). \tag{3.153}$$

Note that in general, that is, without any category specification, the lag 1 conditional expectation (3.152) implies that

$$E[Y_{it}|y_{i,t-1}] = \pi + \rho_M(y_{i,t-1} - \pi), \tag{3.154}$$

where $y_{i,t-1} = [y_{i,t-1,1}, \ldots, y_{i,t-1,j}, \ldots, y_{i,t-1,J-1}]'$ and

$$y_{i,t-1}^{(g)} = \begin{cases} (y_{i,t-1,1}^{(g)}, \ldots, y_{i,t-1,g}^{(g)}, \ldots, y_{i,t-1,,J-1}^{(g)})' = (01'_{g-1}, 1, 01'_{J-1-g})' & \text{for } g = 1, \ldots, J-1; \\ (01_{J-1}) & \text{for } g = J. \end{cases} \tag{3.155}$$

Now because the covariance formula, that is, the right-hand side of (3.151) may be expressed as

$$E[\{Y_{it} - \pi\}\{Y_{iu} - \pi\}'] = E_{Y_{iu}} E_{Y_{i,u+1}} \cdots E_{Y_{i,t-1}} E[\{Y_{it} - \pi\}\{Y_{iu} - \pi\}' | Y_{i,t-1}, \cdots, Y_{iu}], \tag{3.156}$$

by using the operation (3.154), this equation provides the formula for the covariance as

$$\begin{aligned} \text{cov}[Y_{it}, Y'_{iu}] &= E[\{Y_{it} - \pi\}\{Y_{iu} - \pi\}'] \\ &= \rho_M^{t-u} E_{Y_{iu}}[\{Y_{iu} - \pi\}\{Y_{iu} - \pi\}'] \\ &= \rho_M^{t-u} \Sigma(\pi) \\ &= \rho_M^{t-u} \left[\text{diag}[\pi_1, \ldots, \pi_j, \ldots, \pi_{J-1}] - \pi\pi'\right], \end{aligned} \tag{3.157}$$

where, for example, $\rho_M^3 = \rho_M \rho_M \rho_M$.

3.4.1.2 GQL Estimation

Let $\theta^* = [\beta_{10}, \ldots, \beta_{j0}, \ldots, \beta_{J-1,0}]'$ be the $(J-1) \times 1$ vector of regression parameters used to model the multinomial probabilities $\{\pi_j,\ j = 1, \ldots, J-1\}$ as in (3.144). Further let $y_i = [y'_{i1}, \ldots, y'_{it}, \ldots, y'_{iT}]'$ be the repeated multinomial responses of the ith individual over T time periods. Here $y_{it} = [y_{it1}, \ldots, y_{itj}, \ldots, y_{it,J-1}]'$ denotes the multinomial variable with

$$E[Y_{it}] = \pi = (\pi_1, \ldots, \pi_j, \ldots, \pi_{J-1})', \text{ and } \text{var}[Y_{it}] = \Sigma(\pi),$$

as in (3.148) and (3.150), respectively. One may then obtain the mean vector

$$\begin{aligned} E[Y_i] &= E[Y'_{i1}, \ldots, Y'_{it}, \ldots, Y'_{iT}]' \\ &= 1_T \otimes \pi : T(J-1) \times 1, \end{aligned} \tag{3.158}$$

where $\otimes$ denotes the Kronecker product. Next, by (3.157), one may obtain the $T(J-1) \times T(J-1)$ covariance matrix of Y_i as

$$\text{cov}[Y_i] = \begin{pmatrix} \Sigma(\pi) & \rho_M \Sigma(\pi) & \rho_M^2 \Sigma(\pi) & \ldots & \rho_M^{T-1} \Sigma(\pi) \\ \rho_M \Sigma(\pi) & \Sigma(\pi) & \rho_M \Sigma(\pi) & \ldots & \rho_M^{T-2} \Sigma(\pi) \\ \vdots & \vdots & \vdots & & \vdots \\ \rho_M^{T-1} \Sigma(\pi) & \rho_M^{T-2} \Sigma(\pi) & \rho_M^{T-3} \Sigma(\pi) & \ldots & \Sigma(\pi) \end{pmatrix}$$

$$
\begin{aligned}
&= \begin{pmatrix} I_{J-1} & \rho_M & \rho_M^2 & \cdots \rho_M^{T-1} \\ \rho_M & I_{J-1} & \rho_M & \cdots \rho_M^{T-2} \\ \vdots & \vdots & \vdots & \vdots \\ \rho_M^{T-1} & \rho_M^{T-2} & \rho_M^{T-3} & \ldots I_{J-1} \end{pmatrix} \begin{pmatrix} \Sigma(\pi) & 0 & 0 \ldots & 0 \\ 0 & \Sigma(\pi) & 0 \ldots & 0 \\ \vdots & \vdots & \vdots & \vdots \\ 0 & 0 & 0 \ldots & \Sigma(\pi) \end{pmatrix} \\
&= \begin{pmatrix} I_{J-1} & \rho_M & \rho_M^2 & \cdots \rho_M^{T-1} \\ \rho_M & I_{J-1} & \rho_M & \cdots \rho_M^{T-2} \\ \vdots & \vdots & \vdots & \vdots \\ \rho_M^{T-1} & \rho_M^{T-2} & \rho_M^{T-3} & \ldots I_{J-1} \end{pmatrix} [I_T \otimes \Sigma(\pi)] \\
&= \tilde{C}(\rho_M)[I_T \otimes \Sigma(\pi)] \\
&= \tilde{\Sigma}(\pi, \rho_M), \text{ (say).}
\end{aligned} \tag{3.159}
$$

By using $\pi_{(i)} = E[Y_i] = 1_T \otimes \pi$ from (3.158), similar to (3.42), one may write the GQL estimating equation for $\theta^* = [\beta_{10}, \ldots, \beta_{j0}, \ldots, \beta_{J-1,0}]'$ as

$$
\begin{aligned}
&\sum_{i=1}^{K} \frac{\partial \pi'_{(i)}}{\partial \theta^*} \tilde{\Sigma}_i^{-1}(\pi, \rho_M)(\rho)(y_i - \pi_{(i)}) \\
&= \sum_{i=1}^{K} \frac{\partial [1'_T \otimes \pi']}{\partial \theta^*} \left\{ [I_T \otimes \Sigma^{-1}(\pi)] \tilde{C}^{-1}(\rho_M) \right\} (y_i - 1_T \otimes \pi) = 0.
\end{aligned} \tag{3.160}
$$

Next express π_j as

$$
\pi_j = \frac{\exp(\beta_{j0})}{1 + \sum_{g=1}^{J-1} \exp(\beta_{g0})} = \frac{\exp(x'_j \theta^*)}{1 + \sum_{g=1}^{J-1} \exp(x'_g \theta^*)}, \tag{3.161}
$$

and use

$$
\begin{aligned}
\frac{\partial \pi_j}{\partial \theta^*} &= \pi_j x_j - \pi_j \sum_{g=1}^{J-1} x_g \pi_g \\
\frac{\partial \pi'}{\partial \theta^*} &= X' \Sigma(\pi),
\end{aligned} \tag{3.162}
$$

where, corresponding to jth category, x'_j is the jth row of the X matrix defined as

$$
X = \begin{pmatrix} x'_1 \\ \vdots \\ x'_j \\ \vdots \\ x'_{J-1} \end{pmatrix} = I_{J-1}.
$$

Then, the GQL estimating equation (3.160) may be expressed as

$$\begin{aligned}
&\sum_{i=1}^{K}[1'_T \otimes X'\Sigma(\pi)]\left\{[I_T \otimes \Sigma^{-1}(\pi)]\tilde{C}^{-1}(\rho_M)\right\}(y_i - 1_T \otimes \pi) \\
&= \sum_{i=1}^{K}[1'_T \otimes I_{J-1}]\left\{\tilde{C}^{-1}(\rho_M)\right\}(y_i - 1_T \otimes \pi) \\
&= \sum_{i=1}^{K}(\tilde{\omega}_{1M},\ldots,\tilde{\omega}_{tM},\ldots,\tilde{\omega}_{TM})(y_i - 1_T \otimes \pi) \\
&= \sum_{t=1}^{T}\tilde{\omega}_{tM}\begin{pmatrix} K_1(t) \\ \vdots \\ K_j(t) \\ \vdots \\ K_{J-1}(t) \end{pmatrix} - K\left(\sum_{t=1}^{T}\tilde{\omega}_{tM}\right)\begin{pmatrix} \pi_1 \\ \vdots \\ \pi_j \\ \vdots \\ \pi_{J-1} \end{pmatrix} = 0,
\end{aligned} \tag{3.163}$$

where, for a given t, $\tilde{\omega}_{tM}$ is the $(J-1)\times(J-1)$ constant weight matrix (stationary case) for all individuals $i = 1,\ldots,K$, and $K_j(t)$ $(j = 1,\ldots,J-1)$ is the number of individuals those provide jth category response at time t as in the contingency Table 3.17.

Next, because in the present case

$$\frac{\partial \pi}{\partial \theta^{*\prime}} = \Sigma'(\pi)X = \Sigma'(\pi) = \Sigma(\pi),$$

the GQL estimating equation (3.163) for θ^* may be solved iteratively by using

$$\begin{aligned}
\hat{\theta}^*(r+1) = \hat{\theta}^*(r) + &\left[K\left(\sum_{t=1}^{T}\tilde{\omega}_{tM}\right)\Sigma'(\pi)\right]^{-1} \\
\times &\left[\sum_{t=1}^{T}\tilde{\omega}_{tM}\begin{pmatrix} K_1(t) \\ \vdots \\ K_j(t) \\ \vdots \\ K_{J-1}(t) \end{pmatrix} - K\left(\sum_{t=1}^{T}\tilde{\omega}_{tM}\right)\begin{pmatrix} \pi_1 \\ \vdots \\ \pi_j \\ \vdots \\ \pi_{J-1} \end{pmatrix}\right].
\end{aligned} \tag{3.164}$$

3.4.1.2(a) Moment Estimation for ρ_M

The GQL estimation of θ^* by (3.164) requires the dynamic dependence parameters matrix ρ_M to be known, which is, however, unknown in practice. In the longitudinal binary data setup, $\rho_M = \rho$, a scalar dependence or correlation index parameter. For the repeated binary data, this parameter ρ was estimated by using the moment equation (3.93) which utilized all possible lagged responses. This refined approach appears to be complicated in the present longitudinal multinomial data setup. For convenience, we therefore, use a lag 1 response based approximate moment estimating formula to estimate the parameters in the ρ_M matrix. Remark that this approximation was also used in the longitudinal binary data setup by Sutradhar (2011, Chapter 7) for simplicity and it was found that such an approximation has a little or no effect on regression estimation. Turning back to the lag 1 response based moment estimation for ρ_M, one first observes from (3.159) that

$$\mathrm{cov}[Y_{it}, Y_{i,t-1}] = \rho_M \Sigma(\pi) = \rho_M \mathrm{var}[Y_{i,t-1}] \equiv \rho_M \mathrm{var}[Y_{it}], \tag{3.165}$$

which, by indicating lags $(0,1)$, we re-express as

$$\Sigma_1(\pi) = \rho_M \Sigma_0(\pi), \tag{3.166}$$

yielding the moment estimate for ρ_M as

$$\hat{\rho}_M = \hat{\Sigma}_0^{-1}(\pi)\hat{\Sigma}_1(\pi), \tag{3.167}$$

where

$$\hat{\Sigma}_1(\pi) = \frac{1}{K(T-1)} \sum_{i=1}^{K}\sum_{t=2}^{T} \left([(y_{i,t-1,g} - \pi_g)(y_{itj} - \pi_j)]\right) : g,j = 1,\ldots,J-1$$

$$= \frac{1}{K(T-1)} \sum_{t=2}^{T} \left(K_{gj}(t-1,t) - K_g(t-1)\pi_j - K_j(t)\pi_g + K\pi_g\pi_j\right) \tag{3.168}$$

by the cell counts from the contingency Table 3.17 for $g,j = 1,\ldots,J-1$. Also, in (3.167),

$$\hat{\Sigma}_0(\pi) = \frac{1}{KT}\sum_{i=1}^{K}\sum_{t=1}^{T} \begin{pmatrix} [(y_{it1}-\pi_1)^2] & \ldots & -\pi_1\pi_j & \ldots & -\pi_1\pi_{J-1} \\ \vdots & & \vdots & & \vdots \\ -\pi_j\pi_1 & \ldots & [(y_{itj}-\pi_j)^2] & \ldots & -\pi_j\pi_{J-1} \\ \vdots & & \vdots & & \vdots \\ -\pi_{J-1}\pi_1 & \ldots & -\pi_{J-1}\pi_j & \ldots & [(y_{it,J-1}-\pi_{J-1})^2] \end{pmatrix}$$

$$= \frac{1}{KT}\sum_{t=1}^{T} \begin{pmatrix} d_{11}(t) & \ldots & -K\pi_1\pi_j & \ldots & -K\pi_1\pi_{J-1} \\ \vdots & & \vdots & & \vdots \\ -K\pi_j\pi_1 & \ldots & d_{jj}(t) & \ldots & -K\pi_j\pi_{J-1} \\ \vdots & & \vdots & & \vdots \\ -K\pi_{J-1}\pi_1 & \ldots & -K\pi_{J-1}\pi_j & \ldots & d_{J-1,J-1}(t) \end{pmatrix}, \tag{3.169}$$

where $d_{jj}(t) = [K_j(t) - 2K_j(t)\pi_j + \pi_j^2]$, for $j = 1, \ldots, J-1$, by using cell counts from Table 3.16.

3.4.1.2.1 Illustration 3.9: Analysis of Longitudinal Three Mile Island Stress-Level (Three Categories) Data (Covariate Free) Using Auto-correlations Class Based GQL Approach

Consider the Three Mile Island Stress-Level (TMISL) data (Fienberg et al. 1985; Conaway 1989) collected from a psychological study of the mental health effects of the accident at the Three Mile Island nuclear power plant in central Pennsylvania began on March 28, 1979. The study focuses on the changes in the post accident stress level of mothers of young children living within 10 miles of the nuclear plant. The accident was followed by four interviews; winter 1979 (wave 1), spring 1980 (wave 2), fall 1981 (wave 3), and fall 1982 (wave 4). The subjects were classified into one of the three response categories namely low, medium, and high stress level, based on a composite score from a 90-item checklist. There were 267 subjects who completed all four interviews. Respondents were stratified into two groups, those living within 5 miles of the plant (LT5) and those live within 5–10 miles from the plant (GT5). It was of interest to compare the distribution of individuals under three stress levels collected over four different time points. For convenience of discussion and analysis, we reproduce this data set in Table 3.18.

Note that this TMISL data set was analyzed by Fienberg et al. (1985) and reanalyzed by Conaway (1989), among others. Fienberg et al. (1985) have collapsed the trinomial (three category) data into 2 category based dichotomized data and modeled the correlations among such repeated binary responses through a BDL model (see also Sutradhar and Farrell 2007). Thus their model does not deal with correlations of repeated multinomial (trinomial in this case to be specific) responses and do not make the desired comparison among 3 original stress levels. Conaway (1989) has however attempted to model the multinomial correlations but has used a random effects, that is, mixed model approach to compute the correlations. There are at least two major drawbacks with this mixed model approach used in Conaway (1989). First, the random effects based correlations are not able to address the correlations among repeated responses. Second, it is extremely difficult to estimate the parameters involved in the multinomial mixed model. As a remedy, Conaway (1989) has used a conditioning to remove the random effects from the model and estimated the regression parameters exploiting the so-called conditional likelihood. But a close look at this conditioning shows that there was a mistake in constructing the conditional likelihood and this approach does not in fact remove the random effects.

Unlike Fienberg et al. (1985), Conaway (1989), and other existing odds ratio based approaches (Lipsitz et al. 1991, Eqs. (5)–(6), p. 155; Yi and Cook 2002, Eq. (3), p. 1072), in this Sect. 3.4.1 we have modeled the correlations among repeated multinomial responses through an LDCMP model. A nonlinear dynamic

Table 3.18 Three Mile Island Stress-level (TMISL) data with $J = 3$ stress levels (categories) over a period of $T = 4$ time points, and with distance of home as a fixed binary covariate

	Time (t)					
	$t = 1$	$t = 2$	$t = 3$	$t = 4$		
				Stress-level (SL)		
Covariate	SL	SL	SL	Low	Medium	High
Distance $\leq$ 5 Miles	Low	Low	Low	2	0	0
			Medium	2	3	0
			High	0	0	0
		Medium	Low	0	1	0
			Medium	2	4	0
			High	0	0	0
		High	Low	0	0	0
			Medium	0	0	0
			High	0	0	0
	Medium	Low	Low	5	1	0
			Medium	1	4	0
			High	0	0	0
		Medium	Low	3	2	0
			Medium	2	38	4
			High	0	2	3
		High	Low	0	0	0
			Medium	0	2	0
			High	0	1	1
	High	Low	Low	0	0	0
			Medium	0	0	0
			High	0	0	0
		Medium	Low	0	0	0
			Medium	0	4	3
			High	0	1	4
		High	Low	0	0	0
			Medium	1	2	0
			High	0	5	12
Distance > 5 Miles	Low	Low	Low	1	2	0
			Medium	2	0	0
			High	0	0	0
		Medium	Low	1	0	0
			Medium	0	3	0
			High	0	0	0
		High	Low	0	0	0
			Medium	0	0	0
			High	0	0	0

(continued)

Table 3.18 (continued)

	Time (t)					
	$t=1$	$t=2$	$t=3$	$t=4$		
				Stress-level (SL)		
Covariate	SL	SL	SL	Low	Medium	High
	Medium	Low	Low	4	4	0
			Medium	5	15	1
			High	0	0	0
		Medium	Low	2	2	0
			Medium	6	53	6
			High	0	5	1
		High	Low	0	0	0
			Medium	0	1	1
			High	0	3	1
	High	Low	Low	0	0	1
			Medium	0	0	0
			High	0	0	0
		Medium	Low	0	0	0
			Medium	1	13	0
			High	0	0	0
		High	Low	0	0	0
			Medium	0	7	2
			High	0	2	7

model, namely MDL model is used in Sect. 3.4.2 to model the correlations. These models are however developed for covariates free repeated multinomial data. The covariates based LDCMP and MDL models are discussed in Sects. 3.5.1 and 3.5.2, respectively.

Turning back to the TMISL data analysis, we now apply the covariates free LDCMP model and compute the probability for an individual worker to be in any of the three stress level categories. These are computed after taking the correlations among repeated multinomial responses into account. However, for the time being, it is pretended that the distance covariates (distance ≤ 5 miles or >5 miles) do not play any role and hence data under two covariates were merged. Note that because the LDCMP model fitting is based on lag 1 time dependence, for convenience of interpretation, we also provide all possible lag 1 transition counts over time ignoring the covariate, in Tables 3.20(1)–3.20(3). When compared with the individuals in high stress group, the results in Table 3.19 show that initially, that is, at year 1, only a small number of individuals had low stress (23 vs 65), whereas more individuals (179 vs 65) were encountering medium level stress. When marginal counts are compared over the years, the results of Tables 3.20(1)–3.20(3) show that the stress situation was improved in year 2 as the number of individuals in low stress group increased to 53 from 23 but again the situation got worsen at years 3 and 4. These numbers are also reflected from the transitional counts as, for example,

Table 3.19 Contingency table for Three Mile Island Stress-level ($J = 3$ categories) (TMISL) data at initial time $t = 1$

Time ($t = 1$)			
SL (Stress-level) Category			
Low (1)	Medium (2)	High (3)	Total
$K_1(1) = 23$	$K_2(1) = 179$	$K_3(1) = 65$	K=267

Table 3.20 (1): Lag $h^* = 1$ based transitional table from time $t - h^* = 1$ to $t = 2$ for Three Mile Island Stress-level ($J = 3$ categories) (TMISL) data

		2			
Time		SL (j)			
Time	SL (g)	1	2	3	Total
1	1	$K_{11}(1,2) = 12$	$K_{12}(1,2) = 11$	$K_{13}(1,2) = 0$	$K_1(1) = 23$
	2	$K_{21}(1,2) = 40$	$K_{22}(1,2) = 129$	$K_{13}(1,2) = 10$	$K_2(1) = 179$
	3	$K_{31}(1,2) = 1$	$K_{32}(1,2) = 26$	$K_{33}(1,2) = 38$	$K_3(1) = 65$
	Total	$K_1(2) = 53$	$K_2(2) = 166$	$K_3(2) = 48$	$K = 267$

Table 3.20 (2): Lag $h^* = 1$ based transitional table from time $t - h^* = 2$ to $t = 3$ for Three Mile Island Stress-level ($J = 3$ categories) (TMISL) data

		3			
Time		SL (j)			
Time	SL (g)	1	2	3	Total
2	1	$K_{11}(2,3) = 20$	$K_{12}(2,3) = 33$	$K_{13}(2,3) = 0$	$K_1(2) = 53$
	2	$K_{21}(2,3) = 11$	$K_{22}(2,3) = 139$	$K_{13}(2,3) = 16$	$K_2(2) = 166$
	3	$K_{31}(2,3) = 0$	$K_{32}(2,3) = 16$	$K_{33}(23) = 32$	$K_3(2) = 48$
	Total	$K_1(3) = 31$	$K_2(3) = 188$	$K_3(3) = 48$	$K = 267$

Table 3.20 (3): Lag $h^* = 1$ based transitional table from time $t - h^* = 3$ to $t = 4$ for Three Mile Island Stress-level ($J = 3$ categories) (TMISL) data

		4			
Time		SL (j)			
Time	SL (g)	1	2	3	Total
3	1	$K_{11}(3,4) = 18$	$K_{12}(3,4) = 12$	$K_{13}(3,4) = 1$	$K_1(3) = 31$
	2	$K_{21}(3,4) = 22$	$K_{22}(3,4) = 149$	$K_{13}(3,4) = 17$	$K_2(3) = 188$
	3	$K_{31}(3,4) = 0$	$K_{32}(3,4) = 19$	$K_{33}(3,4) = 29$	$K_3(3) = 48$
	Total	$K_1(4) = 40$	$K_2(4) = 180$	$K_3(4) = 47$	$K = 267$

$K_{21}(1,2) = 40$ (from year 1 to 2) was higher than corresponding $K_{21}(2,3)$ (from year 2 to 3) and $K_{21}(3,4) = 2$ (from year 3 to 4). Note that even though the marginal counts over time appear to change to a small extent perhaps because of certain time dependent covariates, we however fit a stationary model in this section as no other covariates were collected except the distance. The transitional counts under separate distance groups (see Tables 3.24(1)–3.24(3) show similar pattern as those in Tables 3.20(1)–3.20(3)). This is expected as the distance is not a time dependent covariate.

However, to compute the stationary probabilities $\pi_j,\ j = 1,2$ with $\pi_3 = 1 - \pi_1 - \pi_3$ under three categories defined by (3.144), we take the lag correlations of the multinomial responses into account by using the lag 1 conditional probability model (3.146). The regression parameters β_{10} and β_{20} involved in $\pi_j,\ j = 1,\ldots,3$, and the lag 1 dynamic dependence parameters

$$\rho_M = \begin{pmatrix} \rho_{11}\ \rho_{12} \\ \rho_{21}\ \rho_{22} \end{pmatrix}$$

defined by (3.153)–(3.154) are computed iteratively. We start the iteration using initial ρ_M as

$$\rho_M(0) = \begin{pmatrix} \rho_{11} = 0\ \rho_{12} = 0 \\ \rho_{21} = 0\ \rho_{22} = 0 \end{pmatrix}$$

and compute the GQL estimate of

$$\theta^* = \begin{pmatrix} \beta_{10} \\ \beta_{20} \end{pmatrix}$$

by using the iterative equation (3.164), and the first step estimate of θ^* in 5 iterations was found to be

$$\hat{\theta}^*(1) = \begin{pmatrix} \hat{\beta}_{10} = -0.3471 \\ \hat{\beta}_{20} = 1.2319 \end{pmatrix}.$$

We then compute the estimate of ρ_M by using the moment estimating formula (3.167) and the first step estimate of ρ_M was found to be

$$\hat{\rho}_M(1) = \begin{pmatrix} \hat{\rho}_{11} = 0.3381\ \ \hat{\rho}_{12} = -0.3699 \\ \hat{\rho}_{21} = -0.0862\ \hat{\rho}_{22} = -0.1936 \end{pmatrix}.$$

These estimates of ρ_M were then used in (3.164) to obtain a second step or an improved estimate of θ^*. This cycle of iterations continued until convergence. The convergence was achieved only in 3 cycles of iterations and the final estimates were found to be

$$\hat{\rho}_M = \begin{pmatrix} \hat{\rho}_{11} = 0.3410 & \hat{\rho}_{12} = -0.3646 \\ \hat{\rho}_{21} = -0.0819 & \hat{\rho}_{22} = -0.2008 \end{pmatrix};$$

and

$$\hat{\theta}^*_{GQL} = \begin{pmatrix} \hat{\beta}_{10,GQL} = -0.4092 \\ \hat{\beta}_{20,GQL} = 1.2089 \end{pmatrix}.$$

There is a noticeable difference between this GQL estimate and the aforementioned step 1 estimate $\hat{\theta}^*(1)$ obtained using independence assumption, that is, using

$$\rho_M(0) = \begin{pmatrix} \rho_{11} = 0 & \rho_{12} = 0 \\ \rho_{21} = 0 & \rho_{22} = 0 \end{pmatrix}.$$

Next, the standard errors for the components of $\hat{\theta}^*_{GQL}$ computed by using

$$\text{cov}[\hat{\theta}^*_{GQL}] = \left[K \left(\sum_{t=1}^{T} \tilde{\omega}_{tM} \right) \Sigma'(\pi) \right]^{-1}$$

(see (3.164)) were found to be

$$\text{s.e.}(\hat{\beta}_{10,GQL}) = 0.1369; \; \text{s.e.}(\hat{\beta}_{20,GQL}) = 0.0416,$$

and using the GQL estimates

$$\hat{\beta}_{10,GQL} = -0.4092; \; \hat{\beta}_{20,GQL} = 1.2089,$$

the stationary multinomial probabilities (GQL) for an individual (that is probabilities for an individual to belong to these three categories) by (3.144), were found to be

$$\hat{\pi}_1 = 0.1325(\text{low stress group}), \; \hat{\pi}_2 = 0.6681(\text{medium stress group}),$$
$$\hat{\pi}_3 = 0.1994(\text{high stress group}),$$

which, as seen from the following Table 3.21, appear to agree well in general with marginal counts, that is, with observed marginal probabilities (OMP) over time. The results of the table also show differences in estimates of probabilities computed based on independence (I) assumption ($\rho_M = 0$).

Remark that by using the GQL estimates for the components of θ^* and the moment estimate of ρ_M, one can also estimate the conditional probabilities by (3.146) to reflect the lag 1 transitions and interpret the results corresponding to the transitional counts shown in any of the Tables 3.20(1)–3.20(3).

3.4.1.3 Likelihood Function

Recall from (3.145) that at time point $t = 1$, the multinomial response $y_{i1} = (y_{i11}, \ldots, y_{i1j}, \ldots, y_{i1,J-1})'$ has the multinomial distribution given by

$$f(y_{i1}) = P((y_{i11}, \ldots, y_{i1j}, \ldots, y_{i1,J-1}) = \frac{1!}{y_{i11}! \ldots y_{i1j}! \ldots y_{i1,J-1}! y_{i1J}!} \Pi_{j=1}^{J} \pi_j^{y_{i1j}}, \quad (3.170)$$

Next, by using (3.146), one may write the conditional distribution of y_{it} given $y_{i,t-1}$ as

$$f(y_{it}|y_{i,t-1}) = \frac{1!}{y_{it1}! \ldots y_{itj}! \ldots y_{it,J-1}! y_{itJ}!} \Pi_{j=1}^{J} \left[\lambda_{it|t-1}^{(j)}(y_{i,t-1})\right]^{y_{itj}}, \quad (3.171)$$

where

$$\lambda_{it|t-1}^{(J)}(y_{i,t-1}) = 1 - \sum_{g=1}^{J-1} \lambda_{it|t-1}^{(g)}(y_{i,t-1}) \text{ with } \lambda_{it|t-1}^{(g)}(y_{i,t-1}) = \pi_g + \rho_g'(y_{i,t-1} - \pi),$$

the past multinomial response $y_{i,t-1}$ is being known as

$$y_{i,t-1} \equiv y_{i,t-1}^{(g)}, \text{ for any } g = 1, \ldots, J.$$

It then follows from (3.170) and (3.171) that the likelihood function (of θ^* and ρ_M) is given by

$$L(\theta^*, \rho_M) = \Pi_{i=1}^{K} \left[f(y_{i1}) \Pi_{t=2}^{T} f(y_{it}|y_{i,t-1})\right], \quad (3.172)$$

which is equivalent to

$$\begin{aligned} L(\theta^*, \rho_M) &= \left[\Pi_{i=1}^{K} f(y_{i1})\right] \\ &\times \Pi_{t=2}^{T} \Pi_{g=1}^{J} \Pi_{i \in g}^{K} \left[f(y_{it}|y_{i,t-1}^{(g)})\right] \\ &= c_0 \left[\Pi_{j=1}^{J} \Pi_{i=1}^{K} \pi_j^{y_{i1j}}\right] \\ &\times \Pi_{t=2}^{T} \Pi_{j=1}^{J} \Pi_{g=1}^{J} \Pi_{i \in g}^{K} \left\{\lambda_{it|t-1}^{(j)}(y_{i,t-1}^{(g)})\right\}^{y_{itj}}, \end{aligned} \quad (3.173)$$

where c_0 is the normalizing constant free from any parameters. Next, by using the abbreviation $\lambda^{(j)}(g) \equiv \lambda_{it|t-1}^{(j)}(y_{i,t-1}^{(g)})$, this log likelihood function is written as

$$\begin{aligned} Log\, L(\theta^*, \rho_M) &= log\, c_0 + \sum_{i=1}^{K} \sum_{j=1}^{J} y_{i1j} log\, \pi_j \\ &+ \sum_{t=2}^{T} \sum_{j=1}^{J} \sum_{g=1}^{J} \sum_{i \in g}^{K} \left[y_{itj} log\, \lambda_{it|t-1}^{(j)}(g)\right], \end{aligned} \quad (3.174)$$

which, by using the cell counts from the contingency Table 3.17, reduces to

$$Log\ L(\theta^*, \rho_M) = log\ c_0 + \sum_{j=1}^{J} K_j(1) log\ \pi_j + \sum_{j=1}^{J}\sum_{g=1}^{J}\left\{log\ \lambda^{(j)}(g)\right\}\left[\sum_{t=2}^{T} K_{gj}(t-1,t)\right], \tag{3.175}$$

where $K_{gj}(t-1,t)$ is the number of individuals with responses belonging to jth category at time t, given that their responses were in the gth category at time $t-1$. Also, in (3.175),

$$\lambda^{(j)}(g) = \begin{cases} \pi_j + \rho_j'(\delta_g - \pi) & \text{for } j = 1,\ldots,J-1;\ g = 1,\ldots,J \\ 1 - \sum_{k=1}^{J-1}\left[\pi_k + \rho_k'(\delta_g - \pi)\right] & \text{for } j = J;\ g = 1,\ldots,J, \end{cases} \tag{3.176}$$

where, similar to (3.155),

$$\delta_g = \begin{cases} [01_{g-1}', 1, 01_{J-1-g}']' & \text{for } g = 1,\ldots,J-1 \\ 01_{J-1} & \text{for } g = J. \end{cases}$$

3.4.1.3.1 Likelihood Estimating Equations

3.4.1.3.1(a) Likelihood Estimating Equation for θ^*

Recall from (3.160)–(3.161) that for

$$\pi_j = \frac{\exp(\beta_{j0})}{1 + \sum_{g=1}^{J-1}\exp(\beta_{g0})} = \frac{\exp(x_j'\theta^*)}{1 + \sum_{g=1}^{J-1}\exp(x_g'\theta^*)},\ j = 1,\ldots,J-1$$

with $x_j' = [01_{j-1}', 1, 01_{J-1-j}']$, the first derivative of π_j with respect to $\theta^* = [\beta_{10},\ldots,\beta_{j0},\ldots,\beta_{J-1,0}]'$ has the formula

$$\frac{\partial \pi_j}{\partial \theta^*} = \begin{cases} \pi_j x_j - \pi_j \sum_{g=1}^{J-1} x_g \pi_g = \pi_j(x_j - \pi) & \text{for } j = 1,\ldots,J-1 \\ \frac{\partial}{\partial \theta^*}[1 - \sum_{j=1}^{J-1}\pi_j] = -\sum_{j=1}^{J-1}\pi_j(x_j - \pi) = -\pi\pi_J & \text{for } j = J, \end{cases} \tag{3.177}$$

where $\pi = (\pi_1,\ldots,\pi_j,\ldots,\pi_{J-1})'$. Thus, one may write

$$\frac{1}{\pi_j}\frac{\partial \pi_j}{\partial \theta^*} = \begin{cases} x_j - \sum_{g=1}^{J-1}\pi_g x_g = x_j - \pi & \text{for } j = 1,\ldots,J-1 \\ -\pi & \text{for } j = J. \end{cases} \tag{3.178}$$

Next by re-expressing $\lambda^{(j)}(g)$ in (3.176) as

$$\lambda^{(j)}(g) = \begin{cases} \pi_j + (\delta_g - \pi)'\rho_j & \text{for } j = 1,\ldots,J-1;\ g = 1,\ldots,J \\ 1 - \sum_{k=1}^{J-1}[\pi_k + (\delta_g - \pi)'\rho_k] & \text{for } j = J;\ g = 1,\ldots,J, \end{cases} \tag{3.179}$$

one, by (3.177), obtains their derivatives with respect to θ^* as

$$\frac{\partial \lambda^{(j)}(g)}{\partial \theta^*} = \begin{cases} \frac{\partial \pi_j}{\partial \theta^*} - \left[\frac{\partial \pi'}{\partial \theta^*}\right] \rho_j & \text{for } j = 1, \ldots, J-1 \\ -\Sigma_{k=1}^{J-1} \left[\frac{\partial \pi_k}{\partial \theta^*} - \left\{\frac{\partial \pi'}{\partial \theta^*}\right\} \rho_k\right] & \text{for } j = J \end{cases}$$
$$= \begin{cases} [\pi_j(x_j - \pi)] - [\Sigma(\pi)]\rho_j & \text{for } j = 1, \ldots, J-1 \\ -\left[\pi\pi_J - \{\Sigma(\pi)\}\Sigma_{k=1}^{J-1}\rho_k\right] & \text{for } j = J, \end{cases} \tag{3.180}$$

for any $g = 1, \ldots, J$, where $\rho_j = (\rho_{j1}, \ldots, \rho_{jc}, \ldots, \rho_{j,J-1})'$ for $j = 1, \ldots, J-1$, and

$$\begin{aligned} \frac{\partial \pi'}{\partial \theta^*} &= \left(\pi_1(x_1 - \pi) \ \ldots \ \pi_j(x_j - \pi) \ \ldots \ \pi_{J-1}(x_{J-1} - \pi)\right) \\ &= \text{diag}[\pi_1, \ldots, \pi_j, \ldots, \pi_{J-1}] - \pi\pi' \\ &= \Sigma(\pi). \end{aligned}$$

Remark that the jth column (or row) of this matrix has the form

$$\frac{\partial \pi_j}{\partial \theta^*} = \pi_j(x_j - \pi) = \begin{pmatrix} -\pi_j\pi_1 \\ \vdots \\ -\pi_j\pi_{j-1} \\ \pi_j(1-\pi_j) \\ -\pi_j\pi_{j+1} \\ \vdots \\ -\pi_j\pi_{J-1} \end{pmatrix}.$$

Now by using the derivatives from (3.178) and (3.180), one may construct the likelihood estimating equations for the components of θ^* from the log likelihood function given by (3.175). To be specific, these equations have the form

$$\begin{aligned} \frac{\partial Log\, L(\theta^*, \rho_M)}{\partial \theta^*} &= \sum_{j=1}^{J} K_j(1) \frac{1}{\pi_j} \frac{\partial \pi_j}{\partial \theta^*} \\ &+ \sum_{j=1}^{J} \sum_{g=1}^{J} \left[\left\{ \sum_{t=2}^{T} K_{gj}(t-1,t) \right\} \frac{1}{\lambda^{(j)}(g)} \frac{\partial \lambda^{(j)}(g)}{\partial \theta^*} \right] \\ &= \sum_{j=1}^{J-1} K_j(1)(x_j - \pi) - K_J(1)\pi \\ &+ \sum_{j=1}^{J-1} \sum_{g=1}^{J} \left[\left\{ \sum_{t=2}^{T} K_{gj}(t-1,t) \right\} \frac{1}{\lambda^{(j)}(g)} \left\{ [\pi_j(x_j - \pi)] - \Sigma(\pi)\rho_j \right\} \right] \end{aligned}$$

$$- \sum_{g=1}^{J} \left[\left\{ \sum_{t=2}^{T} K_{gJ}(t-1,t) \right\} \frac{1}{\lambda^{(J)}(g)} \times \left\{ \pi\pi_J - \Sigma(\pi) \sum_{k=1}^{J-1} \rho_k \right\} \right] = 0. \quad (3.181)$$

In fact, by using some conventional notation, that is,

$$x_J = 01_{J-1}, \text{ and } \rho_J = - \sum_{k=1}^{J-1} \rho_k, \quad (3.182)$$

one can re-express the log likelihood equation (3.181) in a simpler form as

$$\frac{\partial Log\ L(\theta^*, \rho_M)}{\partial \theta^*} = \sum_{j=1}^{J} K_j(1)(x_j - \pi) + \sum_{j=1}^{J} \sum_{g=1}^{J} \left[\left\{ \sum_{t=2}^{T} K_{gj}(t-1,t) \right\} \times \frac{1}{\lambda^{(j)}(g)} \left\{ [\pi_j(x_j - \pi)] - \Sigma(\pi)\rho_j \right\} \right] = 0. \quad (3.183)$$

Remark that the notations in (3.182) are used simply for writing the log likelihood and subsequent equations in an easy and compact way. Thus, it should be clear that ρ_J is not a parameter vector so that $\sum_{j=1}^{J} \rho_j = 0$ has to be satisfied, rather it is simply used for $-\sum_{j=1}^{J-1} \rho_j$ for notational convenience.

For known ρ_M, these likelihood equations in (3.181) or (3.183) may be solved iteratively by using the iterative equations for θ^* given by

$$\hat{\theta}^*(r+1) = \hat{\theta}^*(r) - \left[\left\{ \frac{\partial^2 \text{Log}\ L(\theta^*, \rho_M)}{\partial \theta^{*\prime} \partial \theta^*} \right\}^{-1} \frac{\partial \text{Log}\ L(\theta^*, \rho_M)}{\partial \theta^*} \right]_{|\theta^* = \hat{\theta}^*(r)} ; (J-1) \times 1, \quad (3.184)$$

where the second order derivative matrix has the formula

$$\frac{\partial^2 Log\ L(\theta^*, \rho_M)}{\partial \theta^{*\prime} \partial \theta^*} = - \sum_{j=1}^{J} K_j(1) \left[\frac{\partial \pi}{\partial \theta^{*\prime}} \right] + \sum_{j=1}^{J} \sum_{g=1}^{J} \left[\left\{ \sum_{t=2}^{T} K_{gj}(t-1,t) \right\} \times \left\{ \frac{1}{\lambda^{(j)}(g)} \frac{\partial}{\partial \theta^{*\prime}} \left\{ [\pi_j(x_j - \pi)] - \Sigma(\pi)\rho_j \right\} - \frac{1}{[\lambda^{(j)}(g)]^2} \left\{ [\pi_j(x_j - \pi)] - \Sigma(\pi)\rho_j \right\} \frac{\partial \lambda^{(j)}(g)}{\partial \theta^{*\prime}} \right\} \right] \quad (3.185)$$

Note that the formulas for $\frac{\partial \pi_j}{\partial \theta^{*\prime}} = [\frac{\partial \pi_j}{\partial \theta^*}]'$ and $\frac{\partial \lambda^{(j)}(g)}{\partial \theta^{*\prime}} = [\frac{\partial \lambda^{(j)}(g)}{\partial \theta^*}]'$ are known by (3.180). Thus, to compute the second derivative matrix by (3.185), one needs to compute the formulas for

$$\frac{\partial}{\partial \theta^{*\prime}} \left\{ [\pi_j(x_j - \pi)] - \Sigma(\pi)\rho_j \right\}$$

which may be simplified as

Computation of $\frac{\partial}{\partial \theta^{*\prime}} \left\{ [\pi_j(x_j - \pi)] - \Sigma(\pi)\rho_j \right\}$:

By (3.177) and (3.180) it follows that

$$\begin{aligned}
\frac{\partial}{\partial \theta^{*\prime}} [\pi_j(x_j - \pi)] &= \pi_j(x_j - \pi)(x_j - \pi)' - \pi_j \frac{\partial \pi}{\partial \theta^{*\prime}} \\
&= \pi_j(x_j - \pi)(x_j - \pi)' - \pi_j \left[\frac{\partial \pi}{\partial \theta^{*\prime}} \right]' \\
&= \pi_j(x_j - \pi)(x_j - \pi)' - \pi_j [\Sigma(\pi)]' \\
&= \pi_j(x_j - \pi)(x_j - \pi)' - \pi_j \Sigma(\pi) \\
&= \pi_j \left[(x_j - \pi)(x_j - \pi)' - \Sigma(\pi) \right] = \pi_j M_j(x, \pi), \text{ (say)}. \quad (3.186)
\end{aligned}$$

Now, to compute $\frac{\partial \{\Sigma(\pi)\rho_j\}}{\partial \theta^{*\prime}}$, one may first write

$$\Sigma(\pi)\rho_j = \begin{pmatrix} \sigma_1 & \ldots & \sigma_j & \ldots & \sigma_{J-1} \end{pmatrix} \rho_j = \begin{pmatrix} \sigma_1' \\ \vdots \\ \sigma_j' \\ \vdots \\ \sigma_{J-1}' \end{pmatrix} \rho_j, \quad (3.187)$$

where

$$\sigma_j = \begin{pmatrix} -\pi_j \pi_1 \\ \vdots \\ -\pi_j \pi_{j-1} \\ \pi_j(1 - \pi_j) \\ -\pi_j \pi_{j+1} \\ \vdots \\ -\pi_j \pi_{J-1} \end{pmatrix} = \pi_j(x_j - \pi) = \begin{pmatrix} \sigma_{1j} \\ \vdots \\ \sigma_{j-1,j} \\ \sigma_{jj} \\ \sigma_{j+1,j} \\ \vdots \\ \sigma_{J-1,j} \end{pmatrix},$$

(say), for $j = 1,\ldots,J-1$. Thus, one obtains

$$\frac{\partial\{\Sigma(\pi)\rho_j\}}{\partial\theta^{*\prime}} = \frac{\partial}{\partial\theta^{*\prime}}\begin{pmatrix}\sigma_1' \\ \vdots \\ \sigma_j' \\ \vdots \\ \sigma_{J-1}'\end{pmatrix}\rho_j = \frac{\partial}{\partial\theta^{*\prime}}\begin{pmatrix}\Sigma_{h=1}^{J-1}\sigma_{h1}\rho_{jh} \\ \vdots \\ \Sigma_{h=1}^{J-1}\sigma_{hj}\rho_{jh} \\ \vdots \\ \Sigma_{h=1}^{J-1}\sigma_{h,J-1}\rho_{jh}\end{pmatrix}$$

$$= \frac{\partial}{\partial\theta^{*\prime}}\sum_{h=1}^{J-1}\begin{pmatrix}\sigma_{h1} \\ \vdots \\ \sigma_{hk} \\ \vdots \\ \sigma_{h,J-1}\end{pmatrix}\rho_{jh} = \sum_{h=1}^{J-1}\frac{\partial}{\partial\theta^{*\prime}}\begin{pmatrix}\sigma_{1h} \\ \vdots \\ \sigma_{kh} \\ \vdots \\ \sigma_{J-1,h}\end{pmatrix}\rho_{jh} = \sum_{h=1}^{J-1}\frac{\partial\sigma_h}{\partial\theta^{*\prime}}\rho_{jh} \tag{3.188}$$

$$= \sum_{h=1}^{J-1}\left[\rho_{jh}\otimes\right.$$

$$\left.\begin{pmatrix}-(\pi_h\sigma_{11}+\pi_1\sigma_{1h}) & \ldots & -(\pi_h\sigma_{c1}+\pi_1\sigma_{ch}) & \ldots & -(\pi_h\sigma_{J-1,1}+\pi_1\sigma_{J-1,h}) \\ \vdots & \vdots & \vdots & & \\ -(\pi_h\sigma_{1,h-1}+\pi_{h-1}\sigma_{1h}) & \ldots & -(\pi_h\sigma_{c,h-1}+\pi_{h-1}\sigma_{ch}) & \ldots & -(\pi_h\sigma_{J-1,h-1}+\pi_{h-1}\sigma_{J-1,h}) \\ \{(1-2\pi_h)\sigma_{1h}\} & \ldots & \{(1-2\pi_h)\sigma_{ch}\} & \ldots & \{(1-2\pi_h)\sigma_{J-1,h}\} \\ -(\pi_h\sigma_{1,h+1}+\pi_{h+1}\sigma_{1h}) & \ldots & -(\pi_h\sigma_{c,h+1}+\pi_{h+1}\sigma_{ch}) & \ldots & -(\pi_h\sigma_{J-1,h+1}+\pi_{h+1}\sigma_{J-1,h}) \\ \vdots & \vdots & \vdots & & \\ -(\pi_h\sigma_{1,J-1}+\pi_{J-1}\sigma_{1h}) & \ldots & -(\pi_h\sigma_{c,J-1}+\pi_{J-1}\sigma_{ch}) & \ldots & -(\pi_h\sigma_{J-1,J-1}+\pi_{J-1}\sigma_{J-1,h})\end{pmatrix}\right].$$

Alternatively, a simpler formula for this derivative may be obtained first by taking the derivative of the scalar quantity $\sigma_h'\rho_j$ with respect to $\theta^{*\prime}$ as follows:

$$\begin{aligned}\frac{\partial\sigma_h'\rho_j}{\partial\theta^{*\prime}} &= \frac{\partial\left[\pi_h(x_h-\pi)'\rho_j\right]}{\partial\theta^{*\prime}} : 1\times J-1 \\ &= \frac{\partial\left[\pi_h\left\{\rho_j'(x_h-\pi)\right\}\right]}{\partial\theta^{*\prime}} \\ &= \pi_h(x_h-\pi)'\left\{\rho_j'(x_h-\pi)\right\} - \pi_h\left[\rho_j'\frac{\partial\pi}{\partial\theta^{*\prime}}\right] \\ &= \pi_h(x_h-\pi)'\left\{\rho_j'(x_h-\pi)\right\} - \pi_h\left[\rho_j'\Sigma(\pi)\right], \text{by (3.180)} \\ &= \pi_h\left\{\rho_j'(x_h-\pi)\right\}(x_h-\pi)' - \pi_h\left[\rho_j'\Sigma(\pi)\right] \\ &= \pi_h\rho_j'[(x_h-\pi)(x_h-\pi)' - \Sigma(\pi)] \\ &= \pi_h\left\{\rho_j'M_h(x,\pi)\right\},\end{aligned} \tag{3.189}$$

where $M_h(\cdot)$ is the $(J-1)\times(J-1)$ matrix as in (3.186). Hence, by using (3.189), it follows from (3.187) that

$$\frac{\partial\{\Sigma(\pi)\rho_j\}}{\partial\theta^{*'}} = \begin{pmatrix} \pi_1\rho_j' M_1(x,\pi) \\ \vdots \\ \pi_j\rho_j' M_j(x,\pi) \\ \vdots \\ \pi_{J-1}\rho_j' M_{J-1}(x,\pi) \end{pmatrix}, \ (J-1)\times(J-1). \tag{3.190}$$

By combining (3.190) and (3.186), one finally obtains

$$\frac{\partial}{\partial\theta^{*'}}\left\{[\pi_j(x_j-\pi)] - \Sigma(\pi)\rho_j\right\} = \pi_j M_j(x,\pi) - \begin{pmatrix} \pi_1\rho_j' M_1(x,\pi) \\ \vdots \\ \pi_j\rho_j' M_j(x,\pi) \\ \vdots \\ \pi_{J-1}\rho_j' M_{J-1}(x,\pi) \end{pmatrix}. \tag{3.191}$$

Hence by using component derivative results from (3.191), (3.177), and (3.180) into (3.185), one completes the computation of the second order likelihood derivative matrix $\frac{\partial^2 Log\, L(\theta^*,\rho_M)}{\partial\theta^{*'}\partial\theta^*}$.

Further Alternative Ways to Compute the Derivatives One may find the following derivatives computation useful where the notation $\sum_{g=1}^{J-1} x_g\pi_g$ is retained instead of using its value π. Thus, to compute the general formula for $\frac{\partial^2\pi_j}{\partial\theta^{*'}\partial\theta^*}$, one uses

$$\frac{\partial\pi_j}{\partial\theta^*} = \pi_j x_j - \pi_j\sum_{g=1}^{J-1} x_g\pi_g = \pi_j[x_j - \sum_{g=1}^{J-1} x_g\pi_g] = \sigma_j(x), \text{ (say)}, \tag{3.192}$$

where $x_g = (x_{1g},\ldots,x_{kg},\ldots,x_{J-1,g})'$ is a known $(J-1)\times 1$ design vector involved in the probability formula for the gth category response. It then follows that

$$\begin{aligned}\frac{\partial^2\pi_j}{\partial\theta^{*'}\partial\theta^*} = \frac{\partial\sigma_j(x)}{\partial\theta^{*'}} &= \pi_j[\{x_j - \sum_{g=1}^{J-1} x_g\pi_g\}\{x_j - \sum_{g=1}^{J-1} x_g\pi_g\}'] \\ &- \pi_j\sum_{g=1}^{J-1}\pi_g x_g\{x_g - \sum_{k=1}^{J-1} x_k\pi_k\}' \\ &= \pi_j[\{x_j - \sum_{g=1}^{J-1} x_g\pi_g\}\{x_j - \sum_{g=1}^{J-1} x_g\pi_g\}'] \\ &- \pi_j\left[\sum_{g=1}^{J-1}\pi_g x_g x_g' - \{\sum_{g=1}^{J-1} x_g\pi_g\}\{\sum_{g=1}^{J-1} x_g\pi_g\}'\right]\end{aligned}$$

$$= \pi_j \left[\left(x_j x_j' - \sum_{g=1}^{J-1} \pi_g x_g x_g' \right) \right.$$
$$\left. - 2 \left(x_j \{ \sum_{g=1}^{J-1} x_g \pi_g \}' - \{ \sum_{g=1}^{J-1} x_g \pi_g \} \{ \sum_{g=1}^{J-1} x_g \pi_g \}' \right) \right]. \tag{3.193}$$

In the binary case, that is when $J = 2$, $x_1 = 1$, and $\theta^* = \beta_{10}$, this second order derivative in (3.193) reduces to

$$\pi_1[(1-\pi_1) - 2(\pi_1 - \pi_1^2)] = \pi_1(1-\pi_1)(1-2\pi_1),$$

as expected.

Next to compute the general version of the formula for $\frac{\partial \lambda^{(j)}(g)}{\partial \theta^*}$, one writes

$$\frac{\partial \pi'}{\partial \theta^*} = \frac{\partial}{\partial \theta^*} (\pi_1 \ldots \pi_j \ldots \pi_{J-1})$$
$$= \left[\pi_1 (x_1 - \sum_{g=1}^{J-1} \pi_g x_g) \ \ldots \ \pi_j (x_j - \sum_{g=1}^{J-1} \pi_g x_g) \right.$$
$$\left. \ldots \ \pi_{J-1} (x_{J-1} - \sum_{g=1}^{J-1} \pi_g x_g) \right] : (J-1) \times (J-1)$$
$$= \Sigma(\pi, x), \text{ (say)}, \tag{3.194}$$

which is the same as $\Sigma(\pi)$ in (3.180). More specifically, by writing (3.180) as

$$\frac{\partial \lambda^{(j)}(g)}{\partial \theta^*} = \begin{cases} \sigma_j(x) - [\Sigma(\pi,x)]\rho_j & \text{for } j = 1, \ldots, J-1 \\ -\sum_{k=1}^{J-1} [\sigma_k(x) - \Sigma(\pi,x)\rho_k] & \text{for } j = J, \end{cases} \tag{3.195}$$

one computes the second order derivatives as

$$\frac{\partial^2 \lambda^{(j)}(g)}{\partial \theta^{*\prime} \partial \theta^*} = \frac{\partial \sigma_j(x)}{\partial \theta^{*\prime}} - \left[\frac{\partial \{ \Sigma(\pi,x)\rho_j \}}{\partial \theta^{*\prime}} \right] \text{ for } j = 1, \ldots, J-1$$
$$= \frac{\partial^2 \pi_j}{\partial \theta^{*\prime} \partial \theta^*} - \left[\frac{\partial \{ \Sigma(\pi,x)\rho_j \}}{\partial \theta^{*\prime}} \right], \tag{3.196}$$

where the first term $\frac{\partial^2 \pi_j}{\partial \theta^{*\prime} \partial \theta^*}$ in general form involving x is known from (3.193). The second term may be computed as

$$\frac{\partial \{ \Sigma(\pi,x)\rho_j \}}{\partial \theta^{*\prime}} = \frac{\partial}{\partial \theta^{*\prime}} \left[\left\{ \pi_1 (x_1 - \sum_{g=1}^{J-1} \pi_g x_g) \ \ldots \ \pi_j (x_j - \sum_{g=1}^{J-1} \pi_g x_g) \right. \right.$$
$$\left. \left. \ldots \ \pi_{J-1} (x_{J-1} - \sum_{g=1}^{J-1} \pi_g x_g) \right\} \rho_j \right]$$

$$= \frac{\partial}{\partial \theta^{*\prime}} \sum_{m=1}^{J-1} \left[\pi_m (x_m - \sum_{g=1}^{J-1} \pi_g x_g) \rho_{jm} \right]$$

$$= \sum_{m=1}^{J-1} \left[\pi_m \left\{ \left(x_m x_m' - \sum_{g=1}^{J-1} \pi_g x_g x_g' \right) \right. \right.$$

$$\left. \left. - \; 2 \left(x_m \{ \sum_{g=1}^{J-1} x_g \pi_g \}' - \{ \sum_{g=1}^{J-1} x_g \pi_g \} \{ \sum_{g=1}^{J-1} x_g \pi_g \}' \right) \right\} \rho_{jm} \right], \quad (3.197)$$

by (3.193). Hence all first and second order derivatives with respect to θ^* are computed.

3.4.1.3.1(b) Likelihood Estimating Equation for ρ_M

Let

$$\rho^* = (\rho_1', \ldots, \rho_j', \ldots, \rho_{J-1}')' : (J-1)^2 \times 1; \text{ with } \rho_j = (\rho_{j1}, \ldots, \rho_{jc}, \ldots, \rho_{j,J-1})', \quad (3.198)$$

where ρ_j is the $(J-1) \times 1$ vector of dynamic dependence parameters involved in the conditional linear function in (3.171), i.e., $\lambda_{it|t-1}^{(j)}(y_{i,t-1}) = \pi_j + \rho_j'(y_{i,t-1} - \pi)$. Also recall that these conditional linear functions in (3.171) are re-expressed in (3.176) for computational convenience by using an indication vector for the known past response. That is, the conditional probabilities have the form

$$\lambda^{(j)}(g) = \begin{cases} \pi_j + \rho_j'(\delta_g - \pi) & \text{for } j = 1, \ldots, J-1; \; g = 1, \ldots, J \\ 1 - \sum_{k=1}^{J-1} \left[\pi_k + \rho_k'(\delta_g - \pi) \right] & \text{for } j = J; \; g = 1, \ldots, J. \end{cases} \quad (3.199)$$

Now because π_j is free from ρ_j and $\lambda^{(j)}(g)$ depends on ρ_j through (3.199), it follows from the likelihood function (3.175) that the likelihood estimating equations for ρ_j $(j = 1, \ldots, J-1)$ have the form

$$\frac{\partial Log\, L(\theta^*, \rho_M)}{\partial \rho_j} = \sum_{h=1}^{J} \sum_{g=1}^{J} \left[\left\{ \sum_{t=2}^{T} K_{gh}(t-1,t) \right\} \frac{1}{\lambda^{(h)}(g)} \frac{\partial \lambda^{(h)}(g)}{\partial \rho_j} \right]$$

$$= \sum_{g=1}^{J} \left[\left\{ \sum_{t=2}^{T} K_{gj}(t-1,t) \right\} \frac{1}{\lambda^{(j)}(g)} (\delta_g - \pi) \right]$$

$$- \sum_{g=1}^{J} \left[\left\{ \sum_{t=2}^{T} K_{gJ}(t-1,t) \right\} \frac{1}{\lambda^{(J)}(g)} (\delta_g - \pi) \right] = 0, \quad (3.200)$$

for $j = 1,\ldots,J-1$, leading to the estimating equations for the elements of $\rho^* = (\rho_1',\ldots,\rho_j',\ldots,\rho_{J-1}')'$ as

$$\frac{\partial Log\, L(\theta^*,\rho_M)}{\partial \rho^*} = \begin{pmatrix} \frac{\partial Log\, L(\theta^*,\rho_M)}{\partial \rho_1} \\ \vdots \\ \frac{\partial Log\, L(\theta^*,\rho_M)}{\partial \rho_j} \\ \vdots \\ \frac{\partial Log\, L(\theta^*,\rho_M)}{\partial \rho_{J-1}} \end{pmatrix} = 0 : (J-1)^2 \times 1. \quad (3.201)$$

One may solve these likelihood equations in (3.201) for ρ^* by using the iterative equation

$$\hat{\rho}^*(r+1) = \hat{\rho}^*(r) - \left[\left\{ \frac{\partial^2 \text{Log}\, L(\theta^*,\rho_M)}{\partial \rho^* \partial \rho^{*\prime}} \right\}^{-1} \frac{\partial \text{Log}\, L(\theta^*,\rho_M)}{\partial \rho^*} \right]_{|\rho^*=\hat{\rho}^*(r)}, \quad (3.202)$$

where the $(J-1)^2 \times (J-1)^2$ second derivative matrix is computed by using the formulas

$$\begin{aligned} \frac{\partial^2 \text{Log}\, L(\theta^*,\rho_M)}{\partial \rho_j \partial \rho_j'} &= -\sum_{g=1}^{J} \left[\left\{ \sum_{t=2}^{T} K_{gj}(t-1,t) \right\} \frac{1}{\{\lambda^{(j)}(g)\}^2} (\delta_g - \pi)(\delta_g - \pi)' \right] \\ &\quad - \sum_{g=1}^{J} \left[\left\{ \sum_{t=2}^{T} K_{gJ}(t-1,t) \right\} \frac{1}{\{\lambda^{(J)}(g)\}^2} (\delta_g - \pi)(\delta_g - \pi)' \right], \end{aligned} \quad (3.203)$$

for all $j = 1,\ldots,J-1$, and

$$\frac{\partial^2 \text{Log}\, L(\theta^*,\rho_M)}{\partial \rho_j \partial \rho_k'} = -\sum_{g=1}^{J} \left[\left\{ \sum_{t=2}^{T} K_{gJ}(t-1,t) \right\} \frac{1}{\{\lambda^{(J)}(g)\}^2} (\delta_g - \pi)(\delta_g - \pi)' \right], \quad (3.204)$$

for all $j \neq k; j,k = 1,\ldots,J-1$.

In Sect. 3.4.1.2 we have fitted the LDCMP model (3.146)–(3.147) by using the GQL approach and the estimation methodology was illustrated in Sect. 3.4.1.2.1 by analyzing the TMISL data. Even though the estimation technique was different, because in this Sect. 3.4.1.3 we have fitted the same LDCMP model, we did not apply this technique of computation to the TMISL data. However, in Sect. 3.4.2.2 we will analyze the TMISL data by fitting a different, namely non-linear MDL model.

3.4.2 MDL Model

In this section, we generalize the covariate free BDL model discussed in Sect. 3.2.4, to the multinomial case. Remark that this type of non-linear dynamic logit model is appropriate for the situations where the mean and variance of the responses at a given time are likely to be recursive functions of the past means and variances, respectively. See Sutradhar (2011, Section 7.7.2) for details on such dynamic logit models for binary data with time dependent covariates, whereas we have concentrated on a simpler covariate free stationary binary case in Sect. 3.2.4. Further stationary binary cases with stationary (time independent) covariates were discussed in Sect. 3.3.2. Turning back to the multinomial case, similar to (3.170), we write the probability density for the multinomial variable y_{it} at initial time $t = 1$, that is, for $y_{i1} = (y_{i11}, \ldots, y_{i1j}, \ldots, y_{i1,J-1})'$ as

$$\begin{aligned} f(y_{i1}) &= P((y_{i11}, \ldots, y_{i1j}, \ldots, y_{i1,J-1}) \\ &= \frac{1!}{y_{i11}! \ldots y_{i1j}! \ldots y_{i1,J-1}! y_{i1J}!} \Pi_{j=1}^{J} \pi_j^{y_{i1j}}, \end{aligned} \tag{3.205}$$

where, for $t = 1$, by (3.144), π_j is defined as

$$P[y_{i1} = y_{i1}^{(j)}] = \pi_{(i1)j} \equiv \pi_j = \begin{cases} \frac{\exp(\beta_{j0})}{1+\sum_{g=1}^{J-1}\exp(\beta_{g0})} & \text{for } j = 1, \ldots, J-1 \\ \frac{1}{1+\sum_{g=1}^{J-1}\exp(\beta_{g0})} & \text{for } j = J. \end{cases} \tag{3.206}$$

However, for $t = 2, \ldots, T$, as a generalization of the conditional probability (3.71) for the binary data, we now consider that the conditional probability for the multinomial variable at time t ($t = 2, \ldots, T$) given the responses at time $t-1$ has the dynamic logit form given by

$$\begin{aligned} \eta_{it|t-1}^{(j)}(g) &= P\left(Y_{it} = y_{it}^{(j)} \,\middle|\, Y_{i,t-1} = y_{i,t-1}^{(g)}\right) \\ &= \begin{cases} \frac{\exp\left(\beta_{j0}+\gamma_j' y_{i,t-1}^{(g)}\right)}{1+\sum_{h=1}^{J-1}\exp\left(\beta_{h0}+\gamma_h' y_{i,t-1}^{(g)}\right)}, & \text{for } j = 1, \ldots, J-1; g = 1, \ldots, J \\ \frac{1}{1+\sum_{h=1}^{J-1}\exp\left(\beta_{h0}+\gamma_h' y_{i,t-1}^{(g)}\right)}, & \text{for } j = J; g = 1, \ldots, J, \end{cases} \end{aligned} \tag{3.207}$$

where $\gamma_j = (\gamma_{j1}, \ldots, \gamma_{jh}, \ldots, \gamma_{j,J-1})'$ for $j = 1, \ldots, J-1$, and hence

$$\gamma_j' y_{i,t-1}^{(g)} = \sum_{h=1}^{J-1} \gamma_{jh} y_{i,t-1,h}^{(g)}, \text{ for all } g = 1, \ldots, J.$$

Note that for $\gamma_j = (\gamma_{j1}, \ldots, \gamma_{jh}, \ldots, \gamma_{j,J-1})'$,

$$\gamma = (\gamma_1', \ldots, \gamma_j', \ldots, \gamma_{J-1}')'$$

denotes the vector of dynamic dependence parameters, but they are neither correlation nor odds ratio parameters. However, it is true that the correlations of the repeated multinomial responses will be functions of these γ parameters.

Basic Moment Properties of the MDL Model It follows from (3.148)–(3.150) that for $t = 1$,

$$\begin{aligned} E[Y_{i1}] &= [\pi_1, \ldots, \pi_j, \ldots, \pi_{J-1}]' = \pi : (J-1) \times 1 \\ \mathrm{var}[Y_{i1}] &= \Sigma(\pi) = \mathrm{diag}[\pi_1, \ldots, \pi_j, \ldots, \pi_{J-1}] - \pi\pi'. \end{aligned}$$

For $t = 2, \ldots, T$, by using the initial marginal model (3.206) for $t = 1$ and the conditional probability model (3.207) for $t = 2, \ldots, T$, similar to (3.72)–(3.73), one may derive the recursive relationships for the unconditional mean, variance, and covariance matrices (see also Loredo-Osti and Sutradhar 2012) as

$$\begin{aligned} E[Y_{it}] &= \tilde{\pi}_{(t)} = \eta(J) + \left[\eta_M - \eta(J)1'_{J-1}\right] \tilde{\pi}_{(t-1)} \\ \mathrm{var}[Y_{it}] &= \mathrm{diag}[\tilde{\pi}_{(t)1}, \ldots, \tilde{\pi}_{(t)j}, \ldots, \tilde{\pi}_{(t)(J-1)}] - \tilde{\pi}_{(t)}\tilde{\pi}'_{(t)} \\ &= (\mathrm{cov}(Y_{itj}, Y_{itk})) = (\sigma_{(t)jk}),\ j,k = 1, \ldots, J-1 \\ \mathrm{cov}[Y_{iu}, Y_{it}] &= \mathrm{var}[Y_{iu}][\eta_M - \eta(J)1'_{J-1}]^{t-u}, \text{ for } u < t \\ &= (\mathrm{cov}(Y_{iuj}, Y_{itk})) = (\sigma_{(ut)jk}),\ j,k = 1, \ldots, J-1, \end{aligned} \tag{3.208}$$

where

$$\tilde{\pi}_{(1)} = \pi : (J-1) \times 1,$$

and for example,

$$[\eta_M - \eta(J)1'_{J-1}]^3 = [\eta_M - \eta(J)1'_{J-1}][\eta_M - \eta(J)1'_{J-1}][\eta_M - \eta(J)1'_{J-1}],$$

and where

$$\eta(J) = [\eta^{(1)}(J), \ldots, \eta^{(j)}(J) \ldots, \eta^{(J-1)}(J)]' = \pi : (J-1) \times 1$$

$$\eta_M = \begin{pmatrix} \eta^{(1)}(1) & \cdots & \eta^{(1)}(g) & \cdots & \eta^{(1)}(J-1) \\ \vdots & \vdots & \vdots & \vdots & \vdots \\ \eta^{(j)}(1) & \cdots & \eta^{(j)}(g) & \cdots & \eta^{(j)}(J-1) \\ \vdots & \vdots & \vdots & \vdots & \vdots \\ \eta^{(J-1)}(1) & \cdots & \eta^{(J-1)}(g) & \cdots & \eta^{(J-1)}(J-1) \end{pmatrix} : (J-1) \times (J-1).$$

3.4.2.1 Likelihood Function

Because y_{it} is a multinomial variable at any time point t, it is clear that conditional on $Y_{i,t-1} = y_{i,t-1}^{(g)}$, one may write the conditional distribution of y_{it} as

$$f(y_{it}|y^{(g)}_{i,t-1}) = \frac{1!}{y_{it1}!\ldots y_{itj}!\ldots y_{it,J-1}!y_{itJ}!}\Pi_{j=1}^{J}\left[\eta^{(j)}_{it|t-1}(g)\right]^{y_{itj}}, \ g = 1,\ldots,J \quad (3.209)$$

where $\eta^{(j)}_{it|t-1}(g)$ for $j = 1,\ldots,J$, are given by (3.207). Let γ_M be the $(J-1)\times(J-1)$ dynamic dependence parameters matrix given by

$$\gamma_M = \begin{pmatrix} \gamma'_1 \\ \vdots \\ \gamma'_j \\ \vdots \\ \gamma'_{J-1} \end{pmatrix} : (J-1)\times(J-1), \quad (3.210)$$

and $\theta^* = [\beta_{10},\ldots,\beta_{j0},\ldots,\beta_{J-1,0}]'$ denotes the vector of category index parameters. Similar to the LDCMP model (3.172)–(3.173), one may write the likelihood function under the present MDL model as

$$\begin{aligned} L(\theta^*,\gamma_M) &= \Pi_{i=1}^{K}\left[f(y_{i1})\Pi_{t=2}^{T}f(y_{it}|y_{i,t-1})\right] \\ &= \left[\Pi_{i=1}^{K}f(y_{i1})\right] \\ &\times \Pi_{t=2}^{T}\Pi_{g=1}^{J}\Pi_{i\in g}^{K}\left[f(y_{it}|y^{(g)}_{i,t-1})\right] \\ &= c_0^*\left[\Pi_{j=1}^{J}\Pi_{i=1}^{K}\pi_j^{y_{i1j}}\right] \\ &\times \Pi_{t=2}^{T}\Pi_{j=1}^{J}\Pi_{g=1}^{J}\Pi_{i\in g}^{K}\left\{\eta^{(j)}_{it|t-1}(y^{(g)}_{i,t-1})\right\}^{y_{itj}}, \end{aligned} \quad (3.211)$$

where c_0^* is the normalizing constant free from any parameters. Next, by using the abbreviation $\eta^{(j)}(g) \equiv \eta^{(j)}_{it|t-1}(y^{(g)}_{i,t-1})$, the log likelihood function may be written as

$$\begin{aligned} Log\,L(\theta^*,\gamma_M) &= log\,c_0^* + \sum_{i=1}^{K}\sum_{j=1}^{J}y_{i1j}log\,\pi_j \\ &+ \sum_{t=2}^{T}\sum_{j=1}^{J}\sum_{g=1}^{J}\sum_{i\in g}^{K}\left[y_{itj}log\,\eta^{(j)}_{it|t-1}(g)\right], \end{aligned} \quad (3.212)$$

which, by using the cell counts from the contingency Table 3.17, reduces to

$$\begin{aligned} Log\,L(\theta^*,\gamma_M) &= log\,c_0^* + \sum_{j=1}^{J}K_j(1)log\,\pi_j \\ &+ \sum_{j=1}^{J}\sum_{g=1}^{J}\left\{log\,\eta^{(j)}(g)\right\}\left[\sum_{t=2}^{T}K_{gj}(t-1,t)\right], \end{aligned} \quad (3.213)$$

where $K_{gj}(t-1,t)$ is the number of individuals with responses belonging to jth category at time t, given that their responses were in the gth category at time $t-1$. Note that this log likelihood function is similar to (3.175) for the LDCMP model, but the big difference lies in the definition of the conditional probabilities. That is, unlike the linear conditional probabilities in (3.175), the conditional probabilities in the present case are non-linear and they are given by

$$\eta^{(j)}(g) = \begin{cases} \frac{\exp(x_j'\theta^* + \gamma_j'\delta_g)}{1+\sum_{h=1}^{J-1}\exp(x_h'\theta^* + \gamma_h'\delta_g)} & \text{for } j = 1,\ldots,J-1;\ g = 1,\ldots,J \\ \frac{1}{1+\sum_{h=1}^{J-1}\exp(x_h'\theta^* + \gamma_h'\delta_g)} & \text{for } j = J;\ g = 1,\ldots,J, \end{cases} \tag{3.214}$$

where, similar to (3.176),

$$\delta_g = \begin{cases} [01'_{g-1}, 1, 01'_{J-1-g}]' & \text{for } g = 1,\ldots,J-1 \\ 01_{J-1} & \text{for } g = J. \end{cases}$$

3.4.2.1.1 Likelihood Estimating Equation for θ^*

It follows from the log likelihood function in (3.213) that the likelihood estimating equations for θ^* has the form

$$\begin{aligned} \frac{\partial Log\, L(\theta^*, \gamma_M)}{\partial \theta^*} &= \sum_{j=1}^{J} K_j(1) \frac{1}{\pi_j} \frac{\partial \pi_j}{\partial \theta^*} \\ &+ \sum_{j=1}^{J}\sum_{g=1}^{J}\left[\left\{\sum_{t=2}^{T} K_{gj}(t-1,t)\right\}\frac{1}{\eta^{(j)}(g)}\frac{\partial \eta^{(j)}(g)}{\partial \theta^*}\right] = 0. \end{aligned} \tag{3.215}$$

For given γ_M, these likelihood equations in (3.215) may be solved iteratively by using the iterative equations for θ^* given by

$$\hat{\theta}^*(r+1) = \hat{\theta}^*(r) - \left[\left\{\frac{\partial^2 \text{Log}\, L(\theta^*, \gamma_M)}{\partial \theta^{*\prime}\partial \theta^*}\right\}^{-1} \frac{\partial \text{Log}\, L(\theta^*, \gamma_M)}{\partial \theta^*}\right]_{|\theta^* = \hat{\theta}^*(r)} ;\ (J-1)\times 1, \tag{3.216}$$

where the second order derivative matrix has the formula

$$\begin{aligned} \frac{\partial^2 Log\, L(\theta^*, \gamma_M)}{\partial \theta^{*\prime}\partial \theta^*} &= \sum_{j=1}^{J} K_j(1)\left[\frac{\partial}{\partial \theta^{*\prime}}\left\{\frac{1}{\pi_j}\frac{\partial \pi_j}{\partial \theta^*}\right\}\right] \\ &+ \sum_{j=1}^{J}\sum_{g=1}^{J}\left[\left\{\sum_{t=2}^{T} K_{gj}(t-1,t)\right\}\left\{\frac{1}{\eta^{(j)}(g)}\frac{\partial^2 \eta^{(j)}(g)}{\partial \theta^{*\prime}\partial \theta^*}\right.\right. \end{aligned}$$

$$- \frac{1}{\{\eta^{(j)}(g)\}^2} \frac{\partial \eta^{(j)}(g)}{\partial \theta^*} \frac{\partial \eta^{(j)}(g)}{\partial \theta^{*\prime}} \Bigg\} \Bigg]. \tag{3.217}$$

The first and second order derivatives involved in the estimating equations (3.215)–(3.217) are computed as follows:

Computation of $\frac{1}{\pi_j}\frac{\partial \pi_j}{\partial \theta^*}$ and $\frac{\partial}{\partial \theta^{*\prime}}\left\{\frac{1}{\pi_j}\frac{\partial \pi_j}{\partial \theta^*}\right\}$:
These formulas are the same as in (3.178) under the LDCMP model. That is,

$$\frac{1}{\pi_j}\frac{\partial \pi_j}{\partial \theta^*} = \begin{cases} x_j - \sum_{g=1}^{J-1} \pi_g x_g = x_j - \pi & \text{for } j = 1,\ldots,J-1 \\ -\pi & \text{for } j = J, \end{cases} \tag{3.218}$$

and

$$\begin{aligned} \frac{\partial}{\partial \theta^{*\prime}}\left\{\frac{1}{\pi_j}\frac{\partial \pi_j}{\partial \theta^*}\right\} &= -\frac{\partial \pi}{\partial \theta^{*\prime}} \\ &= -\left[\frac{\partial \pi'}{\partial \theta^*}\right]' = -\Sigma'(\pi) = -\Sigma(\pi), \end{aligned} \tag{3.219}$$

(see (3.180)).

Computation of $\frac{\partial \eta^{(j)}(g)}{\partial \theta^*}$ and $\frac{\partial^2 \eta^{(j)}(g)}{\partial \theta^{*\prime}\partial \theta^*}$:
By (3.214), the first derivative has the formula

$$\begin{aligned} \frac{\partial \eta^{(j)}(g)}{\partial \theta^*} &= \begin{cases} \eta^{(j)}(g)\left[x_j - \sum_{h=1}^{J-1} x_h \eta^{(h)}(g)\right] & \text{for } j = 1,\ldots,J-1;\ g = 1,\ldots,J \\ -\left[\eta^{(J)}(g) \sum_{h=1}^{J-1} x_h \eta^{(h)}(g)\right] & \text{for } j = J;\ g = 1,\ldots,J, \end{cases} \\ &= \begin{cases} \eta^{(j)}(g)\left[x_j - \eta(g)\right] & \text{for } j = 1,\ldots,J-1;\ g = 1,\ldots,J \\ -\left[\eta^{(J)}(g)\eta(g)\right] & \text{for } j = J;\ g = 1,\ldots,J, \end{cases} \end{aligned} \tag{3.220}$$

where

$$\eta(g) = [\eta^{(1)}(g),\ldots,\eta^{(j)}(g),\ldots,\eta^{(J-1)}(g)]'.$$

The formulae for the second order derivatives follow from (3.220) and they are given by

$$\frac{\partial^2 \eta^{(j)}(g)}{\partial \theta^{*\prime}\partial \theta^*} = \begin{cases} \eta^{(j)}(g)\left[(x_j - \eta(g))(x_j - \eta(g))' - \frac{\partial \eta(g)}{\partial \theta^{*\prime}}\right] & \text{for } j = 1,\ldots,J-1 \\ \eta^{(J)}(g)\left[\eta(g)\eta'(g) - \frac{\partial \eta(g)}{\partial \theta^{*\prime}}\right] & \text{for } j = J \end{cases} \tag{3.221}$$

$$\begin{aligned} &= \eta^{(j)}(g)\left[(x_j - \eta(g))(x_j - \eta(g))' - \frac{\partial \eta(g)}{\partial \theta^{*\prime}}\right] \\ &= \eta^{(j)}(g) M_j^*(x, \eta(g)),\ \text{(say), for all } j = 1,\ldots,J;\ g = 1,\ldots,J, \end{aligned} \tag{3.222}$$

by using the notation $x_J = 01_{J-1}$. However, it remains yet to derive the formula for $\frac{\partial \eta(g)}{\partial \theta^{*\prime}}$.

Computation of $\frac{\partial \eta(g)}{\partial \theta^{*\prime}}$:
Notice from (3.220) that

$$\frac{\partial \eta^{(j)}(g)}{\partial \theta^{*\prime}} = \eta^{(j)}(g)(x_j - \eta(g))' : 1 \times (J-1),$$

yielding

$$\frac{\partial \eta(g)}{\partial \theta^{*\prime}} = \frac{\partial}{\partial \theta^{*\prime}} \begin{pmatrix} \eta^{(1)}(g) \\ \vdots \\ \eta^{(j)}(g) \\ \vdots \\ \eta^{(J-1)}(g) \end{pmatrix}$$

$$= \begin{pmatrix} \eta^{(1)}(g)(x_1 - \eta(g))' \\ \vdots \\ \eta^{(j)}(g)(x_j - \eta(g))' \\ \vdots \\ \eta^{(J-1)}(g)(x_{J-1} - \eta(g))' \end{pmatrix} : (J-1) \times (J-1). \quad (3.223)$$

3.4.2.1.2 Likelihood Estimating Equation for γ_M

Let

$$\gamma^* = (\gamma_1', \ldots, \gamma_j', \ldots, \gamma_{J-1}')' : (J-1)^2 \times 1; \text{ where } \gamma_j = (\gamma_{j1}, \ldots, \gamma_{jh}, \ldots, \gamma_{j,J-1})', \quad (3.224)$$

where γ_j is the $(J-1) \times 1$ vector of dynamic dependence parameters involved in the conditional multinomial logit function in (3.207). See also (3.214) for an equivalent but simpler expression for these conditional logit functions. Using this latter form (3.214), by similar calculations as in (3.220), one writes

$$\frac{\partial \eta^{(h)}(g)}{\partial \gamma_j} = \begin{cases} \delta_g \eta^{(j)}(g)[1 - \eta^{(j)}(g)] & \text{for } h = j; h, j = 1, \ldots, J-1 \\ -\delta_g \eta^{(j)}(g) \eta^{(h)}(g) & \text{for } h \neq j; h, j = 1, \ldots, J-1 \\ -\delta_g \eta^{(j)}(g) \eta^{(J)}(g) & \text{for } h = J;\ j = 1, \ldots, J-1, \end{cases} \quad (3.225)$$

for all $g = 1, \ldots, J$. Using these derivatives, it follows from the likelihood function (3.213) that

$$\begin{aligned}
\frac{\partial Log\, L(\theta^*, \gamma_M)}{\partial \gamma_j} &= \sum_{h=1}^{J}\sum_{g=1}^{J}\left[\left\{\sum_{t=2}^{T} K_{gh}(t-1,t)\right\}\frac{1}{\eta^{(h)}(g)}\frac{\partial \eta^{(h)}(g)}{\partial \gamma_j}\right] \\
&= \sum_{g=1}^{J}\left[\left\{\sum_{t=2}^{T} K_{gj}(t-1,t)\right\}\delta_g\left(1-\eta^{(j)}(g)\right)\right] \\
&- \sum_{g=1}^{J}\sum_{h\neq j}^{J}\left[\left\{\sum_{t=2}^{T} K_{gh}(t-1,t)\right\}\frac{1}{\eta^{(h)}(g)}\delta_g\left(\eta^{(j)}(g)\eta^{(h)}(g)\right)\right] \\
&= \sum_{g=1}^{J}\left[\left\{\sum_{t=2}^{T} K_{gj}(t-1,t)\right\}\delta_g\right] \\
&- \sum_{g=1}^{J}\sum_{h=1}^{J}\left[\left\{\sum_{t=2}^{T} K_{gh}(t-1,t)\right\}\delta_g\eta^{(j)}(g)\right] = 0, \qquad (3.226)
\end{aligned}$$

for $j = 1,\ldots,J-1$, leading to the estimating equations for the elements of $\gamma^* = (\gamma_1',\ldots,\gamma_j',\ldots,\gamma_{J-1}')'$ as

$$\frac{\partial Log\, L(\theta^*, \gamma_M)}{\partial \gamma^*} = \begin{pmatrix} \frac{\partial Log\, L(\theta^*,\gamma_M)}{\partial \gamma_1} \\ \vdots \\ \frac{\partial Log\, L(\theta^*,\gamma_M)}{\partial \gamma_j} \\ \vdots \\ \frac{\partial Log\, L(\theta^*,\gamma_M)}{\partial \gamma_{J-1}} \end{pmatrix} = 0 : (J-1)^2 \times 1. \qquad (3.227)$$

One may solve this likelihood equation (3.224) for γ^* by using the iterative equation

$$\hat{\gamma}^*(r+1) = \hat{\gamma}^*(r) - \left[\left\{\frac{\partial^2 \text{Log}\, L(\theta^*, \gamma_M)}{\partial \gamma^* \partial \gamma^{*\prime}}\right\}^{-1}\frac{\partial \text{Log}\, L(\theta^*, \gamma_M)}{\partial \gamma^*}\right]_{|\gamma^*=\hat{\gamma}^*(r)}, \qquad (3.228)$$

where the $(J-1)^2 \times (J-1)^2$ second derivative matrix is computed by using the formulas

$$\frac{\partial^2 \text{Log}\, L(\theta^*, \gamma_M)}{\partial \gamma_j \partial \gamma_j'} = -\sum_{g=1}^{J}\sum_{h=1}^{J}\left[\left\{\sum_{t=2}^{T} K_{gh}(t-1,t)\right\}\eta^{(j)}(g)\left(1-\eta^{(j)}(g)\right)\delta_g\delta_g'\right] \qquad (3.229)$$

for all $j = 1,\ldots,J-1$, and

$$\frac{\partial^2 \text{Log}\, L(\theta^*, \gamma_M)}{\partial \gamma_j \partial \gamma_k'} = \sum_{g=1}^{J}\sum_{h=1}^{J}\left[\left\{\sum_{t=2}^{T} K_{gh}(t-1,t)\right\}\left(\eta^{(j)}(g)\eta^{(k)}(g)\right)\delta_g\delta_g'\right], \qquad (3.230)$$

for all $j \neq k; j,k = 1,\ldots,J-1$.

Table 3.21 Observed and LDCMP model based fitted probabilities (by using GQL approach) under all three stress levels for the TMISL data

			OMP at time t			
Stress level	Probabilities (I)	Probabilities (LDCMP)	1	2	3	4
Low	0.1376	0.1325	0.0861	0.1985	0.1161	0.1498
Medium	0.6676	0.6681	0.6704	0.6217	0.7041	0.6742
High	0.1948	0.1994	0.2435	0.1798	0.1798	0.1760

3.4.2.2 Illustration 3.10: Analysis of Longitudinal TMISL (Three Categories) Data (Covariate Free) Fitting MDL Model Using Likelihood Approach

In Sect. 3.4.1.2.1, we have fitted an LDCMP model to the TMISL data through a GQL inference approach. Because the model was assumed to be covariate free, the multinomial (three category) marginal probabilities at different times were time independent, even though the data exhibit the change in marginal probabilities over time. See, for example, Table 3.21 where these OMP along with estimated stationary marginal probabilities are displayed. In fact the inclusion of the distance covariate in the LDCMP model will also not change the marginal probabilities over time, because this covariate is not time dependent. However, because the MDL model considered in the present section (see (3.206)–(3.207)) is conditionally non-linear, as shown in (3.208), it produces recursive mean, variance, and correlations over time. Thus, even though the model is either covariate free completely or contains time independent covariates, the MDL model is capable of producing time dependent marginal probabilities through the recursive relationship due to non-linearity. The purpose of this section is to illustrate such a non-linear MDL model by applying it to the same TMISL data used in illustration 3.9. Furthermore, for this MDL model, the standard likelihood approach is quite manageable and hence we illustrate the fitting through maximum likelihood estimation (MLE) approach, instead of using the GQL technique.

For easy understanding of the application of the MLE approach, we further simplify the likelihood equations (3.215) for the category based intercept parameters $\theta^* = (\beta_{10}, \beta_{20})'$ and (3.227) for the category based dynamic dependence parameters $\gamma^* = (\gamma_{11}, \gamma_{12}, \gamma_{21}, \gamma_{22})'$ in the context of the present TMISL data. By writing, for example,

$$K_{gj}^* = K_{gj}(1,2) + K_{gj}(2,3) + K_{gj}(3,4),$$

for $g, j = 1, \ldots, 3$, and

$$K_g^* = \sum_{j=1}^{3} K_{gj}^*,$$

for $g = 1,\ldots,3$ the two likelihood equations in (3.215) have the form

$$\begin{aligned} f_1(\theta^*,\gamma^*) &= [K_1(1) - K\pi_1] + [\{K_{11}^* - K_1^*\eta^{(1)}(1)\} + \{K_{21}^* - K_2^*\eta^{(1)}(2)\} \\ &\quad + \{K_{31}^* - K_3^*\eta^{(1)}(3)\}] = 0 \\ f_2(\theta^*,\gamma^*) &= [K_2(1) - K\pi_2] + [\{K_{12}^* - K_1^*\eta^{(2)}(1)\} + \{K_{22}^* - K_2^*\eta^{(2)}(2)\} \\ &\quad + \{K_{32}^* - K_3^*\eta^{(2)}(3)\}] = 0, \end{aligned}$$

and similarly the four likelihood equations for γ^* in (3.227) have the forms

$$\begin{aligned} g_1(\gamma^*,\theta^*) &= K_{11}^* - K_1^*\eta^{(1)}(1) = 0 \\ g_2(\gamma^*,\theta^*) &= K_{21}^* - K_2^*\eta^{(1)}(2) = 0 \\ g_3(\gamma^*,\theta^*) &= K_{12}^* - K_1^*\eta^{(2)}(1) = 0 \\ g_4(\gamma^*,\theta^*) &= K_{22}^* - K_2^*\eta^{(2)}(2) = 0, \end{aligned}$$

respectively. Similarly, the second order derivatives of the likelihood function with respect to θ^* and γ^* were simplified. The second order derivative matrix for θ^*, following (3.217), is given by

$$F(\theta^*,\gamma^*) = \begin{pmatrix} f_{11}(\theta^*,\gamma^*) & f_{12}(\theta^*,\gamma^*) \\ f_{21}(\theta^*,\gamma^*) & f_{22}(\theta^*,\gamma^*) \end{pmatrix},$$

where

$$\begin{aligned} f_{11}(\cdot) &= -K\pi_1(1-\pi_1) - \Big[K_1^*\eta^{(1)}(1)(1-\eta^{(1)}(1)) \\ &\quad + K_2^*\eta^{(1)}(2)(1-\eta^{(1)}(2)) + K_3^*\eta^{(1)}(3)(1-\eta^{(1)}(3))\Big] \\ f_{12}(\cdot) &= K\pi_1\pi_2 + (K_{12}^* + K_{13}^*)\eta^{(1)}(1)\eta^{(2)}(1) \\ &\quad + (K_{22}^* + K_{23}^*)\eta^{(1)}(2)\eta^{(2)}(2) + (K_{31}^* + K_{33}^*)\eta^{(1)}(3)\eta^{(2)}(3) \\ f_{21}(\cdot) &= f_{12}(\cdot) \\ f_{22}(\cdot) &= -K\pi_2(1-\pi_2) - \Big[K_1^*\eta^{(2)}(1)(1-\eta^{(2)}(1)) \\ &\quad + K_2^*\eta^{(2)}(2)(1-\eta^{(2)}(2)) + K_3^*\eta^{(2)}(3)(1-\eta^{(2)}(3))\Big], \end{aligned}$$

and similarly the second order derivative matrix for γ^*, following (3.229)–(3.230), is given by

$$\Gamma(\gamma^*,\theta^*) = \begin{pmatrix} G_1 & G_2 \\ G_2' & G_3 \end{pmatrix},$$

where

$$G_1 = -\begin{pmatrix} K_1^*\eta^{(1)}(1)(1-\eta^{(1)}(1)) & 0 \\ 0 & K_2^*\eta^{(1)}(2)(1-\eta^{(1)}(2)) \end{pmatrix}$$

$$G_2 = \begin{pmatrix} K_1^*\eta^{(1)}(1)\eta^{(2)}(1) & 0 \\ 0 & K_2^*\eta^{(1)}(2)\eta^{(2)}(2) \end{pmatrix}$$

$$G_3 = -\begin{pmatrix} K_1^*\eta^{(2)}(1)(1-\eta^{(2)}(1)) & 0 \\ 0 & K_2^*\eta^{(2)}(2)(1-\eta^{(2)}(2)) \end{pmatrix}.$$

Now by using the iterative equations

$$\hat{\theta}^*(r+1) = \hat{\theta}^*(r) - \left[\{F(\theta^*,\gamma^*)\}^{-1}\begin{pmatrix} f_1(\theta^*,\gamma^*) \\ f_2(\theta^*,\gamma^*) \end{pmatrix}\right]_{|\theta^*=\hat{\theta}^*(r)} : 2\times 1,$$

(see (3.216)) for θ^*, and

$$\hat{\gamma}^*(r+1) = \hat{\gamma}^*(r) - \left[\{\Gamma(\gamma^*,\theta^*)\}^{-1}\begin{pmatrix} g_1(\gamma^*,\theta^*) \\ g_2(\gamma^*,\theta^*) \\ g_3(\gamma^*,\theta^*) \\ g_4(\gamma^*,\theta^*) \end{pmatrix}\right]_{|\gamma^*=\hat{\gamma}^*(r)} : 4\times 1,$$

(see (3.228)) for γ^*, in ten cycles of iterations, we obtained the maximum likelihood estimates (MLE) for the category intercept parameters as

$$\hat{\beta}_{10,MLE} = -1.9117;\ \hat{\beta}_{20,MLE} = 0.3798,$$

and for the lag 1 dynamic dependence parameters as

$$\hat{\gamma}_{11,MLE} = 5.8238,\ \hat{\gamma}_{12,MLE} = 2.4410;\ \hat{\gamma}_{21,MLE} = 3.6455,\ \hat{\gamma}_{22,MLE} = 1.8920.$$

To understand the marginal probabilities (3.208) for three categories over time, we first use the above estimates to compute

$$\begin{aligned}\tilde{\pi}_{(1)} &= [\tilde{\pi}_{(1)1}\ \text{(Low group)}, \tilde{\pi}_{(1)2}\ \text{(Medium group)}]' : 2\times 1 \\ &= \pi : 2\times 1 \\ &= [0.0567,\ 0.5602]',\end{aligned}$$

Table 3.22 Observed marginal probabilities (OMP) and MDL model based fitted marginal probabilities (FMP) ($\tilde{\pi}_{(t)}$ (208)) under all three stress levels for the TMISL data

	OMP at time t				FMP at time $t(\tilde{\pi}_{(t)})$			
Stress level	1	2	3	4	1	2	3	4
Low	0.0861	0.1985	0.1161	0.1498	0.0567	0.1247	0.1624	0.1798
Medium	0.6704	0.6217	0.7041	0.6742	0.5602	0.6828	0.7076	0.7117
High	0.2435	0.1798	0.1798	0.1760	0.3831	0.1925	0.1290	0.1085

with $\tilde{\pi}_{(1)3}$ (High group) $= 1 - \tilde{\pi}_{(1)1} - \tilde{\pi}_{(1)2} = 0.3831$, and the lag 1 based but constant matrix of conditional probabilities η_M as

$$\eta_M = \begin{pmatrix} \eta^{(1)}(1) \; \eta^{(1)}(2) \\ \eta^{(2)}(1) \; \eta^{(2)}(2) \end{pmatrix} : 2 \times 2$$

$$= \begin{pmatrix} 0.4666 \; 0.5240 \\ 0.1366 \; 0.7827 \end{pmatrix},$$

and $\eta(J) = \tilde{\pi}_{(1)} = \pi$. These results are then used in the recursive relationship (3.208) to produce the marginal probabilities $\tilde{\pi}_{(t)}$ (3.208) for three categories over remaining three time points as in Table 3.22.

Notice from the Table 3.22 that the FMP over time indicate that as time progresses the stress decreases. Thus, for Low and Medium group the probabilities are increasing over time, whereas for the High stress level the probabilities are generally decreasing. This fitted pattern shows an excellent agreement with the observed data, that is OMP shown in the same table. Thus as compared to fitting the LDCMP model (see the constant probabilities shown in column 3 in Table 3.21), the MDL model fits the marginal probabilities over time much better.

For the sake of completeness, by using the above estimates, following (3.208), we also provide the covariances or correlations among the elements of the multinomial responses. Thus, for $t = 1, \ldots, 4$, we first provide the variance and covariances of the elements of $\text{var}[Y_{it}] = (\sigma_{(t)jk}),\ j,k = 1,2$, and then the values of correlations

$$\text{corr}[Y_{iuj}, Y_{itk}] = \left(\frac{\sigma_{(ut)jk}}{[\sigma_{(u)jj}\sigma_{(t)kk}]^{\frac{1}{2}}}\right) = (\rho_{(ut)jk}),$$

for $u < t$.

Values of $(\sigma_{(t)jk})$:

$$\text{var}[Y_{i1}] = (\sigma_{(1)jk}) = \begin{pmatrix} 0.0534 & -0.0317 \\ -0.0317 & 0.2464 \end{pmatrix}$$

$$\text{var}[Y_{i2}] = (\sigma_{(2)jk}) = \begin{pmatrix} 0.1091 & -0.0851 \\ -0.0851 & 0.2166 \end{pmatrix}$$

$$\text{var}[Y_{i3}] = (\sigma_{(3)jk}) = \begin{pmatrix} 0.1360 & -0.1149 \\ -0.1149 & 0.2069 \end{pmatrix}$$

$$\text{var}[Y_{i4}] = (\sigma_{(4)jk}) = \begin{pmatrix} 0.1475 & -0.1280 \\ -0.1280 & 0.2052 \end{pmatrix},$$

Values of $(\rho_{(ut)jk})$ **:**

$$\text{corr}[Y_{i1j}, Y_{i2k}] = (\rho_{(12)jk}) = \begin{pmatrix} 0.3019 & -0.0259 \\ -0.1337 & 0.2263 \end{pmatrix}$$

$$\text{corr}[Y_{i1j}, Y_{i3k}] = (\rho_{(13)jk}) = \begin{pmatrix} 0.1120 & 0.0117 \\ -0.0594 & 0.0437 \end{pmatrix}$$

$$\text{corr}[Y_{i1j}, Y_{i4k}] = (\rho_{(14)jk}) = \begin{pmatrix} 0.0436 & 0.0099 \\ -0.0253 & 0.0059 \end{pmatrix}$$

$$\text{corr}[Y_{i2j}, Y_{i3k}] = (\rho_{(23)jk}) = \begin{pmatrix} 0.3925 & -0.0679 \\ -0.2490 & 0.1954 \end{pmatrix}$$

$$\text{corr}[Y_{i2j}, Y_{i4k}] = (\rho_{(24)jk}) = \begin{pmatrix} 0.1574 & 0.0104 \\ -0.1064 & 0.0274 \end{pmatrix}$$

$$\text{corr}[Y_{i3j}, Y_{i4k}] = (\rho_{(34)jk}) = \begin{pmatrix} 0.4230 & -0.0879 \\ -0.3125 & 0.1788 \end{pmatrix}.$$

As expected the multinomial correlations appear to decay as time lag increases.

3.5 Univariate Longitudinal Stationary Multinomial Fixed Effect Regression Models

In Sect. 3.4, we have used first order Markovian type linear (LDCMP) and non-linear dynamic (MDL) models to analyze longitudinal multinomial responses in the absence of any covariates. Thus, even though the original TMISL data based on 3 stress levels displayed in Table 3.18 were collected from 267 workers along with their covariate information on their house distance (less or greater than 5 miles) from the nuclear plant, the LDCMP (Sect. 3.4.1) and MDL (Sect. 3.4.2) models were applied to this data set as an illustration ignoring the covariate (distance) information. However, because finding the covariate effects on categories may be of interest as well, in fact in some cases finding covariate effects may be of primary interest, in this section, we generalize the LDCMP and MDL models from Sects. 3.4.1 and 3.4.2 to accommodate the stationary covariates (time independent). We refer to these generalized models as the LDCMP and MDL regression models.

Table 3.23 Contingency table for $J > 2$ categories at initial time $t = 1$ for individuals belonging to ℓ-th ($\ell = 1, \ldots, p+1$) level of a covariate

	t ($t = 1$)					
	Category					
Covariate level	1	...	j	...	J	Total
1	$K_{[1]1}(1)$	...	$K_{[1]j}(1)$	...	$K_{[1]J}(1)$	$K_{[1]}$
·	...	...	...	...	...	·
ℓ	$K_{[\ell]1}(1)$	...	$K_{[\ell]j}(1)$	...	$K_{[\ell]J}(1)$	$K_{[\ell]}$
·	...	...	...	...	...	·
$p+1$	$K_{[p+1]1}(1)$	...	$K_{[p+1]j}(1)$	...	$K_{[p+1]J}(1)$	$K_{[p+1]}$
Total	$K_1(1)$	...	$K_j(1)$	...	$K_J(1)$	K

Naturally one should be able to apply these regression models to analyze, for example, the original TMISL data in Table 3.18. For convenience, to make the application purpose of the regression models easier and clear, we first extend the general contingency Tables 3.16 and 3.17 for $J > 2$ categories to the regression case with a covariate with $p+1$ levels through Tables 3.23 and 3.24, respectively. Note that these Tables 3.23 and 3.24 also generalize the covariates based contingency Tables 3.8 and 3.9, respectively, for the binary longitudinal data.

To illustrate these Tables 3.23 and 3.24, we turn back to the original TMISL data of Table 3.18 and first, corresponding to Table 3.23, display the marginal counts at initial time $t = 1$ for two levels of the distance (between workplace and home) covariate in Table 3.25. Next, corresponding to Table 3.24, we display three $(T-1)$ lag 1 based transitional contingency Tables 3.26(1)–(3) to be constructed from the TMISL data of Table 3.18. Each table contains the counts under two levels of the distance covariate. Once the multinomial regression models are developed and estimation methods are discussed in Sects. 5.1 and 5.2, they will be fitted, as an illustration, to the TMISL data from Tables 3.25 and 3.26(1)–(3).

3.5.1 Covariates Based Linear Dynamic Conditional Multinomial Probability Models

In this section, we generalize the LDCMP model discussed in Sect. 3.4.1 to examine the effects of covariates as well on the multinomial responses. For convenience we consider one covariate with $p+1$ levels, ℓ being a general level so that $\ell = 1, \ldots, p+1$. For example, in the aforementioned TMISL data, distance covariate has 2 levels, namely distance less than or equal to 5 miles (DLE5) ($\ell = 1$) and the distance greater than 5 miles (DGT5) ($\ell = 2$). Suppose that for $i \in \ell$, in addition to β_{j0}, $\beta_{j\ell}$ denotes the effect of the covariate for the response of the ith individual to be in jth category. Thus, for $t = 1, \ldots, T$, we may write the marginal probabilities as

Table 3.24 Lag h^* ($h^* = 1,\ldots,T-1$) based $[h^*(T-h^*)]$ transitional counts for multinomial responses with $J > 2$ categories, for individuals belonging to ℓ-th ($\ell = 1,\ldots,p+1$) level of the covariate

		Covariate level (ℓ)					
		t ($t = h^*+1,\ldots,T$)					
Time		Category (j)					
Time	Category (g)	1	...	j	...	J	Total
t-h^*	1	$K_{[\ell]11}(t-h^*, t)$	...	$K_{[\ell]1j}(t-h^*, t)$	...	$K_{[\ell]1J}(t-h^*, t)$	$K_{[\ell]1}(t-h^*)$
	.	...	...	...	...	...	.
	g	$K_{[\ell]g1}(t-h^*, t)$	...	$K_{[\ell]gj}(t-h^*, t)$	...	$K_{[\ell]gJ}(t-h^*, t)$	$K_{[\ell]g}(t-h^*)$
	.	...	...	...	...	...	.
	J	$K_{[\ell]J1}(t-h^*, t)$	...	$K_{[\ell]Jj}(t-h^*, t)$	...	$K_{[\ell]JJ}(t-h^*, t)$	$K_{[\ell]J}(t-h^*)$
	Total	$K_{[\ell]1}(t)$	...	$K_{[\ell]j}(t)$	...	$K_{[\ell]J}(t)$	$K_{[\ell]}$

Table 3.25 Contingency table for TMISL data with $J = 3$ categories at initial time $t = 1$ for individuals with covariate level 1 or 2

	t ($t = 1$)			
	Stress level (j)			
Covariate level (ℓ)	Low (1)	Medium (2)	High (3)	Total
Distance $\leq$ 5 Miles (1)	$K_{[1]1}(1) = 14$	$K_{[1]2}(1) = 69$	$K_{[1]3}(1) = 32$	$K_{[1]} = 115$
Distance $>$ 5 Miles (2)	$K_{[2]1}(1) = 9$	$K_{[2]2}(1) = 110$	$K_{[2]3}(1) = 33$	$K_{[2]} = 152$
Total	$K_1(1) = 23$	$K_2(1) = 179$	$K_3(1) = 65$	$K = 267$

Table 3.26 (1): Transitional counts for the TMISL data from time 1 to 2 ($h^* = 1$) for individuals belonging to ℓ-th ($\ell = 1,2$) level of the distance covariate

		Distance $\leq$ 5 Miles (1)			
		t=2			
Time		Stress level (j)			
Time	Stress level (g)	Low (1)	Medium (2)	High (3)	Total
$[t-h^*] = 1$	Low (1)	$K_{[1]11}(1,2) = 7$	$K_{[1]12}(1,2) = 7$	$K_{[1]13}(1,2) = 0$	$K_{[1]1}(1) = 14$
	Medium (2)	$K_{[1]21}(1,2) = 11$	$K_{[1]22}(1,2) = 54$	$K_{[1]23}(1,2) = 4$	$K_{[1]2}(1) = 69$
	High (3)	$K_{[1]31}(1,2) = 0$	$K_{[1]32}(1,2) = 12$	$K_{[1]33}(1,2) = 20$	$K_{[1]3}(1) = 32$
	Total	$K_{[1]1}(2) = 18$	$K_{[1]2}(2) = 73$	$K_{[1]3}(2) = 24$	$K_{[1]} = 115$
		Distance $>$ 5 Miles (2)			
		t=2			
Time		Stress level (j)			
Time	Stress level (g)	Low (1)	Medium (2)	High (3)	Total
$[t-h^*] = 1$	Low (1)	$K_{[2]11}(1,2) = 5$	$K_{[2]12}(1,2) = 4$	$K_{[2]13}(1,2) = 0$	$K_{[2]1}(1) = 9$
	Medium (2)	$K_{[2]21}(1,2) = 29$	$K_{[2]22}(1,2) = 75$	$K_{[2]23}(1,2) = 6$	$K_{[2]2}(1) = 110$
	High (3)	$K_{[2]31}(1,2) = 1$	$K_{[2]32}(1,2) = 14$	$K_{[2]33}(1,2) = 18$	$K_{[2]3}(1) = 33$
	Total	$K_{[2]1}(2) = 35$	$K_{[2]2}(2) = 93$	$K_{[2]3}(2) = 24$	$K_{[2]} = 152$

Table 3.26 (2): Transitional counts for the TMISL data from time 2 to 3 ($h^* = 1$) for individuals belonging to ℓ-th ($\ell = 1, 2$) level of the distance covariate

		Distance ≤ 5 Miles (1)			
		t=3			
Time		Stress level (j)			
Time	Stress level (g)	Low (1)	Medium (2)	High (3)	Total
$[t-h^*]=2$	Low (1)	$K_{[1]11}(2,3)=8$	$K_{[1]12}(2,3)=10$	$K_{[1]13}(2,3)=0$	$K_{[1]1}(2)=18$
	Medium (2)	$K_{[1]21}(2,3)=6$	$K_{[1]22}(2,3)=57$	$K_{[1]23}(2,3)=10$	$K_{[1]2}(2)=73$
	High (3)	$K_{[1]31}(2,3)=0$	$K_{[1]32}(2,3)=5$	$K_{[1]33}(2,3)=19$	$K_{[1]3}(2)=24$
	Total	$K_{[1]1}(3)=14$	$K_{[1]2}(3)=72$	$K_{[1]3}(3)=29$	$K_{[1]}=115$
		Distance > 5 Miles (2)			
		t=3			
Time		Stress level (j)			
Time	Stress level (g)	Low (1)	Medium (2)	High (3)	Total
$[t-h^*]=2$	Low (1)	$K_{[2]11}(2,3)=12$	$K_{[2]12}(2,3)=23$	$K_{[2]13}(2,3)=0$	$K_{[2]1}(2)=35$
	Medium (2)	$K_{[2]21}(2,3)=5$	$K_{[2]22}(2,3)=82$	$K_{[2]23}(2,3)=6$	$K_{[2]2}(2)=93$
	High (3)	$K_{[2]31}(2,3)=0$	$K_{[2]32}(2,3)=11$	$K_{[2]33}(2,3)=13$	$K_{[2]3}(2)=24$
	Total	$K_{[2]1}(3)=17$	$K_{[2]2}(3)=116$	$K_{[2]3}(3)=19$	$K_{[2]}=152$

Table 3.26 (3) Transitional counts for the TMISL data from time 3 to 4 ($h^* = 1$) for individuals belonging to ℓ-th ($\ell = 1, 2$) level of the distance covariate

		Distance ≤ 5 Miles (1)			
		t=4			
Time		Stress level (j)			
Time	Stress level (g)	Low (1)	Medium (2)	High (3)	Total
$[t-h^*]=3$	Low (1)	$K_{[1]11}(3,4)=10$	$K_{[1]12}(3,4)=4$	$K_{[1]13}(3,4)=0$	$K_{[1]1}(3)=14$
	Medium (2)	$K_{[1]21}(3,4)=8$	$K_{[1]22}(3,4)=57$	$K_{[1]23}(3,4)=7$	$K_{[1]2}(3)=72$
	High (3)	$K_{[1]31}(3,4)=0$	$K_{[1]32}(3,4)=9$	$K_{[1]33}(3,4)=20$	$K_{[1]3}(3)=29$
	Total	$K_{[1]1}(4)=18$	$K_{[1]2}(4)=70$	$K_{[1]3}(4)=27$	$K_{[1]}=115$
		Distance > 5 Miles (2)			
		t=4			
Time		Stress level (j)			
Time	Stress level (g)	Low (1)	Medium (2)	High (3)	Total
$[t-h^*]=3$	Low (1)	$K_{[2]11}(3,4)=8$	$K_{[2]12}(3,4)=8$	$K_{[2]13}(3,4)=1$	$K_{[2]1}(3)=17$
	Medium (2)	$K_{[2]21}(3,4)=14$	$K_{[2]22}(3,4)=92$	$K_{[2]23}(3,4)=10$	$K_{[2]2}(3)=116$
	High (3)	$K_{[2]31}(3,4)=0$	$K_{[2]32}(3,4)=10$	$K_{[2]33}(3,4)=9$	$K_{[2]3}(3)=19$
	Total	$K_{[2]1}(4)=22$	$K_{[2]2}(4)=110$	$K_{[2]3}(4)=20$	$K_{[2]}=152$

$$P[y_{it} = y_{it}^{(j)} | i \in \ell] = \pi_{[(i\in\ell]t)j} \equiv \pi_{[\ell]j} (\text{same for all t using stationary assumption})$$
$$= \begin{cases} \frac{\exp(\beta_{j0}+\beta_{j\ell})}{1+\sum_{g=1}^{J-1}\exp(\beta_{g0}+\beta_{g\ell})} & \text{for } j = 1,\ldots,J-1;\ \ell = 1,\ldots,p \\ \frac{1}{1+\sum_{g=1}^{J-1}\exp(\beta_{g0}+\beta_{g\ell})} & \text{for } j = J;\ \ell = 1,\ldots,p, \end{cases} \quad (3.231)$$

and for $\ell = p+1$, these probabilities have the formulas

$$P[y_{it} = y_{it}^{(j)} | i \in (p+1)] = = \pi_{(i\in(p+1)t)j} \equiv \pi_{[p+1]j}$$
$$= \begin{cases} \frac{\exp(\beta_{j0})}{1+\sum_{g=1}^{J-1}\exp(\beta_{g0})} & \text{for } j = 1,\ldots,J-1 \\ \frac{1}{1+\sum_{g=1}^{J-1}\exp(\beta_{g0})} & \text{for } j = J. \end{cases} \quad (3.232)$$

Note that these marginal probabilities are similar to those for the binary case given by (3.89)–(3.90), with a difference that j now ranges from 1 to $J(\geq 2)$, whereas in the binary case $J = 2$. Further note that for notational convenience, one may re-express the probabilities in (3.231)–(3.232) as follows. Let

$$\theta^* = [\beta_1^{*\prime},\ldots,\beta_j^{*\prime},\ldots,\beta_{J-1}^{*}{}'\,]' : (J-1)(p+1)\times 1, \text{ with } \beta_j^* = [\beta_{j0},\ldots,\beta_{j\ell},\ldots,\beta_{jp}]'. \quad (3.233)$$

It then follows that

$$\pi_{[\ell]j} = \frac{\exp(x'_{[\ell]j}\theta^*)}{\sum_{g=1}^{J}\exp(x'_{[\ell]g}\theta^*)}, \quad (3.234)$$

where $x'_{[\ell]j}$ is the jth $(j = 1,\ldots,J)$ row of the $J \times (J-1)(p+1)$ matrix X_ℓ, defined for ℓth level as follows:

$$X_\ell = \begin{pmatrix} x'_{[\ell]1} \\ \vdots \\ x'_{[\ell]j} \\ \vdots \\ x'_{[\ell](J-1)} \\ x'_{[\ell]J} \end{pmatrix}, \quad (3.235)$$

with

$$x'_{[\ell]j} = \begin{cases} \left(01'_{(j-1)(p+1)} \; d'_{[\ell]1} \; 01'_{(J-1-j)(p+1)}\right) & \text{for } j = 1,\ldots,J-1;\; \ell = 1,\ldots,p \\ \left(01'_{(j-1)(p+1)} \; d'_{[\ell]2} \; 01'_{(J-1-j)(p+1)}\right) & \text{for } j = 1,\ldots,J-1;\; \ell = p+1 \\ \left(01'_{(J-1)(p+1)}\right) & \text{for } j = J;\; \ell = 1,\ldots,p+1, \end{cases} \tag{3.236}$$

where

$$d'_{[\ell]m} = \begin{cases} \left(1 \; 01'_{\ell-1} \; 1 \; 01'_{p-\ell}\right) & \text{for } m = 1 \\ \left(1 \; 01'_{p}\right) & \text{for } m = 2. \end{cases} \tag{3.237}$$

Next, to accommodate the covariates, level $(i \in \ell)$ specific conditional probabilities in linear form may be written by modifying the LDCMPs in (3.146)–(3.147), as

$$\begin{aligned} P[Y_{it} = y_{it}^{(j)} | Y_{i,t-1} = y_{i,t-1}^{(g)}, i \in \ell] &= \pi_{(i\in\ell,t)j} + \sum_{h=1}^{J-1} \rho_{jh} \left[y_{i,t-1,h}^{(g)} - \pi_{(i\in\ell,t-1)h}\right] \\ &= \pi_{[\ell]j} + \sum_{h=1}^{J-1} \rho_{jh} \left[y_{i,t-1,h}^{(g)} - \pi_{[\ell]h}\right] \text{ by stationary property (3.144)} \\ &= \pi_{[\ell]j} + \rho'_j \left(y_{i,t-1}^{(g)} - \pi_{[\ell]}\right) \\ &= \lambda_{it|t-1}^{(j)}(g,\ell), \text{ (say), for } g = 1,\ldots,J; j = 1,\ldots,J-1, \end{aligned} \tag{3.238}$$

and

$$P[Y_{it} = y_{it}^{(J)} | Y_{i,t-1} = y_{i,t-1}^{(g)}, i \in \ell] = \lambda_{it|t-1}^{(J)}(g,\ell) = 1 - \sum_{j=1}^{J-1} \lambda_{it|t-1}^{(j)}(g,\ell), \tag{3.239}$$

where

$$\rho_j = (\rho_{j1},\ldots,\rho_{jh},\ldots,\rho_{j,J-1})' : (J-1)\times 1;\; \pi_{[\ell]} = [\pi_{[\ell]1},\ldots,\pi_{[\ell]j},\ldots,\pi_{[\ell],J-1}]' : (J-1)\times 1.$$

3.5.1.1 Likelihood Function and Estimating Equations

When covariates are accommodated, following (3.172), one writes the product multinomial likelihood function (see Poleto et al. 2013 for a more complex missing data setup) as

$$L(\theta^*, \rho_M) = \Pi_{\ell=1}^{p+1} \Pi_{i\in\ell}^{K} \left[f(y_{i1}) \Pi_{t=2}^{T} f(y_{it}|y_{i,t-1})\right]$$

$$= \left[\Pi_{\ell=1}^{p+1}\Pi_{i\in\ell}^{K} f(y_{i1})\right]$$
$$\times \Pi_{t=2}^{T}\Pi_{\ell=1}^{p+1}\Pi_{g=1}^{J}\Pi_{i\in(g,\ell)}^{K}\left[f(y_{it}|y_{i,t-1}^{(g)})\right]$$
$$= d_0^*\left[\Pi_{\ell=1}^{p+1}\Pi_{j=1}^{J}\Pi_{i\in\ell}^{K}\pi_{[\ell]j}^{y_{i1j}}\right]$$
$$\times \Pi_{t=2}^{T}\Pi_{\ell=1}^{p+1}\Pi_{j=1}^{J}\Pi_{g=1}^{J}\Pi_{i\in(g,\ell)}^{K}\left\{\lambda_{it|t-1}^{(j)}(y_{i,t-1}^{(g)})\right\}^{y_{itj}}, \quad (3.240)$$

where θ^* now has the form as in (3.233) but ρ_M has the same form as before that is, as in (3.153), that is,

$$\rho_M = \begin{pmatrix} \rho_1' \\ \vdots \\ \rho_j' \\ \vdots \\ \rho_{J-1}' \end{pmatrix} : (J-1)\times(J-1).$$

In (3.240), d_0^* is the normalizing constant free from any parameters. Next, by using the abbreviation $\lambda^{(j)}(g,\ell)$ for the conditional probabilities in (3.238)–(3.239), that is,

$$\lambda^{(j)}(g,\ell) \equiv \left[\lambda_{it|t-1}^{(j)}(y_{i,t-1}^{(g)})\right]_{|i\in\ell}$$
$$= \begin{cases} \pi_{[\ell]j} + \rho_j'(\delta_{[\ell]g} - \pi_{[\ell]}) & \text{for } j = 1,\ldots,J-1 \\ 1 - \sum_{k=1}^{J-1}\left[\pi_{[\ell]k} + (\delta_{[\ell]g} - \pi_{[\ell]})'\rho_k\right] & \text{for } j = J, \end{cases} \quad (3.241)$$

with

$$\delta_{[\ell]g} = \begin{cases} \left(01_{g-1}' \; 1 \; 01_{J-1-g}'\right)' & \text{for } g = 1,\ldots,J-1;\ \ell = 1,\ldots,p+1 \\ 01_{J-1} & \text{for } g = J;\ \ell = 1,\ldots,p+1, \end{cases} \quad (3.242)$$

the log of the likelihood function (3.240), that is,

$$Log\, L(\theta^*,\rho_M) = log\, d_0^* + \sum_{\ell=1}^{p+1}\sum_{i\in\ell}^{K}\sum_{j=1}^{J} y_{i1j} log\, \pi_{[\ell]j}$$
$$+ \sum_{\ell=1}^{p+1}\sum_{t=2}^{T}\sum_{j=1}^{J}\sum_{g=1}^{J}\sum_{i\in(g,\ell)}^{K}\left[y_{itj} log\, \lambda_{it|t-1}^{(j)}(g,\ell)\right], \quad (3.243)$$

by using the cell counts from the contingency Tables 3.17 and 3.18, may be written as

$$
\begin{aligned}
Log\, L(\theta^*,\rho_M) &= log\, d_0^* + \sum_{\ell=1}^{p+1}\sum_{j=1}^{J} K_{[\ell]j}(1) log\, \pi_{[\ell]j} \\
&+ \sum_{\ell=1}^{p+1}\sum_{j=1}^{J}\sum_{g=1}^{J}\left[\left\{log\, \lambda^{(j)}(g,\ell)\right\}\left\{\sum_{t=2}^{T} K_{[\ell]gj}(t-1,t)\right\}\right], \quad (3.244)
\end{aligned}
$$

where $K_{[\ell]gj}(t-1,t)$ (Table 3.18) is the number of individuals with covariate level ℓ, whose responses were in gth category at time $t-1$ and in jth category at time t.

3.5.1.1.1 Likelihood Estimating Equation for θ^*

It follows from (3.244) that the likelihood estimating equation for θ^* is given by

$$
\begin{aligned}
\frac{\partial Log\, L(\theta^*,\rho_M)}{\partial\theta^*} &= \sum_{\ell=1}^{p+1}\sum_{j=1}^{J} K_{[\ell]j}(1)\frac{1}{\pi_{[\ell]j}}\frac{\partial \pi_{[\ell]j}}{\partial\theta^*} \\
&+ \sum_{\ell=1}^{p+1}\sum_{j=1}^{J}\sum_{g=1}^{J}\left[\left\{\sum_{t=2}^{T} K_{[\ell]gj}(t-1,t)\right\}\frac{1}{\lambda^{(j)}(g,\ell)}\right. \\
&\times \left.\frac{\partial\lambda^{(j)}(g,\ell)}{\partial\theta^*}\right] = 0, \quad (3.245)
\end{aligned}
$$

where, by (3.234), one obtains

$$
\begin{aligned}
\frac{\partial \pi_{[\ell]j}}{\partial\theta^*} &= \pi_{[\ell]j}x_{[\ell]j} - \pi_{[\ell]j}\sum_{g=1}^{J-1} x_{[\ell]g}\pi_{[\ell]g} \\
&= \begin{cases} \pi_{[\ell]j}\left(x_{[\ell]j} - \pi_{[\ell]}\otimes d_{[\ell]1}\right) \text{ for } \ell = 1,\ldots,p;\ j = 1,\ldots,J \\ \pi_{[\ell]j}\left(x_{[\ell]j} - \pi_{[\ell]}\otimes d_{[\ell]2}\right) \text{ for } \ell = p+1;\ j = 1,\ldots,J, \end{cases} \quad (3.246)
\end{aligned}
$$

or equivalently

$$
\frac{1}{\pi_{[\ell]j}}\frac{\partial \pi_{[\ell]j}}{\partial\theta^*} = \begin{cases} \left(x_{[\ell]j} - \pi_{[\ell]}\otimes d_{[\ell]1}\right) \text{ for } \ell = 1,\ldots,p;\ j = 1,\ldots,J \\ \left(x_{[\ell]j} - \pi_{[\ell]}\otimes d_{[\ell]2}\right) \text{ for } \ell = p+1;\ j = 1,\ldots,J, \end{cases} \quad (3.247)
$$

where $x_{[\ell]J} = 01_{(J-1)(p+1)}$. Further, by (3.246), it follows from (3.241) that the first derivative $\frac{\partial\lambda^{(j)}(g,\ell)}{\partial\theta^*}$ in (3.245) has the formula as

$$\frac{\partial \lambda^{(j)}(g,\ell)}{\partial \theta^*} = \begin{cases} \frac{\partial}{\partial \theta^*}\left[\pi_{[\ell]j} + \rho_j'(\delta_{[\ell]g} - \pi_{[\ell]})\right] & \text{for } j = 1,\ldots,J-1 \\ -\frac{\partial}{\partial \theta^*}\left[\sum_{k=1}^{J-1}\{\pi_{[\ell]k} + (\delta_{[\ell]g} - \pi_{[\ell]})'\rho_k\}\right] & \text{for } j = J, \end{cases} \quad (3.248)$$

$$= \begin{cases} \left[\frac{\partial \pi_{[\ell]j}}{\partial \theta^*} - \left\{\frac{\partial \pi'_{[\ell]}}{\partial \theta^*}\right\}\rho_j\right] & \text{for } j = 1,\ldots,J-1 \\ -\sum_{k=1}^{J-1}\left[\frac{\partial \pi_{[\ell]k}}{\partial \theta^*} - \left\{\frac{\partial \pi'_{[\ell]}}{\partial \theta^*}\right\}\rho_k\right] & \text{for } j = J, \end{cases} \quad (3.249)$$

$$= \begin{cases} \pi_{[\ell]j}\left(x_{[\ell]j} - \pi_{[\ell]} \otimes d_{[\ell]1}\right) - [\Sigma(\pi_{[\ell]}) \otimes d_{[\ell]1}]\rho_j & \text{for } \ell = 1,\ldots,p \\ \pi_{[\ell]j}\left(x_{[\ell]j} - \pi_{[\ell]} \otimes d_{[\ell]2}\right) - [\Sigma(\pi_{[\ell]}) \otimes d_{[\ell]2}]\rho_j & \text{for } \ell = p+1, \end{cases} \quad (3.250)$$

for all $j = 1,\ldots,J$, where by using similar conventional notations as that of (3.182), one writes

$$x_{[\ell]J} = 01_{(J-1)(p+1)} \text{ and } \rho_J = -\sum_{k=1}^{J-1}\rho_k.$$

Also in (3.250),

$$\Sigma(\pi_{[\ell]}) = \begin{pmatrix} \pi_{[\ell]1}(1-\pi_{[\ell]1}) & \ldots & -\pi_{[\ell]1}\pi_{[\ell]g} & \ldots & -\pi_{[\ell]1}\pi_{[\ell](J-1)} \\ \vdots & & \vdots & & \vdots \\ -\pi_{[\ell]g}\pi_{[\ell]1} & \ldots & \pi_{[\ell]g}(1-\pi_{[\ell]g}) & \ldots & -\pi_{[\ell]g}\pi_{[\ell](J-1)} \\ \vdots & & \vdots & & \vdots \\ -\pi_{[\ell](J-1)}\pi_{[\ell]1} & \ldots & -\pi_{[\ell](J-1)}\pi_{[\ell]g} & \ldots & \pi_{[\ell](J-1)}(1-\pi_{[\ell](J-1)}) \end{pmatrix}, \quad (3.251)$$

which, similar to (3.150), is the covariance matrix of the multinomial response variable $Y_{i\in\ell,t}$ for the ith individual with covariate level ℓ.

Now for known ρ_M, the likelihood equation in (3.245) for θ^* may be obtained by using the iterative formula

$$\hat{\theta}^*(r+1) = \hat{\theta}^*(r) - \left[\left\{\frac{\partial^2 \text{Log}\, L(\theta^*, \rho_M)}{\partial \theta^{*\prime}\partial \theta^*}\right\}^{-1} \frac{\partial \text{Log}\, L(\theta^*, \rho_M)}{\partial \theta^*}\right]_{|\theta^* = \hat{\theta}^*(r)} ; (J-1)(p+1) \times 1, \quad (3.252)$$

where the second order derivative matrix has the form

$$\frac{\partial^2 Log\, L(\theta^*, \rho_M)}{\partial \theta^{*\prime}\partial \theta^*} = \sum_{\ell=1}^{p+1}\sum_{j=1}^{J} K_{[\ell]j}(1)\left[\frac{\partial}{\partial \theta^{*\prime}}\left\{\frac{1}{\pi_{[\ell]j}}\frac{\partial \pi_{[\ell]j}}{\partial \theta^*}\right\}\right]$$

$$+ \sum_{\ell=1}^{p+1}\sum_{j=1}^{J}\sum_{g=1}^{J}\left[\left\{\sum_{t=2}^{T} K_{[\ell]gj}(t-1,t)\right\}\left\{\frac{1}{\lambda^{(j)}(g,\ell)}\frac{\partial^2 \lambda^{(j)}(g,\ell)}{\partial \theta^{*\prime}\partial \theta^*}\right.\right.$$

$$-\left.\left.\frac{1}{\{\lambda^{(j)}(g,\ell)\}^2}\frac{\partial\lambda^{(j)}(g,\ell)}{\partial\theta^*}\frac{\partial\lambda^{(j)}(g,\ell)}{\partial\theta^{*\prime}}\right\}\right]. \tag{3.253}$$

To compute this derivative matrix, first we notice that the formulas for $\lambda^{(j)}(g,\ell)$ and its first order derivative with respect to θ^* are given by (3.241) and (3.250), respectively. Also the formula for $\frac{1}{\pi_{[\ell]j}}\frac{\partial\pi_{[\ell]j}}{\partial\theta^*}$ is given in (3.247). We then turn back to (3.253) and construct the necessary second order derivatives as follows.

Computation of $\frac{\partial}{\partial\theta^{*\prime}}\left\{\frac{1}{\pi_{[\ell]j}}\frac{\partial\pi_{[\ell]j}}{\partial\theta^*}\right\}$ **:**
By (3.247), for all $j=1,\ldots,J$, we write

$$\frac{\partial}{\partial\theta^{*\prime}}\left\{\frac{1}{\pi_{[\ell]j}}\frac{\partial\pi_{[\ell]j}}{\partial\theta^*}\right\}=\begin{cases}\frac{\partial}{\partial\theta^{*\prime}}\left(x_{[\ell]j}-\pi_{[\ell]}\otimes d_{[\ell]1}\right) & \text{for } \ell=1,\ldots,p\\ \frac{\partial}{\partial\theta^{*\prime}}\left(x_{[\ell]j}-\pi_{[\ell]}\otimes d_{[\ell]2}\right) & \text{for } \ell=p+1,\end{cases} \tag{3.254}$$

which by (3.246) yields

$$\begin{aligned}\frac{\partial}{\partial\theta^{*\prime}}\left\{\frac{1}{\pi_{[\ell]j}}\frac{\partial\pi_{[\ell]j}}{\partial\theta^*}\right\}&=-\begin{pmatrix}d_{[\ell]1}\otimes[\sigma'_{[\ell]1}\otimes d'_{[\ell]1}]\\ \vdots\\ d_{[\ell]1}\otimes[\sigma'_{[\ell]j}\otimes d'_{[\ell]1}]\\ \vdots\\ d_{[\ell]1}\otimes[\sigma'_{[\ell](J-1)}\otimes d'_{[\ell]1}]\end{pmatrix}:(J-1)(p+1)\times(J-1)(p+1)\\ &=-\Sigma_1^*(\pi_{[\ell]}),\ \text{(say), for } \ell=1,\ldots,p;\ j=1,\ldots,J,\end{aligned} \tag{3.255}$$

and

$$\begin{aligned}\frac{\partial}{\partial\theta^{*\prime}}\left\{\frac{1}{\pi_{[\ell]j}}\frac{\partial\pi_{[\ell]j}}{\partial\theta^*}\right\}&=-\begin{pmatrix}d_{[\ell]2}\otimes[\sigma'_{[\ell]1}\otimes d'_{[\ell]2}]\\ \vdots\\ d_{[\ell]2}\otimes[\sigma'_{[\ell]j}\otimes d'_{[\ell]2}]\\ \vdots\\ d_{[\ell]2}\otimes[\sigma'_{[\ell](J-1)}\otimes d'_{[\ell]2}]\end{pmatrix}:(J-1)(p+1)\times(J-1)(p+1)\\ &=-\Sigma_2^*(\pi_{[\ell]}),\ \text{(say), for } \ell=p+1;\ j=1,\ldots,J,\end{aligned} \tag{3.256}$$

where $\sigma'_{[\ell]j}$ is the jth row of the $\Sigma(\pi_{[\ell]})$ matrix given in (3.251), that is,

$$\begin{pmatrix}\sigma'_{[\ell]1}\\ \vdots\\ \sigma'_{[\ell]j}\\ \vdots\\ \sigma'_{[\ell](J-1)}\end{pmatrix}=\Sigma(\pi_{[\ell]}). \tag{3.257}$$

Computation of $\frac{\partial}{\partial \theta^{*\prime}}\left\{\frac{\partial \lambda^{(j)}(g,\ell)}{\partial \theta^*}\right\}$:
This derivative, by (3.250), for all $j = 1,\ldots,J$, is computed as

$$\frac{\partial \lambda^{(j)}(g,\ell)}{\partial \theta^*} = \begin{cases} \frac{\partial}{\partial \theta^{*\prime}}\left\{\pi_{[\ell]j}\left(x_{[\ell]j} - \pi_{[\ell]} \otimes d_{[\ell]1}\right) - [\Sigma(\pi_{[\ell]}) \otimes d_{[\ell]1}]\rho_j\right\} & \text{for } \ell = 1,\ldots,p \\ \frac{\partial}{\partial \theta^{*\prime}}\left\{\pi_{[\ell]j}\left(x_{[\ell]j} - \pi_{[\ell]} \otimes d_{[\ell]2}\right) - [\Sigma(\pi_{[\ell]}) \otimes d_{[\ell]2}]\rho_j\right\} & \text{for } \ell = p+1. \end{cases} \tag{3.258}$$

By combining (3.246) and (3.255)–(3.256), the derivatives for the first components may be written as

$$\begin{aligned} \frac{\partial}{\partial \theta^{*\prime}}\left\{\pi_{[\ell]j}\left(x_{[\ell]j} - \pi_{[\ell]} \otimes d_{[\ell]1}\right)\right\} &= \pi_{[\ell]j}\left[\left(x_{[\ell]j} - \pi_{[\ell]} \otimes d_{[\ell]1}\right)\left(x_{[\ell]j} - \pi_{[\ell]} \otimes d_{[\ell]1}\right)'\right] \\ &\quad -\pi_{[\ell]j}\Sigma_1^*(\pi_{[\ell]}) \\ &= \pi_{[\ell]j}\left[\left(x_{[\ell]j} - \pi_{[\ell]} \otimes d_{[\ell]1}\right)\left(x_{[\ell]j} - \pi_{[\ell]} \otimes d_{[\ell]1}\right)' - \Sigma_1^*(\pi_{[\ell]})\right] \\ &= \pi_{[\ell]j} M_{j,1}^*(x, \pi_{[\ell]}), \text{ for } \ell = 1,\ldots,p; j = 1,\ldots,J, \end{aligned} \tag{3.259}$$

and

$$\begin{aligned} \frac{\partial}{\partial \theta^{*\prime}}\left\{\pi_{[\ell]j}\left(x_{[\ell]j} - \pi_{[\ell]} \otimes d_{[\ell]2}\right)\right\} &= \pi_{[\ell]j}\left[\left(x_{[\ell]j} - \pi_{[\ell]} \otimes d_{[\ell]2}\right)\left(x_{[\ell]j} - \pi_{[\ell]} \otimes d_{[\ell]2}\right)'\right] \\ &\quad -\pi_{[\ell]j}\Sigma_2^*(\pi_{[\ell]}) \\ &= \pi_{[\ell]j}\left[\left(x_{[\ell]j} - \pi_{[\ell]} \otimes d_{[\ell]2}\right)\left(x_{[\ell]j} - \pi_{[\ell]} \otimes d_{[\ell]2}\right)' - \Sigma_2^*(\pi_{[\ell]})\right] \\ &= \pi_{[\ell]j} M_{j,2}^*(x, \pi_{[\ell]}), \text{ for } \ell = p+1; j = 1,\ldots,J. \end{aligned} \tag{3.260}$$

Note that these derivatives in (3.259) and (3.260) have similar form to that of (3.186) for the covariate free case, but they are different. In the manner similar to (3.190), we now compute the formulas for $\frac{\partial}{\partial \theta^{*\prime}}\left\{[\Sigma(\pi_{[\ell]}) \otimes d_{[\ell]1}]\rho_j\right\}$ and $\frac{\partial}{\partial \theta^{*\prime}}\left\{[\Sigma(\pi_{[\ell]}) \otimes d_{[\ell]2}]\rho_j\right\}$ as follows.

Computation of $\frac{\partial}{\partial \theta^{*\prime}}\left\{[\Sigma(\pi_{[\ell]}) \otimes d_{[\ell]1}]\rho_j\right\}$ and $\frac{\partial}{\partial \theta^{*\prime}}\left\{[\Sigma(\pi_{[\ell]}) \otimes d_{[\ell]2}]\rho_j\right\}$:
Because

$$\frac{\partial}{\partial \theta^{*\prime}} \{[\Sigma(\pi_{[\ell]}) \otimes d_{[\ell]1}]\rho_j\} = \frac{\partial}{\partial \theta^{*\prime}} \begin{pmatrix} [\{\sigma'_{[\ell]1} \otimes d_{[\ell]1}\}\rho_j] \\ \vdots \\ [\{\sigma'_{[\ell]h} \otimes d_{[\ell]1}\}\rho_j] \\ \vdots \\ [\{\sigma'_{[\ell](J-1)} \otimes d_{[\ell]1}\}\rho_j] \end{pmatrix}, \tag{3.261}$$

with

$$\begin{aligned} \sigma'_{\ell]h} &= = [-\pi_{[\ell]h}\pi_{[\ell]1} \ldots \pi_{[\ell]h}(1-\pi_{[\ell]h}) \ldots - \pi_{[\ell]h}\pi_{[\ell](J-1)}] \\ &= \pi_{[\ell]h}[\delta_{[\ell]h} - \pi_{[\ell]}]', \end{aligned} \tag{3.262}$$

$\delta_{[\ell]h} = \left(01'_{h-1}\ 1\ 01'_{J-1-h}\right)'$ is being given in (3.242) for $h = 1,\ldots,J-1$; $\ell = 1,\ldots,p+1$, one may compute the derivatives in (3.261) by using

$$\begin{aligned} &\frac{\partial}{\partial \theta^{*\prime}}[\{\sigma'_{[\ell]h} \otimes d_{[\ell]1}\}\rho_j] = \frac{\partial}{\partial \theta^{*\prime}}\left[\{\pi_{[\ell]h}(\delta_{[\ell]h} - \pi_{[\ell]})' \otimes d_{[\ell]1}\}\rho_j\right] \\ &= \frac{\partial}{\partial \theta^{*\prime}}\left[\pi_{[\ell]h}\{\rho'_j \otimes d_{[\ell]1}\}(\delta_{[\ell]h} - \pi_{[\ell]})\right] \\ &= \{(\rho'_j \otimes d_{[\ell]1})(\delta_{[\ell]h} - \pi_{[\ell]})\} \otimes \left\{\pi_{[\ell]h}\left(x_{[\ell]h} - \pi_{[\ell]} \otimes d_{[\ell]1}\right)'\right\} \\ &- \left[\pi_{[\ell]h}\{\rho'_j \otimes d_{[\ell]1}\}\left\{\Sigma(\pi_{[\ell]}) \otimes d'_{[\ell]1}\right\}\right] \\ &= \pi_{[\ell]h}\{\rho'_j \otimes d_{[\ell]1}\}\left[\{(\delta_{[\ell]h} - \pi_{[\ell]})\} \otimes \left\{\left(x_{[\ell]h} - \pi_{[\ell]} \otimes d_{[\ell]1}\right)'\right\}\right. \\ &- \left.\left\{\Sigma(\pi_{[\ell]}) \otimes d'_{[\ell]1}\right\}\right] \\ &= \pi_{[\ell]h}\{\rho'_j \otimes d_{[\ell]1}\}[Q^*_{h,1}(x, \pi_{[\ell]})] : (p+1) \times (J-1)(p+1). \end{aligned} \tag{3.263}$$

By using (3.263) in (3.261) for all $h = 1,\ldots,J-1$, one obtains

$$\begin{aligned} \frac{\partial}{\partial \theta^{*\prime}} \{[\Sigma(\pi_{[\ell]}) \otimes d_{[\ell]1}]\rho_j\} &= \begin{pmatrix} \pi_{[\ell]1}\left\{\rho'_j \otimes d_{[\ell]1}\right\}[Q^*_{1,1}(x, \pi_{[\ell]})] \\ \vdots \\ \pi_{[\ell]h}\left\{\rho'_j \otimes d_{[\ell]1}\right\}[Q^*_{h,1}(x, \pi_{[\ell]})] \\ \vdots \\ \pi_{[\ell](J-1)}\left\{\rho'_j \otimes d_{[\ell]1}\right\}[Q^*_{(J-1),1}(x, \pi_{[\ell]})] \end{pmatrix} \\ &= \Omega^*_1(\pi_{[\ell]}). \end{aligned} \tag{3.264}$$

Similarly, one obtains

$$\frac{\partial}{\partial \theta^{*'}} \{[\Sigma(\pi_{[\ell]}) \otimes d_{[\ell]2}]\rho_j\} = \begin{pmatrix} \pi_{[\ell]1} \left\{\rho_j' \otimes d_{[\ell]2}\right\} [Q^*_{1,2}(x, \pi_{[\ell]})] \\ \vdots \\ \pi_{[\ell]h} \left\{\rho_j' \otimes d_{[\ell]2}\right\} [Q^*_{h,2}(x, \pi_{[\ell]})] \\ \vdots \\ \pi_{[\ell](J-1)} \left\{\rho_j' \otimes d_{[\ell]2}\right\} [Q^*_{(J-1),2}(x, \pi_{[\ell]})] \end{pmatrix}$$
$$= \Omega_2^*(\pi_{[\ell]}), \tag{3.265}$$

where

$$Q^*_{h,2}(x, \pi_{[\ell]}) = \left[\{(\delta_{[\ell]h} - \pi_{[\ell]})\} \otimes \left\{(x_{[\ell]h} - \pi_{[\ell]} \otimes d_{[\ell]1})'\right\} - \left\{\Sigma(\pi_{[\ell]}) \otimes d'_{[\ell]1}\right\}\right].$$

Next by using (3.259) and (3.264) into (3.258) one obtains the desired derivatives for $j = 1, \ldots, J$; $\ell = 1, \ldots, p$, and similarly by using (3.260) and (3.265) into (3.258) one obtains the derivatives for $j = 1, \ldots, J$; $\ell = p+1$. It completes the computation for the derivatives in (3.258). Now by using (3.254) and (3.258), one completes the calculation for the second order likelihood derivative matrix (3.253).

3.5.1.1.2 Likelihood Estimating Equation for ρ_M

The likelihood estimation of ρ_M is equivalent to estimate $\rho_j : (J-1) \times 1$, for $j = 1, \ldots, J-1$, by maximizing the log likelihood function $Log\ L(\theta^*, \rho_M)$ given in (3.244). Next, because $\pi_{[\ell]j}$ is free of ρ_j, the likelihood estimating equation for ρ_j has the form given by

$$\frac{\partial Log\ L(\theta^*, \rho_M)}{\partial \rho_j} = \sum_{\ell=1}^{p+1} \sum_{h=1}^{J} \sum_{g=1}^{J} \left[\left\{\sum_{t=2}^{T} K_{[\ell]gh}(t-1, t)\right\} \frac{1}{\lambda^{(h)}(g, \ell)} \times \frac{\partial \lambda^{(h)}(g, \ell)}{\partial \rho_j}\right] = 0, \tag{3.266}$$

where, by (3.241), one obtains

$$\frac{\partial \lambda^{(h)}(g, \ell)}{\partial \rho_j} = \begin{cases} \frac{\partial}{\partial \rho_j} \left[\pi_{[\ell]h} + \rho_h'(\delta_{[\ell]g} - \pi_{[\ell]})\right] & \text{for } h = 1, \ldots, J-1 \\ -\frac{\partial}{\partial \rho_j} \left[\sum_{k=1}^{J-1} \left\{\pi_{[\ell]k} + (\delta_{[\ell]g} - \pi_{[\ell]})'\rho_k\right\}\right] & \text{for } h = J, \end{cases} \tag{3.267}$$

$$= \begin{cases} \left[\delta_{[\ell]g} - \pi_{[\ell]}\right] & \text{for } h = j; h, j = 1, \ldots, J-1 \\ 0 & \text{for } h \neq j; h, j = 1, \ldots, J-1 \\ -\left[\delta_{[\ell]g} - \pi_{[\ell]}\right] & \text{for } h = J; j = 1, \ldots, J-1. \end{cases} \tag{3.268}$$

It then follows from (3.266) that

$$\frac{\partial Log\, L(\theta^*,\rho_M)}{\partial \rho_j} = \sum_{\ell=1}^{p+1}\sum_{g=1}^{J}\left[\left\{\sum_{t=2}^{T} K_{[\ell]gj}(t-1,t)\right\}\frac{1}{\lambda^{(j)}(g,\ell)}(\delta_{[\ell]g}-\pi_{[\ell]})\right]$$
$$-\sum_{\ell=1}^{p+1}\sum_{g=1}^{J}\left[\left\{\sum_{t=2}^{T} K_{[\ell]gJ}(t-1,t)\right\}\frac{1}{\lambda^{(J)}(g,\ell)}(\delta_{[\ell]g}-\pi_{[\ell]})\right] = 0, \tag{3.269}$$

for $j = 1,\ldots,J-1$. Note that this likelihood equation is quite similar to that of (3.200) for the covariate free multinomial case. This is because, unlike the form of θ^*, the ρ_j parameter is not covariate level (ℓ) dependent. For this reason, (3.269) and (3.200) look similar except that by adjusting the quantities for the ℓth level covariate, an additional summation over $\ell = 1,\ldots,p+1$ is taken to construct (3.269). Consequently, the second order $(J-1)^2 \times (J-1)^2$ derivative matrices can easily be written following (3.203) and (3.204), and they are given by

$$\frac{\partial^2 \mathrm{Log}\, L(\theta^*,\rho_M)}{\partial \rho_j \partial \rho_j'} = -\sum_{\ell=1}^{p+1}\sum_{g=1}^{J}\left[\left\{\sum_{t=2}^{T} K_{[\ell]gj}(t-1,t)\right\}\frac{1}{\{\lambda^{(j)}(g,\ell)\}^2}(\delta_{[\ell]g}-\pi_{[\ell]})(\delta_{[\ell]g}-\pi_{[\ell]})'\right]$$
$$-\sum_{\ell=1}^{p+1}\sum_{g=1}^{J}\left[\left\{\sum_{t=2}^{T} K_{[\ell]gJ}(t-1,t)\right\}\frac{1}{\{\lambda^{(J)}(g,\ell)\}^2}\right.$$
$$\times\left.\left[(\delta_{[\ell]g}-\pi_{[\ell]})(\delta_{[\ell]g}-\pi_{[\ell]})'\right]\right], \tag{3.270}$$

for all $j = 1,\ldots,J-1$, and

$$\frac{\partial^2 \mathrm{Log}\, L(\theta^*,\rho_M)}{\partial \rho_j \partial \rho_k'} = -\sum_{\ell=1}^{p+1}\sum_{g=1}^{J}\left[\left\{\sum_{t=2}^{T} K_{[\ell]gJ}(t-1,t)\right\}\frac{1}{\{\lambda^{(J)}(g,\ell)\}^2}\right.$$
$$\times\left.\left[(\delta_{[\ell]g}-\pi_{[\ell]})(\delta_{[\ell]g}-\pi_{[\ell]})'\right]\right], \tag{3.271}$$

for all $j \neq k; j,k = 1,\ldots,J-1$.

Next by writing $\rho^* = (\rho_1',\ldots,\rho_j',\ldots,\rho_{J-1}')'$, the likelihood equations for this stacked vector of parameters, that is,

$$\frac{\partial Log\, L(\theta^*,\rho_M)}{\partial \rho^*} = \begin{pmatrix} \frac{\partial Log\, L(\theta^*,\rho_M)}{\partial \rho_1} \\ \vdots \\ \frac{\partial Log\, L(\theta^*,\rho_M)}{\partial \rho_j} \\ \vdots \\ \frac{\partial Log\, L(\theta^*,\rho_M)}{\partial \rho_{J-1}} \end{pmatrix} = 0 : (J-1)^2 \times 1. \tag{3.272}$$

may be solved by using the iterative equation

$$\hat{\rho}^*(r+1) = \hat{\rho}^*(r) - \left[\left\{ \frac{\partial^2 \mathrm{Log}\, L(\theta^*, \rho_M)}{\partial \rho^* \partial \rho^{*\prime}} \right\}^{-1} \frac{\partial \mathrm{Log}\, L(\theta^*, \rho_M)}{\partial \rho^*} \right]_{|\rho^* = \hat{\rho}^*(r)}, \tag{3.273}$$

where

$$\frac{\partial^2 Log\, L(\theta^*, \rho_M)}{\partial \rho^* \partial \rho^{*\prime}} = \begin{pmatrix} \frac{\partial^2 Log\, L(\theta^*,\rho_M)}{\partial \rho_1 \partial \rho_1'} & \cdots & \frac{\partial^2 Log\, L(\theta^*,\rho_M)}{\partial \rho_1 \partial \rho_j'} & \cdots & \frac{\partial^2 Log\, L(\theta^*,\rho_M)}{\partial \rho_1 \partial \rho_{J-1}'} \\ \vdots & & \vdots & & \vdots \\ \frac{\partial^2 Log\, L(\theta^*,\rho_M)}{\partial \rho_j \partial \rho_1'} & \cdots & \frac{\partial^2 Log\, L(\theta^*,\rho_M)}{\partial \rho_j \partial \rho_j'} & \cdots & \frac{\partial^2 Log\, L(\theta^*,\rho_M)}{\partial \rho_j \partial \rho_{J-1}'} \\ \vdots & & \vdots & & \vdots \\ \frac{\partial^2 Log\, L(\theta^*,\rho_M)}{\partial \rho_{J-1} \partial \rho_1'} & \cdots & \frac{\partial^2 Log\, L(\theta^*,\rho_M)}{\partial \rho_{J-1} \partial \rho_j'} & \cdots & \frac{\partial^2 Log\, L(\theta^*,\rho_M)}{\partial \rho_{J-1} \partial \rho_{J-1}'} \end{pmatrix}. \tag{3.274}$$

3.5.2 Covariates Based Multinomial Dynamic Logit Models

In this nonlinear dynamic modeling approach, we assume that the marginal probabilities at initial time $t = 1$ have the same form as (3.231)–(3.232) under the covariates based linear dynamic conditional multinomial probability (CBLDCMP) model. Thus, we write

$$P[y_{i1} = y_{i1}^{(j)} | i \in \ell] = \pi_{[(i \in \ell]1)j} \equiv \pi_{[\ell]j}$$
$$= \begin{cases} \frac{\exp(\beta_{j0} + \beta_{j\ell})}{1 + \sum_{g=1}^{J-1} \exp(\beta_{g0} + \beta_{g\ell})} & \text{for } j = 1, \ldots, J-1;\ \ell = 1, \ldots, p \\ \frac{1}{1 + \sum_{g=1}^{J-1} \exp(\beta_{g0} + \beta_{g\ell})} & \text{for } j = J;\ \ell = 1, \ldots, p \\ \frac{\exp(\beta_{j0})}{1 + \sum_{g=1}^{J-1} \exp(\beta_{g0})} & \text{for } j = 1, \ldots, J-1; \ell = p+1 \\ \frac{1}{1 + \sum_{g=1}^{J-1} \exp(\beta_{g0})} & \text{for } j = J; \ell = p+1. \end{cases} \tag{3.275}$$

Next for $t = 2, \ldots, T$, we write the conditional probabilities also in logit form given by

$$P[Y_{it} = y_{it}^{(j)} | Y_{i,t-1} = y_{i,t-1}^{(g)}, i \in \ell]$$

$$= \begin{cases} \frac{\exp(\beta_{j0}+\beta_{j\ell}+\gamma_j' y_{i,t-1}^{(g)})}{1+\sum_{h=1}^{J-1}\exp(\beta_{h0}+\beta_{h\ell}+\gamma_h' y_{i,t-1}^{(g)})} & \text{for } j=1,\ldots,J-1;\ \ell=1,\ldots,p \\ \frac{\exp(\beta_{j0}+\gamma_j' y_{i,t-1}^{(g)})}{1+\sum_{h=1}^{J-1}\exp(\beta_{h0}+\gamma_h' y_{i,t-1}^{(g)})} & \text{for } j=1,\ldots,J-1;\ell=p+1 \\ \frac{1}{1+\sum_{h=1}^{J-1}\exp(\beta_{h0}+\beta_{h\ell}+\gamma_h' y_{i,t-1}^{(g)})} & \text{for } j=J;\ \ell=1,\ldots,p \\ \frac{1}{1+\sum_{h=1}^{J-1}\exp(\beta_{h0}+\gamma_h' y_{i,t-1}^{(g)})} & \text{for } j=J;\ell=p+1. \end{cases}$$

$$= \eta_{it|t-1}^{(j)}(g,\ell), \text{ (say), for } g=1,\ldots,J, \tag{3.276}$$

where

$$\gamma_j = (\gamma_{j1},\ldots,\gamma_{jh},\ldots,\gamma_{j,J-1})' : (J-1)\times 1.$$

Note that these conditional probabilities are similar to those given in (3.207) for the covariate free case, but they have now extended form to accommodate properly the regression effects of the covariates under all J categories. Further note that by using the notations

$$\theta^* = [\beta_1^{*\prime},\ldots,\beta_j^{*\prime},\ldots,\beta_{J-1}^{*}{}']' : (J-1)(p+1)\times 1, \text{ with } \beta_j^* = [\beta_{j0},\ldots,\beta_{j\ell},\ldots,\beta_{jp}]',$$

and

$$x_{[\ell]j}' = \begin{cases} \left(01_{(j-1)(p+1)}' \ d_{[\ell]1}' \ 01_{(J-1-j)(p+1)}'\right) & \text{for } j=1,\ldots,J-1;\ \ell=1,\ldots,p \\ \left(01_{(j-1)(p+1)}' \ d_{[\ell]2}' \ 01_{(J-1-j)(p+1)}'\right) & \text{for } j=1,\ldots,J-1;\ \ell=p+1 \\ \left(01_{(J-1)(p+1)}'\right) & \text{for } j=J;\ \ell=1,\ldots,p+1, \end{cases}$$

with

$$d_{[\ell]m}' = \begin{cases} \left(1\ 01_{\ell-1}' \ 1\ 01_{p-\ell}'\right) & \text{for } m=1 \\ \left(1\ 01_p'\right) & \text{for } m=2, \end{cases}$$

from (3.233)–(3.237), and

$$\begin{aligned} \delta_{[\ell]g} &= y_{i,t-1}^{(g)} \\ &= \begin{cases} \left(01_{g-1}' \ 1\ 01_{J-1-g}'\right)' & \text{for } g=1,\ldots,J-1;\ \ell=1,\ldots,p+1 \\ 01_{J-1} & \text{for } g=J;\ \ell=1,\ldots,p+1, \end{cases} \end{aligned}$$

from (3.242), we may re-express the above logit form marginal probabilities, by

$$\pi_{[\ell]j} = \frac{\exp(x'_{[\ell]j}\theta^*)}{1+\sum_{g=1}^{J-1}\exp(x'_{[\ell]g}\theta^*)}, \tag{3.277}$$

for all $j = 1,\ldots,J$, and $\ell = 1,\ldots,p+1$, and the logit form conditional probabilities, by

$$\eta^{(j)}(g,\ell) = \begin{cases} \frac{\exp\left(x'_{[\ell]j}\theta^*+\gamma'_j\delta_{[\ell]g}\right)}{1+\sum_{h=1}^{J-1}\exp\left(x'_{[\ell]h}\theta^*+\gamma'_h\delta_{[\ell]g}\right)} & \text{for } j=1,\ldots,J-1;\ \ell=1,\ldots,p+1 \\ \frac{1}{1+\sum_{h=1}^{J-1}\exp\left(x'_{[\ell]h}\theta^*+\gamma'_h\delta_{[\ell]g}\right)} & \text{for } j=J;\ \ell=1,\ldots,p+1, \end{cases} \tag{3.278}$$

for a given $g = 1,\ldots,J$.

As far as the fitting of this covariates based multinomial dynamic logit (CBMDL) model (3.277)–(3.278) to a given data set is concerned, similar to the MDL model, one may develop the likelihood estimation approach as follows.

3.5.2.1 Likelihood Function

By (3.277)–(3.278), similar to the likelihood function under the CBLDCMP model (3.240), discussed in the last section, we write the likelihood function under the present CBMDL model as

$$\begin{aligned} L(\theta^*,\gamma_M) &= \Pi_{\ell=1}^{p+1}\Pi_{i\in\ell}^{K}\left[f(y_{i1})\Pi_{t=2}^{T}f(y_{it}|y_{i,t-1})\right] \\ &= \left[\Pi_{\ell=1}^{p+1}\Pi_{i\in\ell}^{K}f(y_{i1})\right] \\ &\times \Pi_{t=2}^{T}\Pi_{\ell=1}^{p+1}\Pi_{g=1}^{J}\Pi_{i\in(g,\ell)}^{K}\left[f(y_{it}|y_{i,t-1}^{(g)})\right] \\ &= d_0^{**}\left[\Pi_{\ell=1}^{p+1}\Pi_{j=1}^{J}\Pi_{i\in\ell}^{K}\pi_{[\ell]j}^{y_{i1j}}\right] \\ &\times \Pi_{t=2}^{T}\Pi_{\ell=1}^{p+1}\Pi_{j=1}^{J}\Pi_{g=1}^{J}\Pi_{i\in(g,\ell)}^{K}\left\{\eta_{it|t-1}^{(j)}(y_{i,t-1}^{(g)})\right\}^{y_{itj}}, \end{aligned} \tag{3.279}$$

where d_0^{**} is the normalizing constant free from any parameters, and γ_M is the $(J-1)\times(J-1)$ matrix of dynamic dependence parameters given by

$$\gamma_M = \begin{pmatrix} \gamma'_1 \\ \vdots \\ \gamma'_j \\ \vdots \\ \gamma'_{J-1} \end{pmatrix} : (J-1)\times(J-1).$$

Next, similar to the linear dynamic model case (3.243)–(3.244), that is, by replacing the conditional probabilities $\lambda^{(j)}(g,\ell)$ with $\eta^{(j)}(g,\ell)$, the log of the likelihood function is written as

$$Log\ L(\theta^*,\gamma_M) = log\ d_0^{**} + \sum_{\ell=1}^{p+1}\sum_{i\in\ell}^{K}\sum_{j=1}^{J} y_{i1j} log\ \pi_{[\ell]j}$$
$$+ \sum_{\ell=1}^{p+1}\sum_{t=2}^{T}\sum_{j=1}^{J}\sum_{g=1}^{J}\sum_{i\in(g,\ell)}^{K}\left[y_{itj} log\ \eta_{it|t-1}^{(j)}(g,\ell)\right], \quad (3.280)$$

which, by using the cell counts from the contingency Tables 3.17 and 3.18, may be written as

$$Log\ L(\theta^*,\gamma_M) = log\ d_0^{**} + \sum_{\ell=1}^{p+1}\sum_{j=1}^{J} K_{[\ell]j}(1) log\ \pi_{[\ell]j}$$
$$+ \sum_{\ell=1}^{p+1}\sum_{j=1}^{J}\sum_{g=1}^{J}\left[\left\{log\ \eta^{(j)}(g,\ell)\right\}\left\{\sum_{t=2}^{T} K_{[\ell]gj}(t-1,t)\right\}\right], \quad (3.281)$$

where $K_{[\ell]gj}(t-1,t)$ (Table 3.18) is the number of individuals with covariate level ℓ, whose responses were in gth category at time $t-1$ and in jth category at time t.

3.5.2.1.1 Likelihood Estimating Equation for θ^*

By using (3.281), the likelihood estimating equation for θ^* may be written as

$$\frac{\partial Log\ L(\theta^*,\gamma_M)}{\partial\theta^*} = \sum_{\ell=1}^{p+1}\sum_{j=1}^{J} K_{[\ell]j}(1)\frac{1}{\pi_{[\ell]j}}\frac{\partial\pi_{[\ell]j}}{\partial\theta^*}$$
$$+ \sum_{\ell=1}^{p+1}\sum_{j=1}^{J}\sum_{g=1}^{J}\left[\left\{\sum_{t=2}^{T} K_{[\ell]gj}(t-1,t)\right\}\frac{1}{\eta^{(j)}(g,\ell)}\right.$$
$$\left.\times\ \frac{\partial\eta^{(j)}(g,\ell)}{\partial\theta^*}\right] = 0. \quad (3.282)$$

For given γ_M, this likelihood equation in (3.282) may be solved iteratively by using the iterative equation for θ^* given by

$$\hat{\theta}^*(r+1) = \hat{\theta}^*(r) - \left[\left\{\frac{\partial^2 \text{Log}\ L(\theta^*,\gamma_M)}{\partial\theta^{*\prime}\partial\theta^*}\right\}^{-1}\frac{\partial \text{Log}\ L(\theta^*,\gamma_M)}{\partial\theta^*}\right]_{|\theta^*=\hat{\theta}^*(r)};\ (J-1)(p+1)\times 1, \quad (3.283)$$

where the second order derivative matrix has the formula

$$\frac{\partial^2 Log\, L(\theta^*,\gamma_M)}{\partial\theta^{*\prime}\partial\theta^*} = \sum_{\ell=1}^{p+1}\sum_{j=1}^{J} K_{[\ell]j}(1)\left[\frac{\partial}{\partial\theta^{*\prime}}\left\{\frac{1}{\pi_{[\ell]j}}\frac{\partial\pi_{[\ell]j}}{\partial\theta^*}\right\}\right]$$
$$+\sum_{\ell=1}^{p+1}\sum_{j=1}^{J}\sum_{g=1}^{J}\left[\left\{\sum_{t=2}^{T}K_{[\ell]gj}(t-1,t)\right\}\left\{\frac{1}{\eta^{(j)}(g,\ell)}\frac{\partial^2\eta^{(j)}(g,\ell)}{\partial\theta^{*\prime}\partial\theta^*}\right.\right.$$
$$\left.\left.-\frac{1}{\{\eta^{(j)}(g,\ell)\}^2}\frac{\partial\eta^{(j)}(g,\ell)}{\partial\theta^*}\frac{\partial\eta^{(j)}(g,\ell)}{\partial\theta^{*\prime}}\right\}\right]. \quad (3.284)$$

The first and second order derivatives involved in the estimating equations (3.282)–(3.284) are computed as follows:

Computation of $\frac{1}{\pi_{[\ell]j}}\frac{\partial\pi_{[\ell]j}}{\partial\theta^*}$ and $\frac{\partial}{\partial\theta^{*\prime}}\left\{\frac{1}{\pi_{[\ell]j}}\frac{\partial\pi_{[\ell]j}}{\partial\theta^*}\right\}$:
These formulas, in particular, the formulas for $\frac{1}{\pi_{[\ell]j}}\frac{\partial\pi_{[\ell]j}}{\partial\theta^*}$ are the same as (3.247), and the formulas for $\frac{\partial}{\partial\theta^{*\prime}}\left\{\frac{1}{\pi_{[\ell]j}}\frac{\partial\pi_{[\ell]j}}{\partial\theta^*}\right\}$ are as in (3.255)–(3.256) under the LDCMP model.

Computation of $\frac{\partial\eta^{(j)}(g,\ell)}{\partial\theta^*}$ and $\frac{\partial^2\eta^{(j)}(g,\ell)}{\partial\theta^{*\prime}\partial\theta^*}$:
Note that the conditional probabilities $\eta^{(j)}(g,\ell)$ given by (3.278) for the MDL model are different than those of $\lambda^{(j)}(g,\ell)$ given in (3.241) under the LDCMP model. Thus their derivatives will be different. However, because $\eta^{(j)}(g,\ell)$ is a generalization of the conditional probabilities $\eta^{(j)}(g)$ (3.214) under the covariate free MDL model, the first and second order derivatives of $\eta^{(j)}(g,\ell)$ can be obtained in the fashion similar to those of $\eta^{(j)}(g)$ given by (3.220)–(3.221). Hence, for all $g = 1,\ldots,J;\ j = 1,\ldots,J$, it follows from (3.278) that

$$\frac{\partial\eta^{(j)}(g,\ell)}{\partial\theta^*} = \begin{cases}\eta^{(j)}(g,\ell)\left[x_{[\ell]j}-\Sigma_{h=1}^{J-1}x_{[\ell]h}\eta^{(h)}(g,\ell)\right] & \text{for } \ell=1,\ldots,p\\ -\left[\eta^{(J)}(g,\ell)\Sigma_{h=1}^{J-1}x_{[\ell]h}\eta^{(h)}(g,\ell)\right] & \text{for } \ell=p+1\end{cases} \quad (3.285)$$

$$= \begin{cases}\eta^{(j)}(g,\ell)\left[x_{[\ell]j}-\eta(g,\ell)\otimes d_{[\ell]1}\right] \text{ for } \ell=1,\ldots,p\\ \eta^{(j)}(g,\ell)\left[x_{[\ell]j}-\eta(g,\ell)\otimes d_{[\ell]2}\right] \text{ for } \ell=p+1,\end{cases} \quad (3.286)$$

where

$$\eta(g,\ell) = [\eta^{(1)}(g,\ell),\ldots,\eta^{(j)}(g,\ell),\ldots,\eta^{(J-1)}(g,\ell)]'.$$

The formulae for the second order derivatives follow from (3.286) and they are given by

$$\frac{\partial^2 \eta^{(j)}(g,\ell)}{\partial \theta^{*\prime} \partial \theta^*}$$
$$= \begin{cases} \eta^{(j)}(g,\ell)\left[(x_{[\ell]j} - \eta(g,\ell) \otimes d_{[\ell]1})(x_{[\ell]j} - \eta(g,\ell) \otimes d_{[\ell]1})' - \frac{\partial \eta(g,\ell)}{\partial \theta^{*\prime}}\right] & \text{for } \ell = 1,\ldots,p \\ \eta^{(j)}(g,\ell)\left[(x_{[\ell]j} - \eta(g,\ell) \otimes d_{[\ell]2})(x_{[\ell]j} - \eta(g,\ell) \otimes d_{[\ell]1})' - \frac{\partial \eta(g,\ell)}{\partial \theta^{*\prime}}\right] & \text{for } \ell = p+1, \end{cases} \tag{3.287}$$
$$= \eta^{(j)}(g,\ell) M^*_{[\ell]j}(x, \eta(g,\ell)), \text{ (say)}, \tag{3.288}$$

by using the notation $x_J = 01_{J-1}$. In (3.287)–(3.288), the derivative $\frac{\partial \eta(g,\ell)}{\partial \theta^{*\prime}}$ is computed as follows.

Computation of $\frac{\partial \eta(g,\ell)}{\partial \theta^{*\prime}}$:
Notice from (3.286) that

$$\frac{\partial \eta^{(j)}(g,\ell)}{\partial \theta^{*\prime}} = \begin{cases} \eta^{(j)}(g,\ell)\left[x_{[\ell]j} - \eta(g,\ell) \otimes d_{[\ell]1}\right]' & \text{for } \ell = 1,\ldots,p;\ j = 1,\ldots,J \\ \eta^{(j)}(g,\ell)\left[x_{[\ell]j} - \eta(g,\ell) \otimes d_{[\ell]2}\right]' & \text{for } \ell = p+1;\ j = 1,\ldots,J, \end{cases}$$

yielding

$$\frac{\partial \eta(g,\ell)}{\partial \theta^{*\prime}} = \frac{\partial}{\partial \theta^{*\prime}} \begin{pmatrix} \eta^{(1)}(g,\ell) \\ \vdots \\ \eta^{(j)}(g,\ell) \\ \vdots \\ \eta^{(J-1)}(g,\ell) \end{pmatrix}$$
$$= \begin{pmatrix} \eta^{(1)}(g,\ell)\left[x_{[\ell]1} - \eta(g,\ell) \otimes d_{[\ell]1}\right]' \\ \vdots \\ \eta^{(j)}(g,\ell)\left[x_{[\ell]j} - \eta(g,\ell) \otimes d_{[\ell]1}\right]' \\ \vdots \\ \eta^{(J-1)}(g,\ell)\left[x_{[\ell](J-1)} - \eta(g,\ell) \otimes d_{[\ell]1}\right]' \end{pmatrix}, \text{ for } \ell = 1,\ldots,p, \tag{3.289}$$

and

$$\frac{\partial \eta(g,\ell)}{\partial \theta^{*\prime}} = \begin{pmatrix} \eta^{(1)}(g,\ell)\left[x_{[\ell]1} - \eta(g,\ell) \otimes d_{[\ell]2}\right]' \\ \vdots \\ \eta^{(j)}(g,\ell)\left[x_{[\ell]j} - \eta(g,\ell) \otimes d_{[\ell]2}\right]' \\ \vdots \\ \eta^{(J-1)}(g,\ell)\left[x_{[\ell](J-1)} - \eta(g,\ell) \otimes d_{[\ell]2}\right]' \end{pmatrix}, \text{ for } \ell = p+1. \tag{3.290}$$

3.5.2.1.2 Likelihood Estimating Equation for γ_M

Let

$$\gamma^* = (\gamma_1', \ldots, \gamma_j', \ldots, \gamma_{J-1}')' : (J-1)^2 \times 1; \text{ where } \gamma_j = (\gamma_{j1}, \ldots, \gamma_{jh}, \ldots, \gamma_{j,J-1})', \tag{3.291}$$

where γ_j is the $(J-1) \times 1$ vector of dynamic dependence parameters involved in the conditional multinomial logit function in (3.278). By similar calculations as in (3.225), it follows from (3.278) that

$$\frac{\partial \eta^{(h)}(g,\ell)}{\partial \gamma_j} = \begin{cases} \delta_{[\ell]g}\eta^{(j)}(g,\ell)[1-\eta^{(j)}(g,\ell)] & \text{for } h=j; h,j=1,\ldots,J-1 \\ -\delta_{[\ell]g}\eta^{(j)}(g,\ell)\eta^{(h)}(g,\ell) & \text{for } h \neq j; h,j=1,\ldots,J-1 \\ -\delta_{[\ell]g}\eta^{(j)}(g,\ell)\eta^{(J)}(g,\ell) & \text{for } h=J;\ j=1,\ldots,J-1, \end{cases} \tag{3.292}$$

where $g = 1, \ldots, J$, and $\ell = 1, \ldots, p+1$.

Using these derivatives, by similar calculations as in (3.293), it follows from the likelihood function (3.281) that

$$\frac{\partial Log\, L(\theta^*, \gamma_M)}{\partial \gamma_j} = \sum_{\ell=1}^{p+1}\sum_{g=1}^{J}\left[\left\{\sum_{t=2}^{T} K_{[\ell]gj}(t-1,t)\right\}\delta_{[\ell]g}\right] - \sum_{\ell=1}^{p+1}\sum_{g=1}^{J}\sum_{h=1}^{J}\left[\left\{\sum_{t=2}^{T} K_{[\ell]gh}(t-1,t)\right\}\delta_{[\ell]g}\eta^{(j)}(g,\ell)\right] = 0, \tag{3.293}$$

for $j = 1, \ldots, J-1$, leading to the estimating equations for the elements of $\gamma^* = (\gamma_1', \ldots, \gamma_j', \ldots, \gamma_{J-1}')'$ as

$$\frac{\partial Log\, L(\theta^*, \gamma_M)}{\partial \gamma^*} = \begin{pmatrix} \frac{\partial Log\, L(\theta^*, \gamma_M)}{\partial \gamma_1} \\ \vdots \\ \frac{\partial Log\, L(\theta^*, \gamma_M)}{\partial \gamma_j} \\ \vdots \\ \frac{\partial Log\, L(\theta^*, \gamma_M)}{\partial \gamma_{J-1}} \end{pmatrix} = 0 : (J-1)^2 \times 1. \tag{3.294}$$

One may now solve this likelihood equation (3.294) for γ^* by using the iterative equation

$$\hat{\gamma}^*(r+1) = \hat{\gamma}^*(r) - \left[\left\{\frac{\partial^2 \text{Log}\, L(\theta^*, \gamma_M)}{\partial \gamma^* \partial \gamma^{*\prime}}\right\}^{-1} \frac{\partial \text{Log}\, L(\theta^*, \gamma_M)}{\partial \gamma^*}\right]_{|\gamma^* = \hat{\gamma}^*(r)}, \tag{3.295}$$

where the $(J-1)^2 \times (J-1)^2$ second derivative matrix is computed by using the formulas

$$\frac{\partial^2 \text{Log}\, L(\theta^*, \gamma_M)}{\partial \gamma_j \partial \gamma_j'} = -\sum_{\ell=1}^{p+1} \sum_{g=1}^{J} \sum_{h=1}^{J} \left[\left\{ \sum_{t=2}^{T} K_{[\ell]gh}(t-1,t) \right\} \eta^{(j)}(g,\ell) \left(1-\eta^{(j)}(g,\ell)\right) \delta_{[\ell]g} \delta_{[\ell]g}' \right] \quad (3.296)$$

for all $j = 1, \ldots, J-1$, and

$$\frac{\partial^2 \text{Log}\, L(\theta^*, \gamma_M)}{\partial \gamma_j \partial \gamma_k'} = \sum_{\ell=1}^{p+1} \sum_{g=1}^{J} \sum_{h=1}^{J} \left[\left\{ \sum_{t=2}^{T} K_{[\ell]gh}(t-1,t) \right\} \left(\eta^{(j)}(g,\ell) \eta^{(k)}(g,\ell) \right) \delta_{[\ell]g} \delta_{[\ell]g}' \right], \quad (3.297)$$

for all $j \neq k; j,k = 1, \ldots, J-1$.

3.5.2.2 Illustration 3.11: Analysis of Longitudinal TMISL (Three Categories) Data by Fitting CBMDL Model with Distance as a Covariate Using the Likelihood Approach

Recall that in illustration 3.9 in Sect. 3.4.1.2.1, the TMISL data analysis results were presented where an LDCMP model was fitted to the data by using a GQL approach. In Sect. 3.4.2.2 (illustration 3.10), the same data were fitted by using the MDL model, and as results in Table 3.22 show, it was found that the MDL model fits the data much better. The MDL model provides recursive means over time that reflected the change in marginal probabilities well. However, the MDL model was fitted for simplicity ignoring the distance covariate. But as it is also of interest to find the effect of the distance on the stress level responses over time, in this section, we fit the CBMDL model discussed in Sect. 5.2.

For the purpose, following the model (3.275)–(3.276), we first simplify the marginal and conditional probability formulas using the distance as a covariate. Note that in the TMISL data, distance is a binary covariate with $\ell = 1,2$. To be specific, the level $\ell = 1$ would represent the group of workers commuting distance ≤ 5 miles, and $\ell = 2$ would represent the other group commuting distance > 5 miles. Thus, by (3.275)–(3.276), the marginal probabilities at time $t = 1$ and conditional probabilities at $t = 2,3,4$, corresponding to these two levels of distance have the formulas as follows:

Group 1 (Distance $\leq$ 5 miles):

Marginal probabilities:

$$\pi_{[1]1} = \frac{\exp(\beta_{10}+\beta_{11})}{1+\sum_{g=1}^{2}\exp(\beta_{g0}+\beta_{g1})}, \quad \pi_{[1]2} = \frac{\exp(\beta_{20}+\beta_{21})}{1+\sum_{g=1}^{2}\exp(\beta_{g0}+\beta_{g1})},$$

$$\pi_{[1]3} = \frac{1}{1+\sum_{g=1}^{2}\exp(\beta_{g0}+\beta_{g1})}.$$

Conditional probabilities:
From stress level 1 to 1,2,3:

$$\eta^{(1)}(1,1) = \frac{\exp(\beta_{10}+\beta_{11}+\gamma_{11})}{1+\sum_{h=1}^{2}\exp(\beta_{h0}+\beta_{h1}+\gamma_{h1})},\ \eta^{(2)}(1,1) = \frac{\exp(\beta_{20}+\beta_{21}+\gamma_{21})}{1+\sum_{h=1}^{2}\exp(\beta_{h0}+\beta_{h1}+\gamma_{h1})},$$
$$\eta^{(3)}(1,1) = \frac{1}{1+\sum_{h=1}^{2}\exp(\beta_{h0}+\beta_{h1}+\gamma_{h1})};$$

From stress level 2 to 1,2,3:

$$\eta^{(1)}(2,1) = \frac{\exp(\beta_{10}+\beta_{11}+\gamma_{12})}{1+\sum_{h=1}^{2}\exp(\beta_{h0}+\beta_{h1}+\gamma_{h2})},\ \eta^{(2)}(2,1) = \frac{\exp(\beta_{20}+\beta_{21}+\gamma_{22})}{1+\sum_{h=1}^{2}\exp(\beta_{h0}+\beta_{h1}+\gamma_{h2})},$$
$$\eta^{(3)}(2,1) = \frac{1}{1+\sum_{h=1}^{2}\exp(\beta_{h0}+\beta_{h1}+\gamma_{h2})};$$

From stress level 3 to 1,2,3:

$$\eta^{(1)}(3,1) = \frac{\exp(\beta_{10}+\beta_{11})}{1+\sum_{h=1}^{2}\exp(\beta_{h0}+\beta_{h1})},\ \eta^{(2)}(3,1) = \frac{\exp(\beta_{20}+\beta_{21})}{1+\sum_{h=1}^{2}\exp(\beta_{h0}+\beta_{h1})},$$
$$\eta^{(3)}(3,1) = \frac{1}{1+\sum_{h=1}^{2}\exp(\beta_{h0}+\beta_{h1})}.$$

Group 2 (Distance > 5 miles):
Marginal probabilities:

$$\pi_{[2]1} = \frac{\exp(\beta_{10})}{1+\sum_{g=1}^{2}\exp(\beta_{g0})},\ \pi_{[2]2} = \frac{\exp(\beta_{20})}{1+\sum_{g=1}^{2}\exp(\beta_{g0})},$$
$$\pi_{[2]3} = \frac{1}{1+\sum_{g=1}^{2}\exp(\beta_{g0})}.$$

Conditional probabilities:
From stress level 1 to 1,2,3:

$$\eta^{(1)}(1,2) = \frac{\exp(\beta_{10}+\gamma_{11})}{1+\sum_{h=1}^{2}\exp(\beta_{h0}+\gamma_{h1})},\ \eta^{(2)}(1,2) = \frac{\exp(\beta_{20}+\gamma_{21})}{1+\sum_{h=1}^{2}\exp(\beta_{h0}+\gamma_{h1})},$$
$$\eta^{(3)}(1,2) = \frac{1}{1+\sum_{h=1}^{2}\exp(\beta_{h0}+\gamma_{h1})};$$

From stress level 2 to 1,2,3:

$$\eta^{(1)}(2,2) = \frac{\exp(\beta_{10}+\gamma_{12})}{1+\sum_{h=1}^{2}\exp(\beta_{h0}+\gamma_{h2})},\ \eta^{(2)}(2,2) = \frac{\exp(\beta_{20}+\gamma_{22})}{1+\sum_{h=1}^{2}\exp(\beta_{h0}+\gamma_{h2})},$$

$$\eta^{(3)}(2,2) = \frac{1}{1+\sum_{h=1}^{2}\exp(\beta_{h0}+\gamma_{h2})};$$

From stress level 3 to 1,2,3:

$$\eta^{(1)}(3,2) = \frac{\exp(\beta_{10})}{1+\sum_{h=1}^{2}\exp(\beta_{h0})},\ \eta^{(2)}(3,2) = \frac{\exp(\beta_{20})}{1+\sum_{h=1}^{2}\exp(\beta_{h0})},$$

$$\eta^{(3)}(3,2) = \frac{1}{1+\sum_{h=1}^{2}\exp(\beta_{h0})}.$$

Unlike in the illustration 3.10, β_{j1} for $j = 1,2$, represent the distance covariate effect on the multinomial responses belonging to jth category, when $\beta_{31} = 0$, and hence θ^* has four components. That is,

$$\theta^* = (\beta_{10}, \beta_{11}, \beta_{20}, \beta_{21})'.$$

However when compared to the covariate free case in 3.10 illustration, dynamic dependence parameter vector $\gamma^* = (\gamma_{11}, \gamma_{12}, \gamma_{21}, \gamma_{22})'$ remains the same, but their estimating equations would be different. Now by writing, for example,

$$K^*_{[\ell]gj} = K_{[\ell]gj}(1,2) + K_{[\ell]gj}(2,3) + K_{[\ell]gj}(3,4),$$

for $\ell = 1,2$; $g, j = 1,\ldots,3$, and

$$K^*_{[\ell]g} = \sum_{j=1}^{3} K^*_{[\ell]gj},$$

for $g = 1,\ldots,3$, the four likelihood equations in (3.282) may be simplified as

$$f_1(\theta^*,\gamma^*) = \sum_{\ell=1}^{2}[K_{[\ell]1}(1) - K_{[\ell]}\pi_{[\ell]1}] + \sum_{\ell=1}^{2}\Big[\{K^*_{[\ell]11} - K^*_{[\ell]1}\eta^{(1)}(1,\ell)\}$$
$$+ \sum_{\ell=1}^{2}\{K^*_{[\ell]21} - K^*_{[\ell]2}\eta^{(1)}(2,\ell)\} + \sum_{\ell=1}^{2}\{K^*_{[\ell]31} - K^*_{[\ell]3}\eta^{(1)}(3,\ell)\}\Big] = 0$$

$$f_2(\theta^*,\gamma^*) = [K_{[1]1}(1) - K_{[1]}\pi_{[1]1}] + \Big[\{K^*_{[1]11} - K^*_{[1]1}\eta^{(1)}(1,1)\}$$
$$+ \{K^*_{[1]21} - K^*_{[1]2}\eta^{(1)}(2,1)\} + \{K^*_{[1]31} - K^*_{[1]3}\eta^{(1)}(3,1)\}\Big] = 0$$

$$f_3(\theta^*,\gamma^*) = \sum_{\ell=1}^{2}[K_{[\ell]2}(1) - K_{[\ell]}\pi_{[\ell]2}] + \sum_{\ell=1}^{2}\Big[\{K^*_{[\ell]12} - K^*_{[\ell]1}\eta^{(2)}(1,\ell)\}$$
$$+ \sum_{\ell=1}^{2}\{K^*_{[\ell]22} - K^*_{[\ell]2}\eta^{(2)}(2,\ell)\} + \sum_{\ell=1}^{2}\{K^*_{[\ell]32} - K^*_{[\ell]3}\eta^{(2)}(3,\ell)\}\Big] = 0$$
$$f_4(\theta^*,\gamma^*) = [K_{[1]2}(1) - K_{[1]}\pi_{[1]2}] + \Big[\{K^*_{[1]12} - K^*_{[1]1}\eta^{(2)}(1,1)\}$$
$$+ \{K^*_{[1]22} - K^*_{[1]2}\eta^{(2)}(2,1)\} + \{K^*_{[1]32} - K^*_{[1]3}\eta^{(2)}(3,1)\}\Big] = 0,$$

and similarly the four likelihood equations for γ^* in (3.294) have the forms

$$g_1(\gamma^*,\theta^*) = \sum_{\ell=1}^{2}[K^*_{[\ell]11} - K^*_{[\ell]1}\eta^{(1)}(1,\ell)] = 0$$
$$g_2(\gamma^*,\theta^*) = \sum_{\ell=1}^{2}[K^*_{[\ell]21} - K^*_{[\ell]2}\eta^{(1)}(2,\ell)] = 0$$
$$g_3(\gamma^*,\theta^*) = \sum_{\ell=1}^{2}[K^*_{[\ell]12} - K^*_{[\ell]1}\eta^{(2)}(1,\ell)] = 0$$
$$g_4(\gamma^*,\theta^*) = \sum_{\ell=1}^{2}[K^*_{[\ell]22} - K^*_{[\ell]2}\eta^{(2)}(2,\ell)] = 0,$$

respectively. Similarly, the second order derivatives of the likelihood function with respect to θ^* and γ^* were simplified. The second order derivative matrix for θ^*, following (3.284), is given by

$$F(\theta^*,\gamma^*) = \begin{pmatrix} f_{11}(\theta^*,\gamma^*) & f_{12}(\theta^*,\gamma^*) & f_{13}(\theta^*,\gamma^*) & f_{14}(\theta^*,\gamma^* \\ f_{21}(\theta^*,\gamma^*) & f_{22}(\theta^*,\gamma^*) & f_{23}(\theta^*,\gamma^*) & f_{24}(\theta^*,\gamma^*) \\ f_{31}(\theta^*,\gamma^*) & f_{32}(\theta^*,\gamma^*) & f_{33}(\theta^*,\gamma^*) & f_{34}(\theta^*,\gamma^* \\ f_{41}(\theta^*,\gamma^*) & f_{42}(\theta^*,\gamma^*) & f_{43}(\theta^*,\gamma^*) & f_{44}(\theta^*,\gamma^*) \end{pmatrix},$$

where

$$f_{11}(\cdot) = -\sum_{\ell=1}^{2}\Big[K_{[\ell]}\pi_{[\ell]1}(1-\pi_{[\ell]1}) + \Big\{K^*_{[\ell]1}\eta^{(1)}(1,\ell)(1-\eta^{(1)}(1,\ell))$$
$$+ K^*_{[\ell]2}\eta^{(1)}(2,\ell)(1-\eta^{(1)}(2,\ell)) + K^*_{[\ell]3}\eta^{(1)}(3,\ell)(1-\eta^{(1)}(3,\ell))\Big\}\Big]$$
$$f_{12}(\cdot) = -\Big[K_{[1]}\pi_{[1]1}(1-\pi_{[1]1}) + \Big\{K^*_{[1]1}\eta^{(1)}(1,1)(1-\eta^{(1)}(1,1))$$

$$+ \; K^*_{[1]2}\eta^{(1)}(2,1)(1-\eta^{(1)}(2,1)) + K^*_{[1]3}\eta^{(1)}(3,1)(1-\eta^{(1)}(3,1))\Big\}\Big]$$

$$f_{13}(\cdot) = \sum_{\ell=1}^{2}\Big[K_{[\ell]}\pi_{[\ell]1}\pi_{[\ell]2} + (K^*_{[\ell]12}+K^*_{[\ell]13})\eta^{(1)}(1,\ell)\eta^{(2)}(1,\ell)$$

$$+ \; (K^*_{[\ell]22}+K^*_{[\ell]23})\eta^{(1)}(2,\ell)\eta^{(2)}(2,\ell) + (K^*_{[\ell]31}+K^*_{[\ell]33})\eta^{(1)}(3,\ell)\eta^{(2)}(3,\ell)\Big]$$

$$f_{14}(\cdot) = \Big[K_{[1]}\pi_{[1]1}\pi_{[1]2} + (K^*_{[1]12}+K^*_{[1]13})\eta^{(1)}(1,1)\eta^{(2)}(1,1)$$

$$+ \; (K^*_{[1]22}+K^*_{[1]23})\eta^{(1)}(2,1)\eta^{(2)}(2,1) + (K^*_{[1]31}+K^*_{[1]33})\eta^{(1)}(3,1)\eta^{(2)}(3,1)\Big]$$

$$f_{21}(\cdot) = f_{12}(\cdot)$$

$$f_{22}(\cdot) = f_{12}(\cdot)$$

$$f_{23}(\cdot) = f_{14}(\cdot)$$

$$f_{24}(\cdot) = f_{14}(\cdot)$$

$$f_{31}(\cdot) = f_{13}(\cdot)$$

$$f_{32}(\cdot) = f_{23}(\cdot)$$

$$f_{33}(\cdot) = -\sum_{\ell=1}^{2}\Big[K_{[\ell]}\pi_{[\ell]2}(1-\pi_{[\ell]2}) + \Big\{K^*_{[\ell]1}\eta^{(2)}(1,\ell)(1-\eta^{(2)}(1,\ell))$$

$$+ \; K^*_{[\ell]2}\eta^{(2)}(2,\ell)(1-\eta^{(2)}(2,\ell)) + K^*_{[\ell]3}\eta^{(2)}(3,\ell)(1-\eta^{(2)}(3,\ell))\Big\}\Big]$$

$$f_{34}(\cdot) = -\Big[K_{[1]}\pi_{[1]2}(1-\pi_{[1]2}) + \Big\{K^*_{[1]1}\eta^{(2)}(1,1)(1-\eta^{(2)}(1,1))$$

$$+ \; K^*_{[1]2}\eta^{(2)}(2,1)(1-\eta^{(2)}(2,1)) + K^*_{[1]3}\eta^{(2)}(3,1)(1-\eta^{(2)}(3,1))\Big\}\Big]$$

$$f_{41}(\cdot) = f_{14}(\cdot)$$

$$f_{42}(\cdot) = f_{24}(\cdot)$$

$$f_{43}(\cdot) = f_{34}(\cdot)$$

$$f_{44}(\cdot) = f_{34}(\cdot),$$

and similarly the second order derivative matrix for γ^*, following (3.296)–(3.297), is given by

$$\Gamma(\gamma^*,\theta^*) = \begin{pmatrix} G_1 & G_2 \\ G_2' & G_3 \end{pmatrix},$$

where

$$G_1 = -\begin{pmatrix} \Sigma_{\ell=1}^{2}[K^*_{[\ell]1}\eta^{(1)}(1,\ell)(1-\eta^{(1)}(1,\ell))] & 0 \\ 0 & \Sigma_{\ell=1}^{2}[K^*_{[\ell]2}\eta^{(1)}(2,\ell)(1-\eta^{(1)}(2,\ell))] \end{pmatrix}$$

$$G_2 = \begin{pmatrix} \Sigma_{\ell=1}^{2}[K^*_{[\ell]1}\eta^{(1)}(1,\ell)\eta^{(2)}(1,\ell)] & 0 \\ 0 & \Sigma_{\ell=1}^{2}[K^*_{[\ell]2}\eta^{(1)}(2,\ell)\eta^{(2)}(2,\ell)] \end{pmatrix}$$

$$G_3 = -\begin{pmatrix} \Sigma_{\ell=1}^{2}[K^*_{[\ell]1}\eta^{(2)}(1,\ell)(1-\eta^{(2)}(1,\ell))] & 0 \\ 0 & \Sigma_{\ell=1}^{2}[K^*_{[\ell]2}\eta^{(2)}(2,\ell)(1-\eta^{(2)}(2,\ell))] \end{pmatrix}.$$

Now by using the iterative equations

$$\hat{\theta}^*(r+1) = \hat{\theta}^*(r) - \left[\{F(\theta^*,\gamma^*)\}^{-1} \begin{pmatrix} f_1(\theta^*,\gamma^*) \\ f_2(\theta^*,\gamma^*) \\ f_3(\theta^*,\gamma^*) \\ f_4(\theta^*,\gamma^*) \end{pmatrix} \right]_{|\theta^*=\hat{\theta}^*(r)} \quad : 4\times 1,$$

(see (3.283)) for θ^*, and

$$\hat{\gamma}^*(r+1) = \hat{\gamma}^*(r) - \left[\{\Gamma(\gamma^*,\theta^*)\}^{-1} \begin{pmatrix} g_1(\gamma^*,\theta^*) \\ g_2(\gamma^*,\theta^*) \\ g_3(\gamma^*,\theta^*) \\ g_4(\gamma^*,\theta^*) \end{pmatrix} \right]_{|\gamma^*=\hat{\gamma}^*(r)} \quad : 4\times 1,$$

(see (3.295)) for γ^*, in ten cycles of iterations, we obtained the maximum likelihood estimates (MLE) for the category intercept and regression parameters as

$$\hat{\beta}_{10,MLE} = -1.6962,\ \hat{\beta}_{11,MLE} = -0.3745;\ \hat{\beta}_{20,MLE} = 0.6265, \hat{\beta}_{21,MLE} = -0.5196,$$

and for the lag 1 dynamic dependence parameters as

$$\hat{\gamma}_{11,MLE} = 5.7934,\ \hat{\gamma}_{12,MLE} = 2.4007;\ \hat{\gamma}_{21,MLE} = 3.6463,\ \hat{\gamma}_{22,MLE} = 1.8790.$$

The aforementioned regression and dynamic dependence parameter estimates may now be used to compute the recursive means (multinomial probabilities) over time at distance covariate level ($\ell = 1,2$) following (3.208). More specifically, for distance group $\ell (= 1,2)$, the recursive marginal probabilities have the formula

$$\begin{aligned} E[Y_{i\in\ell,t}] = \tilde{\pi}_{[t,\ell]} &= \eta(J,\ell) + \left[\eta_M(\ell) - \eta(J,\ell)1'_{J-1}\right]\tilde{\pi}_{[t-1,\ell]} \\ &= [\tilde{\pi}_{[t,\ell]1},\ldots,\tilde{\pi}_{[t,\ell]j},\ldots,\tilde{\pi}_{[t,\ell](J-1)}]' : (J-1)\times 1, \end{aligned}$$

where

$$\tilde{\pi}_{[1,\ell]} = [\pi_{[\ell]1},\ldots,\pi_{[\ell]j},\ldots,\pi_{[\ell](J-1)}]' = \pi_{[\ell]}$$
$$\eta(J,\ell) = [\eta^{(1)}(J,\ell),\ldots,\eta^{(j)}(J,\ell)\ldots,\eta^{(J-1)}(J,\ell)]' = \tilde{\pi}_{[1,\ell]} : (J-1)\times(J-1)$$
$$\eta_M(\ell) = \begin{pmatrix} \eta^{(1)}(1,\ell) & \cdots & \eta^{(1)}(g,\ell) & \cdots & \eta^{(1)}(J-1,\ell) \\ \vdots & \vdots & \vdots & \vdots & \vdots \\ \eta^{(j)}(1,\ell) & \cdots & \eta^{(j)}(g,\ell) & \cdots & \eta^{(j)}(J-1,\ell) \\ \vdots & \vdots & \vdots & \vdots & \vdots \\ \eta^{(J-1)}(1,\ell) & \cdots & \eta^{(J-1)}(g,\ell) & \cdots & \eta^{(J-1)}(J-1,\ell) \end{pmatrix} : (J-1)\times(J-1).$$

For the TMISL data $J = 3$. For two distance groups, the constant vectors and matrices are estimated as
Group 1: Distance ≤ 5 miles
Mean vector at $t = 1$:

$$\begin{aligned}\tilde{\pi}_{(1,1)} &= [\tilde{\pi}_{(1,1)1} \text{ (Low group)}, \tilde{\pi}_{(1,1)2} \text{ (Medium group)}]' : 2\times 1 \\ &= \pi_{[1]} : 2\times 1 \\ &= [0.0563,\ 0.4970]',\end{aligned}$$

with $\tilde{\pi}_{(1,1)3}$ (High group) $= 1 - \tilde{\pi}_{(1,1)1} - \tilde{\pi}_{(1,1)2} = 0.4466$.
Constant conditional probabilities at any time:

$$\begin{aligned}\eta_M(1) &= \begin{pmatrix} \eta^{(1)}(1,1) & \eta^{(1)}(2,1) \\ \eta^{(2)}(1,1) & \eta^{(2)}(2,1) \end{pmatrix} : 2\times 2 \\ &= \begin{pmatrix} 0.4839 & 0.5043 \\ 0.1424 & 0.7541 \end{pmatrix},\end{aligned}$$

and $\eta(J,1) = \tilde{\pi}_{(1,1)} = \pi_{[1]}$.
Group 2: Distance > 5 miles
Mean vector at $t = 1$:

$$\begin{aligned}\tilde{\pi}_{(1,2)} &= [\tilde{\pi}_{(1,2)1} \text{ (Low group)}, \tilde{\pi}_{(1,2)2} \text{ (Medium group)}]' : 2\times 1 \\ &= \pi_{[2]} : 2\times 1 \\ &= [0.0600,\ 0.6126]',\end{aligned}$$

with $\tilde{\pi}_{(1,2)3}$ (High group) $= 1 - \tilde{\pi}_{(1,2)1} - \tilde{\pi}_{(1,2)2} = 0.3274$.
Constant conditional probabilities at any time :

$$\eta_M(2) = \begin{pmatrix} \eta^{(1)}(1,2) & \eta^{(1)}(2,2) \\ \eta^{(2)}(1,2) & \eta^{(2)}(2,2) \end{pmatrix} : 2\times 2$$

Table 3.27 MDL model based fitted marginal probabilities (FMP) ($\tilde{\pi}_{(t,\ell)}$ for $\ell = 1,2$, under all three stress levels for the TMISL data

	FMP at time $t(\tilde{\pi}_{(t,1)})$[Distance $\leq$ 5 miles]				FMP at time $t(\tilde{\pi}_{(t,2)})$[Distance $>$ 5 miles]			
Stress level	1	2	3	4	1	2	3	4
Low	0.0563	0.1232	0.1628	0.1826	0.0600	0.1270	0.1612	0.1757
Medium	0.4970	0.6253	0.6587	0.6676	0.6126	0.7252	0.7419	0.7427
High	0.4466	0.2515	0.1785	0.1498	0.3274	0.1478	0.0969	0.0816

$$= \begin{pmatrix} 0.4501 & 0.5423 \\ 0.1312 & 0.8033 \end{pmatrix},$$

and $\eta(J,2) = \tilde{\pi}_{(1,2)} = \pi_{[2]}$.

These results are then used in the aforementioned recursive relationship for both distance groups ($\ell = 1,2$) to compute the marginal probabilities $\tilde{\pi}_{(t,\ell)}$ for three categories over remaining tree time points. These fitted recursive marginal probabilities for both distance groups are shown in Table 3.27.

These probabilities clearly reveal differences between the stress levels under two distance groups. For example, even though the probabilities in the high level stress group decrease as time progresses under both distance groups, these probabilities remain much higher in the short distance group as expected. As far as the other two stress levels are concerned, the probabilities increase as time progresses under both distance groups. Furthermore, relatively more workers appear to have medium stress under both distance groups, with smaller proportion in the short distance group as compared to the long distance group.

Note that to compute the correlations among the multinomial responses, one may use the aforementioned regression and dynamic dependence parameter estimates in (3.208) for each of the two distance groups. For $t = 1,\ldots,4$, we first provide the variance and covariances of the elements of $\text{var}[Y_{i\in\ell,t}] = (\sigma_{([\ell],t)jk})$, $\ell = 1,2;\ j,k = 1,2$, and then the values of correlations

$$\text{corr}[Y_{i\in\ell,uj}, Y_{i\in\ell,tk}] = (\frac{\sigma_{([\ell],ut)jk}}{[\sigma_{([\ell],u)jj}\sigma_{([\ell],t)kk}]^{\frac{1}{2}}}) = (\rho_{([\ell],ut)jk}),$$

for $u < t$. **Group 1: Distance $\leq$ 5 miles**
Values of $(\sigma_{([1],t)jk})$:

$$\text{var}[Y_{i\in 1,1}] = (\sigma_{([1],1)jk}) = \begin{pmatrix} 0.0531 & -0.0280 \\ -0.0280 & 0.2500 \end{pmatrix}$$

$$\text{var}[Y_{i\in 1,2}] = (\sigma_{([1],2)jk}) = \begin{pmatrix} 0.1080 & -0.0770 \\ -0.0770 & 0.2343 \end{pmatrix}$$

$$\mathrm{var}[Y_{i\in 1,3}] = (\sigma_{([1],3)jk}) = \begin{pmatrix} 0.1363 & -0.1072 \\ -0.1072 & 0.2248 \end{pmatrix}$$

$$\mathrm{var}[Y_{i\in 1,4}] = (\sigma_{([1],4)jk}) = \begin{pmatrix} 0.1492 & -0.1219 \\ -0.1219 & 0.2219 \end{pmatrix},$$

Values of $(\rho_{([1],ut)jk})$:

$$\mathrm{corr}[Y_{i\in 1,1j}, Y_{i\in 1,2k}] = (\rho_{([1],12)jk}) = \begin{pmatrix} 0.2972 & -0.0235 \\ -0.0618 & 0.2556 \end{pmatrix}$$

$$\mathrm{corr}[Y_{i\in 1,1j}, Y_{i\in 1,3k}] = (\rho_{([1],13)jk}) = \begin{pmatrix} 0.1129 & 0.0116 \\ -0.0211 & 0.0634 \end{pmatrix}$$

$$\mathrm{corr}[Y_{i\in 1,1j}, Y_{i\in 1,4k}] = (\rho_{([1],14)jk}) = \begin{pmatrix} 0.0462 & 0.0106 \\ -0.0080 & 0.0150 \end{pmatrix}$$

$$\mathrm{corr}[Y_{i\in 1,2j}, Y_{i\in 1,3k}] = (\rho_{([1],23)jk}) = \begin{pmatrix} 0.3759 & -0.0674 \\ -0.1748 & 0.2336 \end{pmatrix}$$

$$\mathrm{corr}[Y_{i\in 1,2j}, Y_{i\in 1,4k}] = (\rho_{([1],24)jk}) = \begin{pmatrix} 0.1530 & 0.0008 \\ -0.0693 & 0.0487 \end{pmatrix}$$

$$\mathrm{corr}[Y_{i\in 1,3j}, Y_{i\in 1,4k}] = (\rho_{([1],34)jk}) = \begin{pmatrix} 0.4031 & -0.0911 \\ -0.2414 & 0.2174 \end{pmatrix}.$$

Group 2: Distance > 5 miles
Values of $(\sigma_{([2],t)jk})$:

$$\mathrm{var}[Y_{i\in 2,1}] = (\sigma_{([2],1)jk}) = \begin{pmatrix} 0.0564 & -0.0368 \\ -0.0368 & 0.2373 \end{pmatrix}$$

$$\mathrm{var}[Y_{i\in 2,2}] = (\sigma_{([2],2)jk}) = \begin{pmatrix} 0.1109 & -0.0921 \\ -0.0921 & 0.1993 \end{pmatrix}$$

$$\mathrm{var}[Y_{i\in 2,3}] = (\sigma_{([2],3)jk}) = \begin{pmatrix} 0.1352 & -0.1196 \\ -0.1196 & 0.1915 \end{pmatrix}$$

$$\mathrm{var}[Y_{i\in 2,4}] = (\sigma_{([2],4)jk}) = \begin{pmatrix} 0.1448 & -0.1305 \\ -0.1219 & 0.1911 \end{pmatrix},$$

Values of $(\rho_{([2],ut)jk})$:

$$\mathrm{corr}[Y_{i\in 2,1j}, Y_{i\in 2,2k}] = (\rho_{([2],12)jk}) = \begin{pmatrix} 0.3109 & -0.0283 \\ -0.1912 & 0.1961 \end{pmatrix}$$

$$\text{corr}[Y_{i\in 2,1j}, Y_{i\in 2,3k}] = (\rho_{([2],13)jk}) = \begin{pmatrix} 0.1122 & 0.0113 \\ -0.0842 & 0.0278 \end{pmatrix}$$

$$\text{corr}[Y_{i\in 2,1j}, Y_{i\in 2,4k}] = (\rho_{([2],14)jk}) = \begin{pmatrix} 0.0414 & 0.0089 \\ -0.0340 & 0.0003 \end{pmatrix}$$

$$\text{corr}[Y_{i\in 2,2j}, Y_{i\in 2,3k}] = (\rho_{([2],23)jk}) = \begin{pmatrix} 0.4061 & -0.0664 \\ -0.3042 & 0.1610 \end{pmatrix}$$

$$\text{corr}[Y_{i\in 2,2j}, Y_{i\in 2,4k}] = (\rho_{([2],24)jk}) = \begin{pmatrix} 0.1584 & 0.0116 \\ -0.1276 & 0.0125 \end{pmatrix}$$

$$\text{corr}[Y_{i\in 2,3j}, Y_{i\in 2,4k}] = (\rho_{([2],34)jk}) = \begin{pmatrix} 0.4369 & -0.0820 \\ -0.3609 & 0.1464 \end{pmatrix}.$$

As expected the multinomial correlations appear to decay as time lag increases, under both distance groups.

3.6 Cumulative Logits Model for Univariate Ordinal Longitudinal Data With One Covariate

In this section, we generalize the ordinal categorical data analysis from the cross-sectional (see Chap. 2, Sect. 2.3) to the longitudinal setup. Similar to Sect. 2.3, we consider a single covariate case with $p+1$ levels for simplicity, and an individual belong to a group based on the covariate level. For example, when gender covariate is considered, there are 2 levels, and individual i either can belong to group 1 or 2. In general when an individual i belongs to ℓ-th level or group, one writes $i \in \ell$, where $\ell = 1, \ldots, p+1$. As an extension of Sect. 2.3, we however now collect the ordinal responses over a period of time T. To be specific, similar to Sect. 3.5, the $J-1$ dimensional response at time t for the i $(i \in \ell)$ individual may be denoted as

$$y_{i\in\ell,t} = [y_{i\in\ell,t1}, \ldots, y_{i\in\ell,tj}, \ldots, y_{i\in\ell,t(J-1)}]'$$

and if this response belongs to jth category, then one writes

$$y_{i\in\ell,t} = y^{(j)}_{i\in\ell,t} = [01'_{j-1}, 1, 01'_{J-1-j}]' \tag{3.298}$$

with a big difference that categories are now ordinal. It is of interest to develop a longitudinal categorical model similar to Sect. 3.5 but by accommodating the ordinal nature of the categories. Similar to Sect. 3.5, we consider both LDCP and MDL type models. The LDCP type model is discussed in Sect. 3.6.1 and the MDL type model in Sect. 3.6.2.

Table 3.28 Contingency table for $J > 2$ ordinal categories at initial time $t = 1$ for individuals belonging to ℓ-th $(\ell = 1,\ldots,p+1)$ level of a covariate

	t $(t = 1)$					
	Ordinal categories					
Covariate level	1	...	j	...	J	Total
1	$K_{[1]1}(1)$	...	$K_{[1]j}(1)$	...	$K_{[1]J}(1)$	$K_{[1]}$
.	...	...	...	...	...	.
ℓ	$K_{[\ell]1}(1)$	...	$K_{[\ell]j}(1)$	...	$K_{[\ell]J}(1)$	$K_{[\ell]}$
.	...	...	...	...	...	.
$p+1$	$K_{[p+1]1}(1)$	...	$K_{[p+1]j}(1)$	...	$K_{[p+1]J}(1)$	$K_{[p+1]}$
Total	$K_1(1)$	...	$K_j(1)$	...	$K_J(1)$	K

Table 3.29 (a): Binary response $b^{(j)}_{i\in(\ell,c)}(1)$ generated at cut point $j = 1,\ldots,J-1$ along with its probability for individual $i \in \ell$

	$b^{(j)}_{i\in(\ell,c)}(1)$	
Group (g^*) based on cut point j	Low $(g^* = 1)$	High $(g^* = 2)$
Response	0	1
Probability	$F_{[\ell]j}(1)$	$1 - F_{[\ell]j}(1)$

Table 3.29 (b): Cumulative counts as responses at cut points $j = 1,\ldots,J-1$, reflecting the cumulative probabilities (3.300)–(3.301), under covariate level ℓ

	Binomial response		
Cut point	**Low group** $(g^* = 1)$	**High group** $(g^* = 2)$	**Total**
1	$K^*_{[\ell]1} = \sum_{c=1}^{1} K_{[\ell]c}$	$K_{[\ell]} - K^*_{[\ell]1}$	$K_{[\ell]}$
.	.	.	.
j	$K^*_{[\ell]j} = \sum_{c=1}^{j} K_{[\ell]c}$	$K_{[\ell]} - K^*_{[\ell]j}$	$K_{[\ell]}$
.	.	.	.
$J-1$	$K^*_{[\ell](J-1)} = \sum_{c=1}^{J-1} K_{[\ell]c}$	$K_{[\ell]} - K^*_{[\ell](J-1)}$	$K_{[\ell]}$

The data will look similar to those in Table 3.23 for initial time $t = 1$ and as in Table 3.24 for transitional counts from time $t-h$ to t, h being the time lag in the longitudinal setup. However, now the categories are ordinal. For clarity, we reproduce Table 3.23 here as Tables 3.28, 3.29(a) and 3.29(b), indicating that the categories are ordinal.

In the ordinal categorical setup, it is meaningful to model the odds ratios through cumulative logits. Recall from Chap. 2, more specifically from Sects. 2.3.1.2 and 2.3.1.3, that with a cut point at jth category, one may use the binary variable at initial time point $t = 1$ as

$$b_{i\in(\ell,c)}^{(j)}(1) = \begin{cases} 1 \text{ for the i-th individual responded in category } c > j \\ 0 \text{ for the i-th individual responded in category } c \leq j, \end{cases} \tag{3.299}$$

with probabilities

$$\begin{aligned} P[b_{i\in(\ell,c)}^{(j)}(1) = 1] &= \sum_{c=j+1}^{J} \pi_{[\ell]c}(1) = 1 - F_{[\ell]j}(1) = \pi_{[\ell]j}^{*}(1) \\ &= \begin{cases} \frac{\exp(\alpha_{j0}+\alpha_{j\ell})}{1+\exp(\alpha_{j0}+\alpha_{j\ell})} & \text{for } \ell = 1,\ldots,p \\ \frac{\exp(\alpha_{j0})}{1+\exp(\alpha_{j0})} & \text{for } \ell = p+1, \end{cases} \end{aligned} \tag{3.300}$$

and

$$\begin{aligned} P[b_{i\in(\ell,c)}^{(j)}(1) = 0] &= \sum_{c=1}^{j} \pi_{[\ell]c}(1) = F_{[\ell]j}(1) = 1 - \pi_{[\ell]j}^{*}(1) \\ &= = \begin{cases} \frac{1}{1+\exp(\alpha_{j0}+\alpha_{j\ell})} & \text{for } \ell = 1,\ldots,p \\ \frac{1}{1+\exp(\alpha_{j0})} & \text{for } \ell = p+1, \end{cases} \end{aligned} \tag{3.301}$$

respectively, where $\pi_{[\ell]c}(1)$ is the probability for the ith individual to be in category c at time point $t = 1$. That is

$$\pi_{[\ell]c}(1) = Pr[y_{i\in\ell,1} = y_{i\in\ell,1}^{(c)}]$$

with $y_{i\in\ell,1}^{(c)}$ as in (3.298). These binary variables along with their probabilities at time $t = 1$ are displayed in Table 3.29(a) for convenience. Further, based on this binary characteristic of a response from Table 3.29(a), the cumulative counts computed from Table 3.28 are displayed in Table 3.29(b) at all possible $J-1$ cut points.

Next to study the transitional counts over time, we first reproduce the Table 3.24 in its own form in Table 3.30 but indicating that the categories are now ordinal, and in two other cumulative forms in Tables 3.31 and 3.32. In order to reflect two ways (based on past and present times) cumulative logits, one requires to cumulate the transitional counts displayed in Table 3.30. This cumulation is shown in Tables 3.31 and 3.32 at various possible cut points. Following these two latter tables, we now define a lag 1 conditional binary probability model as follows. Tables for other lags can be constructed similarly. We will consider both LDCP (see (3.24) in Sect. 3.2.2.1) and BDL (see (3.71) in Sect. 3.2.4.1) type models.

Table 3.30 Lag h^* $(h^* = 1,\ldots,T-1)$ based $[h^*(T-h^*)]$ transitional counts for multinomial responses with $J > 2$ ordinal categories, for individuals belonging to ℓ-th $(\ell = 1,\ldots,p+1)$ level of the covariate

		Covariate level (ℓ)						
		t $(t = h^*+1,\ldots,T)$						
Time		Ordinal category (j)						
Time	Category (g)	1	...	j	...	J	Total
t-h^*	1	$K_{[\ell]11}(t-h^*, t)$	...	$K_{[\ell]1j}(t-h^*, t)$	...	$K_{[\ell]1J}(t-h^*, t)$	$K_{[\ell]1}(t-h^*)$
	.	...	...	...	...	...	.
	g	$K_{[\ell]g1}(t-h^*, t)$	...	$K_{[\ell]gj}(t-h^*, t)$	...	$K_{[\ell]gJ}(t-h^*, t)$	$K_{[\ell]g}(t-h^*)$
	.	...	...	...	...	...	.
	J	$K_{[\ell]J1}(t-h^*, t)$	...	$K_{[\ell]Jj}(t-h^*, t)$	...	$K_{[\ell]JJ}(t-h^*, t)$	$K_{[\ell]J}(t-h^*)$
	Total	$K_{[\ell]1}(t)$	...	$K_{[\ell]j}(t)$	...	$K_{[\ell]J}(t)$	$K_{[\ell]}$

Table 3.31 Bivariate binary responses $(b^{(g)}_{i\in(\ell,c_1)}(t-1), b^{(j)}_{i\in(\ell,c_2)}(t))$ along with their conditional probabilities $\tilde{\lambda}^{(j^*)}_{[\ell],gj}(g^*)$ $j^* = 1,2; g^* = 1,2$, for the ith individual based on cut points g at time $t-1$ and j at time t

			t $(t = 2,\ldots,T)$	
	Time		Category j^* based on cut point j	
Covariate level	Time	Category g^*	1	2
ℓ	t-1	1	(0,0)	(0,1)
			$\tilde{\lambda}^{(1)}_{[\ell],gj}(1)$	$\tilde{\lambda}^{(2)}_{[\ell],gj}(1)$
		2	(1,0)	(1,1)
			$\tilde{\lambda}^{(1)}_{[\ell],gj}(2)$	$\tilde{\lambda}^{(2)}_{[\ell],gj}(2)$

Table 3.32 Transitional counts from time $t-1$ to t, computed from Table 3.30 by reflecting the cut points (g, j) based individual probabilities from Table 3.31

	j^* at t		
g^* at $t-1$	$j^* = 1$	$j^* = 2$	Total
$g^* = 1$	$\sum_{c_2=1}^{j}\sum_{c_1=1}^{g} K_{[\ell]c_1c_2}(t-1,t)$	$\sum_{c_2=j+1}^{J}\sum_{c_1=1}^{g} K_{[\ell]c_1c_2}(t-1,t)$	$K^*_{[\ell]1}(t-1;\ g)$
$g^* = 2$	$\sum_{c_2=1}^{j}\sum_{c_1=g+1}^{J} K_{[\ell]c_1c_2}(t-1,t)$	$\sum_{c_2=j+1}^{J}\sum_{c_1=g+1}^{J} K_{[\ell]c_1c_2}(t-1,t)$	$K^*_{[\ell]2}(t-1;\ g)$
Total	$K^*_{[\ell]1}(t;\ j)$	$K^*_{[\ell]2}(t;\ j)$	$K_{[\ell]}$

3.6.1 LDCP Model with Cut Points g at Time t − 1 and j at Time t

Similar to (3.299), for $t = 2, \ldots, T$, define two binary variables $b^{(g)}_{i\in(\ell,c_1)}(t-1)$ and $b^{(j)}_{i\in(\ell,c_2)}(t)$ at times $t-1$ and t, respectively, where g and j denote the cut points such that $g, j = 1, \ldots, J-1$. We now write an LDCP model

$$
\begin{aligned}
P[b^{(j)}_{i\in(\ell,c_2)}(t) = 1 | b^{(g)}_{i\in(\ell,c_1)}(t-1)] &= [\pi^*_{[\ell]j}(1)] + \tilde{\rho}_{gj}\left[b^{(g)}_{i\in(\ell,c_1)}(t-1) - \pi^*_{[\ell]g}(1)\right] \\
&= \tilde{\lambda}^{(2)}_{[\ell],gj}(b^{(g)}_{i\in(\ell,c_1)}(t-1)) \\
&= \begin{cases} \tilde{\lambda}^{(2)}_{[\ell],gj}(1) \text{ for } b^{(g)}_{i\in(\ell,c_1)}(t-1) = 0 \\ \tilde{\lambda}^{(2)}_{[\ell],gj}(2) \text{ for } b^{(g)}_{i\in(\ell,c_1)}(t-1) = 1, \end{cases}
\end{aligned}
\tag{3.302}
$$

and

$$
\begin{aligned}
&P[b^{(j)}_{i\in(\ell,c_2)}(t) = 0 | b^{(g)}_{i\in(\ell,c_1)}(t-1)] = 1 - \tilde{\lambda}^{(2)}_{[\ell],gj}(b^{(g)}_{i\in(\ell,c_1)}(t-1)) \\
&= \begin{cases} \tilde{\lambda}^{(1)}_{[\ell],gj}(1) = 1 - \tilde{\lambda}^{(2)}_{[\ell],gj}(1) \text{ for } b^{(g)}_{i\in(\ell,c_1)}(t-1) = 0 \\ \tilde{\lambda}^{(1)}_{[\ell],gj}(2) = 1 - \tilde{\lambda}^{(2)}_{[\ell],gj}(2) \text{ for } b^{(g)}_{i\in(\ell,c_1)}(t-1) = 1. \end{cases}
\end{aligned}
\tag{3.303}
$$

Note that there is an implicit connection between the multinomial linear conditional probabilities $\lambda^{(c_2)}_{it|t-1}(c_1,\ell)$ in (3.238) and the cumulative conditional binary probabilities in (3.302). For example, it is reasonable to relate them as

$$
\begin{aligned}
\tilde{\lambda}^{(2)}_{[\ell],gj}(1) &= \frac{1}{g}\sum_{c_1=1}^{g}\sum_{c_2=j+1}^{J}\lambda^{(c_2)}_{it|t-1}(c_1,\ell) \\
\tilde{\lambda}^{(2)}_{[\ell],gj}(2) &= \frac{1}{J-g}\sum_{c_1=g+1}^{J}\sum_{c_2=j+1}^{J}\lambda^{(c_2)}_{it|t-1}(c_1,\ell),
\end{aligned}
$$

but their explicit relations are not needed as one is interested to understand the logit ratios only, which can be done through fitting the dynamic (over time) cut points based cumulative logits model. The above four conditional probabilities at a given cut point were presented in Table 3.31. By the same token, in Table 3.32, we displayed the transitional counts computed from Table 3.30 by reflecting the cut points based individual probabilities given in Table 3.32.

3.6.1.1 Fitting Bivariate Binary Mapping Based LDCP Model: A Pseudo-Likelihood Estimation Approach

Recall that in Chap. 2, more specifically in Sect. 2.3.1.2, a binary mapping based likelihood function was constructed in a cross-sectional setup for the estimation of the cut points that lead to the estimation of the logit ratios. That likelihood function from (2.179) still can be used here but as a segment only for time $t = 1$. More specifically, for

$$\alpha = [\alpha_1^{*\prime}, \ldots, \alpha_j^{*\prime}, \ldots, \alpha_{J-1}^{*}{}^{\prime}]^{\prime}, \text{ with } \alpha_j^* = [\alpha_{j0}, \alpha_{j1}, \ldots, \alpha_{j\ell}, \ldots, \alpha_{jp}]^{\prime},$$

we label $L(\alpha)$ from (2.179) as $L_1(\alpha)$ for $t = 1$ case, and by writing

$$b_{i\in(\ell,c)}^{(j)}(1),\ F_{[\ell]j}(1);\ \text{and}\ K_{[\ell]c}(1)$$

for

$$b_{i\in(\ell,c)}^{(j)},\ F_{[\ell]j};\ \text{and}\ K_{[\ell]c},$$

we compute $L_1(\alpha)$ as

$$\begin{aligned}
L_1(\alpha) &= \Pi_{\ell=1}^{p+1} \Pi_{j=1}^{J-1} \Pi_{[i\in(\ell,h)|j,\ell]}^{K_{[\ell]}} \left[\{F_{[\ell]j}(1)\}^{1-b_{i\in(\ell,h)(1)}^{(j)}} \right] \left[\{1 - F_{[\ell]j}(1)\}^{b_{i\in(\ell,h)}^{(j)}(1)} \right] \\
&= \Pi_{\ell=1}^{p+1} \Pi_{j=1}^{J-1} \left[\{F_{[\ell]j(1)}\}^{\Sigma_{c=1}^{j} K_{[\ell]c}(1)} \right] \left[\{1 - F_{[\ell]j}(1)\}^{\Sigma_{c=j+1}^{J} K_{[\ell]c}(1)} \right] \\
&= \Pi_{\ell=1}^{p+1} \Pi_{j=1}^{J-1} \left[\{F_{[\ell]j}(1)\}^{\Sigma_{c=1}^{j} K_{[\ell]c}(1)} \right] \left[\{1 - F_{[\ell]j}(1)\}^{K_{[\ell]} - \Sigma_{c=1}^{j} K_{[\ell]c}(1)} \right] \\
&= \Pi_{\ell=1}^{p+1} \Pi_{j=1}^{J-1} \left[\{F_{[\ell]j}(1)\}^{K_{[\ell]j}^*(1)} \right] \left[\{1 - F_{[\ell]j}(1)\}^{K_{[\ell]} - K_{[\ell]j}^*(1)} \right] \\
&= \Pi_{\ell=1}^{p+1} \Pi_{j=1}^{J-1} \left[\{1 - \pi_{[\ell]j}^*(1)\}^{K_{[\ell]j}^*(1)} \right] \left[\{\pi_{[\ell]j}^*(1)\}^{K_{[\ell]} - K_{[\ell]j}^*(1)} \right]. \qquad (3.304)
\end{aligned}$$

Next by using the conditional probabilities from (3.302)–(3.303), for $t = 2, \ldots, T$, and by using the transitional counts from Table 3.25, we write the conditional likelihood, namely $L_{t|t-1}(\alpha, \tilde{\rho}_M)$ where $\tilde{\rho}_M$ represents all $(J-1)^2$ dynamic dependence parameters $\{\tilde{\rho}_{gj}\}$ $(g, j = 1, \ldots, J-1)$, as

$$\begin{aligned}
&L_{t|t-1}(\alpha, \tilde{\rho}_M) \\
&= \Pi_{\ell=1}^{p+1} \Pi_{g=1}^{J-1} \Pi_{j=1}^{J-1} \Pi_{g^*=1}^{2} \Pi_{[i\in(\ell,c_2,g^*)|j,g,\ell]}^{K_{[\ell]}} \left[\{\tilde{\lambda}_{[\ell],gj}^{(2)}(g^*)\}^{b_{i\in(\ell,c_2,)}^{(j)}(t)} \{\tilde{\lambda}_{[\ell],gj}^{(1)}(g^*)\}^{1-b_{i\in(\ell,c_2)}^{(j)}(t)} \right] \\
&= \Pi_{\ell=1}^{p+1} \Pi_{g=1}^{J-1} \Pi_{j=1}^{J-1} \Pi_{g^*=1}^{2} \left[\{\tilde{\lambda}_{[\ell],gj}^{(1)}(g^*)\}^{K_{[\ell]g^*1}^*(t-1,t;g,j)} \{\tilde{\lambda}_{[\ell],gj}^{(2)}(g^*)\}^{K_{[\ell]g^*2}^*(t-1,t;g,j)} \right], \qquad (3.305)
\end{aligned}$$

where, by Table 3.28,

$$K_{[\ell]11}^*(t-1,t;g,j) = \sum_{c_2=1}^{j} \sum_{c_1=1}^{g} K_{[\ell]c_1c_2}(t-1,t);\ K_{[\ell]12}^*(t-1,t;g,j) = \sum_{c_2=j+1}^{J} \sum_{c_1=1}^{g} K_{[\ell]c_1c_2}(t-1,t),$$

$$K^*_{[\ell]21}(t-1,t;g,j) = \sum_{c_2=1}^{j}\sum_{c_1=g+1}^{J} K_{[\ell]c_1c_2}(t-1,t);\ K^*_{[\ell]22}(t-1,t;g,j) = \sum_{c_2=j+1}^{J}\sum_{c_1=g+1}^{J} K_{[\ell]c_1c_2}(t-1,t).$$

Now by combining (3.304) and (3.305), for all $t = 1,\ldots,T$, we may write the desired likelihood function as

$$L(\alpha,\tilde{\rho}_M) = \Pi_{\ell=1}^{p+1}\Pi_{j=1}^{J-1}\Big[\left(\{F_{[\ell]j}(1)\}^{K^*_{[\ell]j}(1)}\right)\left(\{1-F_{[\ell]j}(1)\}^{K_{[\ell]}-K^*_{[\ell]j}(1)}\right)$$
$$\times\ \Pi_{t=2}^{T}\Pi_{g=1}^{J-1}\Pi_{g^*=1}^{2}\left(\{\tilde{\lambda}^{(1)}_{[\ell],gj}(g^*)\}^{K^*_{[\ell]g^*1}(t-1,t;g,j)}\{\tilde{\lambda}^{(2)}_{[\ell],gj}(g^*)\}^{K^*_{[\ell]g^*2}(t-1,t;g,j)}\right)\Big]. \quad (3.306)$$

3.6.1.1.1 Pseudo-Likelihood Estimating Equation for α

For convenience, we use the log likelihood function, which by (3.306) produces the estimating equation for α as

$$\frac{\partial Log\,L(\alpha,\tilde{\rho}_M)}{\partial\alpha} = \sum_{\ell=1}^{p+1}\sum_{j=1}^{J-1}\left[(K_{[\ell]}-K^*_{[\ell]j}(1))\frac{\partial}{\partial\alpha}\{log\,\pi^*_{[\ell]j}(1)\}+K^*_{[\ell]j}(1)\frac{\partial}{\partial\alpha}\{log\,(1-\pi^*_{[\ell]j}(1))\}\right]$$
$$+\sum_{\ell=1}^{p+1}\sum_{j=1}^{J-1}\sum_{g=1}^{J-1}\sum_{g^*=1}^{2}\sum_{t=2}^{T}\Big[K^*_{[\ell]g^*1}(t-1,t;g,j)\frac{\partial}{\partial\alpha}log\,\{\tilde{\lambda}^{(1)}_{[\ell],gj}(g^*)\}$$
$$+\ K^*_{[\ell]g^*2}(t-1,t;g,j)\frac{\partial}{\partial\alpha}log\,\{\tilde{\lambda}^{(2)}_{[\ell],gj}(g^*)\}\Big]=0$$
$$\equiv I+II=0\,(\text{say}). \quad (3.307)$$

Notice that the first term in (3.307) corresponding to time $t = 1$ may easily be computed by following the notations from (2.181)–(2.184) in Chap. 2. More specifically, by using

$$\pi^*_{[\ell]j}(1) = \frac{\exp(x'_{[\ell]j}\alpha)}{1+\exp(x'_{[\ell]j}\alpha)}$$
$$1-\pi^*_{[\ell]j}(1) = \frac{1}{1+\exp(x'_{[\ell]j}\alpha)}, \quad (3.308)$$

where $x'_{[\ell]j}$ is the jth $(j=1,\ldots,J-1)$ row of the $(J-1)\times(J-1)(p+1)$ matrix X_ℓ, defined for ℓth level as

$$X_\ell = \begin{pmatrix} x'_{[\ell]1} \\ x'_{[\ell]2} \\ \cdot \\ x'_{[\ell](J-1)} \end{pmatrix}$$

$$= \begin{pmatrix} 1\ 01'_{\ell-1}, 1, 01'_{p-\ell} & 0 & 01'_p & \cdot & 0 & 01'_p \\ 0 & 01'_p & 1\ 01'_{\ell-1}, 1, 01'_{p-\ell} & \cdot & 0 & 01'_p \\ \cdot & \cdot & \cdot & \cdot & \cdot\ \cdot & \cdot \\ 0 & 01'_p & 0 & 01'_p & \cdot & 1\ 01'_{\ell-1}, 1, 01'_{p-\ell} \end{pmatrix} \text{ for } \ell = 1, \ldots, p,$$

$$X_{p+1} = \begin{pmatrix} x'_{[p+1]1} \\ x'_{[p+1]2} \\ \cdot \\ x'_{[p+1](J-1)} \end{pmatrix} = \begin{pmatrix} 1\ 01'_p & 0\ 01'_p & \cdot & 0\ 01'_p \\ 0\ 01'_p & 1\ 01'_p & \cdot & 0\ 01'_p \\ \cdot\ \cdot & \cdot\ \cdot & \cdot & \cdot\ \cdot \\ 0\ 01'_p & 0\ 01'_p & \cdot & 1\ 01'_p \end{pmatrix}, \tag{3.309}$$

the first term in (3.307) has the formula

$$I \equiv \sum_{\ell=1}^{p+1} X'_\ell \left[y^*_{[\ell]}(1) - K_{[\ell]} \pi^*_{[\ell]}(1) \right], \tag{3.310}$$

where the observation and corresponding probability vectors at $t = 1$ are written as

$$\begin{aligned} y^*_{[\ell]}(1) &= [K_{[\ell]} - K^*_{[\ell]1}(1), \ldots, K_{[\ell]} - K^*_{[\ell]j}(1), \ldots, K_{[\ell]} - K^*_{[\ell](J-1)}(1)]' \text{ and} \\ \pi^*_{[\ell]}(1) &\equiv [\pi^*_{[\ell]1}(1), \ldots, \pi^*_{[\ell]j}(1), \ldots, \pi^*_{[\ell](J-1)}(1)]'. \end{aligned} \tag{3.311}$$

To compute the second term in (3.307), first write the conditional probabilities by (3.302)–(3.303), as

$$\begin{aligned} \tilde{\lambda}^{(2)}_{[\ell],gj}(1) &= \pi^*_{[\ell]j}(1) - \tilde{\rho}_{gj} \pi^*_{[\ell]g}(1) \\ \tilde{\lambda}^{(1)}_{[\ell],gj}(1) &= 1 - [\pi^*_{[\ell]j}(1) - \tilde{\rho}_{gj} \pi^*_{[\ell]g}(1)] \\ \tilde{\lambda}^{(2)}_{[\ell],gj}(2) &= \pi^*_{[\ell]j}(1) + \tilde{\rho}_{gj}\{1 - \pi^*_{[\ell]g}(1)\}, \text{ and} \\ \tilde{\lambda}^{(1)}_{[\ell],gj}(2) &= 1 - [\pi^*_{[\ell]j}(1) + \tilde{\rho}_{gj}\{1 - \pi^*_{[\ell]g}(1)\}]. \end{aligned} \tag{3.312}$$

The computation for the derivatives of these conditional probabilities with respect to α is straightforward. To be specific,

$$\begin{aligned} \frac{\partial \tilde{\lambda}^{(2)}_{[\ell],gj}(1)}{\partial \alpha} = \frac{\partial \tilde{\lambda}^{(2)}_{[\ell],gj}(2)}{\partial \alpha} &= \pi^*_{[\ell]j}(1)[1 - \pi^*_{[\ell]j}(1)] x_{[\ell]j} \\ &- \rho_{gj} \pi^*_{[\ell]g}(1)[1 - \pi^*_{[\ell]g}(1)] x_{[\ell]g}, \end{aligned}$$

and

$$\frac{\partial \tilde{\lambda}^{(1)}_{[\ell],gj}(1)}{\partial \alpha} = \frac{\partial \tilde{\lambda}^{(1)}_{[\ell],gj}(2)}{\partial \alpha} = -\left[\frac{\partial \tilde{\lambda}^{(2)}_{[\ell],gj}(1)}{\partial \alpha} \right].$$

Now compute *II* using these derivatives and combine this formula with that of *I* given in (3.310) to simplify the likelihood equation for α given by (3.307). The simplified likelihood equation has the form

$$\begin{aligned}
\frac{\partial Log\, L(\alpha,\rho_M)}{\partial \alpha} &= \sum_{\ell=1}^{p+1}\left[X'_\ell\left\{y^*_{[\ell]}(1) - K_{[\ell]}\pi^*_{[\ell]}(1)\right\}\right.\\
&+ \sum_{j=1}^{J-1}\sum_{g=1}^{J-1}\left[\left\{-\frac{\sum_{t=2}^{T}K^*_{[\ell]11}(t-1,t;g,j)}{\tilde{\lambda}^{(1)}_{[\ell],gj}(1)} + \frac{\sum_{t=2}^{T}K^*_{[\ell]12}(t-1,t;g,j)}{\tilde{\lambda}^{(2)}_{[\ell],gj}(1)}\right.\right.\\
&\left.\left. - \frac{\sum_{t=2}^{T}K^*_{[\ell]21}(t-1,t;g,j)}{\tilde{\lambda}^{(1)}_{[\ell],gj}(2)} + \frac{\sum_{t=2}^{T}K^*_{[\ell]22}(t-1,t;g,j)}{\tilde{\lambda}^{(2)}_{[\ell],gj}(2)}\right\}\right]\\
&\times \left.\left\{\pi^*_{[\ell]j}(1)\{1-\pi^*_{[\ell]j}(1)\}x_{[\ell]j} - \rho_{gj}\pi^*_{[\ell]g}(1)\{1-\pi^*_{[\ell]g}(1)\}x_{[\ell]g}\right\}\right]\\
&= f_1(\alpha) + f_2(\alpha) = f(\alpha) = 0. \qquad (3.313)
\end{aligned}$$

Let $\hat{\alpha}$ be the solution of $f(\alpha) = 0$ in (3.313). Assuming that $\hat{\alpha}_0$ is not a solution for $f(\alpha) = 0$ but a trial estimate, and hence $f(\hat{\alpha}_0) \neq 0$, the iterative equation for $\hat{\alpha}$ is obtained as

$$\hat{\alpha} = \hat{\alpha}_0 - \left[\{f'(\alpha)\}^{-1}f(\alpha)\right]|_{\alpha=\hat{\alpha}_0}, \qquad (3.314)$$

where

$$f'(\alpha) = f'_1(\alpha) + f'_2(\alpha) = \frac{\partial f_1(\alpha)}{\partial \alpha'} + \frac{\partial f_2(\alpha)}{\partial \alpha'}$$

is computed as follows.

Because

$$\frac{\partial \pi^*_{[\ell]j}(1)}{\partial \alpha'} = \pi^*_{[\ell]j}(1)(1-\pi^*_{[\ell]j}(1))x'_{[\ell]j},$$

it then follows that

$$\begin{aligned}
\frac{\partial \pi^*_{[\ell]}(1)}{\partial \alpha'} &= \text{diag}[\pi^*_{[\ell]1}(1)(1-\pi^*_{[\ell]1}(1)),\ldots,\pi^*_{[\ell](J-1)}(1)(1-\pi^*_{[\ell](J-1)}(1))]X_\ell\\
&= D_{\pi^*_{[\ell]}(1)}X_\ell. \qquad (3.315)
\end{aligned}$$

Consequently, one obtains

$$\begin{aligned}
f'_1(\alpha) &= \frac{\partial f_1(\alpha)}{\partial \alpha'}\\
&= -\sum_{\ell=1}^{p+1}K_{[\ell]}X'_\ell D_{\pi^*_{[\ell]}(1)}X_\ell. \qquad (3.316)
\end{aligned}$$

Next, by (3.313),

$$
\begin{aligned}
f_2'(\alpha) &= \frac{\partial f_2(\alpha)}{\partial \alpha'} \\
&= \sum_{\ell=1}^{p+1}\sum_{j=1}^{J-1}\sum_{g=1}^{J-1}\left\{-\frac{\sum_{t=2}^{T} K^*_{[\ell]11}(t-1,t;g,j)}{\tilde{\lambda}^{(1)}_{[\ell],gj}(1)}+\frac{\sum_{t=2}^{T} K^*_{[\ell]12}(t-1,t;g,j)}{\tilde{\lambda}^{(2)}_{[\ell],gj}(1)}\right. \\
&\quad \left.-\frac{\sum_{t=2}^{T} K^*_{[\ell]21}(t-1,t;g,j)}{\tilde{\lambda}^{(1)}_{[\ell],gj}(2)}+\frac{\sum_{t=2}^{T} K^*_{[\ell]22}(t-1,t;g,j)}{\tilde{\lambda}^{(2)}_{[\ell],gj}(2)}\right\} \\
&\quad \times\left[\left\{\pi^*_{[\ell]j}(1)(1-\pi^*_{[\ell]j}(1))(1-2\pi^*_{[\ell]j}(1))\right\}x_{[\ell]j}x'_{[\ell]j}\right. \\
&\quad \left.-\rho_{gj}\left\{\pi^*_{[\ell]g}(1)(1-\pi^*_{[\ell]g}(1))(1-2\pi^*_{[\ell]g}(1))\right\}x_{[\ell]g}x'_{[\ell]g}\right] \\
&\quad -\sum_{\ell=1}^{p+1}\sum_{j=1}^{J-1}\sum_{g=1}^{J-1}\left\{\frac{\sum_{t=2}^{T} K^*_{[\ell]11}(t-1,t;g,j)}{\{\tilde{\lambda}^{(1)}_{[\ell],gj}(1)\}^2}+\frac{\sum_{t=2}^{T} K^*_{[\ell]12}(t-1,t;g,j)}{\{\tilde{\lambda}^{(2)}_{[\ell],gj}(1)\}^2}\right. \\
&\quad \left.+\frac{\sum_{t=2}^{T} K^*_{[\ell]21}(t-1,t;g,j)}{\{\tilde{\lambda}^{(1)}_{[\ell],gj}(2)\}^2}+\frac{\sum_{t=2}^{T} K^*_{[\ell]22}(t-1,t;g,j)}{\{\tilde{\lambda}^{(2)}_{[\ell],gj}(2)\}^2}\right\} \\
&\quad \times\left[\left\{\pi^*_{[\ell]j}(1)\{1-\pi^*_{[\ell]j}(1)\}x_{[\ell]j}-\rho_{gj}\pi^*_{[\ell]g}(1)\{1-\pi^*_{[\ell]g}(1)\}x_{[\ell]g}\right\}\right. \\
&\quad \left.\times\left\{\pi^*_{[\ell]j}(1)\{1-\pi^*_{[\ell]j}(1)\}x_{[\ell]j}-\rho_{gj}\pi^*_{[\ell]g}(1)\{1-\pi^*_{[\ell]g}(1)\}x_{[\ell]g}\right\}'\right] \qquad (3.317)
\end{aligned}
$$

3.6.1.1.2 Pseudo-Likelihood Estimating Equation for $\tilde{\rho}_M$

The $\tilde{\rho}_M$ parameters matrix is written for the cut points based dynamic dependence parameters, that is, $\tilde{\rho}_M = (\tilde{\rho}_{gj})$ where both g and j refer to cut points and they range from 1 to $J-1$. Finding the estimating equation for $\tilde{\rho}_M$ means finding the estimating equations for $\tilde{\rho}_{gj}$ for all $g, j = 1, \ldots, J-1$. This is done as follows.

Because the first term in the likelihood function (3.306) does not contain any $\tilde{\rho}_{gj}$ parameters, by similar calculations as in (3.307), one obtains the likelihood equations for $\tilde{\rho}_{gj}$ as

$$
\begin{aligned}
\frac{\partial Log\, L(\alpha)}{\partial \tilde{\rho}_{gj}} &= \sum_{\ell=1}^{p+1}\left\{[\sum_{t=2}^{T} K^*_{[\ell]11}(t-1,t;g,j)]\frac{\pi^*_{[\ell]g}}{\tilde{\lambda}^{(1)}_{[\ell],gj}(1)}-[\sum_{t=2}^{T} K^*_{[\ell]12}(t-1,t;g,j)]\frac{\pi^*_{[\ell]g}}{\tilde{\lambda}^{(2)}_{[\ell],gj}(1)}\right. \\
&\quad -[\sum_{t=2}^{T} K^*_{[\ell]21}(t-1,t;g,j)]\frac{1-\pi^*_{[\ell]g}}{\tilde{\lambda}^{(1)}_{[\ell],gj}(2)}
\end{aligned}
$$

$$+ \ [\sum_{t=2}^{T} K^*_{[\ell]22}(t-1,t;g,j)] \frac{1-\pi^*_{[\ell]g}}{\tilde{\lambda}^{(2)}_{[\ell],gj}(2)} \Bigg\} = 0, \tag{3.318}$$

for all $g, j = 1, \ldots, J-1$. By using

$$\tilde{\rho} = (\tilde{\rho}'_1, \ldots, \tilde{\rho}'_g, \ldots, \tilde{\rho}'_{J-1})' \text{ with } \tilde{\rho}'_g = (\tilde{\rho}_{g1}, \ldots, \tilde{\rho}_{gj}, \ldots, \tilde{\rho}_{g,J-1}),$$

the $(J-1)^2$ estimating equations in (3.318) may be solved iteratively by using the formula

$$\hat{\tilde{\rho}}(r+1) = \hat{\tilde{\rho}}(r) - \left[\left\{ \frac{\partial^2 Log\, L(\alpha, \tilde{\rho}_M)}{\partial \tilde{\rho}' \partial \tilde{\rho}} \right\}^{-1} \frac{\partial Log\, L(\alpha, \tilde{\rho}_M)}{\partial \tilde{\rho}} \right]_{|\tilde{\rho} = \hat{\tilde{\rho}}(r)}, \tag{3.319}$$

where the first order derivative vector $\frac{\partial Log\, L(\alpha, \tilde{\rho}_M)}{\partial \tilde{\rho}}$ may be constructed by stacking the scalar derivatives from (3.318). The computation of the second order derivative matrix follows from the following two general second order derivatives:

$$\frac{\partial^2 Log\, L(\alpha)}{\partial \tilde{\rho}_{gj} \partial \tilde{\rho}_{gj}} = -\sum_{\ell=1}^{p+1} \Bigg\{ [\sum_{t=2}^{T} K^*_{[\ell]11}(t-1,t;g,j)] \left(\frac{\pi^*_{[\ell]g}}{\tilde{\lambda}^{(1)}_{[\ell],gj}(1)} \right)^2 + [\sum_{t=2}^{T} K^*_{[\ell]12}(t-1,t;g,j)] \left(\frac{\pi^*_{[\ell]g}}{\tilde{\lambda}^{(2)}_{[\ell],gj}(1)} \right)^2$$
$$+ \ [\sum_{t=2}^{T} K^*_{[\ell]21}(t-1,t;g,j)] \left(\frac{1-\pi^*_{[\ell]g}}{\tilde{\lambda}^{(1)}_{[\ell],gj}(2)} \right)^2$$
$$+ \ [\sum_{t=2}^{T} K^*_{[\ell]22}(t-1,t;g,j)] \left(\frac{1-\pi^*_{[\ell]g}}{\tilde{\lambda}^{(2)}_{[\ell],gj}(2)} \right)^2 \Bigg\}, \tag{3.320}$$

and

$$\frac{\partial^2 Log\, L(\alpha)}{\partial \tilde{\rho}_{g'j'} \partial \tilde{\rho}_{gj}} = 0, \text{ for all } g = g', j' \neq j; g \neq g', j' \neq j; g \neq g', j' = j; g \neq g', j' \neq j. \tag{3.321}$$

3.6.1.2 Fitting Bivariate Binary Mapping Based LDCP Model: A Conditional GQL Estimation Approach

In the last section, we have discussed the likelihood estimation for the parameters involved in the LDCP model. In this section, it is shown how one can use the quasi-likelihood approach for the estimation of parameters under these models.

We observe from the likelihood function (3.306) (see also Table 3.32) that at time point $t = 1$, there are $J-1$ binomial responses, namely

$$\{y_{[\ell]j}(1) = K_{[\ell]} - K^*_{[\ell]j}(1), \text{ for } j = 1, \ldots, J-1,\} \tag{3.322}$$

with parameters $K_{[\ell]}$ and $\pi^*_{[\ell]j}(1)$. However, for $t = 2, \ldots, T$, there are $2(J-1)^2$ binomial responses, namely

$$\{K^*_{[\ell]g^*2}(t-1, t; g, j), \text{ for } g, j = 1, \ldots, J-1,\} \tag{3.323}$$

with parameters $K^*_{[\ell]g^*}(t-1;\, g)$ and $\tilde{\lambda}^{(2)}_{[\ell],gj}(g^*)$.

3.6.1.2.1 CGQL Estimation for α

For known $\{\tilde{\rho}_{gj},\, g, j = 1, \ldots, J-1\}$, we now construct a Conditional GQL (CGQL) estimating equation for α as

$$\sum_{\ell=1}^{p+1}\sum_{j=1}^{J-1}\left[K_{[\ell]}\frac{\partial \pi^*_{[\ell]j}(1)}{\partial \alpha}\left\{K_{[\ell]}\pi^*_{[\ell]j}(1)[1-\pi^*_{[\ell]j}(1)]\right\}^{-1}[y_{[\ell]j}(1) - K_{[\ell]}\pi^*_{[\ell]j}(1)]\right]$$
$$+\sum_{\ell=1}^{p+1}\sum_{g=1}^{J-1}\sum_{j=1}^{J-1}\sum_{t=2}^{T}\sum_{g^*=1}^{2}\left[K^*_{[\ell]g^*}(t-1;\, g)\frac{\partial \tilde{\lambda}^{(2)}_{[\ell],gj}(g^*)}{\partial \alpha}\left\{K^*_{[\ell]g^*}(t-1;\, g)\tilde{\lambda}^{(2)}_{[\ell],gj}(g^*)\tilde{\lambda}^{(1)}_{[\ell],gj}(g^*)\right\}^{-1}\right.$$
$$\left.\times\ [K^*_{[\ell]g^*2}(t-1, t;\, g, j) - K^*_{[\ell]g^*}(t-1;\, g)\tilde{\lambda}^{(2)}_{[\ell],gj}(g^*)]\right] = 0. \tag{3.324}$$

Now because

$$\begin{aligned}
\frac{\partial \pi^*_{[\ell]j}(1)}{\partial \alpha} &= \left[\pi^*_{[\ell]j}(1)(1-\pi^*_{[\ell]j}(1))\right] x_{[\ell]j} \text{ and} \\
\frac{\partial \tilde{\lambda}^{(2)}_{[\ell],gj}(g^*)}{\partial \alpha} &= \left[\pi^*_{[\ell]j}(1)(1-\pi^*_{[\ell]j}(1))\right] x_{[\ell]j} \\
&\quad - \tilde{\rho}_{gj}\left[\pi^*_{[\ell]g}(1)(1-\pi^*_{[\ell]g}(1))\right] x_{[\ell]g}
\end{aligned} \tag{3.325}$$

for both $g^* = 1, 2$, the CGQL estimating equation (3.324) reduces to

$$\sum_{\ell=1}^{p+1} X'_\ell\left[y^*_{[\ell]}(1) - K_{[\ell]}\pi^*_{[\ell]}(1)\right]$$
$$+\sum_{\ell=1}^{p+1}\sum_{g=1}^{J-1}\sum_{j=1}^{J-1}\sum_{t=2}^{T}\sum_{g^*=1}^{2}\left[\left\{\pi^*_{[\ell]j}(1)(1-\pi^*_{[\ell]j}(1))\right\}x_{[\ell]j} - \rho_{gj}\left\{\pi^*_{[\ell]g}(1)(1-\pi^*_{[\ell]g}(1))\right\}x_{[\ell]g}\right]$$
$$\times\left[\left\{\tilde{\lambda}^{(2)}_{[\ell],gj}(g^*)\tilde{\lambda}^{(1)}_{[\ell],gj}(g^*)\right\}^{-1}[K^*_{[\ell]g^*2}(t-1, t;\, g, j) - K^*_{[\ell]g^*}(t-1;\, g)\tilde{\lambda}^{(2)}_{[\ell],gj}(g^*)]\right]$$

$$
\begin{aligned}
&= \sum_{\ell=1}^{p+1} X'_\ell \left[y^*_{[\ell]}(1) - K_{[\ell]}\pi^*_{[\ell]}(1) \right] \\
&+ \sum_{\ell=1}^{p+1}\sum_{g=1}^{J-1}\sum_{j=1}^{J-1} \left[\left\{ \pi^*_{[\ell]j}(1)(1-\pi^*_{[\ell]j}(1)) \right\} x_{[\ell]j} - \rho_{gj} \left\{ \pi^*_{[\ell]g}(1)(1-\pi^*_{[\ell]g}(1)) \right\} x_{[\ell]g} \right] \\
&\times \left[\left\{ \tilde{\lambda}^{(2)}_{[\ell],gj}(1)\tilde{\lambda}^{(1)}_{[\ell],gj}(1) \right\}^{-1} [\sum_{t=2}^{T} K^*_{[\ell]12}(t-1,t;\, g,j) - \sum_{t=2}^{T} K^*_{[\ell]1}(t-1;\, g)\tilde{\lambda}^{(2)}_{[\ell],gj}(1)] \right. \\
&+ \left. \left\{ \tilde{\lambda}^{(2)}_{[\ell],gj}(2)\tilde{\lambda}^{(1)}_{[\ell],gj}(2) \right\}^{-1} [\sum_{t=2}^{T} K^*_{[\ell]22}(t-1,t;\, g,j) - \sum_{t=2}^{T} K^*_{[\ell]2}(t-1;\, g)\tilde{\lambda}^{(2)}_{[\ell],gj}(2)] \right] \\
&= f_1(\alpha) + \tilde{f}_2(\alpha) = \tilde{f}(\alpha) = 0. \qquad (3.326)
\end{aligned}
$$

To solve (3.326) for the CGQL estimate of α, similar to the iterative equation (3.314) used in the likelihood approach, one may use the iterative equation given by

$$\hat{\alpha} = \hat{\alpha}_0 - \left[\{\tilde{f}'(\alpha)\}^{-1} \tilde{f}(\alpha) \right] |_{\alpha=\hat{\alpha}_0}, \qquad (3.327)$$

where $\tilde{f}'(\alpha) = f'_1(\alpha) + \tilde{f}'_2(\alpha)$ with $f'_1(\alpha)$ same as in (3.316) under the likelihood approach, that is,

$$f'_1(\alpha) = -\sum_{\ell=1}^{p+1} K_{[\ell]} X'_\ell D_{\pi^*_{[\ell]}(1)} X_\ell,$$

and $\tilde{f}'_2(\alpha)$, by (3.324), is computed as

$$
\begin{aligned}
\tilde{f}'_2(\alpha) &- \sum_{\ell=1}^{p+1}\sum_{g=1}^{J-1}\sum_{j=1}^{J-1}\sum_{t=2}^{T}\sum_{g^*=1}^{2} \left[K^*_{[\ell]g^*}(t-1;\, g) \frac{\partial \tilde{\lambda}^{(2)}_{[\ell],gj}(g^*)}{\partial \alpha} \left\{ K^*_{[\ell]g^*}(t-1;\, g)\tilde{\lambda}^{(2)}_{[\ell],gj}(g^*)\tilde{\lambda}^{(1)}_{[\ell],gj}(g^*) \right\}^{-1} \right. \\
&\times \left. [K^*_{[\ell]g^*2}(t-1,t;\, g,j) - K^*_{[\ell]g^*}(t-1;\, g)\tilde{\lambda}^{(2)}_{[\ell],gj}(g^*)] \right] \frac{\partial \tilde{\lambda}^{(2)}_{[\ell],gj}(g^*)}{\partial \alpha'} \\
&= \sum_{\ell=1}^{p+1}\sum_{g=1}^{J-1}\sum_{j=1}^{J-1} \left[\left\{ \pi^*_{[\ell]j}(1)(1-\pi^*_{[\ell]j}(1))x_{[\ell]j} - \tilde{\rho}_{gj}\pi^*_{[\ell]g}(1)(1-\pi^*_{[\ell]g}(1))x_{[\ell]g} \right\} \right. \\
&\times \left. \left\{ \pi^*_{[\ell]j}(1)(1-\pi^*_{[\ell]j}(1))x_{[\ell]j} - \tilde{\rho}_{gj}\pi^*_{[\ell]g}(1)(1-\pi^*_{[\ell]g}(1))x_{[\ell]g} \right\}' \right] \\
&\times \left[\left\{ \tilde{\lambda}^{(2)}_{[\ell],gj}(1)\tilde{\lambda}^{(1)}_{[\ell],gj}(1) \right\}^{-1} [\sum_{t=2}^{T} K^*_{[\ell]12}(t-1,t;\, g,j) - \sum_{t=2}^{T} K^*_{[\ell]1}(t-1;\, g)\tilde{\lambda}^{(2)}_{[\ell],gj}(1)] \right. \\
&+ \left. \left\{ \tilde{\lambda}^{(2)}_{[\ell],gj}(2)\tilde{\lambda}^{(1)}_{[\ell],gj}(2) \right\}^{-1} [\sum_{t=2}^{T} K^*_{[\ell]22}(t-1,t;\, g,j) - \sum_{t=2}^{T} K^*_{[\ell]2}(t-1;\, g)\tilde{\lambda}^{(2)}_{[\ell],gj}(2)] \right]. \qquad (3.328)
\end{aligned}
$$

3.6.1.2.2 Moment Estimation for $\{\tilde{\rho}_{gj}\}$

Note that by using (3.300)–(3.301), it follows from the LDCP model (3.302) that for any $t = 1,\ldots,T$,

$$\begin{aligned} E[b^{(j)}_{i\in(\ell,c)}(t)] &= \pi^*_{[\ell]j} \\ \text{var}[b^{(j)}_{i\in(\ell,c)}(t)] &= \pi^*_{[\ell]j}[1-\pi^*_{[\ell]j}], \end{aligned} \tag{3.329}$$

and

$$\begin{aligned} \text{cov}[b^{(g)}_{i\in(\ell,c_1)}(t-1), b^{(j)}_{i\in(\ell,c_2)}(t)] &= E[\{b^{(g)}_{i\in(\ell,c_1)}(t-1)-\pi^*_{[\ell]g}\}\{b^{(j)}_{i\in(\ell,c_2)}(t)-\pi^*_{[\ell]j}\}] \\ &= \tilde{\rho}_{gj}E[b^{(g)}_{i\in(\ell,c_1)}(t-1)-\pi^*_{[\ell]g}]^2 \\ &= \tilde{\rho}_{gj}\pi^*_{[\ell]g}[1-\pi^*_{[\ell]g}]. \end{aligned} \tag{3.330}$$

Consequently, for $g, j = 1,\ldots,J-1$, by using

$$b^{*(j)}_{i\in(\ell,c)}(t) = \frac{b^{(j)}_{i\in(\ell,c)}(t)-\pi^*_{[\ell]j}}{[\pi^*_{[\ell]j}(1-\pi^*_{[\ell]j})]^{\frac{1}{2}}},$$

one may develop a moment estimating equation for $\tilde{\rho}_{gj}$ as

$$\hat{\tilde{\rho}}_{gj} = \frac{\sum_{\ell=1}^{p+1}\sum_{i=1}^{K_{[\ell]}}\sum_{t=2}^{T} b^{*(j)}_{i\in(\ell,c_2)}(t) b^{*(g)}_{i\in(\ell,c_1)}(t-1)/[(T-1)\sum_{\ell=1}^{p+1}K_{[\ell]}]}{\sum_{\ell=1}^{p+1}\sum_{i=1}^{K_{[\ell]}}\sum_{t=1}^{T}[b^{*(g)}_{i\in(\ell,c_1)}(t)]^2/[T\sum_{\ell=1}^{p+1}K_{[\ell]}]}. \tag{3.331}$$

Note that to compute (3.331), it is convenient to use the following formulas:

$$\begin{aligned} &\sum_{i=1}^{K_{[\ell]}}\sum_{t=2}^{T} b^{*(j)}_{i\in(\ell,c_2)}(t) b^{*(g)}_{i\in(\ell,c_1)}(t-1) \\ &= \sum_{t=2}^{T} K^*_{[\ell]22}(t-1,t;g,j)\left[\left\{\frac{(1-\pi^*_{[\ell]j})}{\pi^*_{[\ell]j}}\right\}^{\frac{1}{2}}\left\{\frac{(1-\pi^*_{[\ell]g})}{\pi^*_{[\ell]g}}\right\}^{\frac{1}{2}}\right] \\ &- \sum_{t=2}^{T} K^*_{[\ell]21}(t-1,t;g,j)\left[\left\{\frac{\pi^*_{[\ell]j}}{(1-\pi^*_{[\ell]j})}\right\}^{\frac{1}{2}}\left\{\frac{(1-\pi^*_{[\ell]g})}{\pi^*_{[\ell]g}}\right\}^{\frac{1}{2}}\right] \\ &- \sum_{t=2}^{T} K^*_{[\ell]12}(t-1,t;g,j)\left[\left\{\frac{(1-\pi^*_{[\ell]j})}{\pi^*_{[\ell]j}}\right\}^{\frac{1}{2}}\left\{\frac{\pi^*_{[\ell]g}}{(1-\pi^*_{[\ell]g})}\right\}^{\frac{1}{2}}\right] \end{aligned}$$

$$+\sum_{t=2}^{T} K^*_{[\ell]11}(t-1,t;g,j)\left[\left\{\frac{\pi^*_{[\ell]j}}{(1-\pi^*_{[\ell]j})}\right\}^{\frac{1}{2}}\left\{\frac{\pi^*_{[\ell]g}}{(1-\pi^*_{[\ell]g})}\right\}^{\frac{1}{2}}\right], \quad (3.332)$$

and

$$\sum_{i=1}^{K_{[\ell]}}\sum_{t=1}^{T}[b^{*(g)}_{i\in(\ell,c_1)}(t)]^2 = \sum_{t=1}^{T} K^*_{[\ell]2}(t,g)\left[\frac{(1-\pi^*_{[\ell]g})}{\pi^*_{[\ell]g}}\right] + \sum_{t=1}^{T} K^*_{[\ell]1}(t,g)\left[\frac{\pi^*_{[\ell]g}}{(1-\pi^*_{[\ell]g})}\right]. \quad (3.333)$$

3.6.1.3 Fitting the LDCMP Model Subject to Order Restriction of the Categories: A Pseudo-Likelihood Approach

In this approach, there is no need for any new modeling for the cut points based marginal binary probabilities defined by (3.300)–(3.301) for time point $t = 1$, and conditional probabilities for the lag 1 dynamic relationship between two binary variables defined by (3.302)–(3.303) for the time points $t = 2,\ldots,T$. More specifically, these marginal and conditional probabilities are written in terms of the original multinomial probabilities given in (3.231)–(3.234), and (3.241), respectively. Thus, the marginal probabilities in (3.300)–(3.301) are written as

$$\begin{aligned} P[b^{(j)}_{i\in(\ell,c)}(1)=1] &= \sum_{c=j+1}^{J}\pi_{[\ell]c}(1) \\ &= \frac{\sum_{c=j+1}^{J}\exp(x'_{[\ell]c}\theta^*)}{\sum_{u=1}^{J}\exp(x'_{[\ell]u}\theta^*)} \\ &= \pi^*_{[\ell]j}(1) \end{aligned} \quad (3.334)$$

and

$$\begin{aligned} P[b^{(j)}_{i\in(\ell,c)}(1)=0] &= \sum_{c=1}^{j}\pi_{[\ell]c}(1) \\ &= \frac{\sum_{c=1}^{j}\exp(x'_{[\ell]c}\theta^*)}{\sum_{u=1}^{J}\exp(x'_{[\ell]u}\theta^*)} \\ &= 1-\pi^*_{[\ell]j}(1). \end{aligned} \quad (3.335)$$

In the same token, unlike (3.302)–(3.303), by using (3.241), the conditional probabilities are now written as

$$P[b^{(j)}_{i\in(\ell,c_2)}(t)=1|b^{(g)}_{i\in(\ell,c_1)}(t-1)] = \tilde{\lambda}^{(2)}_{[\ell],gj}(b^{(g)}_{i\in(\ell,c_1)}(t-1))$$
$$= \begin{cases} \tilde{\lambda}^{(2)}_{[\ell],gj}(1) \text{ for } b^{(g)}_{i\in(\ell,c_1)}(t-1)=0 \\ \tilde{\lambda}^{(2)}_{[\ell],gj}(2) \text{ for } b^{(g)}_{i\in(\ell,c_1)}(t-1)=1, \end{cases} \tag{3.336}$$

where

$$\tilde{\lambda}^{(2)}_{[\ell],gj}(1) = \frac{1}{g}\sum_{c_1=1}^{g}\sum_{c_2=j+1}^{J}\lambda^{(c_2)}(c_1,\ell) \tag{3.337}$$

$$\tilde{\lambda}^{(2)}_{[\ell],gj}(2) = \frac{1}{J-g}\sum_{c_1=g+1}^{J}\sum_{c_2=j+1}^{J}\lambda^{(c_2)}(c_1,\ell), \text{ with} \tag{3.338}$$

$$\lambda^{(c_2)}(c_1,\ell) = \begin{cases} \pi_{[\ell]c_2} + \rho'_{c_2}(\delta_{[\ell]c_1} - \pi_{[\ell]}) & \text{for } c_2 = 1,\ldots,J-1 \\ 1-\sum_{c=1}^{J-1}\left[\pi_{[\ell]c} + (\delta_{[\ell]c_1} - \pi_{[\ell]})'\rho_c\right] & \text{for } c_2 = J, \end{cases} \tag{3.339}$$

where

$$\delta_{[\ell]c_1} = \begin{cases} \left(01'_{c_1-1} \; 1 \; 01'_{J-1-c_1}\right)' & \text{for } c_1 = 1,\ldots,J-1 \\ 01_{J-1} & \text{for } c_1 = J. \end{cases}$$

By applying (3.336), one can compute the remaining conditional probabilities as

$$P[b^{(j)}_{i\in(\ell,c_2)}(t)=0|b^{(g)}_{i\in(\ell,c_1)}(t-1)] = 1-\tilde{\lambda}^{(2)}_{[\ell],gj}(b^{(g)}_{i\in(\ell,c_1)}(t-1))$$
$$= \begin{cases} \tilde{\lambda}^{(1)}_{[\ell],gj}(1) = 1-\tilde{\lambda}^{(2)}_{[\ell],gj}(1) \text{ for } b^{(g)}_{i\in(\ell,c_1)}(t-1)=0 \\ \tilde{\lambda}^{(1)}_{[\ell],gj}(2) = 1-\tilde{\lambda}^{(2)}_{[\ell],gj}(2) \text{ for } b^{(g)}_{i\in(\ell,c_1)}(t-1)=1. \end{cases} \tag{3.340}$$

Next, the likelihood function for θ^* and ρ_M still has the same form as in (3.306), that is,

$$L(\theta^*,\rho_M) = \Pi_{\ell=1}^{p+1}\Pi_{j=1}^{J-1}\left[\left(\{1-\pi^*_{[\ell]j}(1)\}^{K^*_{[\ell]j}(1)}\right)\left(\{\pi^*_{[\ell]j}(1)\}^{K_{[\ell]}-K^*_{[\ell]j}(1)}\right)\right.$$
$$\left.\times\ \Pi_{t=2}^{T}\Pi_{g=1}^{J-1}\Pi_{g^*=1}^{2}\left(\{\tilde{\lambda}^{(1)}_{[\ell],gj}(g^*)\}^{K^*_{[\ell]g^*1}(t-1,t;g,j)}\{\tilde{\lambda}^{(2)}_{[\ell],gj}(g^*)\}^{K^*_{[\ell]g^*2}(t-1,t;g,j)}\right)\right], \tag{3.341}$$

but the marginal and conditional probabilities in (3.341) are now computed from (3.334)–(3.340).

3.6.1.3.1 Pseudo-Likelihood Estimating Equation for θ^*

Following derivatives will be necessary to compute the desired likelihood estimating equations. Note that here we are interested to estimate β_{c0} and $\beta_{c\ell}$ $(c = 1,\ldots,J-1; \ell = 1,\ldots,p)$ involved in the multinomial probabilities $\pi_{[\ell]c}$ given in (3.231)–(3.232). These probabilities for computational convenience were expressed in (3.234) as

$$\pi_{[\ell]c} = \frac{\exp(x'_{[\ell]c}\theta^*)}{\sum_{g=1}^{J}\exp(x'_{[\ell]g}\theta^*)},$$

where

$$\theta^* = [\beta_1^{*\prime},\ldots,\beta_c^{*\prime},\ldots,\beta_{J-1}^{*\prime}]' : (J-1)(p+1)\times 1, \text{ with } \beta_c^* = [\beta_{c0},\ldots,\beta_{c\ell},\ldots,\beta_{cp}]'.$$

Denote the derivatives

$$\frac{\partial \pi_{[\ell]c}}{\partial \theta^*}, \ \frac{1}{\pi_{[\ell]c}}\frac{\partial \pi_{[\ell]c}}{\partial \theta^*}, \text{ and } \frac{\partial \lambda^{(c_2)}(c_1,\ell)}{\partial \theta^*},$$

computed in (3.246), (3.247), and (3.250); by

$$\pi_{[\ell]c}p_{[\ell]c}, \ p_{[\ell]c}, \text{ and } \lambda_{(1)}^{(c_2)}(c_1,\ell),$$

respectively. That is, by (3.246),

$$\begin{aligned}\frac{\partial \pi_{[\ell]c}}{\partial \theta^*} &= \begin{cases}\pi_{[\ell]c}\left(x_{[\ell]c} - \pi_{[\ell]}\otimes d_{[\ell]1}\right) & \text{for } \ell = 1,\ldots,p;\ c = 1,\ldots,J\\ \pi_{[\ell]c}\left(x_{[\ell]c} - \pi_{[\ell]}\otimes d_{[\ell]2}\right) & \text{for } \ell = p+1;\ c = 1,\ldots,J,\end{cases}\\ &= \pi_{[\ell]c}p_{[\ell]c},\end{aligned}$$

and by (3.250),

$$\begin{aligned}\frac{\partial \lambda^{(c_2)}(c_1,\ell)}{\partial \theta^*} &= \begin{cases}\pi_{[\ell]c_2}\left(x_{[\ell]c_2} - \pi_{[\ell]}\otimes d_{[\ell]1}\right) - [\Sigma(\pi_{[\ell]})\otimes d_{[\ell]1}]\rho_{c_2} & \text{for } c_2 = 1,\ldots,J; \ell = 1,\ldots,p\\ \pi_{[\ell]c_2}\left(x_{[\ell]c_2} - \pi_{[\ell]}\otimes d_{[\ell]2}\right) - [\Sigma(\pi_{[\ell]})\otimes d_{[\ell]2}]\rho_{c_2} & \text{for } c_2 = 1,\ldots,J; \ell = p+1,\end{cases}\\ &= \lambda_{(1)}^{(c_2)}(c_1,\ell), \text{ for all } c_1 = 1,\ldots,J.\end{aligned}$$

It then follows by (3.334) that for cut point j, one obtains

$$\begin{aligned}\frac{\partial \pi^*_{[\ell]j}(1)}{\partial \theta^*} &= \sum_{c=j+1}^{J}\frac{\partial \pi_{[\ell]c}}{\partial \theta^*}\\ &= \sum_{c=j+1}^{J}\pi_{[\ell]c}p_{[\ell]c} = p^*_{[\ell]j}(\theta^*),\end{aligned} \tag{3.342}$$

where $x_{[\ell]c}$ for all $c = 1,\ldots,J; \ell = 1,\ldots,p+1$, is defined by (3.235). Also it follows by (3.337), (3.338), and (3.340) that for cut points (g, j), one obtains

$$\frac{\partial \tilde{\lambda}^{(2)}_{[\ell],gj}(1)}{\partial \theta^*} = \frac{1}{g}\sum_{c_1=1}^{g}\sum_{c_2=j+1}^{J}\lambda^{(c_2)}_{(1)}(c_1,\ell) = \xi_{[\ell]gj}(1,2;\theta^*)$$

$$\frac{\partial \tilde{\lambda}^{(2)}_{[\ell],gj}(2)}{\partial \theta^*} = \frac{1}{J-g}\sum_{c_1=g+1}^{J}\sum_{c_2=j+1}^{J}\lambda^{(c_2)}_{(1)}(c_1,\ell) = \xi_{[\ell]gj}(2,2;\theta^*)$$

$$\frac{\partial \tilde{\lambda}^{(1)}_{[\ell],gj}(1)}{\partial \theta^*} = -\frac{1}{g}\sum_{c_1=1}^{g}\sum_{c_2=j+1}^{J}\lambda^{(c_2)}_{(1)}(c_1,\ell) = \xi_{[\ell]gj}(1,1;\theta^*) = -\xi_{[\ell]gj}(1,2;\theta^*)$$

$$\frac{\partial \tilde{\lambda}^{(1)}_{[\ell],gj}(2)}{\partial \theta^*} = -\frac{1}{J-g}\sum_{c_1=g+1}^{J}\sum_{c_2=j+1}^{J}\lambda^{(c_2)}_{(1)}(c_1,\ell) = \xi_{[\ell]gj}(2,1;\theta^*)$$
$$= -\xi_{[\ell]gj}(2,2;\theta^*). \tag{3.343}$$

Consequently, by (3.341) and by similar calculations as in (3.313), one obtains the pseudo-likelihood estimating equation for θ^* as

$$\frac{\partial Log\, L(\theta^*,\rho_M)}{\partial \theta^*} = \sum_{\ell=1}^{p+1}\sum_{j=1}^{J-1}\left[\left\{(K_{[\ell]} - K^*_{[\ell]j}(1))\left(\frac{p^*_{[\ell]j}(\theta^*)}{\pi^*_{[\ell]j}(1)}\right) - K^*_{[\ell]j}(1)\left(\frac{p^*_{[\ell]j}(\theta^*)}{1-\pi^*_{[\ell]j}(1)}\right)\right\}\right.$$
$$+\sum_{g=1}^{J-1}\left\{-\sum_{t=2}^{T}K^*_{[\ell]11}(t-1,t;g,j)\frac{\xi_{[\ell]gj}(1,2;\theta^*)}{\tilde{\lambda}^{(1)}_{[\ell],gj}(1)} + \sum_{t=2}^{T}K^*_{[\ell]12}(t-1,t;g,j)\frac{\xi_{[\ell]gj}(1,2;\theta^*)}{\tilde{\lambda}^{(2)}_{[\ell],gj}(1)}\right.$$
$$\left.\left. - \sum_{t=2}^{T}K^*_{[\ell]21}(t-1,t;g,j)\frac{\xi_{[\ell]gj}(2,2;\theta^*)}{\tilde{\lambda}^{(1)}_{[\ell],gj}(2)} + \sum_{t=2}^{T}K^*_{[\ell]22}(t-1,t;g,j)\frac{\xi_{[\ell]gj}(2,2;\theta^*)}{\tilde{\lambda}^{(2)}_{[\ell],gj}(2)}\right\}\right]$$
$$= h_1(\theta^*) + h_2(\theta^*) = h(\theta^*) = 0. \tag{3.344}$$

This likelihood equation (3.344) may be solved iteratively by using

$$\hat{\theta}^*(r+1) = \hat{\theta}^*(r) - \left[\{h^{(1)}(\theta^*)\}^{-1}h(\theta^*)\right]|_{\theta^*=\hat{\theta}^*(r)}, \tag{3.345}$$

to obtain the final likelihood estimate $\hat{\theta}^*$. In (3.345), $h^{(1)}(\theta^*) = \frac{\partial h(\theta^*)}{\partial \theta^{*\prime}}$.

Computation of $\frac{\partial h(\theta^*)}{\partial \theta^{*\prime}}$ **:**
By (3.344),

$$h^{(1)}(\theta^*) = \frac{\partial Log\, L(\theta^*,\rho_M)}{\partial \theta^{*\prime}}$$

$$
\begin{aligned}
&= \sum_{\ell=1}^{p+1}\sum_{j=1}^{J-1}\left[\left\{(K_{[\ell]}-K^*_{[\ell]j}(1))\left(\frac{p^{*(1)}_{[\ell]j}(\theta^*,\theta^*)}{\pi^*_{[\ell]j}(1)}-\frac{p^*_{[\ell]j}(\theta^*)p^{*'}_{[\ell]j}(\theta^*)}{[\pi^*_{[\ell]j}(1)]^2}\right)\right.\right.\\
&- K^*_{[\ell]j}(1)\left.\left(\frac{p^*_{[\ell]j}(\theta^*)p^{*'}_{[\ell]j}(\theta^*)}{[1-\pi^*_{[\ell]j}(1)]^2}+\frac{p^{*(1)}_{[\ell]j}(\theta^*,\theta^*)}{1-\pi^*_{[\ell]j}(1)}\right)\right\}\\
&+ \sum_{g=1}^{J-1}\left[-\left\{\sum_{t=2}^{T}K^*_{[\ell]11}(t-1,t;g,j)\left(\frac{\xi^{(1)}_{[\ell]gj}(1,2;\theta^*,\theta^*)}{\tilde{\lambda}^{(1)}_{[\ell],gj}(1)}-\frac{\xi_{[\ell]gj}(1,2;\theta^*)\xi'_{[\ell]gj}(1,2;\theta^*)}{[\tilde{\lambda}^{(1)}_{[\ell],gj}(1)]^2}\right)\right\}\right.\\
&+ \left\{\sum_{t=2}^{T}K^*_{[\ell]12}(t-1,t;g,j)\left(\frac{\xi^{(1)}_{[\ell]gj}(1,2;\theta^*,\theta^*)}{\tilde{\lambda}^{(2)}_{[\ell],gj}(1)}-\frac{\xi_{[\ell]gj}(1,2;\theta^*)\xi'_{[\ell]gj}(1,2;\theta^*)}{[\tilde{\lambda}^{(2)}_{[\ell],gj}(1)]^2}\right)\right\}\\
&- \left\{\sum_{t=2}^{T}K^*_{[\ell]21}(t-1,t;g,j)\left(\frac{\xi^{(1)}_{[\ell]gj}(2,2;\theta^*,\theta^*)}{\tilde{\lambda}^{(1)}_{[\ell],gj}(2)}-\frac{\xi_{[\ell]gj}(2,2;\theta^*)\xi'_{[\ell]gj}(2,2;\theta^*)}{[\tilde{\lambda}^{(1)}_{[\ell],gj}(2)]^2}\right)\right\}\\
&+ \left.\left.\left\{\sum_{t=2}^{T}K^*_{[\ell]22}(t-1,t;g,j)\left(\frac{\xi^{(1)}_{[\ell]gj}(2,2;\theta^*,\theta^*)}{\tilde{\lambda}^{(2)}_{[\ell],gj}(2)}-\frac{\xi_{[\ell]gj}(2,2;\theta^*)\xi'_{[\ell]gj}(2,2;\theta^*)}{[\tilde{\lambda}^{(2)}_{[\ell],gj}(2)]^2}\right)\right\}\right]\right],
\end{aligned}
\tag{3.346}
$$

where

$$
\begin{aligned}
p^{*(1)}_{[\ell]j}(\theta^*,\theta^*) &= \frac{\partial p^*_{[\ell]j}(\theta^*)}{\partial\theta^{*'}}\\
&= \sum_{c=j+1}^{J}\frac{\partial\pi_{[\ell]c}p_{[\ell]c}}{\partial\theta^{*'}},\ \text{by (3.342)}\\
&= \sum_{c=j+1}^{J}\left[\pi_{[\ell]c}\left\{p_{[\ell]c}p'_{[\ell]c}-\Sigma^*(\pi_{[\ell]})\right\}\right],
\end{aligned}
\tag{3.347}
$$

where, by (3.342),

$$
p_{[\ell]c} \equiv \begin{cases} \left(x_{[\ell]c}-\pi_{[\ell]}\otimes d_{[\ell]1}\right) \text{ for } \ell=1,\ldots,p\\ \left(x_{[\ell]c}-\pi_{[\ell]}\otimes d_{[\ell]2}\right) \text{ for } \ell=p+1,\end{cases}
$$

and by (3.255)–(3.256),

$$
\Sigma^*(\pi_{[\ell]}) \equiv \begin{cases} \Sigma^*_1(\pi_{[\ell]}) \text{ for } \ell=1,\ldots,p\\ \Sigma^*_2(\pi_{[\ell]}) \text{ for } \ell=p+1.\end{cases}
\tag{3.348}
$$

Furthermore, in (3.346), by (3.343),

$$\xi^{(1)}_{[\ell]gj}(1,2;\theta^*,\theta^*) = \frac{\partial \xi_{[\ell]gj}(1,2;\theta^*)}{\partial \theta^{*\prime}}$$
$$= \frac{1}{g}\sum_{c_1=1}^{g}\sum_{c_2=j+1}^{J}\frac{\partial \lambda^{(c_2)}_{(1)}(c_1,\ell)}{\partial \theta^{*\prime}}$$
$$= \frac{1}{g}\sum_{c_1=1}^{g}\sum_{c_2=j+1}^{J}\left[\pi_{[\ell]c_2}M^*_{c_2}(x,\pi_{[\ell]}) - \Omega^*(\pi_{[\ell]})\right], \tag{3.349}$$

$$\xi^{(1)}_{[\ell]gj}(2,2;\theta^*,\theta^*) = \frac{\partial \xi_{[\ell]gj}(2,2;\theta^*)}{\partial \theta^{*\prime}}$$
$$= \frac{1}{J-g}\sum_{c_1=g+1}^{J}\sum_{c_2=j+1}^{J}\frac{\partial \lambda^{(c_2)}_{(1)}(c_1,\ell)}{\partial \theta^{*\prime}}$$
$$= \frac{1}{J-g}\sum_{c_1=g+1}^{J}\sum_{c_2=j+1}^{J}\left[\pi_{[\ell]c_2}M^*_{c_2}(x,\pi_{[\ell]}) - \Omega^*(\pi_{[\ell]})\right], \tag{3.350}$$

where, by (3.259)–(3.260),

$$M^*_{c_2}(x,\pi_{[\ell]}) \equiv \begin{cases} M^*_{c_2,1}(x,\pi_{[\ell]}) \text{ for } \ell = 1,\ldots,p \\ M^*_{c_2,2}(x,\pi_{[\ell]}) \text{ for } \ell = p+1, \end{cases} \tag{3.351}$$

and by (3.264)–(3.265),

$$\Omega^*(\pi_{[\ell]}) \equiv \begin{cases} \Omega^*_1(\pi_{[\ell]}) \text{ for } \ell = 1,\ldots,p \\ \Omega^*_2(\pi_{[\ell]}) \text{ for } \ell = p+1. \end{cases} \tag{3.352}$$

3.6.1.3.2 Pseudo-Likelihood Estimating Equation for ρ_M

The likelihood estimation of ρ_M is equivalent to estimate $\rho_c : (J-1)\times 1$, for $c = 1,\ldots,J-1$, by maximizing the log likelihood function $Log\ L(\theta^*,\rho_M)$ given in (3.341). Note that for a given cut point j, either $c \le j$ or $c > j$ holds. Next, because $\pi^*_{[\ell]j}$ is free of ρ_c, for any c and j, the pseudo-likelihood estimating equation for ρ_c can be computed as

$$\frac{\partial Log\ L(\theta^*,\rho_M)}{\partial \rho_c} = \sum_{\ell=1}^{p+1}\sum_{j=1}^{J-1}\sum_{g=1}^{J-1}\left[\sum_{t=2}^{T}K^*_{[\ell]11}(t-1,t;g,j)\left\{\frac{\xi^*_{[\ell]gj}(1,1;\rho_c)}{\tilde{\lambda}^{(1)}_{[\ell],gj}(1)}\right\}\right.$$
$$+\sum_{t=2}^{T}K^*_{[\ell]12}(t-1,t;g,j)\left\{\frac{\xi^*_{[\ell]gj}(1,2;\rho_c)}{\tilde{\lambda}^{(2)}_{[\ell],gj}(1)}\right\}$$

$$+ \sum_{t=2}^{T} K^*_{[\ell]21}(t-1,t;g,j) \left\{ \frac{\xi^*_{[\ell]gj}(2,1;\rho_c)}{\tilde{\lambda}^{(1)}_{[\ell],gj}(2)} \right\}$$

$$+ \sum_{t=2}^{T} K^*_{[\ell]22}(t-1,t;g,j) \left\{ \frac{\xi^*_{[\ell]gj}(2,2;\rho_c)}{\tilde{\lambda}^{(2)}_{[\ell],gj}(2)} \right\} \Bigg] = 0, \tag{3.353}$$

where, for example,

$$\xi^*_{[\ell]gj}(1,1;\rho_c) = \frac{\partial \tilde{\lambda}^{(1)}_{[\ell],gj}(1)}{\partial \rho_c}, \tag{3.354}$$

for a general $c \leq j$ or $c > j$, j being the cut point at time t. Next, it follows by (3.337), (3.338), and (3.340) that for cut points (g, j), one obtains

$$\begin{aligned}
\frac{\partial \tilde{\lambda}^{(2)}_{[\ell],gj}(1)}{\partial \rho_c} &= \frac{1}{g} \sum_{c_1=1}^{g} \left[\sum_{c_2=j+1}^{J} \frac{\partial \lambda^{(c_2)}(c_1,\ell)}{\partial \rho_c} \right] = \xi^*_{[\ell]gj}(1,2;\rho_c) \\
&= \frac{1}{g} \sum_{c_1=1}^{g} \left[\frac{\partial}{\partial \rho_c} \sum_{c_2=j+1}^{J-1} \{\pi_{[\ell]c_2} + (\delta_{[\ell]c_1} - \pi_{[\ell]})' \rho_{c_2}\} \right. \\
&\quad \left. + \frac{\partial}{\partial \rho_c} \left\{ 1 - \sum_{h=1}^{J-1} (\pi_{[\ell]h} + (\delta_{[\ell]c_1} - \pi_{[\ell]})' \rho_h) \right\} \right] \\
&= \begin{cases} -\frac{1}{g} \sum_{c_1=1}^{g} [\delta_{[\ell]c_1} - \pi_{[\ell]}] & \text{for } c \leq j \\ 0 & \text{for } j < c \leq (J-1), \end{cases}
\end{aligned} \tag{3.355}$$

and

$$\begin{aligned}
\frac{\partial \tilde{\lambda}^{(2)}_{[\ell],gj}(2)}{\partial \rho_c} &= \frac{1}{J-g} \sum_{c_1=g+1}^{J} \left[\sum_{c_2=j+1}^{J} \frac{\partial \lambda^{(c_2)}(c_1,\ell)}{\partial \rho_c} \right] = \xi^*_{[\ell]gj}(2,2;\rho_c) \\
&= \frac{1}{J-g} \sum_{c_1=g+1}^{J} \left[\frac{\partial}{\partial \rho_c} \sum_{c_2=j+1}^{J-1} \{\pi_{[\ell]c_2} + (\delta_{[\ell]c_1} - \pi_{[\ell]})' \rho_{c_2}\} \right. \\
&\quad \left. + \frac{\partial}{\partial \rho_c} \left\{ 1 - \sum_{h=1}^{J-1} (\pi_{[\ell]h} + (\delta_{[\ell]c_1} - \pi_{[\ell]})' \rho_h) \right\} \right] \\
&= \begin{cases} -\frac{1}{J-g} \sum_{c_1=g+1}^{J} [\delta_{[\ell]c_1} - \pi_{[\ell]}] & \text{for } c \leq j \\ 0 & \text{for } j < c \leq (J-1). \end{cases}
\end{aligned} \tag{3.356}$$

Using the above two derivatives, the derivatives for the remaining two complementary conditional probabilities are easily obtained as

$$\frac{\partial \tilde{\lambda}^{(1)}_{[\ell],gj}(1)}{\partial \rho_c} = -\frac{\partial \tilde{\lambda}^{(2)}_{[\ell],gj}(1)}{\partial \rho_c} = \xi^*_{[\ell]gj}(1,1;\rho_c)$$

$$= \begin{cases} \frac{1}{g}\sum_{c_1=1}^{g}[\delta_{[\ell]c_1} - \pi_{[\ell]}] & \text{for } c \leq j \\ 0 & \text{for } j < c \leq (J-1), \text{ and} \end{cases} \tag{3.357}$$

$$\frac{\partial \tilde{\lambda}^{(1)}_{[\ell],gj}(2)}{\partial \rho_c} = -\frac{\partial \tilde{\lambda}^{(2)}_{[\ell],gj}(2)}{\partial \rho_c} = \xi^*_{[\ell]gj}(2,1;\rho_c)$$

$$= \begin{cases} \frac{1}{J-g}\sum_{c_1=g+1}^{J}[\delta_{[\ell]c_1} - \pi_{[\ell]}] & \text{for } c \leq j \\ 0 & \text{for } j < c \leq (J-1). \end{cases} \tag{3.358}$$

Thus, the computation for the estimating equation (3.353) is complete, yielding the estimating equation for $\rho^* = (\rho'_1, \ldots, \rho'_j, \ldots, \rho'_{J-1})'$, (i.e., for the elements of ρ_M) as

$$\frac{\partial Log\, L(\theta^*, \rho_M)}{\partial \rho^*} = \begin{pmatrix} \frac{\partial Log\, L(\theta^*,\rho_M)}{\partial \rho_1} \\ \vdots \\ \frac{\partial Log\, L(\theta^*,\rho_M)}{\partial \rho_c} \\ \vdots \\ \frac{\partial Log\, L(\theta^*,\rho_M)}{\partial \rho_{J-1}} \end{pmatrix} = 0 : (J-1)^2 \times 1. \tag{3.359}$$

This estimating equation may be solved by using the iterative equation

$$\hat{\rho}^*(r+1) = \hat{\rho}^*(r) - \left[\left\{\frac{\partial^2 \text{Log}\, L(\theta^*, \rho_M)}{\partial \rho^* \partial \rho^{*\prime}}\right\}^{-1} \frac{\partial \text{Log}\, L(\theta^*, \rho_M)}{\partial \rho^*}\right]_{|\rho^* = \hat{\rho}^*(r)}, \tag{3.360}$$

where

$$\frac{\partial^2 Log\, L(\theta^*, \rho_M)}{\partial \rho^* \partial \rho^{*\prime}} = \begin{pmatrix} \frac{\partial^2 Log\, L(\theta^*,\rho_M)}{\partial \rho_1 \partial \rho'_1} & \cdots & \frac{\partial^2 Log\, L(\theta^*,\rho_M)}{\partial \rho_1 \partial \rho'_c} & \cdots & \frac{\partial^2 Log\, L(\theta^*,\rho_M)}{\partial \rho_1 \partial \rho'_{J-1}} \\ \vdots & & \vdots & & \vdots \\ \frac{\partial^2 Log\, L(\theta^*,\rho_M)}{\partial \rho_c \partial \rho'_1} & \cdots & \frac{\partial^2 Log\, L(\theta^*,\rho_M)}{\partial \rho_c \partial \rho'_c} & \cdots & \frac{\partial^2 Log\, L(\theta^*,\rho_M)}{\partial \rho_c \partial \rho'_{J-1}} \\ \vdots & & \vdots & & \vdots \\ \frac{\partial^2 Log\, L(\theta^*,\rho_M)}{\partial \rho_{J-1} \partial \rho'_1} & \cdots & \frac{\partial^2 Log\, L(\theta^*,\rho_M)}{\partial \rho_{J-1} \partial \rho'_j} & \cdots & \frac{\partial^2 Log\, L(\theta^*,\rho_M)}{\partial \rho_{J-1} \partial \rho'_{J-1}} \end{pmatrix}. \tag{3.361}$$

The second order derivatives involved in (3.361) may be computed by using the first order derivatives from (3.355)–(3.358) into (3.353). To be specific, two general second order derivatives are:

$$\frac{\partial^2 Log\,L(\theta^*,\rho_M)}{\partial\rho_c\partial\rho_c'} = -\sum_{\ell=1}^{p+1}\sum_{j=1}^{J-1}\sum_{g=1}^{J-1}\left[\sum_{t=2}^{T}K^*_{[\ell]11}(t-1,t;g,j)\left\{\frac{[\xi^*_{[\ell]gj}(1,1;\rho_c){\xi^*}'_{[\ell]gj}(1,1;\rho_c)]}{[\tilde{\lambda}^{(1)}_{[\ell],gj}(1)]^2}\right\}\right.$$
$$+\sum_{t=2}^{T}K^*_{[\ell]12}(t-1,t;g,j)\left\{\frac{[\xi^*_{[\ell]gj}(1,2;\rho_c){\xi^*}'_{[\ell]gj}(1,2;\rho_c)]}{[\tilde{\lambda}^{(2)}_{[\ell],gj}(1)]^2}\right\}$$
$$+\sum_{t=2}^{T}K^*_{[\ell]21}(t-1,t;g,j)\left\{\frac{[\xi^*_{[\ell]gj}(2,1;\rho_c){\xi^*}'_{[\ell]gj}(2,1;\rho_c)]}{[\tilde{\lambda}^{(1)}_{[\ell],gj}(2)]^2}\right\}$$
$$\left.+\sum_{t=2}^{T}K^*_{[\ell]22}(t-1,t;g,j)\left\{\frac{[\xi^*_{[\ell]gj}(2,2;\rho_c){\xi^*}'_{[\ell]gj}(2,2;\rho_c)]}{[\tilde{\lambda}^{(2)}_{[\ell],gj}(2)]^2}\right\}\right] \quad (3.362)$$

and

$$\frac{\partial^2 Log\,L(\theta^*,\rho_M)}{\partial\rho_c\partial\rho_d'} = -\sum_{\ell=1}^{p+1}\sum_{j=1}^{J-1}\sum_{g=1}^{J-1}\left[\sum_{t=2}^{T}K^*_{[\ell]11}(t-1,t;g,j)\left\{\frac{[\xi^*_{[\ell]gj}(1,1;\rho_c){\xi^*}'_{[\ell]gj}(1,1;\rho_d)]}{[\tilde{\lambda}^{(1)}_{[\ell],gj}(1)]^2}\right\}\right.$$
$$+\sum_{t=2}^{T}K^*_{[\ell]12}(t-1,t;g,j)\left\{\frac{[\xi^*_{[\ell]gj}(1,2;\rho_c){\xi^*}'_{[\ell]gj}(1,2;\rho_d)]}{[\tilde{\lambda}^{(2)}_{[\ell],gj}(1)]^2}\right\}$$
$$+\sum_{t=2}^{T}K^*_{[\ell]21}(t-1,t;g,j)\left\{\frac{[\xi^*_{[\ell]gj}(2,1;\rho_c){\xi^*}'_{[\ell]gj}(2,1;\rho_d)]}{[\tilde{\lambda}^{(1)}_{[\ell],gj}(2)]^2}\right\}$$
$$\left.+\sum_{t=2}^{T}K^*_{[\ell]22}(t-1,t;g,j)\left\{\frac{[\xi^*_{[\ell]gj}(2,2;\rho_c){\xi^*}'_{[\ell]gj}(2,2;\rho_d)]}{[\tilde{\lambda}^{(2)}_{[\ell],gj}(2)]^2}\right\}\right], \quad (3.363)$$

where, for example,

$$[\xi^*_{[\ell]gj}(1,1;\rho_c){\xi^*}'_{[\ell]gj}(1,1;\rho_d)]$$
$$= \begin{cases} \frac{1}{g^2}\sum_{c_1=1}^{g}[\delta_{[\ell]c_1}-\pi_{[\ell]}]\sum_{c_1=1}^{g}[\delta_{[\ell]c_1}-\pi_{[\ell]}]' & \text{for } c\le j, \text{ and } d\le j \\ 0 & \text{otherwise.}\end{cases} \quad (3.364)$$

3.6.2 *MDL Model with Cut Points g at Time t − 1 and j at Time t*

3.6.2.1 Fitting Bivariate Binary Mapping Based MDL Model: A Pseudo-Likelihood Approach

There is no difference for the probabilities at initial time $t = 1$ between the LDCP and this BDL models. These probabilities at $t = 1$ are given by (3.300) and (3.301). However, at time points $t = 2,\ldots,T$, instead of linear forms given by (3.302)–(3.303), the conditional binary probabilities now have the logit form given by

$$P[b^{(j)}_{i\in(\ell,c_2)}(t) = 1|b^{(g)}_{i\in(\ell,c_1)}(t-1)]$$
$$= \begin{cases} \frac{\exp(\alpha_{j0}+\alpha_{j\ell}+\tilde{\gamma}_{gj}b^{(g)}_{i\in(\ell,c_1)}(t-1))}{1+\exp(\alpha_{j0}+\alpha_{j\ell}+\tilde{\gamma}_{gj}b^{(g)}_{i\in(\ell,c_1)}(t-1))} & \text{for } \ell = 1,\ldots,p \\ \frac{\exp(\alpha_{j0}+\tilde{\gamma}_{gj}b^{(g)}_{i\in(\ell,c_1)}(t-1))}{1+\exp(\alpha_{j0}+\tilde{\gamma}_{jg}b^{(g)}_{i\in(\ell,c_1)}(t-1))} & \text{for } \ell = p+1, \end{cases} \tag{3.365}$$
$$= \tilde{\eta}^{(2)}_{[\ell],gj}(b^{(g)}_{i\in(\ell,c_1)}(t-1)),$$

yielding

$$\tilde{\eta}^{(2)}_{[\ell],gj}(1) = \begin{cases} \frac{\exp(\alpha_{j0}+\alpha_{j\ell})}{1+\exp(\alpha_{j0}+\alpha_{j\ell})} & \text{for } \ell = 1,\ldots,p \\ \frac{\exp(\alpha_{j0})}{1+\exp(\alpha_{j0})} & \text{for } \ell = p+1, \end{cases} \tag{3.366}$$

$$\tilde{\eta}^{(2)}_{[\ell],gj}(2) = \begin{cases} \frac{\exp(\alpha_{j0}+\alpha_{j\ell}+\tilde{\gamma}_{gj})}{1+\exp(\alpha_{j0}+\alpha_{j\ell}+\tilde{\gamma}_{gj})} & \text{for } \ell = 1,\ldots,p \\ \frac{\exp(\alpha_{j0}+\tilde{\gamma}_{jg})}{1+\exp(\alpha_{j0}+\tilde{\gamma}_{gj})} & \text{for } \ell = p+1, \end{cases} \tag{3.367}$$

and

$$P[b^{(j)}_{i\in(\ell,c_2)}(t) = 0|b^{(g)}_{i\in(\ell,c_1)}(t-1)]$$
$$= \begin{cases} \frac{1}{1+\exp(\alpha_{j0}+\alpha_{j\ell}+\tilde{\gamma}_{gj}b^{(g)}_{i\in(\ell,c_1)}(t-1))} & \text{for } \ell = 1,\ldots,p \\ \frac{1}{1+\exp(\alpha_{j0}+\tilde{\gamma}_{gj}b^{(g)}_{i\in(\ell,c_1)}(t-1))} & \text{for } \ell = p+1, \end{cases} \tag{3.368}$$
$$= 1-\tilde{\eta}^{(2)}_{[\ell],gj}(b^{(g)}_{i\in(\ell,c_1)}(t-1)),$$

yielding

$$\tilde{\eta}^{(1)}_{[\ell],gj}(1) = \begin{cases} \frac{1}{1+\exp(\alpha_{j0}+\alpha_{j\ell})} & \text{for } \ell = 1,\ldots,p \\ \frac{1}{1+\exp(\alpha_{j0})} & \text{for } \ell = p+1, \end{cases} \tag{3.369}$$

$$\tilde{\eta}^{(1)}_{[\ell],gj}(2) = \begin{cases} \frac{1}{1+\exp(\alpha_{j0}+\alpha_{j\ell}+\tilde{\gamma}_{gj})} & \text{for } \ell = 1,\ldots,p \\ \frac{1}{1+\exp(\alpha_{j0}+\gamma_{gj})} & \text{for } \ell = p+1. \end{cases} \tag{3.370}$$

Let $\tilde{\gamma}_M = (\tilde{\gamma}_{gj})$ denote the $(J-1)\times(J-1)$ matrix of dynamic dependence parameters under the BDL model.

Then simply by replacing the conditional probabilities, for example, $\tilde{\lambda}^{(1)}_{[\ell],gj}(1)$ with $\tilde{\eta}^{(1)}_{[\ell],gj}(1)$, in (3.306), one writes the likelihood function under the BDL model as

$$L(\alpha,\tilde{\gamma}_M) = \Pi_{\ell=1}^{p+1}\Pi_{j=1}^{J-1}\left[\left(\{1-\pi^*_{[\ell]j}(1)\}^{K^*_{[\ell]j}(1)}\right)\left(\{\pi^*_{[\ell]j}(1)\}^{K_{[\ell]}-K^*_{[\ell]j}(1)}\right)\right.$$
$$\left.\times\ \Pi_{t=2}^{T}\Pi_{g=1}^{J-1}\Pi_{g^*=1}^{2}\left(\{\tilde{\eta}^{(1)}_{[\ell],gj}(g^*)\}^{K^*_{[\ell]g^*1}(t-1,t;g,j)}\{\tilde{\eta}^{(2)}_{[\ell],gj}(g^*)\}^{K^*_{[\ell]g^*2}(t-1,t;g,j)}\right)\right], \tag{3.371}$$

where $\pi^*_{[\ell]j}(1)$ has the same formula as in (3.308), that is,

$$\pi^*_{[\ell]j}(1) = \frac{\exp(x'_{[\ell]j}\alpha)}{1+\exp(x'_{[\ell]j}\alpha)}$$
$$1-\pi^*_{[\ell]j}(1) = \frac{1}{1+\exp(x'_{[\ell]j}\alpha)},$$

but unlike $\tilde{\lambda}^{(j^*)}_{[\ell],gj}(g^*)$ for $g^* = 1,2; j^* = 1,2$ in (3.312), $\tilde{\eta}^{(j^*)}_{[\ell],gj}(g^*)$ for $g^* = 1,2; j^* = 1,2$ have the formulas

$$\tilde{\eta}^{(2)}_{[\ell],gj}(1) = \frac{\exp(x'_{[\ell]j}\alpha)}{1+\exp(x'_{[\ell]j}\alpha)},\ \tilde{\eta}^{(2)}_{[\ell],gj}(2) = \frac{\exp(x'_{[\ell]j}\alpha+\tilde{\gamma}_{gj})}{1+\exp(x'_{[\ell]j}\alpha+\tilde{\gamma}_{gj})},$$
$$\tilde{\eta}^{(1)}_{[\ell],gj}(1) = \frac{1}{1+\exp(x'_{[\ell]j}\alpha)},\ \tilde{\eta}^{(1)}_{[\ell],gj}(2) = \frac{1}{1+\exp(x'_{[\ell]j}\alpha+\tilde{\gamma}_{gj})}. \tag{3.372}$$

3.6.2.1.1 Pseudo-Likelihood Estimating Equation for α

By similar calculations as in (3.307) and (3.313), one obtains the likelihood equation for α as

$$\frac{\partial Log\ L(\alpha,\tilde{\gamma}_M)}{\partial\alpha} = \sum_{\ell=1}^{p+1}\left[X'_\ell\left\{y^*_{[\ell]}(1) - K_{[\ell]}\pi^*_{[\ell]}(1)\right\}\right.$$
$$+\sum_{j=1}^{J-1}\sum_{g=1}^{J-1}\left\{-\sum_{t=2}^{T}K^*_{[\ell]11}(t-1,t;g,j)\{1-\tilde{\eta}^{(1)}_{[\ell],gj}(1)\} + \sum_{t=2}^{T}K^*_{[\ell]12}(t-1,t;g,j)\{1-\tilde{\eta}^{(2)}_{[\ell],gj}(1)\}\right.$$

$$- \sum_{t=2}^{T} K^*_{[\ell]21}(t-1,t;g,j)\{1-\tilde{\eta}^{(1)}_{[\ell],gj}(2)\} + \sum_{t=2}^{T} K^*_{[\ell]22}(t-1,t;g,j)\{1-\tilde{\eta}^{(2)}_{[\ell],gj}(2)\} \Big\} x_{[\ell]j} \Big]$$

$$= f_1(\alpha) + f_2^*(\alpha) = f^*(\alpha) = 0. \tag{3.373}$$

Let $\hat{\alpha}$ be the solution of $f^*(\alpha) = 0$ in (3.373). Assuming that $\hat{\alpha}_0$ is not a solution for $f^*(\alpha) = 0$ but a trial estimate, and hence $f^*(\hat{\alpha}_0) \neq 0$, the iterative equation for $\hat{\alpha}$ is obtained as

$$\hat{\alpha} = \hat{\alpha}_0 - \left[\{f^{*\prime}(\alpha)\}^{-1} f^*(\alpha)\right] |_{\alpha=\hat{\alpha}_0}, \tag{3.374}$$

where

$$f^{*\prime}(\alpha) = f_1'(\alpha) + f^{*\prime}_2(\alpha) = \frac{\partial f_1(\alpha)}{\partial \alpha'} + \frac{\partial f_2^*(\alpha)}{\partial \alpha'}$$

is computed as follows.

Note that $f_1'(\alpha)$ has the same formula as in (3.316), that is,

$$f_1'(\alpha) = \frac{\partial f_1(\alpha)}{\partial \alpha'} = -\sum_{\ell=1}^{p+1} K_{[\ell]} X_\ell' D_{\pi^*_{[\ell]}(1)} X_\ell.$$

Next, by (3.372), it follows from (3.373) that

$$\begin{aligned} f^{*\prime}_2(\alpha) &= \frac{\partial f_2^*(\alpha)}{\partial \alpha'} \\ &- \sum_{\ell=1}^{p+1} \sum_{j=1}^{J-1} \sum_{g=1}^{J-1} \Bigg[\Bigg\{ \sum_{t=2}^{T} K^*_{[\ell]11}(t-1,t;g,j)[\tilde{\eta}^{(1)}_{[\ell],gj}(1)\{1-\tilde{\eta}^{(1)}_{[\ell],gj}(1)\}] \\ &+ \sum_{t=2}^{T} K^*_{[\ell]12}(t-1,t;g,j)[\tilde{\eta}^{(2)}_{[\ell],gj}(1)\{1-\tilde{\eta}^{(2)}_{[\ell],gj}(1)\}] \\ &+ \sum_{t=2}^{T} K^*_{[\ell]21}(t-1,t;g,j)[\tilde{\eta}^{(1)}_{[\ell],gj}(2)\{1-\tilde{\eta}^{(1)}_{[\ell],gj}(2)\}] \\ &+ \sum_{t=2}^{T} K^*_{[\ell]22}(t-1,t;g,j)[\tilde{\eta}^{(2)}_{[\ell],gj}(2)\{1-\tilde{\eta}^{(2)}_{[\ell],gj}(2)\}] \Bigg\} x_{[\ell]j} x'_{[\ell]j} \Bigg]. \end{aligned} \tag{3.375}$$

3.6.2.1.2 Pseudo-Likelihood Estimating Equation for $\tilde{\gamma}_M$

Because $\tilde{\gamma}_{gj}$ is involved in the conditional probabilities as shown in (3.372), similar to (3.373), we write the likelihood estimating equations for $\tilde{\gamma}_{gj}$ as

$$\frac{\partial Log\, L(\alpha,\tilde{\gamma}_M)}{\partial \tilde{\gamma}_{gj}} = \sum_{\ell=1}^{p+1} \left\{ -\sum_{t=2}^{T} K^*_{[\ell]11}(t-1,t;g,j)\{1-\tilde{\eta}^{(1)}_{[\ell],gj}(1)\} \right.$$
$$+ \sum_{t=2}^{T} K^*_{[\ell]12}(t-1,t;g,j)\{1-\tilde{\eta}^{(2)}_{[\ell],gj}(1)\}$$
$$- \sum_{t=2}^{T} K^*_{[\ell]21}(t-1,t;g,j)\{1-\tilde{\eta}^{(1)}_{[\ell],gj}(2)\}$$
$$\left. + \sum_{t=2}^{T} K^*_{[\ell]22}(t-1,t;g,j)\{1-\tilde{\eta}^{(2)}_{[\ell],gj}(2)\} \right\} = 0. \quad (3.376)$$

By using

$$\tilde{\gamma} = (\tilde{\gamma}'_1,\ldots,\tilde{\gamma}'_g,\ldots,\tilde{\gamma}'_{J-1})' \text{ with } \tilde{\gamma}'_g = (\tilde{\gamma}_{g1},\ldots,\tilde{\gamma}_{gj},\ldots,\tilde{\gamma}_{g,J-1}),$$

the $(J-1)^2$ estimating equations in (3.376) may be solved iteratively by using the formula

$$\hat{\tilde{\gamma}}(r+1) = \hat{\tilde{\gamma}}(r) - \left[\left\{ \frac{\partial^2 Log\, L(\alpha,\tilde{\gamma}_M)}{\partial \tilde{\gamma}' \partial \tilde{\gamma}} \right\}^{-1} \frac{\partial Log\, L(\alpha,\tilde{\gamma}_M)}{\partial \tilde{\gamma}} \right]_{|\tilde{\gamma}=\hat{\tilde{\gamma}}(r)}, \quad (3.377)$$

where the first order derivative vector $\frac{\partial Log\, L(\alpha,\tilde{\gamma}_M)}{\partial \tilde{\gamma}}$ may be constructed by stacking the scalar derivatives from (3.376). The computation of the second order derivative matrix follows from the following two general second order derivatives:

$$\frac{\partial^2 Log\, L(\alpha)}{\partial \tilde{\gamma}_{gj} \partial \tilde{\gamma}_{gj}} = -\sum_{\ell=1}^{p+1} \left\{ [\sum_{t=2}^{T} K^*_{[\ell]11}(t-1,t;g,j)][\tilde{\eta}^{(1)}_{[\ell],gj}(1)\{1-\tilde{\eta}^{(1)}_{[\ell],gj}(1)\}] \right.$$
$$+ [\sum_{t=2}^{T} K^*_{[\ell]12}(t-1,t;g,j)][\tilde{\eta}^{(2)}_{[\ell],gj}(1)\{1-\tilde{\eta}^{(2)}_{[\ell],gj}(1)\}]$$
$$+ [\sum_{t=2}^{T} K^*_{[\ell]21}(t-1,t;g,j)][\tilde{\eta}^{(1)}_{[\ell],gj}(2)\{1-\tilde{\eta}^{(1)}_{[\ell],gj}(2)\}]$$
$$\left. + [\sum_{t=2}^{T} K^*_{[\ell]22}(t-1,t;g,j)][\tilde{\eta}^{(2)}_{[\ell],gj}(2)\{1-\tilde{\eta}^{(2)}_{[\ell],gj}(2)\}] \right\}, \quad (3.378)$$

and

$$\frac{\partial^2 Log\, L(\alpha)}{\partial \tilde{\gamma}_{g'j'} \partial \tilde{\gamma}_{gj}} = 0, \text{ for all } g=g', j' \neq j; g \neq g', j' \neq j; g \neq g', j'=j; g \neq g', j' \neq j. \quad (3.379)$$

3.6.2.2 Fitting the MDL Model Subject to Order Restriction of the Categories: A Pseudo-Likelihood Approach

In Sect. 3.5.2, MDL models were fitted by assuming that the categories are nominal. In this section we fit the same MDL model (3.275)–(3.276) but by assuming that the categories are ordinal. For nominal categories, recall from (3.277) and (3.278) that the marginal probabilities at initial time $t = 1$, are given by

$$\pi_{[\ell]j}(1) = \frac{\exp(x'_{[\ell]j}\theta^*)}{1 + \sum_{g=1}^{J-1}\exp(x'_{[\ell]g}\theta^*)}, \tag{3.380}$$

for all $j = 1,\ldots,J$, and $\ell = 1,\ldots,p+1$; and the conditional probabilities at time t conditional on the response at time $t-1$ (for $t = 2,\ldots,T$) are given by

$$\eta_{t|t-1}^{(j)}(g,\ell) = \begin{cases} \frac{\exp\left(x'_{[\ell]j}\theta^* + \gamma'_j\delta_{[\ell]g}\right)}{1+\sum_{h=1}^{J-1}\exp\left(x'_{[\ell]h}\theta^* + \gamma'_h\delta_{[\ell]g}\right)} & \text{for } j = 1,\ldots,J-1;\ \ell = 1,\ldots,p+1 \\ \frac{1}{1+\sum_{h=1}^{J-1}\exp\left(x'_{[\ell]h}\theta^* + \gamma'_h\delta_{[\ell]g}\right)} & \text{for } j = J;\ \ell = 1,\ldots,p+1, \end{cases} \tag{3.381}$$

for a given $g = 1,\ldots,J$. In (3.380) and (3.381),

$$\theta^* = [\beta_1^{*\prime},\ldots,\beta_j^{*\prime},\ldots,\beta_{J-1}^{*\prime}]' : (J-1)(p+1)\times 1, \text{ with } \beta_j^* = [\beta_{j0},\ldots,\beta_{j\ell},\ldots,\beta_{jp}]',$$

represents the vector of parameters for the MDL model for nominal categorical data, and $x_{[\ell]j}$ is the design covariate vector defined as in (3.277).

Now because categories are considered to be ordinal, similar to the bivariate binary mapping based LDCP model (see (3.334) and (3.337)–(3.338)), for given cut points j at time t and g at time point $t-1$, we write the marginal and conditional probabilities in cumulative form as

$$\begin{aligned} \pi^*_{[\ell]j}(1) &= \sum_{c=j+1}^{J}\pi_{[\ell]c}(1) \\ &= \frac{\sum_{c=j+1}^{J}\exp(x'_{[\ell]c}\theta^*)}{\sum_{h=1}^{J}\exp(x'_{[\ell]h}\theta^*)}, \end{aligned} \tag{3.382}$$

with $\pi_{[\ell]c}(1)$ as in (3.380), and

$$\tilde{\eta}^{(2)}_{[\ell],gj}(1) = \frac{1}{g}\sum_{c_1=1}^{g}\sum_{c_2=j+1}^{J}\eta_{t|t-1}^{(c_2)}(c_1,\ell) \tag{3.383}$$

$$\tilde{\eta}^{(2)}_{[\ell],gj}(2) = \frac{1}{J-g}\sum_{c_1=g+1}^{J}\sum_{c_2=j+1}^{J}\eta_{t|t-1}^{(c_2)}(c_1,\ell) \tag{3.384}$$

with $\eta^{(c_2)}_{t|t-1}(c_1,\ell)$ as in (3.381). Note that as we are dealing with stationary correlations case, the conditional probabilities in (3.383)–(3.384) remain the same for all $t = 2,\ldots,T$, and hence the subscript $t|t-1$ may be suppressed. Next by using the marginal (at $t = 1$) and conditional probabilities (at $t|t-1; t = 2,\ldots,T,$) from (3.382)–(3.384), and the transitional count data corresponding to cut points (g, j), one writes the pseudo-likelihood function

$$L(\theta^*,\gamma_M) = \Pi_{\ell=1}^{p+1}\Pi_{j=1}^{J-1}\left[\left(\{1-\pi^*_{[\ell]j}(1)\}^{K^*_{[\ell]j}(1)}\right)\left(\{\pi^*_{[\ell]j}(1)\}^{K_{[\ell]}-K^*_{[\ell]j}(1)}\right)\right.$$
$$\left.\times\ \Pi_{t=2}^{T}\Pi_{g=1}^{J-1}\Pi_{g^*=1}^{2}\left(\{\tilde{\eta}^{(1)}_{[\ell],gj}(g^*)\}^{K^*_{[\ell]g^*1}(t-1,t;g,j)}\{\tilde{\eta}^{(2)}_{[\ell],gj}(g^*)\}^{K^*_{[\ell]g^*2}(t-1,t;g,j)}\right)\right], \quad (3.385)$$

which is similar but different than the likelihood function (3.341) under the LDCP model.

3.6.2.2.1 Pseudo-Likelihood Estimating Equation for θ^*

The following derivatives are required to construct the desired likelihood equation. The derivative of $\pi^*_{[\ell]j}(1)$ with respect to θ^* is the same as (3.342) under the LCDMP model. That is,

$$\frac{\partial\pi^*_{[\ell]j}(1)}{\partial\theta^*} = \sum_{c=j+1}^{J}\frac{\partial\pi_{[\ell]c}}{\partial\theta^*} = \sum_{c=j+1}^{J}\pi_{[\ell]c}p_{[\ell]c} = p^*_{[\ell]j}(\theta^*).$$

However, to compute the derivatives of the cumulative probabilities such as $\tilde{\eta}^{(2)}_{[\ell],gj}(1)$ (3.383) with respect to θ^*, by (3.286) under the MDL model, we first write

$$\frac{\partial\eta^{(j)}(g,\ell)}{\partial\theta^*} = \begin{cases}\eta^{(j)}(g,\ell)\left[x_{[\ell]j}-\eta(g,\ell)\otimes d_{[\ell]1}\right] & \text{for } \ell=1,\ldots,p;\ j=1,\ldots,J\\ \eta^{(j)}(g,\ell)\left[x_{[\ell]j}-\eta(g,\ell)\otimes d_{[\ell]2}\right] & \text{for } \ell=p+1;\ j=1,\ldots,J,\end{cases} \quad (3.386)$$

$$= \eta^{(j)}_{(1)}(g,\ell),\ \text{(say)}, \quad (3.387)$$

where

$$\eta(g,\ell) = [\eta^{(1)}(g,\ell),\ldots,\eta^{(j)}(g,\ell),\ldots,\eta^{(J-1)}(g,\ell)]'.$$

By (3.383)–(3.384), we then obtain

$$\frac{\partial\tilde{\eta}^{(2)}_{[\ell],gj}(1)}{\partial\theta^*} = \frac{1}{g}\sum_{c_1=1}^{g}\sum_{c_2=j+1}^{J}\frac{\partial\eta^{(c_2)}(c_1,\ell)}{\partial\theta^*}$$

$$= \frac{1}{g}\sum_{c_1=1}^{g}\sum_{c_2=j+1}^{J}\eta_{(1)}^{(c_2)}(c_1,\ell) = \zeta_{[\ell]gj}(1,2;\theta^*)$$

$$\frac{\partial\tilde{\eta}_{[\ell],gj}^{(2)}(2)}{\partial\theta^*} = \frac{1}{J-g}\sum_{c_1=g+1}^{J}\sum_{c_2=j+1}^{J}\frac{\partial\eta^{(c_2)}(c_1,\ell)}{\partial\theta^*}$$

$$= \frac{1}{J-g}\sum_{c_1=g+1}^{J}\sum_{c_2=j+1}^{J}\eta_{(1)}^{(c_2)}(c_1,\ell) = \zeta_{[\ell]gj}(2,2;\theta^*)$$

$$\frac{\partial\tilde{\eta}_{[\ell],gj}^{(1)}(1)}{\partial\theta^*} = -\zeta_{[\ell]gj}(1,2;\theta^*) = \zeta_{[\ell]gj}(1,1;\theta^*)$$

$$\frac{\partial\tilde{\eta}_{[\ell],gj}^{(1)}(1)}{\partial\theta^*} = -\zeta_{[\ell]gj}(2,2;\theta^*) = \zeta_{[\ell]gj}(2,1;\theta^*), \quad (3.388)$$

yielding, by (3.385), the likelihood equation for θ^* as

$$\frac{\partial Log\, L(\theta^*,\gamma_M)}{\partial\theta^*} = \sum_{\ell=1}^{p+1}\sum_{j=1}^{J-1}\left[\left\{(K_{[\ell]}-K^*_{[\ell]j}(1))\left(\frac{p^*_{[\ell]j}(\theta^*)}{\pi^*_{[\ell]j}(1)}\right) - K^*_{[\ell]j}(1)\left(\frac{p^*_{[\ell]j}(\theta^*)}{1-\pi^*_{[\ell]j}(1)}\right)\right\}\right.$$
$$+\sum_{g=1}^{J-1}\left\{-\sum_{t=2}^{T}K^*_{[\ell]11}(t-1,t;g,j)\frac{\zeta_{[\ell]gj}(1,2;\theta^*)}{\tilde{\eta}_{[\ell],gj}^{(1)}(1)} + \sum_{t=2}^{T}K^*_{[\ell]12}(t-1,t;g,j)\frac{\zeta_{[\ell]gj}(1,2;\theta^*)}{\tilde{\eta}_{[\ell],gj}^{(2)}(1)}\right.$$
$$\left.\left.-\sum_{t=2}^{T}K^*_{[\ell]21}(t-1,t;g,j)\frac{\zeta_{[\ell]gj}(2,2;\theta^*)}{\tilde{\eta}_{[\ell],gj}^{(1)}(2)} + \sum_{t=2}^{T}K^*_{[\ell]22}(t-1,t;g,j)\frac{\zeta_{[\ell]gj}(2,2;\theta^*)}{\tilde{\eta}_{[\ell],gj}^{(2)}(2)}\right\}\right]$$
$$= \tilde{h}_1(\theta^*)+\tilde{h}_2(\theta^*) = \tilde{h}(\theta^*) = 0. \quad (3.389)$$

This likelihood equation (3.389) may be solved iteratively by using

$$\hat{\theta}^*(r+1) = \hat{\theta}^*(r) - \left[\{\tilde{h}^{(1)}(\theta^*)\}^{-1}\tilde{h}(\theta^*)\right]|_{\theta^*=\hat{\theta}^*(r)}, \quad (3.390)$$

to obtain the final likelihood estimate $\hat{\theta}^*$. In (3.390), $\tilde{h}^{(1)}(\theta^*) = \frac{\partial\tilde{h}(\theta^*)}{\partial\theta^{*\prime}}$.

Computation of $\frac{\partial\tilde{h}(\theta^*)}{\partial\theta^{*\prime}}$ **:**
By (3.389),

$$h^{(1)}(\theta^*) = \frac{\partial Log\, L(\theta^*,\rho_M)}{\partial\theta^{*\prime}}$$
$$= \sum_{\ell=1}^{p+1}\sum_{j=1}^{J-1}\left[\left\{(K_{[\ell]}-K^*_{[\ell]j}(1))\left(\frac{p^{*(1)}_{[\ell]j}(\theta^*,\theta^*)}{\pi^*_{[\ell]j}(1)} - \frac{p^*_{[\ell]j}(\theta^*)p^{*\prime}_{[\ell]j}(\theta^*)}{[\pi^*_{[\ell]j}(1)]^2}\right)\right.\right.$$

$$- K^*_{[\ell]j}(1)\left(\frac{p^*_{[\ell]j}(\theta^*)p^{*'}_{[\ell]j}(\theta^*)}{[1-\pi^*_{[\ell]j}(1)]^2} + \frac{p^{*(1)}_{[\ell]j}(\theta^*,\theta^*)}{1-\pi^*_{[\ell]j}(1)}\right)\Bigg\}$$

$$+ \sum_{g=1}^{J-1}\Bigg[-\Bigg\{\sum_{t=2}^{T} K^*_{[\ell]11}(t-1,t;g,j)\left(\frac{\zeta^{(1)}_{[\ell]gj}(1,2;\theta^*,\theta^*)}{\tilde{\eta}^{(1)}_{[\ell],gj}(1)} - \frac{\zeta_{[\ell]gj}(1,2;\theta^*)\zeta'_{[\ell]gj}(1,2;\theta^*)}{[\tilde{\eta}^{(1)}_{[\ell],gj}(1)]^2}\right)\Bigg\}$$

$$+ \Bigg\{\sum_{t=2}^{T} K^*_{[\ell]12}(t-1,t;g,j)\left(\frac{\zeta^{(1)}_{[\ell]gj}(1,2;\theta^*,\theta^*)}{\tilde{\eta}^{(2)}_{[\ell],gj}(1)} - \frac{\zeta_{[\ell]gj}(1,2;\theta^*)\zeta'_{[\ell]gj}(1,2;\theta^*)}{[\tilde{\eta}^{(2)}_{[\ell],gj}(1)]^2}\right)\Bigg\}$$

$$- \Bigg\{\sum_{t=2}^{T} K^*_{[\ell]21}(t-1,t;g,j)\left(\frac{\zeta^{(1)}_{[\ell]gj}(2,2;\theta^*,\theta^*)}{\tilde{\eta}^{(1)}_{[\ell],gj}(2)} - \frac{\zeta_{[\ell]gj}(2,2;\theta^*)\zeta'_{[\ell]gj}(2,2;\theta^*)}{[\tilde{\eta}^{(1)}_{[\ell],gj}(2)]^2}\right)\Bigg\}$$

$$+ \Bigg\{\sum_{t=2}^{T} K^*_{[\ell]22}(t-1,t;g,j)\left(\frac{\zeta^{(1)}_{[\ell]gj}(2,2;\theta^*,\theta^*)}{\tilde{\eta}^{(2)}_{[\ell],gj}(2)} - \frac{\zeta_{[\ell]gj}(2,2;\theta^*)\zeta'_{[\ell]gj}(2,2;\theta^*)}{[\tilde{\eta}^{(2)}_{[\ell],gj}(2)]^2}\right)\Bigg\}\Bigg]\Bigg], \quad (3.391)$$

where $p^{*(1)}_{[\ell]j}(\theta^*,\theta^*)$ is given by (3.347)–(3.348), and the remaining two second order derivative matrices in (3.391) are given by

$$\zeta^{(1)}_{[\ell]gj}(1,2;\theta^*,\theta^*) = \frac{\partial \zeta_{[\ell]gj}(1,2;\theta^*)}{\partial \theta^{*'}} = \frac{1}{g}\sum_{c_1=1}^{g}\sum_{c_2=j+1}^{J}\frac{\partial \eta^{(c_2)}_{(1)}(c_1,\ell)}{\partial \theta^{*'}}, \quad (3.392)$$

$$\zeta^{(1)}_{[\ell]gj}(2,2;\theta^*,\theta^*) = \frac{\partial \zeta_{[\ell]gj}(2,2;\theta^*)}{\partial \theta^{*'}} = \frac{1}{J-g}\sum_{c_1=g+1}^{J}\sum_{c_2=j+1}^{J}\frac{\partial \eta^{(c_2)}_{(1)}(c_1,\ell)}{\partial \theta^{*'}}, \quad (3.393)$$

where, for

$$\eta^{(c_2)}_{(1)}(c_1,\ell) = \begin{cases} \eta^{(c_2)}(c_1,\ell)\left[x_{[\ell]c_2} - \eta(c_1,\ell)\otimes d_{[\ell]1}\right] & \text{for } \ell = 1,\ldots,p \\ \eta^{(c_2)}(c_1,\ell)\left[x_{[\ell]c_2} - \eta(c_1,\ell)\otimes d_{[\ell]2}\right] & \text{for } \ell = p+1, \end{cases} \quad (3.394)$$

(see (3.386)–(3.387)) with

$$\eta(c_1,\ell) = [\eta^{(1)}(c_1,\ell),\ldots,\eta^{(j)}(c_1,\ell),\ldots,\eta^{(J-1)}(c_1,\ell)]',$$

the second order derivative $\frac{\partial \eta^{(c_2)}_{(1)}(c_1,\ell)}{\partial \theta^{*'}}$ by (3.287)–(3.288) has the formula

$$\frac{\partial \eta^{(c_2)}_{(1)}(c_1,\ell)}{\partial \theta^{*'}} = \eta^{(c_2)}(c_1,\ell)M^*_{[\ell]c_2}(x,\eta(c_1,\ell))$$

$$= \begin{cases} \eta^{(c_2)}(c_1,\ell)\left[(x_{[\ell]c_2} - \eta(c_1,\ell)\otimes d_{[\ell]1})(x_{[\ell]c_2} - \eta(c_1,\ell)\otimes d_{[\ell]1})' - \frac{\partial \eta(c_1,\ell)}{\partial \theta^{*'}}\right] & \text{for } \ell = 1,\ldots,p \\ \eta^{(c_2)}(c_1,\ell)\left[(x_{[\ell]c_2} - \eta(c_1,\ell)\otimes d_{[\ell]2})(x_{[\ell]c_2} - \eta(c_1,\ell)\otimes d_{[\ell]1})' - \frac{\partial \eta(c_1,\ell)}{\partial \theta^{*'}}\right] & \text{for } \ell = p+1, \end{cases}$$

with $\frac{\partial \eta(c_1,\ell)}{\partial \theta^{*'}}$ given as in (3.290).

3.6.2.2.2 Pseudo-Likelihood Estimating Equation for γ_M

The likelihood estimation of γ_M is equivalent to estimate $\gamma_c : (J-1) \times 1$, for $c = 1,\ldots,J-1$, by maximizing the log likelihood function $Log\,L(\theta^*,\gamma_M)$ computed from (3.385). Note that for a given cut point j, either $c \le j$ or $c > j$ holds. Next, because $\pi^*_{[\ell]j}(1)$ is free of γ_c, for any c and j, the pseudo-likelihood estimating equation for γ_c can be computed as

$$\frac{\partial Log\,L(\theta^*,\gamma_M)}{\partial \gamma_c} = \sum_{\ell=1}^{p+1}\sum_{j=1}^{J-1}\sum_{g=1}^{J-1}\left[\sum_{t=2}^{T} K^*_{[\ell]11}(t-1,t;g,j)\left\{\frac{\zeta^*_{[\ell]gj}(1,1;\gamma_c)}{\tilde{\eta}^{(1)}_{[\ell],gj}(1)}\right\}\right.$$

$$+ \sum_{t=2}^{T} K^*_{[\ell]12}(t-1,t;g,j)\left\{\frac{\zeta^*_{[\ell]gj}(1,2;\gamma_c)}{\tilde{\eta}^{(2)}_{[\ell],gj}(1)}\right\}$$

$$+ \sum_{t=2}^{T} K^*_{[\ell]21}(t-1,t;g,j)\left\{\frac{\zeta^*_{[\ell]gj}(2,1;\rho_c)}{\tilde{\eta}^{(1)}_{[\ell],gj}(2)}\right\}$$

$$\left. + \sum_{t=2}^{T} K^*_{[\ell]22}(t-1,t;g,j)\left\{\frac{\zeta^*_{[\ell]gj}(2,2;\gamma_c)}{\tilde{\eta}^{(2)}_{[\ell],gj}(2)}\right\}\right] = 0, \tag{3.395}$$

where, for example,

$$\zeta^*_{[\ell]gj}(1,2;\gamma_c) = \frac{\partial \tilde{\eta}^{(2)}_{[\ell],gj}(1)}{\partial \gamma_c}, \tag{3.396}$$

for a general $c \le j$ or $c > j$, j being the cut point at time t. More specifically, because

$$\frac{\partial \eta^{(h)}(g,\ell)}{\partial \gamma_j} = \begin{cases} \delta_{[\ell]g}\eta^{(j)}(g,\ell)[1-\eta^{(j)}(g,\ell)] & \text{for } h = j; h,j = 1,\ldots,J-1 \\ -\delta_{[\ell]g}\eta^{(j)}(g,\ell)\eta^{(h)}(g,\ell) & \text{for } h \ne j; h,j = 1,\ldots,J-1 \\ -\delta_{[\ell]g}\eta^{(j)}(g,\ell)\eta^{(J)}(g,\ell) & \text{for } h = J;\ j = 1,\ldots,J-1, \end{cases}$$

by (3.225), the derivatives of the conditional probabilities in (3.395), that is, the formulas for $\zeta^*_{[\ell]gj}(\cdot,\cdot;\gamma_c)$, at cut point (g,j), are given by

$$\frac{\partial \tilde{\eta}^{(2)}_{[\ell],gj}(1)}{\partial \gamma_c} = \frac{1}{g}\sum_{c_1=1}^{g}\left[\sum_{c_2=j+1}^{J}\frac{\partial \eta^{(c_2)}(c_1,\ell)}{\partial \gamma_c}\right] = \zeta^*_{[\ell]gj}(1,2;\gamma_c)$$

$$= \begin{cases} -\frac{1}{g}\sum_{c_1=1}^{g}\delta_{[\ell]c_1}\eta^{(c)}(c_1,\ell)\sum_{c_2=j+1}^{J}\eta^{(c_2)}(c_1,\ell) & \text{for } c \le j \\ \frac{1}{g}\sum_{c_1=1}^{g}\delta_{[\ell]c_1}\eta^{(c)}(c_1,\ell)\left[1-\sum_{c_2=j+1}^{J}\eta^{(c_2)}(c_1,\ell)\right] & \text{for } j < c \le (J-1), \end{cases} \tag{3.397}$$

$$\frac{\partial \tilde{\eta}^{(2)}_{[\ell],gj}(2)}{\partial \gamma_c} = \frac{1}{J-g}\sum_{c_1=g+1}^{J}\left[\sum_{c_2=j+1}^{J}\frac{\partial \eta^{(c_2)}(c_1,\ell)}{\partial \gamma_c}\right] = \zeta^*_{[\ell]gj}(2,2;\gamma_c)$$

$$= \begin{cases} -\frac{1}{J-g}\sum_{c_1=g+1}^{J}\delta_{[\ell]c_1}\eta^{(c)}(c_1,\ell)\sum_{c_2=j+1}^{J}\eta^{(c_2)}(c_1,\ell) & \text{for } c \le j \\ \frac{1}{J-g}\sum_{c_1=g+1}^{J}\delta_{[\ell]c_1}\eta^{(c)}(c_1,\ell)\left[1-\sum_{c_2=j+1}^{J}\eta^{(c_2)}(c_1,\ell)\right] & \text{for } j < c \le (J-1), \end{cases} \tag{3.398}$$

$$\frac{\partial \tilde{\eta}^{(1)}_{[\ell],gj}(1)}{\partial \gamma_c} = -\frac{\partial \tilde{\eta}^{(2)}_{[\ell],gj}(1)}{\partial \gamma_c} = -\zeta^*_{[\ell]gj}(1,2;\gamma_c) = \zeta^*_{[\ell]gj}(1,1;\gamma_c), \tag{3.399}$$

and

$$\frac{\partial \tilde{\eta}^{(1)}_{[\ell],gj}(2)}{\partial \gamma_c} = -\frac{\partial \tilde{\eta}^{(2)}_{[\ell],gj}(2)}{\partial \gamma_c} = -\zeta^*_{[\ell]gj}(2,2;\gamma_c) = \zeta^*_{[\ell]gj}(1,1;\gamma_c). \tag{3.400}$$

Thus, the computation for the estimating equation (3.395) is complete, yielding the estimating equation for $\gamma^* = (\gamma_1',\ldots,\gamma_j',\ldots,\gamma_{J-1}')'$, (i.e., for the elements of γ_M) as

$$\frac{\partial Log\, L(\theta^*,\gamma_M)}{\partial \gamma^*} = \begin{pmatrix} \frac{\partial Log\, L(\theta^*,\gamma_M)}{\partial \gamma_1} \\ \vdots \\ \frac{\partial Log\, L(\theta^*,\gamma_M)}{\partial \gamma_c} \\ \vdots \\ \frac{\partial Log\, L(\theta^*,\gamma_M)}{\partial \gamma_{J-1}} \end{pmatrix} = 0 : (J-1)^2 \times 1. \tag{3.401}$$

This estimating equation may be solved by using the iterative equation

$$\hat{\gamma}^*(r+1) = \hat{\gamma}^*(r) - \left[\left\{\frac{\partial^2 \text{Log}\, L(\theta^*,\gamma_M)}{\partial \gamma^* \partial \gamma^{*\prime}}\right\}^{-1}\frac{\partial \text{Log}\, L(\theta^*,\gamma_M)}{\partial \gamma^*}\right]_{|\gamma^*=\hat{\gamma}^*(r)}, \tag{3.402}$$

where

$$\frac{\partial^2 Log\, L(\theta^*,\gamma_M)}{\partial \gamma^* \partial \gamma^{*\prime}} = \begin{pmatrix} \frac{\partial^2 Log\, L(\theta^*,\gamma_M)}{\partial \gamma_1 \partial \gamma_1'} & \cdots & \frac{\partial^2 Log\, L(\theta^*,\gamma_M)}{\partial \gamma_1 \partial \gamma_c'} & \cdots & \frac{\partial^2 Log\, L(\theta^*,\gamma_M)}{\partial \gamma_1 \partial \gamma_{J-1}'} \\ \vdots & & \vdots & & \vdots \\ \frac{\partial^2 Log\, L(\theta^*,\gamma_M)}{\partial \gamma_c \partial \gamma_1'} & \cdots & \frac{\partial^2 Log\, L(\theta^*,\gamma_M)}{\partial \gamma_c \partial \gamma_c'} & \cdots & \frac{\partial^2 Log\, L(\theta^*,\gamma_M)}{\partial \gamma_c \partial \gamma_{J-1}'} \\ \vdots & & \vdots & & \vdots \\ \frac{\partial^2 Log\, L(\theta^*,\gamma_M)}{\partial \gamma_{J-1} \partial \gamma_1'} & \cdots & \frac{\partial^2 Log\, L(\theta^*,\gamma_M)}{\partial \gamma_{J-1} \partial \gamma_j'} & \cdots & \frac{\partial^2 Log\, L(\theta^*,\gamma_M)}{\partial \gamma_{J-1} \partial \gamma_{J-1}'} \end{pmatrix}. \tag{3.403}$$

The second order derivatives involved in (3.403) may be computed by using the first order derivatives from (3.397)–(3.400) into (3.395). To be specific, two general second order derivatives are:

$$\begin{aligned} \frac{\partial^2 Log\, L(\theta^*,\gamma_M)}{\partial \gamma_c \partial \gamma_c'} &= \sum_{\ell=1}^{p+1}\sum_{j=1}^{J-1}\sum_{g=1}^{J-1}\left[\sum_{t=2}^{T} K^*_{[\ell]11}(t-1,t;g,j)\right. \\ &\times \left\{-\frac{[\zeta^*_{[\ell]gj}(1,1;\gamma_c)\zeta^{*\prime}_{[\ell]gj}(1,1;\gamma_c)]}{[\tilde{\eta}^{(1)}_{[\ell],gj}(1)]^2} + \frac{[\zeta^{**}_{[\ell]gj}(1,1;\gamma_c,\gamma_c)]}{[\tilde{\eta}^{(1)}_{[\ell],gj}(1)]}\right\} \\ &+ \sum_{t=2}^{T} K^*_{[\ell]12}(t-1,t;g,j)\left\{-\frac{[\zeta^*_{[\ell]gj}(1,2;\gamma_c)\zeta^{*\prime}_{[\ell]gj}(1,2;\gamma_c)]}{[\tilde{\eta}^{(2)}_{[\ell],gj}(1)]^2} + \frac{[\zeta^{**}_{[\ell]gj}(1,2;\gamma_c,\gamma_c)]}{[\tilde{\eta}^{(2)}_{[\ell],gj}(1)]}\right\} \\ &+ \sum_{t=2}^{T} K^*_{[\ell]21}(t-1,t;g,j)\left\{-\frac{[\zeta^*_{[\ell]gj}(2,1;\gamma_c)\zeta^{*\prime}_{[\ell]gj}(2,1;\gamma_c)]}{[\tilde{\eta}^{(1)}_{[\ell],gj}(2)]^2} + \frac{[\zeta^{**}_{[\ell]gj}(2,1;\gamma_c,\gamma_c)]}{[\tilde{\eta}^{(1)}_{[\ell],gj}(2)]}\right\} \\ &+ \sum_{t=2}^{T} K^*_{[\ell]22}(t-1,t;g,j)\left\{-\frac{[\zeta^*_{[\ell]gj}(2,2;\gamma_c)\zeta^{*\prime}_{[\ell]gj}(2,2;\gamma_c)]}{[\tilde{\eta}^{(2)}_{[\ell],gj}(2)]^2}\right. \\ &\left.\left. + \frac{[\zeta^{**}_{[\ell]gj}(2,2;\gamma_c,\gamma_c)]}{[\tilde{\eta}^{(2)}_{[\ell],gj}(2)]}\right\}\right] \end{aligned} \tag{3.404}$$

and

$$\begin{aligned} \frac{\partial^2 Log\, L(\theta^*,\gamma_M)}{\partial \gamma_c \partial \gamma_d'} &= \sum_{\ell=1}^{p+1}\sum_{j=1}^{J-1}\sum_{g=1}^{J-1}\left[\sum_{t=2}^{T} K^*_{[\ell]11}(t-1,t;g,j)\right. \\ &\times \left\{-\frac{[\zeta^*_{[\ell]gj}(1,1;\gamma_c)\zeta^{*\prime}_{[\ell]gj}(1,1;\gamma_d)]}{[\tilde{\eta}^{(1)}_{[\ell],gj}(1)]^2} + \frac{[\zeta^{**}_{[\ell]gj}(1,1;\gamma_c,\gamma_d)]}{[\tilde{\eta}^{(1)}_{[\ell],gj}(1)]}\right\} \end{aligned}$$

$$+ \sum_{t=2}^{T} K^*_{[\ell]12}(t-1,t;g,j) \left\{ -\frac{[\zeta^*_{[\ell]gj}(1,2;\gamma_c)\zeta^{*\prime}_{[\ell]gj}(1,2;\gamma_d)]}{[\tilde{\eta}^{(2)}_{[\ell],gj}(1)]^2} + \frac{[\zeta^{**}_{[\ell]gj}(1,2;\gamma_c,\gamma_d)]}{[\tilde{\eta}^{(2)}_{[\ell],gj}(1)]} \right\}$$

$$+ \sum_{t=2}^{T} K^*_{[\ell]21}(t-1,t;g,j) \left\{ -\frac{[\zeta^*_{[\ell]gj}(2,1;\gamma_c)\zeta^{*\prime}_{[\ell]gj}(2,1;\gamma_d)]}{[\tilde{\eta}^{(1)}_{[\ell],gj}(2)]^2} + \frac{[\zeta^{**}_{[\ell]gj}(2,1;\gamma_c,\gamma_d)]}{[\tilde{\eta}^{(1)}_{[\ell],gj}(2)]} \right\}$$

$$+ \sum_{t=2}^{T} K^*_{[\ell]22}(t-1,t;g,j) \left\{ -\frac{[\zeta^*_{[\ell]gj}(2,2;\gamma_c)\zeta^{*\prime}_{[\ell]gj}(2,2;\gamma_d)]}{[\tilde{\eta}^{(2)}_{[\ell],gj}(2)]^2} \right.$$

$$\left. + \frac{[\zeta^{**}_{[\ell]gj}(2,2;\gamma_c,\gamma_d)]}{[\tilde{\eta}^{(2)}_{[\ell],gj}(2)]} \right\} \Bigg], \tag{3.405}$$

where, for example,

$$\zeta^{**}_{[\ell]gj}(1,1;\gamma_c,\gamma_c) = \frac{\partial \zeta^*_{[\ell]gj}(1,1;\gamma_c)}{\partial \gamma_c'}$$

$$\zeta^{**}_{[\ell]gj}(1,1;\gamma_c,\gamma_d) = \frac{\partial \zeta^*_{[\ell]gj}(1,1;\gamma_c)}{\partial \gamma_d'}, \text{ for } c \neq d,\ c,d = 1,\ldots,J-1. \tag{3.406}$$

The second order derivative matrices in (3.404) may be computed as follows. By using the basic derivatives for conditional probabilities from (3.225) into (3.397), one obtains

$$\zeta^{**}_{[\ell]gj}(1,2;\gamma_c,\gamma_c)$$

$$= \frac{\partial}{\partial \gamma_c'} \begin{cases} -\frac{1}{g}\sum_{c_1=1}^{g} \delta_{[\ell]c_1} \eta^{(c)}(c_1,\ell) \sum_{c_2=j+1}^{J} \eta^{(c_2)}(c_1,\ell) & \text{for } c \leq j \\ \frac{1}{g}\sum_{c_1=1}^{g} \delta_{[\ell]c_1} \eta^{(c)}(c_1,\ell) \left[1 - \sum_{c_2=j+1}^{J} \eta^{(c_2)}(c_1,\ell)\right] & \text{for } j < c \leq (J-1) \end{cases}$$

$$= \begin{cases} -\frac{1}{g}\sum_{c_1=1}^{g} \delta_{[\ell]c_1} \delta'_{[\ell]c_1} \eta^{(c)}(c_1,\ell) \left[\{1-2\eta^{(c)}(c_1,\ell)\} \sum_{c_2=j+1}^{J} \eta^{(c_2)}(c_1,\ell)\right] & \text{for } c \leq j \\ \frac{1}{g}\sum_{c_1=1}^{g} \delta_{[\ell]c_1} \delta'_{[\ell]c_1} \eta^{(c)}(c_1,\ell) & \\ \times \left[\{1-\eta^{(c)}(c_1,\ell)\} - \{1-2\eta^{(c)}(c_1,\ell)\} \sum_{c_2=j+1}^{J} \eta^{(c_2)}(c_1,\ell)\right] & \text{for } j < c \leq (J-1), \end{cases} \tag{3.407}$$

$$\zeta^{**}_{[\ell]gj}(2,2;\gamma_c,\gamma_c)$$

$$= \frac{\partial}{\partial \gamma_c'} \begin{cases} -\frac{1}{J-g}\sum_{c_1=g+1}^{J} \delta_{[\ell]c_1} \eta^{(c)}(c_1,\ell) \sum_{c_2=j+1}^{J} \eta^{(c_2)}(c_1,\ell) & \text{for } c \leq j \\ \frac{1}{J-g}\sum_{c_1=g+1}^{J} \delta_{[\ell]c_1} \eta^{(c)}(c_1,\ell) \left[\{1 - \sum_{c_2=j+1}^{J} \eta^{(c_2)}(c_1,\ell)\right] & \text{for } j < c \leq (J-1) \end{cases}$$

$$= \begin{cases} -\frac{1}{J-g}\sum_{c_1=g+1}^{J}\delta_{[\ell]c_1}\delta'_{[\ell]c_1}\eta^{(c)}(c_1,\ell)\left[\{1-2\eta^{(c)}(c_1,\ell)\}\sum_{c_2=j+1}^{J}\eta^{(c_2)}(c_1,\ell)\right] & \text{for } c \leq j \\ \frac{1}{J-g}\sum_{c_1=g+1}^{J}\delta_{[\ell]c_1}\delta'_{[\ell]c_1}\eta^{(c)}(c_1,\ell) & \\ \times\left[\{1-\eta^{(c)}(c_1,\ell)\}-\{1-2\eta^{(c)}(c_1,\ell)\}\sum_{c_2=j+1}^{J}\eta^{(c_2)}(c_1,\ell)\right] & \text{for } j < c \leq (J-1), \end{cases} \tag{3.408}$$

and

$$\begin{aligned} \zeta^{**}_{[\ell]gj}(1,1;\gamma_c,\gamma_c) &= -\zeta^{**}_{[\ell]gj}(1,2;\gamma_c,\gamma_c) \\ \zeta^{**}_{[\ell]gj}(2,1;\gamma_c,\gamma_c) &= -\zeta^{**}_{[\ell]gj}(2,2;\gamma_c,\gamma_c). \end{aligned} \tag{3.409}$$

Similarly the second order derivative matrices in (3.405) may be computed by using the basic derivatives for conditional probabilities from (3.225) into (3.397). That is,

$$\zeta^{**}_{[\ell]gj}(1,2;\gamma_c,\gamma_d) \tag{3.410}$$

$$= \frac{\partial}{\partial\gamma'_d}\begin{cases} -\frac{1}{g}\sum_{c_1=1}^{g}\delta_{[\ell]c_1}\eta^{(c)}(c_1,\ell)\sum_{c_2=j+1}^{J}\eta^{(c_2)}(c_1,\ell) & \text{for } c \leq j \\ \frac{1}{g}\sum_{c_1=1}^{g}\delta_{[\ell]c_1}\eta^{(c)}(c_1,\ell)\left[1-\sum_{c_2=j+1}^{J}\eta^{(c_2)}(c_1,\ell)\right] & \text{for } j < c \leq (J-1) \end{cases}$$

$$= \begin{cases} \frac{2}{g}\sum_{c_1=1}^{g}\delta_{[\ell]c_1}\delta'_{[\ell]c_1}\eta^{(c)}(c_1,\ell)\eta^{(d)}(c_1,\ell)\left[\sum_{c_2=j+1}^{J}\eta^{(c_2)}(c_1,\ell)\right] & \text{for } c \leq j;\ d \leq j \\ -\frac{1}{g}\sum_{c_1=1}^{g}\delta_{[\ell]c_1}\delta'_{[\ell]c_1}\eta^{(c)}(c_1,\ell)\eta^{(d)}(c_1,\ell)\left[1-2\sum_{c_2=j+1}^{J}\eta^{(c_2)}(c_1,\ell)\right] & \text{for } c \leq j;\ d > j \\ -\frac{1}{g}\sum_{c_1=1}^{g}\delta_{[\ell]c_1}\delta'_{[\ell]c_1}\eta^{(c)}(c_1,\ell)\eta^{(d)}(c_1,\ell)\left[1-2\sum_{c_2=j+1}^{J}\eta^{(c_2)}(c_1,\ell)\right] & \text{for } c > j;\ d \leq j \\ -\frac{2}{g}\sum_{c_1=1}^{g}\delta_{[\ell]c_1}\delta'_{[\ell]c_1}\eta^{(c)}(c_1,\ell)\eta^{(d)}(c_1,\ell)\left[1-\sum_{c_2=j+1}^{J}\eta^{(c_2)}(c_1,\ell)\right] & \text{for } c > j;\ d > j, \end{cases}$$

$$\zeta^{**}_{[\ell]gj}(2,2;\gamma_c,\gamma_d) \tag{3.411}$$

$$= \frac{\partial}{\partial\gamma'_d}\begin{cases} -\frac{1}{J-g}\sum_{c_1=g+1}^{J}\delta_{[\ell]c_1}\eta^{(c)}(c_1,\ell)\sum_{c_2=j+1}^{J}\eta^{(c_2)}(c_1,\ell) & \text{for } c \leq j \\ \frac{1}{J-g}\sum_{c_1=g+1}^{J}\delta_{[\ell]c_1}\eta^{(c)}(c_1,\ell)\left[1-\sum_{c_2=j+1}^{J}\eta^{(c_2)}(c_1,\ell)\right] & \text{for } j < c \leq (J-1) \end{cases}$$

$$= \begin{cases} \frac{2}{J-g}\sum_{c_1=g+1}^{J}\delta_{[\ell]c_1}\delta'_{[\ell]c_1}\eta^{(c)}(c_1,\ell)\eta^{(d)}(c_1,\ell)\left[\sum_{c_2=j+1}^{J}\eta^{(c_2)}(c_1,\ell)\right] & \text{for } c \leq j;\ d \leq j \\ -\frac{1}{J-g}\sum_{c_1=g+1}^{J}\delta_{[\ell]c_1}\delta'_{[\ell]c_1}\eta^{(c)}(c_1,\ell)\eta^{(d)}(c_1,\ell)\left[1-2\sum_{c_2=j+1}^{J}\eta^{(c_2)}(c_1,\ell)\right] & \text{for } c \leq j;\ d > j \\ -\frac{1}{J-g}\sum_{c_1=g+1}^{J}\delta_{[\ell]c_1}\delta'_{[\ell]c_1}\eta^{(c)}(c_1,\ell)\eta^{(d)}(c_1,\ell)\left[1-2\sum_{c_2=j+1}^{J}\eta^{(c_2)}(c_1,\ell)\right] & \text{for } c > j;\ d \leq j \\ -\frac{2}{J-g}\sum_{c_1=g+1}^{J}\delta_{[\ell]c_1}\delta'_{[\ell]c_1}\eta^{(c)}(c_1,\ell)\eta^{(d)}(c_1,\ell)\left[1-\sum_{c_2=j+1}^{J}\eta^{(c_2)}(c_1,\ell)\right] & \text{for } c > j;\ d > j, \end{cases}$$

and

$$\begin{aligned} \zeta^{**}_{[\ell]gj}(1,1;\gamma_c,\gamma_d) &= -\zeta^{**}_{[\ell]gj}(1,2;\gamma_c,\gamma_d) \\ \zeta^{**}_{[\ell]gj}(2,1;\gamma_c,\gamma_d) &= -\zeta^{**}_{[\ell]gj}(2,2;\gamma_c,\gamma_d). \end{aligned} \tag{3.412}$$

References

Agresti, A. (1989). A survey of models for repeated ordered categorical response data. *Statistics in Medicine*, *8*, 1209–1224.

Agresti, A. (1990). *Categorical Data Analysis* (1st ed.). New York: Wiley.

Agresti, A. (2002). *Categorical Data Analysis* (2nd ed.). New York: Wiley.

Amemiya, T. (1985). *Advanced Econometrics*. Cambridge, MA: Harvard University Press.

Conaway, M. R. (1989). Analysis of repeated categorical measurements with conditional likelihood methods. *Journal of the American Statistical Association*, *84*, 53–62.

Farrell, P. J. & Sutradhar, B. C. (2006). A non-linear conditional probability model for generating correlated binary data. *Statistics and Probability Letters*, *76*, 353–361.

Fienberg, S. E., Bromet, E. J., Follmann, D., Lambert, D., & May, S. M. (1985). Longitudinal analysis of categorical epidemiological data: A study of three mile island. *Enviromental Health Perspectives*, *63*, 241–248.

Honore, B. E. & Kyriazidou, E (2000). Panel data discrete choice models with lagged dependent variables. *Econometica*, *68*, 839–874.

Liang, K.-Y. & Zeger, S. L. (1986). Longitudinal data analysis using generalized linear models. *Biometrika*, *73*, 13–22.

Lipsitz, S. R., Laird, N. M., & Harrington, D. P. (1991). Generalized estimating equations for correlated binary data: Using the odds ratio as a measure of association. *Biometrika*, *78*, 153–160.

Manski, C. F. (1987).Semi-parametric analysis of random effects linear models from binary panel data. *Econometrica*. 55, 357–362.

Oman, S, D. & Zucker, D. M. (2001). Modelling and generating correlated binary variables. *Biometrika*, *88*, 287–290.

Park, C. G., Park, T., & Shin, D. W. (1996). A simple method for generating correlated binary variates. *The American Statistician*, *50*, 306–310.

Poleto, F. Z., Singer, J. M., & Paulino, C. D. (2013). A product-multinomial framework for categorical data analysis with missing responses. *Brazilian Journal of Probability and Statistics* (Accepted). doi:10.1214/12-BJPS198

Prentice, R. L. (1988). Correlated binary regression with covariates specific to each binary observation. *Biometrics*, *44*, 1033–1048.

Qaqish, B. F. (2003). A family of multivariate binary distributions for simulating correlated binary variables with specified marginal means and correlations. *Biometrika*, *90*, 455–463.

Sutradhar, B. C. (2003). An overview on regression models for discrete longitudinal responses. *Statistical Science*, *18*, 377–393.

Sutradhar, B. C. (2010a). Inferences in generalized linear longitudinal mixed models. *Canadian Journal of Statistics*, *38*, 174–196 (Special issue).

Sutradhar, B. C. (2010b). Generalized Quasi-likelihood (GQL) Inference. *StatProb: The Encyclopedia Sponsored by Statistics and Probability Societies*. Freely available at http://statprob.com/encyclopedia/GeneralizedQuasiLikelihoodGQLInferences.html

Sutradhar, B. C. (2011). *Dynamic Mixed Models for Familial Longitudinal Data*. New York: Springer.

Sutradhar, B. C. & Farrell, P. J. (2007). On optimal lag 1 dependence estimation for dynamic binary models with application to asthma data. *Sankhya, B*, *69*, 448–467.

Sutradhar, B. C., Bari, W., & Das, K. (2010). On probit versus logit dynamic mixed models for binary panel data. *Journal of Statistical Computation and Simulation*, *80*, 421–441.

Sutradhar, B. C., Rao, R. P., & Pandit, V. N. (2008). Generalized method of moments and generalized quasi-likelihood inferences in binary panel data models. *Sankhya, B*, *70*, 34–62.

Yi, G. Y. & Cook, R. J. (2002). Marginal methods for incomplete longitudinal data arising in clusters. *Journal of the American Statistical Association*, *97*, 1071–1080.

Zeger, S. L., Liang, K.-Y., & Albert, P. S. (1988). Models for longitudinal data: A generalized estimating equations approach. *Biometrics*, *44*, 1049–1060.

Zeger, S. L., Liang, K.-Y., & Self, S. G. (1985). The analysis of binary longitudinal data with time dependent covariates. *Biometrika*, *72*, 31–38.

Chapter 4
Regression Models For Univariate Longitudinal Non-stationary Categorical Data

4.1 Model Background

In Chap. 3, specifically in Sects. 3.4.1 and 3.4.2, we have studied covariates free LDCMP (linear dynamic conditional multinomial probability) and MDL (multinomial dynamic logit) models. Because the models were free from covariates, the underlying correlation structures (see (3.157) for LDCMP model, and (3.208) for BDL model) are free from covariates and hence stationary. These correlations depend only on lags. These models were extended in Sects. 3.5.1 and 3.5.2 to the cases involving covariates, but the covariates were time independent. Consequently, these models also have stationary correlation structure. See these stationary correlation structures for the binary (2 category) case given in Sect. 3.3.1.1 ($\tilde{C}(\rho)$) for the LDCP model and (3.128) for the BDL model. In this chapter, we deal with a general situation where the covariates collected from an individual over time may be time dependent. Time dependent covariates cause non-stationary correlations which makes the inference procedures relatively difficult as compared to the stationary covariates cases, which is, however, not discussed in the literature adequately for the multinomial response models. For differences in inferences between the stationary and non-stationary binary models, one may refer to Chap. 7 in Sutradhar (2011).

Turning back to the multinomial models with time dependent covariates, for convenience we re-express (3.4) here from Chap. 3 to begin the discussion on non-stationary multinomial models. Thus, in the non-stationary case, we formulate the marginal probability for y_{it} to belong to the jth category as

$$P[y_{it} = y_{it}^{(j)} = \delta_{itj}] = \pi_{(it)j} = \begin{cases} \frac{\exp(\beta_{j0}+\beta_j' w_{it})}{1+\sum_{g=1}^{J-1}\exp(\beta_{g0}+\beta_g' w_{it})} & \text{for } j = 1,\ldots,J-1 \\ \frac{1}{1+\sum_{g=1}^{J-1}\exp(\beta_{g0}+\beta_g' w_{it})} & \text{for } j = J, \end{cases} \quad (4.1)$$

B.C. Sutradhar, *Longitudinal Categorical Data Analysis*, Springer Series in Statistics, DOI 10.1007/978-1-4939-2137-9_4

where $\beta_j = [\beta_{j1}, \ldots, \beta_{js}, \ldots, \beta_{jp}]'$ for $j = 1, \ldots, J-1$, is the regression effects of the time dependent covariates w_{it}, with $w_{it} = [w_{it1}, \ldots, w_{its}, \ldots, w_{itp}]'$. Note that some of the p covariates may be time independent. This marginal probability in (4.1) yields the marginal mean vector and covariance matrix for the multinomial response $y_{it} = (y_{it1}, \ldots, y_{itj}, \ldots, y_{it,J-1})'$ at time t as follows: The mean vector is given by

$$E[Y_{it}] = \sum_{g=1}^{J-1} y_{it}^{(g)} P[Y_{it} = y_{it}^{(g)}] = \sum_{g=1}^{J-1} y_{it}^{(g)} \pi_{(it)g}$$
$$= [\pi_{(it)1}, \ldots, \pi_{(it)j}, \ldots, \pi_{(it)(J-1)}]' = \pi_{(it)} : (J-1) \times 1, \tag{4.2}$$

for all $t = 1, \ldots, T$, and by similar calculations as in (3.149)–(3.150), the covariance matrix has the form

$$\Sigma_{(i,tt)}(\beta) = \text{var}[Y_{it}] = \text{diag}[\pi_{(it)1}, \ldots, \pi_{(it)j}, \ldots, \pi_{(it)(J-1)}] - \pi_{(it)}\pi'_{(it)} : (J-1) \times (J-1), \tag{4.3}$$

for all $t = 1, \ldots, T$; and $i = 1, \ldots, K$, where β denotes all regression parameters, that is,

$$\beta \equiv (\beta_1^{*'}, \ldots, \beta_j^{*'}, \ldots, \beta_{J-1}^{*}{}')', \text{ where } \beta_j^* = (\beta_{j0}, \beta_j')'.$$

As far as the correlation properties of the repeated multinomial responses $y_{i1}, \ldots, y_{it}, \ldots, y_{iT}$ are concerned, it is likely that they will be pair-wise correlated. These pair-wise correlations along with the mean and variance structures (4.2)–(4.3) must be exploited to obtain efficient estimates for the regression parameter vectors $\{\beta_j^*, j = 1, \ldots, J-1\}$ involved in the marginal probability model (4.1). However, as the modeling for correlations for the longitudinal multinomial responses is difficult, some authors such as Lipsitz et al. (1994), Williamson et al. (1995), and Chen et al. (2009) have used an odds ratio based 'working' correlations approach to estimate the regression parameters. This odds ratio based GEE (generalized estimating equations) approach encounters estimation breakdown and/or inefficiency problems similar to those for the longitudinal binary cases (Sutradhar 2011, Chapter 7). Nevertheless for the sake of completeness, we discuss this odds ratio approach in brief in Sect. 4.2. The difficulties encountered by this approach are also pointed out.

As opposed to the 'working' correlations approach, we consider parametric modeling for the non-stationary correlations for multinomial responses, and discuss a conditionally linear dynamic probability model and its fitting in Sect. 4.3; and a non-linear dynamic logit model and its fitting in Sect. 4.4. Note that these linear and non-linear dynamic models are similar to those LDCMP and MDL models discussed in Sects. 3.4.1 and 3.4.2. But these models in the last chapter were developed for time independent covariates, whereas in the present chapter, that is, in Sects. 4.3 and 4.4, we use the time dependent covariates leading to non-stationary correlations among the multinomial responses. For convenience we will refer to these models in this chapter as the non-stationary LDCMP (NSLDCMP) and non-stationary MDL (NSMDL) models, respectively.

4.2 GEE Approach Using 'Working' Structure/Model for Odds Ratio Parameters

Let $y_i = (y'_{i1}, \ldots, y'_{it}, \ldots, y'_{iT})'$ be the $T(J-1) \times 1$ vector of observations for the ith individual with its mean $\pi_i = (\pi'_{i1}, \ldots, \pi'_{it}, \ldots, \pi'_{iT})'$, where y_{it} and π_{it} are $J-1$ dimensional observation and probability vectors as defined in (4.2). Further, let $\Sigma_i(\beta, \tau)$ be the $T(J-1) \times T(J-1)$ covariance matrix of y_i, where β represents all $\beta_1^*, \ldots, \beta_j^*, \ldots, \beta_{J-1}^*$, and τ represents the so-called correlations or log odds ratio parameters. This covariance matrix for the ith individual may be expressed as

$$\Sigma_i(\beta,\tau) = \begin{pmatrix} \Sigma_{(i,11)}(\beta) & \ldots & \Sigma_{(i,1u)}(\beta,\tau) & \ldots & \Sigma_{(i,1t)}(\beta,\tau) & \ldots & \Sigma_{(i,1T)}(\beta,\tau) \\ \vdots & & \vdots & & \vdots & & \vdots \\ \Sigma_{(i,u1)}(\beta,\tau) & \ldots & \Sigma_{(i,uu)}(\beta) & \ldots & \Sigma_{(i,ut)}(\beta,\tau) & \ldots & \Sigma_{(i,uT)}(\beta,\tau) \\ \vdots & & \vdots & & \vdots & & \vdots \\ \Sigma_{(i,t1)}(\beta,\tau) & \ldots & \Sigma_{(i,tu)}(\beta,\tau) & \ldots & \Sigma_{(i,tt)}(\beta) & \ldots & \Sigma_{(i,tT)}(\beta,\tau) \\ \vdots & & \vdots & & \vdots & & \vdots \\ \Sigma_{(i,T1)}(\beta,\tau) & \ldots & \Sigma_{(i,Tu)}(\beta,\tau) & \ldots & \Sigma_{(i,Tt)}(\beta,\tau) & \ldots & \Sigma_{(i,TT)}(\beta) \end{pmatrix}, \tag{4.4}$$

where $\Sigma_{(i,tt)}(\beta)$ is given by (4.3) for all $t = 1, \ldots, T$, and by writing

$$\text{cov}[Y_{iug}, Y_{itj}] = \sigma_{(i,ut)gj}(\beta, \tau),$$

the covariance matrix $\Sigma_{(i,ut)}(\beta, \tau)$ for $u \neq t$, involved in (4.4) may be expressed as

$$\begin{aligned} \Sigma_{(i,ut)}(\beta,\tau) &= \left(\sigma_{(i,ut)gj}(\beta,\tau)\right) = \left(P(Y_{iug} = 1, Y_{itj} = 1) - \pi_{(iu)g}\pi_{(it)j}\right) \\ &= \left(\pi_{(i,ut)gj} - \pi_{(iu)g}\pi_{(it)j}\right), \end{aligned} \tag{4.5}$$

where $y_{iug} = 1$ indicates that the ith individual at time u is in the ℓth category, similarly $y_{itj} = 1$ represents that the ith individual at time t is in the jth category. In (4.4)–(4.5), τ represents all odds ratios involved in the joint probabilities $\pi_{(i,ut)gj}$, these odds ratios for the ith individual being defined as

$$\tau_{i(ut)gj} = \frac{P(Y_{iug} = 1, Y_{itj} = 1)P(Y_{iug} = 0, Y_{itj} = 0)}{P(Y_{iug} = 1, Y_{itj} = 0)P(Y_{iug} = 0, Y_{itj} = 1)}, \tag{4.6}$$

(e.g., Lipsitz et al. 1991).

It is however not easy to model these odds ratios in (4.6) for their estimation. Many researchers such as Lipsitz et al. (1991), Williamson et al. (1995), Yi and Cook (2002), Chen et al. (2009, 2010) have used a so-called working model (see (4.10) below) for these odds ratio parameters and estimated them. Let $\hat{\tau}_w$ represent such 'working (w)' model based estimate for τ. This estimate $\hat{\tau}_w$ is then used to estimate the joint probabilities $\pi_{(i,ut)gj}$ in (4.5). In the next step, the regression parameter vector β involved in the multinomial probabilities is estimated by solving the GEE

$$\sum_{i=1}^{K} \frac{\partial \mu_i'}{\partial \beta} \Sigma_i^{-1}(\beta, \hat{\tau}_w)(y_i - \mu_i) = 0, \tag{4.7}$$

(Liang and Zeger 1986).

Remark that as opposed to (4.4), in Chap. 3, we have used the i free constant $\Sigma(\pi)$ matrix for var$[Y_{it}]$ and $\tilde{\Sigma}(\pi,\rho)$ (3.159) for var$[Y_i]$, under the covariates free stationary LDCMP model. When covariates are present but stationary, these covariance matrices were denoted by $\Sigma(\pi_{[\ell]})$ and $\tilde{\Sigma}(\pi_{[\ell]},\rho)$, that is,

$$\text{var}[Y_{it}|i \in \ell] = \Sigma(\pi_{[\ell]}), \text{ and } \text{var}[Y_i|i \in \ell] = \tilde{\Sigma}(\pi_{[\ell]},\rho),$$

under the covariates based LDCMP model, ℓ being the ℓth level of the covariate.

4.2.1 'Working' Model 1 for Odds Ratios (τ)

To use the odds ratio based covariance matrix in β estimation such as in (4.7), one needs to compute the joint probability in terms of odds ratios. This follows from the relationship (4.6), that is,

$$\tau_{i(ut)gj} = \frac{\pi_{(i,ut)gj}[1 - \pi_{(iu)g} - \pi_{(it)j} + \pi_{(i,ut)gj}]}{[\pi_{(iu)g} - \pi_{(i,ut)gj}][\pi_{(it)j} - \pi_{(i,ut)gj}]}, \tag{4.8}$$

yielding

$$\pi_{(i,ut)gj} = \begin{cases} \frac{f_{i(ut)gj} - [f^2_{i(ut)gj} - 4\tau_{i(ut)gj}(\tau_{i(ut)gj}-1)\pi_{i(ug)}\pi_{(it)j}]^{\frac{1}{2}}}{2(\tau_{i(ut)gj}-1)} & (\tau_{i(ut)gj} \neq 1), \\ \pi_{(iu)g}\pi_{(it)j} & (\tau_{i(ut)gj} = 1), \end{cases} \tag{4.9}$$

where

$$f_{i(ut)gj} = 1 - (1 - \tau_{i(ut)gj})(\pi_{(iu)g} + \pi_{(it)j}).$$

But as the odds ratios $\tau_{i(ut)\ell j}$ are unknown, it is not possible to compute the joint probabilities by (4.9). As a remedy, some authors such as Lipsitz et al. 1991, Eqs. (5)–(6), p. 155, Williamson et al. 1995, Eq. (3) (see also Yi and Cook 2002, Eq. (3), p. 1072) have used 'working (w)' odds ratios $\tau_{i(ut)gj,w}$, say, instead of the true parameters in (4.8), and assumed that these 'working' odds ratio parameters maintain a linear relationship with category and time effects as

$$log\ \tau_{i(ut)gj,w} = \varphi + \varphi_g + \varphi_j + \varphi_{gj} + w_{it}^{*\prime}\xi^*, \tag{4.10}$$

where $w^*_{it} : q \times 1$, (say), is a suitable subset of the covariate vector w_{it} in (4.1), those are considered to be responsible to correlate y_{iuj} and y_{itj}. The selection of this subset also appears to be arbitrary. In (4.10), φ, φ_g, φ_j, φ_{gj}, and ξ^*, are so-called working parameters, which generate 'working' odds ratios (through (4.10), whereas true odds ratios are given by (4.8). In Sect. 4.3, we consider the modeling of the joint probabilities $\pi_{i(ut)gj}$ through the modeling of correlations or equivalently conditional probabilities. Similar modeling of conditional probabilities was also done in Chap. 3 but for either covariate free or time independent covariate cases.

4.2.1.1 Estimation of 'Working' Odds Ratios and Drawbacks

The existing studies such as Yi and Cook (2002, Section 3.2) treat the 'working' parameters

$$\varphi^* = [\varphi,\ \varphi_1, \ldots, \varphi_j, \ldots, \varphi_{J-1},\ \varphi_{11}, \ldots, \varphi_{gj}, \ldots, \varphi_{(J-1)(J-1)},\ \xi^{*'}]' : J(J-1)+q+1 \times 1$$

as a set of 'working' association parameters and estimate them by solving a second order GEE (generalized estimating equation) (Fitzmaurice and Laird 1993) constructed based on a distance measure between pair-wise multinomial responses and their 'working' means. To be specific, let

$$s_{iut} = [y_{iu1}y_{it1}, \ldots, y_{iug}y_{itj}, \ldots, y_{iu,J-1}y_{it,J-1}]' : (J-1)^2 \times 1, \text{ for } u < t,\ t = 2, \ldots, T, \tag{4.11}$$

and

$$s_i = [s'_{i12}, \ldots, s'_{iut}, \ldots, s'_{i,T-1,T}]' : \frac{T(T-1)(J-1)^2}{2} \times 1. \tag{4.12}$$

Note that if the true model for odds ratios (indexed by τ) was known, one would then have computed the $E[S_{iut}]$ and $E[S_i]$ by using the true joint probability $P(Y_{iug} = 1, Y_{itj} = 1)$ given by

$$\pi_{(i,ut)gj}(\beta, \tau) = E[Y_{iug}Y_{itj} | \text{true model indexed by } \tau], \tag{4.13}$$

(see (4.9)). However, because the true joint probabilities are unknown, the GEE approach, by using (4.10) in (4.9), computes the 'working' joint probabilities as

$$\pi_{(i,ut)gj,w}(\beta, \tau_w(\varphi^*)) = E[Y_{iug}Y_{itj}]$$
$$= \begin{cases} \frac{f_{i(ut)gj,w} - [f^2_{i(ut)gj,w} - 4\tau_{i(ut)gj,w}(\tau_{i(ut)gj,w}-1)\pi_{i(ug)}\pi_{(it)j}]^{\frac{1}{2}}}{2(\tau_{i(ut)gj,w}-1)} & (\tau_{i(ut)gj,w} \neq 1), \\ \pi_{(iu)g}\pi_{(it)j} & (\tau_{i(ut)gj,w} = 1), \end{cases} \tag{4.14}$$

with

$$f_{i(ut)gj,w} = 1 - (1 - \tau_{i(ut)gj,w})(\pi_{(iu)g} + \pi_{(it)j}),$$

and constructs an estimating equation for φ^*, given by

$$\sum_{i=1}^{K} \frac{\partial \xi_w{}'(\beta,\varphi^*)}{\partial \varphi^*} \Omega_{i,w}^{-1}(s_i - \xi_w(\beta,\varphi^*)) = 0, \tag{4.15}$$

where

$$\xi_w(\beta,\varphi^*) = [\xi'_{i12,w}(\beta,\varphi^*),\ldots,\xi'_{iut,w}(\beta,\varphi^*),\ldots,\xi'_{i,T-1,T,w}(\beta,\varphi^*)]',$$

with

$$\xi_{iut,w}(\beta,\varphi^*) = E[\{Y_{iu1}Y_{it1},\ldots,Y_{iug}Y_{itj},\ldots,Y_{iu,J-1}Y_{it,J-1}\}|\text{ models (4.10),(4.14)}]'$$
$$= [\pi_{(i,ut)11,w}(\beta,\tau_w(\varphi^*)),\ldots,\pi_{(i,ut)gj,w}(\beta,\tau_w(\varphi^*)),\ldots,\pi_{(i,ut)(J-1),(J-1),w}(\beta,\tau_w(\varphi^*))]'.$$

In (4.15), $\Omega_{i,w}$ is a 'working' covariance matrix of S_i, for which Yi and Cook (2002, Section 3.2) have used the formula

$$\begin{aligned}\Omega_{i,w} = \text{cov}[S_i] = \text{diag}[&\pi_{(i,12)11,w}(\beta,\tau(\varphi^*))s\{1-\pi_{(i,12)11,w}(\beta,\tau_w(\varphi^*))\},\ldots,\\ &\pi_{(i,ut)gj,w}(\beta,\tau_w(\varphi^*))\{1-\pi_{(i,ut)gj,w}(\beta,\tau_w(\varphi^*))\},\ldots,\\ &\pi_{(i,T-1,T)(J-1),(J-1),w}(\beta,\tau_w(\varphi^*))\{1-\pi_{(i,T-1,T)(J-1),(J-1),w}(\beta,\tau_w(\varphi^*))\}],\end{aligned} \tag{4.16}$$

to avoid the computation of third and fourth order moments. Remark that while the use of such a 'working' covariance matrix lacks justification to produce efficient estimates, there is, however, a more serious problem in using the GEE (2.15) for the estimation of φ. This is because, the distance function $(s_i - \xi_w(\beta,\varphi^*))$ does not produce an unbiased equation, as s_i's are generated from a model involving true τ. That is,

$$E[S_i - \xi(\beta,\tau)] = 0, \tag{4.17}$$

whereas

$$E[S_i - \xi_w(\beta,\varphi^*] \neq 0. \tag{4.18}$$

Consequently, the second order GEE (4.15) would produce $\hat{\varphi}^*$ which however may not be unbiased for φ^*, rather

$$\hat{\varphi}^* \to \varphi_0^*(\tau), \text{ (say)}$$

(see Sutradhar and Das 1999; Crowder 1995). Thus, $\hat{\tau}_w(\hat{\varphi}^*)$ obtained by (4.15) and (4.10) will be inconsistent for τ unless true τ satisfies the relation (4.10) which is, however, unlikely to happen. This, in turn, makes the $\hat{\tau}_w(\cdot)$ based GEE (4.7) for β useless.

As opposed to 'working' models, in the next section, we introduce a non-stationary parametric model, namely the non-stationary linear dynamic conditional multinomial probability (NSLDCMP) model.

4.3 NSLDCMP Model

Recall from Chap. 3 (more specifically from Sect. 3.5.1) that when covariates are time independent (referred to as the stationary case), it is possible to make a transition counts table such as Table 3.24 for individuals belonging to ℓ-th ($\ell = 1,\ldots,p+1$) level of a covariate, and use them for model fitting and inferences. For example, in Table 3.24, $K_{[\ell]gj}(t-h^*,t)$ denotes the number of individuals with covariate information at level ℓ who were under category g at time $t-h^*$ and in category j at time t. To reflect these transitional counts, conditional probabilities in linear form (see (3.238)) were modeled as

$$P[Y_{it} = y_{it}^{(j)} | Y_{i,t-1} = y_{i,t-1}^{(g)}, i \in \ell] = \pi_{(i\in\ell,t)j} + \sum_{h=1}^{J-1} \rho_{jh} \left[y_{i,t-1,h}^{(g)} - \pi_{(i\in\ell,t-1)h} \right]$$

$$= \pi_{[\ell]j} + \sum_{h=1}^{J-1} \rho_{jh} \left[y_{i,t-1,h}^{(g)} - \pi_{[\ell]h} \right]$$

$$= \lambda_{it|t-1}^{(j)}(g,\ell), \text{ for } g = 1,\ldots,J; j = 1,\ldots,J-1, \tag{4.19}$$

showing that $\pi_{(i\in\ell,t)j} = \pi_{[\ell]j}$ (see (3.231)–(3.232) for their formulas), that is, the covariates in marginal and conditional probabilities are time independent.

In the present linear non-stationary setup, by using a general p-dimensional time dependent covariates w_{it} as in (4.1), we define the marginal probabilities at time $t(t = 1,\ldots,T)$ as

$$P[y_{it} = y_{it}^{(j)} = \delta_{itj}] = \pi_{(it)j} = \begin{cases} \frac{\exp(\beta_{j0}+\beta_j' w_{it})}{1+\sum_{g=1}^{J-1}\exp(\beta_{g0}+\beta_g' w_{it})} & \text{for } j = 1,\ldots,J-1 \\ \frac{1}{1+\sum_{g=1}^{J-1}\exp(\beta_{g0}+\beta_g' w_{it})} & \text{for } j = J, \end{cases}$$

and for $t = 2,\ldots,T$, the lag 1 based LDCM probabilities as

$$\begin{aligned} P[Y_{it} = y_{it}^{(j)} | Y_{i,t-1} = y_{i,t-1}^{(g)}] &= \pi_{(it)j} + \sum_{h=1}^{J-1} \rho_{jh} \left[y_{i,t-1,h}^{(g)} - \pi_{(i,t-1)h} \right] \\ &= \pi_{(it)j} + \rho_j' \left(y_{i,t-1}^{(g)} - \pi_{(i,t-1)} \right) \\ &= \lambda_{it|t-1}^{(j)}(g), \text{ for } g = 1,\ldots,J; j = 1,\ldots,J-1 \\ P[Y_{it} = y_{it}^{(J)} | Y_{i,t-1} = y_{i,t-1}^{(g)}] &= 1 - \sum_{j=1}^{J-1} \lambda_{it|t-1}^{(j)}(g), \text{ for } g = 1,\ldots,J, \end{aligned} \tag{4.20}$$

where

$$\rho_j = (\rho_{j1},\ldots,\rho_{jh},\ldots,\rho_{j,J-1})' : (J-1)\times 1$$

$$y_{i,t-1}^{(g)} = \begin{cases} (y_{i,t-1,1}^{(g)},\ldots,y_{i,t-1,g}^{(g)},\ldots,y_{i,t-1,,J-1}^{(g)})' = (01'_{g-1},1,01'_{J-1-g})' & \text{for } g=1,\ldots,J-1; \\ (01_{J-1}) & \text{for } g=J. \end{cases}$$

$$\pi_{(it)} = (\pi_{(it)1},\ldots,\pi_{(it)j},\ldots,\pi_{(it)(J-1)})' : (J-1)\times 1.$$

4.3.1 *Basic Properties of the LDCMP Model (4.20)*

4.3.1.1 Marginal Expectation

Notice from (4.20) that for $t=1$,

$$\begin{aligned} E[Y_{i1}] &= \sum_{g=1}^{J} y_{i1}^{(g)} P[Y_{i1} = y_{i1}^{(g)}] = \sum_{g=1}^{J} y_{i1}^{(g)} \pi_{(i1)g} \\ &= [\pi_{(i1)1},\ldots,\pi_{(i1)j},\ldots,\pi_{(i1)(J-1)}]' = \pi_{(i1)} : (J-1)\times 1. \end{aligned} \tag{4.21}$$

Next, for $t=2,\ldots,T$, the conditional probabilities produce

$$\begin{aligned} E[Y_{it}|y_{i,t-1}^{(g)}] &= \begin{pmatrix} \pi_{it)1} + \rho_1'(y_{i,t-1}^{(g)} - \pi_{(i,t-1)}) \\ \pi_{(it)2} + \rho_2'(y_{i,t-1}^{(g)} - \pi_{(i,t-1)}) \\ \cdots \\ \pi_{(it)j} + \rho_j'(y_{i,t-1}^{(g)} - \pi_{(i,t-1)}) \\ \cdots \\ \pi_{(it)(J-1)} + \rho_{J-1}'(y_{i,t-1}^{(g)} - \pi_{(i,t-1)}) \end{pmatrix} \\ &= \pi_{(it)} + \rho_M(y_{i,t-1}^{(g)} - \pi_{(i,t-1)}),\ g=1,\ldots,J, \end{aligned} \tag{4.22}$$

where ρ_M is the $(J-1)\times(J-1)$ linear dependence parameters matrix given by

$$\rho_M = \begin{pmatrix} \rho_1' \\ \vdots \\ \rho_j' \\ \vdots \\ \rho_{J-1}' \end{pmatrix} : (J-1)\times(J-1). \tag{4.23}$$

Note that in general, that is, without any category specification, the lag 1 conditional expectation (4.22) implies that

$$E[Y_{it}|y_{i,t-1}] = \pi_{(it)} + \rho_M(y_{i,t-1} - \pi_{(i,t-1)}). \tag{4.24}$$

Next because

$$E[Y_{it}] = E_{Y_{i1}} E_{Y_{i2}} \cdots E_{Y_{i,t-1}} E[Y_{it} | y_{i,t-1}],$$

it follows by (4.24) that

$$\begin{aligned} E[Y_{it}] &= \pi_{(it)} + E_{Y_{i1}} [\rho_M^{t-1} (Y_{i1} - \pi_{(i1)})] \\ &= \pi_{(it)}. \end{aligned} \tag{4.25}$$

In (4.25), $\rho_M^3 = \rho_M \rho_M \rho_M$, for example.

This marginal mean vector in (4.25) also can be computed as

$$\begin{aligned} E[Y_{it}] &= \sum_{g=1}^{J-1} y_{it}^{(g)} P[Y_{it} = y_{it}^{(g)}] = \sum_{g=1}^{J-1} y_{it}^{(g)} \pi_{(it)g} \\ &= [\pi_{(it)1}, \ldots, \pi_{(it)j}, \ldots, \pi_{(it)(J-1)}]' = \pi_{(it)} : (J-1) \times 1, \end{aligned} \tag{4.26}$$

4.3.1.2 Marginal Covariance Matrix

By using similar idea as in (4.26), one may compute the marginal covariance matrix at time t as follows. Because for $j \neq k$, the jth and kth categories are mutually exclusive, it follows that

$$E[Y_{itj} Y_{itk}] = P[Y_{itj} = 1, Y_{itk} = 1] = P[Y_{it} = y_{it}^{(j)}, Y_{it} = y_{it}^{(k)}] = 0. \tag{4.27}$$

For $j = k$ one obtains

$$E[Y_{itj}^2] = E[Y_{itj}] = P[Y_{itj} = 1] = 1P[Y_{it} = y_{it}^{(j)}] + 0 \sum_{g \neq j}^{J} P[Y_{it} = y_{it}^{(g)}] = \pi_{(it)j}. \tag{4.28}$$

Consequently, by combining (4.27) and (4.28), one computes the covariance matrix as

$$\begin{aligned} \text{var}[Y_{it}] &= E[\{Y_{it} - \pi_{(it)}\}\{Y_{it} - \pi_{(it)}\}'] \\ &= E[Y_{it} Y_{it}'] - \pi_{(it)} \pi_{(it)}' \\ &= \text{diag}[\pi_{(it)1}, \ldots, \pi_{(it)j}, \ldots, \pi_{(it)(J-1)}] - \pi_{(it)} \pi_{(it)}' \\ &= \Sigma_{(i,tt)}(\beta), \end{aligned} \tag{4.29}$$

as in (4.3).

4.3.1.3 Auto-covariance Matrices

For $u < t$, the auto-covariance matrix is written as

$$\text{cov}[Y_{it}, Y'_{iu}] = E[\{Y_{it} - \pi_{(it)}\}\{Y_{iu} - \pi_{(iu)}\}']. \tag{4.30}$$

Now because the covariance formula, that is, the right-hand side of (4.30) may be expressed as

$$E[\{Y_{it} - \pi_{(it)}\}\{Y_{iu} - \pi_{(iu)}\}'] = E_{Y_{iu}} E_{Y_{i,u+1}} \cdots E_{Y_{i,t-1}} E[\{Y_{it} - \pi_{(it)}\}\{Y_{iu} - \pi_{(iu)}\}' | Y_{i,t-1}, \cdots, Y_{iu}], \tag{4.31}$$

by using the operation as in (4.24)–(4.25), this equation provides the formula for the covariance matrix as

$$\begin{aligned}
\text{cov}[Y_{it}, Y'_{iu}] &= E[\{Y_{it} - \pi_{(it)}\}\{Y_{iu} - \pi_{(iu)}\}'] \\
&= \rho_M^{t-u} E_{Y_{iu}}[\{Y_{iu} - \pi_{(iu)}\}\{Y_{iu} - \pi_{(iu)}\}'] \\
&= \rho_M^{t-u} \text{var}[Y_{iu}] \\
&= \rho_M^{t-u} \left[\text{diag}[\pi_{(iu)1}, \ldots, \pi_{(iu)j}, \ldots, \pi_{(iu)(J-1)}] - \pi_{(iu)}\pi'_{(iu)} \right] \\
&= \Sigma_{(i,ut)}(\beta, \rho_M), \text{ (say)},
\end{aligned} \tag{4.32}$$

where, for example, $\rho_M^3 = \rho_M \rho_M \rho_M$.

4.3.2 GQL Estimation of the Parameters

Similar to Sect. 3.4.1.2 (of Chap. 3), we estimate all regression parameters β by solving a GQL estimating equation, and the conditionally linear dynamic dependence parameters ρ_M by using the method of moments. The GQL estimating equation for β is constructed as follows.

Let

$$y_i = [y'_{i1}, \ldots, y'_{it}, \ldots, y'_{iT}]' : T(J-1) \times 1$$

be the repeated multinomial responses of the ith individual over T time periods. Here $y_{it} = [y_{it1}, \ldots, y_{itj}, \ldots, y_{it,J-1}]'$ denotes the multinomial response of the ith individual collected at time t. The expectation and the covariance matrix of this response vector are given by

$$\begin{aligned}
E[Y_i] &= E[Y'_{i1}, \ldots, Y'_{it}, \ldots, Y'_{iT}]' \\
&= [\pi'_{(i1)}, \ldots, \pi'_{(it)}, \ldots, \pi'_{(iT)}]' : T(J-1) \times 1 \\
&= \pi_{(i)}
\end{aligned} \tag{4.33}$$

and

$$\mathrm{cov}[Y_i] = \Sigma_{(i)}(\beta,\rho_M) \tag{4.34}$$

$$= \begin{pmatrix} \Sigma_{(i,11)}(\beta) & \ldots & \Sigma_{(i,1u)}(\beta,\rho_M) & \ldots & \Sigma_{(i,1t)}(\beta,\rho_M) & \ldots & \Sigma_{(i,1T)}(\beta,\rho_M) \\ \vdots & & \vdots & & \vdots & & \vdots \\ \Sigma_{(i,u1)}(\beta,\rho_M) & \ldots & \Sigma_{(i,uu)}(\beta) & \ldots & \Sigma_{(i,ut)}(\beta,\rho_M) & \ldots & \Sigma_{(i,uT)}(\beta,\rho_M) \\ \vdots & & \vdots & & \vdots & & \vdots \\ \Sigma_{(i,t1)}(\beta,\rho_M) & \ldots & \Sigma_{(i,tu)}(\beta,\rho_M) & \ldots & \Sigma_{(i,tt)}(\beta) & \ldots & \Sigma_{(i,tT)}(\beta,\rho_M) \\ \vdots & & \vdots & & \vdots & & \vdots \\ \Sigma_{(i,T1)}(\beta,\rho_M) & \ldots & \Sigma_{(i,Tu)}(\beta,\rho_M) & \ldots & \Sigma_{(i,Tt)}(\beta,\rho_M) & \ldots & \Sigma_{(i,TT)}(\beta) \end{pmatrix},$$

where

$$\Sigma_{(i,tt)}(\beta) = \mathrm{diag}[\pi_{(it)1},\ldots,\pi_{(it)j},\ldots,\pi_{(it)(J-1)}] - \pi_{(it)}\pi'_{(it)},$$

by (4.29), and

$$\Sigma_{(i,ut)}(\beta,\rho_M) = \rho_M^{t-u}\left[\mathrm{diag}[\pi_{(iu)1},\ldots,\pi_{(iu)j},\ldots,\pi_{(iu)(J-1)}] - \pi_{(iu)}\pi'_{(iu)}\right],$$

by (4.32), for $u < t$. Also

$$\Sigma_{(i,tu)}(\beta,\rho_M) = \Sigma'_{(i,ut)}(\beta,\rho_M).$$

Following Sutradhar (2003, Section 3) (see also Sutradhar 2011), using the aforementioned notation (4.33)–(4.34), for known ρ_M, one may now construct the GQL estimating equation for

$$\beta \equiv (\beta_1^{*\prime},\ldots,\beta_j^{*\prime},\ldots,\beta_{J-1}^{*\prime})' : (J-1)(p+1)\times 1, \text{ where } \beta_j^* = (\beta_{j0},\beta_j')',$$

as

$$\sum_{i=1}^{K} \frac{\partial \pi'_{(i)}}{\partial \beta} \Sigma_{(i)}^{-1}(\beta,\rho_M)(y_i - \pi_{(i)}) = 0, \tag{4.35}$$

where for

$$\pi'_{(it)} = [\pi_{(it)1},\ldots,\pi_{(it)j},\ldots,\pi_{(it)(J-1)}]$$

with

$$\pi_{(it)j} = \begin{cases} \frac{\exp(\beta_{j0}+\beta'_j w_{it})}{1+\sum_{g=1}^{J-1}\exp(\beta_{g0}+\beta'_g w_{it})} & \text{for } j=1,\ldots,J-1 \\ \frac{1}{1+\sum_{g=1}^{J-1}\exp(\beta_{g0}+\beta'_g w_{it})} & \text{for } j=J \end{cases}$$

$$= \begin{cases} \frac{\exp(\left(1\ w'_{it}\right)\beta^*_j)}{1+\sum_{g=1}^{J-1}\exp(\left(1\ w'_{it}\right)\beta^*_g)} & \text{for } j=1,\ldots,J-1 \\ \frac{1}{1+\sum_{g=1}^{J-1}\exp(\left(1\ w'_{it}\right)\beta^*_g)} & \text{for } j=J \end{cases}$$

$$= \begin{cases} \frac{\exp(w^{*'}_{it}\beta^*_j)}{1+\sum_{g=1}^{J-1}\exp(w^{*'}_{it}\beta^*_g)} & \text{for } j=1,\ldots,J-1 \\ \frac{1}{1+\sum_{g=1}^{J-1}\exp(w^{*'}_{it}\beta^*_g)} & \text{for } j=J \end{cases}$$

one computes the derivative $\frac{\partial \pi'_{(i)}}{\partial \beta}$ as

$$\frac{\partial \pi'_{(i)}}{\partial \beta} = [\frac{\partial \pi'_{(i1)}}{\partial \beta},\ldots,\frac{\partial \pi'_{(it)}}{\partial \beta},\ldots,\frac{\partial \pi'_{(iT)}}{\partial \beta}] : (J-1)(p+1)\times(J-1)T, \tag{4.36}$$

where

$$\frac{\partial \pi_{(it)j}}{\partial \beta^*_j} = \pi_{(it)j}[1-\pi_{(it)j}]w^*_{it}$$
$$\frac{\partial \pi_{(it)j}}{\partial \beta^*_k} = -[\pi_{(it)j}\pi_{(it)k}]w^*_{it}, \tag{4.37}$$

yielding

$$\frac{\partial \pi_{(it)j}}{\partial \beta} = \begin{pmatrix} -\pi_{(it)1}\pi_{(it)j} \\ \vdots \\ \pi_{(it)j}[1-\pi_{(it)j}] \\ \vdots \\ -\pi_{(it)(J-1)}\pi_{(it)j} \end{pmatrix} \otimes w^*_{it} : (J-1)(p+1)\times 1$$
$$= \left[\pi_{(it)j}(\delta_j - \pi_{(it)})\right] \otimes w^*_{it}, \tag{4.38}$$

with $\delta_j = [01'_{j-1}, 1, 01'_{J-1-j}]'$ for $j=1,\ldots,J-1$. Thus,

$$\frac{\partial \pi'_{(it)}}{\partial \beta} = \Sigma_{(i,tt)}(\beta)\otimes w^*_{it} : (J-1)(p+1)\times(J-1). \tag{4.39}$$

By using (4.39) in (4.36), one obtains the $(J-1)(p+1) \times (J-1)T$ derivative matrix as

$$\frac{\partial \pi'_{(i)}}{\partial \beta} = \left(\Sigma_{(i,11)}(\beta) \otimes w^*_{i1} \cdots \Sigma_{(i,tt)}(\beta) \otimes w^*_{it} \cdots \Sigma_{(i,TT)}(\beta) \otimes w^*_{iT} \right)$$
$$= D'_i(w^*_i, \Sigma_{(i)}(\beta)) : (J-1)(p+1) \times (J-1)T, \text{ (say).} \tag{4.40}$$

Consequently, by using (4.40) in (4.35), we now solve the GQL estimating equation

$$\sum_{i=1}^{K} D'_i(w^*_i, \Sigma_{(i)}(\beta)) \Sigma^{-1}_{(i)}(\beta, \rho_M)(y_i - \pi_{(i)}) = 0, \tag{4.41}$$

for β. By treating β in $D'_i(w^*_i, \Sigma_{(i)}(\beta))$ and $\Sigma_{(i)}(\beta, \rho_M)$ as known from a previous iteration, this estimating equation (4.41) is solved iteratively by using

$$\hat{\beta}(r+1) = \hat{\beta}(r) + \left[\left\{ \sum_{i=1}^{K} D'_i(w^*_i, \Sigma_{(i)}(\beta)) \Sigma^{-1}_{(i)}(\beta, \rho_M) D_i(w^*_i, \Sigma_{(i)}(\beta)) \right\}^{-1} \right.$$
$$\left. \times \left\{ \sum_{i=1}^{K} D'_i(w^*_i, \Sigma_{(i)}(\beta)) \Sigma^{-1}_{(i)}(\beta, \rho_M)(y_i - \pi_{(i)}) \right\} \right]_{|\beta = \hat{\beta}(r)}, \tag{4.42}$$

until convergence.

Note that it is necessary to estimate ρ_M in order to use the iterative equation (4.42). An unbiased (hence consistent under some mild conditions) estimator of ρ_M may be obtained by using the method of moments as follows.

4.3.2.1 Moment Estimation for ρ_M

For $u(=t-1) < t$, it follows from (4.34) that

$$\begin{aligned} \text{cov}[Y_{it}, Y_{i,t-1}] &= \Sigma_{(i,(t-1)t)}(\beta, \rho_M) \\ &= \rho_M \Sigma_{(i,(t-1)(t-1))}(\beta) \\ &= \rho_M \text{var}[Y_{i,t-1}]. \end{aligned} \tag{4.43}$$

Consequently, one may obtain a moment estimate of ρ_M as

$$\hat{\rho}_M = \left[\sum_{i=1}^{K} \hat{\Sigma}_{(i,(t-1)(t-1))}(\beta) \right]^{-1} \sum_{i=1}^{K} \hat{\Sigma}_{(i,(t-1)t)}(\beta, \rho_M), \tag{4.44}$$

where

$$\hat{\Sigma}_{(i,(t-1)t)}(\beta,\rho_M) = \frac{1}{T-1}\sum_{t=2}^{T}[(y_{i,t-1,g}-\pi_{(i,t-1)g})(y_{itj}-\pi_{(it)j})] : g,j=1,\ldots,J-1$$

$$\hat{\Sigma}_{(i,(t-1)(t-1))}(\beta) = \frac{1}{T-1}\sum_{t=2}^{T}[(y_{i,t-1,g}-\pi_{(i,t-1)g})(y_{i,t-1,j}-\pi_{(i,t-1)j})] : g,j=1,\ldots,J-1. \quad (4.45)$$

4.3.3 Likelihood Estimation of the Parameters

Using the notation from (4.20), similar to Chap. 3, more specifically Sect. 3.4.1.3, one writes the likelihood function for β and ρ_M as

$$L(\beta,\rho_M) = \Pi_{i=1}^{K}\left[f(y_{i1})\Pi_{t=2}^{T}f(y_{it}|y_{i,t-1})\right], \quad (4.46)$$

where

$$f(y_{i1}) \propto \Pi_{j=1}^{J}\pi_{(i1)j}^{y_{i1j}},$$

$$f(y_{it}|y_{i,t-1}) \propto \Pi_{j=1}^{J}\Pi_{g=1}^{J}\left[\lambda_{it|t-1}^{(j)}(y_{i,t-1}^{(g)})\right]^{y_{itj}}, \text{ for } t=2,\ldots,T, \quad (4.47)$$

where

$$\lambda_{it|t-1}^{(J)}(y_{i,t-1}^{(g)}) = 1-\sum_{k=1}^{J-1}\lambda_{it|t-1}^{(k)}(y_{i,t-1}^{(g)}) \text{ with } \lambda_{it|t-1}^{(k)}(y_{i,t-1}^{(g)}) = \pi_{(it)k}+\rho_k'(y_{i,t-1}^{(g)}-\pi_{(i,t-1)}).$$

The likelihood function in (4.46) may be re-expressed as

$$L(\beta,\rho_M) = c_0\left[\Pi_{i=1}^{K}\Pi_{j=1}^{J}\pi_{(i1)j}^{y_{i1j}}\right] \times \Pi_{i=1}^{K}\Pi_{t=2}^{T}\Pi_{j=1}^{J}\Pi_{g=1}^{J}\left\{\lambda_{it|t-1}^{(j)}(y_{i,t-1}^{(g)})\right\}^{y_{itj}}, \quad (4.48)$$

where c_0 is the normalizing constant free from any parameters. Next, by using the abbreviation $\lambda_{it|t-1}^{(j)}(y_{i,t-1}^{(g)}) \equiv \lambda_{it|t-1}^{(j)}(g)$, the log likelihood function is written as

$$Log\, L(\beta,\rho_M) = log\, c_0 + \sum_{i=1}^{K}\sum_{j=1}^{J} y_{i1j} log\, \pi_{(i1)j} + \sum_{i=1}^{K}\sum_{t=2}^{T}\sum_{g=1}^{J}\sum_{j=1}^{J}\left[y_{itj} log\, \lambda_{it|t-1}^{(j)}(g)\right]. \quad (4.49)$$

For convenience, the conditional probabilities in (4.49) may be expressed as

$$\lambda^{(j)}_{it|t-1}(g) = \begin{cases} \pi_{(it)j} + \rho'_j(\delta_g - \pi_{(i,t-1)}) & \text{for } j = 1,\ldots,J-1;\ g = 1,\ldots,J \\ 1 - \Sigma_{k=1}^{J-1}\left[\pi_{(it)k} + \rho'_k(\delta_g - \pi_{(i,t-1)})\right] & \text{for } j = J;\ g = 1,\ldots,J, \end{cases} \tag{4.50}$$

where, similar to (3.155),

$$\delta_g = \begin{cases} [01'_{g-1}, 1, 01'_{J-1-g}]' & \text{for } g = 1,\ldots,J-1 \\ 01_{J-1} & \text{for } g = J. \end{cases}$$

4.3.3.1 Likelihood Estimating Equation for β

To compute the likelihood equation for β, we first compute the derivatives $\frac{\partial \pi_{(i1)j}}{\partial \beta}$ and $\frac{\partial \lambda^{(j)}_{it|t-1}(g)}{\partial \beta}$ for all $j = 1,\ldots,J$, as follows.

Formula for $\frac{\partial \pi_{(i1)j}}{\partial \beta}$

$$\begin{aligned} \frac{\partial \pi_{(i1)j}}{\partial \beta} &= \begin{cases} \left[\pi_{(i1)j}(\delta_j - \pi_{(i1)})\right] \otimes w^*_{i1} & \text{for } j = 1,\ldots,J-1 \\ \left[\pi_{(i1)J}(01_{J-1} - \pi_{(i1)})\right] \otimes w^*_{i1} & \text{for } j = J \end{cases} \\ &= \left[\pi_{(i1)j}(\delta_j - \pi_{(i1)})\right] \otimes w^*_{i1}, \text{ for all } j = 1,\ldots,J, \end{aligned} \tag{4.51}$$

with

$$\delta_j = \begin{cases} [01'_{j-1}, 1, 01'_{J-1-j}]' & \text{for } j = 1,\ldots,J-1 \\ 01_{J-1} & \text{for } j = J. \end{cases}$$

Formula for $\frac{\partial \lambda^{(j)}_{it|t-1}(g)}{\partial \beta}$ for $t = 2,\ldots,T$ and all $g = 1,\ldots,J$

$$\frac{\partial \lambda^{(j)}_{it|t-1}(g)}{\partial \beta} = \frac{\partial}{\partial \beta}\begin{cases} \pi_{(it)j} + \rho'_j(\delta_g - \pi_{(i,t-1)}) & \text{for } j = 1,\ldots,J-1 \\ 1 - \Sigma_{k=1}^{J-1}\left[\pi_{(it)k} + \rho'_k(\delta_g - \pi_{(i,t-1)})\right] & \text{for } j = J, \end{cases}$$

$$= \frac{\partial}{\partial \beta}\begin{cases} \pi_{(it)j} - \pi'_{(i,t-1)}\rho_j & \text{for } j = 1,\ldots,J-1 \\ -\Sigma_{k=1}^{J-1}\left[\pi_{(it)k} - \pi'_{(i,t-1)}\rho_k\right] & \text{for } j = J, \end{cases}$$

$$= \begin{cases} \left[\{\pi_{(it)j}(\delta_j - \pi_{(it)})\} \otimes w^*_{it}\right] + \left[\Sigma_{(i,t-1,t-1)}(\beta) \otimes w^*_{i,t-1}\right]\rho_j & \text{for } j = 1,\ldots,J-1 \\ \left[\{\pi_{(it)J}(\delta_J - \pi_{(it)})\} \otimes w^*_{it}\right] + \left[\Sigma_{(i,t-1,t-1)}(\beta) \otimes w^*_{i,t-1}\right]\Sigma_{k=1}^{J-1}\rho_k & \text{for } j = J, \end{cases} \tag{4.52}$$

by (4.38)–(4.39). By using $\rho_J = \sum_{k=1}^{J-1} \rho_k$, this derivative in (4.52), for convenience, may be expressed as

$$\frac{\partial \lambda^{(j)}_{it|t-1}(g)}{\partial \beta} = \left[\{\pi_{(it)j}(\delta_j - \pi_{(it)})\} \otimes w^*_{it}\right] + \left[\Sigma_{(i,t-1,t-1)}(\beta) \otimes w^*_{i,t-1}\right] \rho_j, \qquad (4.53)$$

for all $j = 1, \ldots, J$; $t = 2, \ldots, T$, and $g = 1, \ldots, J$.

Now by using (4.51) and (4.53), one derives the likelihood equation for β from (4.49) as

$$\begin{aligned}\frac{\partial Log\, L(\beta, \rho_M)}{\partial \beta} &= \sum_{i=1}^{K} \sum_{j=1}^{J} \frac{y_{i1j}}{\pi_{(i1)j}} \left[\pi_{(i1)j}(\delta_j - \pi_{(i1)})\right] \otimes w^*_{i1} \\ &+ \sum_{i=1}^{K} \sum_{t=2}^{T} \sum_{g=1}^{J} \sum_{j=1}^{J} \left[\frac{y_{itj}}{\lambda^{(j)}_{it|t-1}(g)} \left[(\{\pi_{(it)j}(\delta_j - \pi_{(it)})\} \otimes w^*_{it}) \right.\right. \\ &+ \left.\left. \left(\Sigma_{(i,t-1,t-1)}(\beta) \otimes w^*_{i,t-1}\right) \rho_j\right]\right] = 0. \qquad (4.54)\end{aligned}$$

This equation is solved for β estimate iteratively by using the iterative formula

$$\begin{aligned}\hat{\beta}(r+1) = \hat{\beta}(r) - &\left[\left\{ \frac{\partial^2 Log\, L(\beta, \rho_M)}{\partial \beta' \partial \beta} \right\}^{-1} \right. \\ &\times \left. \left\{ \frac{\partial Log\, L(\beta, \rho_M)}{\partial \beta} \right\} \right]_{|\beta = \hat{\beta}(r)}, \qquad (4.55)\end{aligned}$$

until convergence. Similar to the derivation of the iterative equation (4.42) under the GQL approach, we compute the second order derivative $\frac{\partial^2 Log\, L(\beta, \rho_M)}{\partial \beta' \partial \beta}$ by treating β involved in the first derivative formulas $\frac{\partial \pi_{(i1)j}}{\partial \beta}$ and $\frac{\partial \lambda^{(j)}_{it|t-1}(g)}{\partial \beta}$, as known, from the previous iteration. This provides a simpler formula for the second order derivative as given by

$$\begin{aligned}\frac{\partial^2 Log\, L(\beta, \rho_M)}{\partial \beta' \partial \beta} &= -\sum_{i=1}^{K} \sum_{t=2}^{T} \sum_{g=1}^{J} \sum_{j=1}^{J} \left[\frac{y_{itj}}{\{\lambda^{(j)}_{it|t-1}(g)\}^2} \right. \\ &\times \left[(\{\pi_{(it)j}(\delta_j - \pi_{(it)})\} \otimes w^*_{it}) + \left(\Sigma_{(i,t-1,t-1)}(\beta) \otimes w^*_{i,t-1}\right) \rho_j\right] \\ &\times \left. \left[(\{\pi_{(it)j}(\delta_j - \pi_{(it)})\} \otimes w^*_{it}) + \left(\Sigma_{(i,t-1,t-1)}(\beta) \otimes w^*_{i,t-1}\right) \rho_j\right]' \right] \qquad (4.56)\end{aligned}$$

4.3.3.2 Likelihood Estimating Equation for ρ_M

Recall from (4.23) that

$$\rho_M = \begin{pmatrix} \rho_1' \\ \vdots \\ \rho_j' \\ \vdots \\ \rho_{J-1}' \end{pmatrix} : (J-1) \times (J-1).$$

Thus, to compute the likelihood equation from (4.49) for ρ_M, we first compute the derivatives $\frac{\partial \lambda^{(j)}_{it|t-1}(g)}{\partial \rho_k}$ for $j = 1, \ldots, J$, and $k = 1, \ldots, J-1$, as follows.

Formula for $\frac{\partial \lambda^{(j)}_{it|t-1}(g)}{\partial \rho_j}$ **for** $t = 2, \ldots, T;\ g = 1, \ldots, J;$ **and** $k = 1, \ldots, J-1$

By (4.50),

$$\frac{\partial \lambda^{(j)}_{it|t-1}(g)}{\partial \rho_k} = \frac{\partial}{\partial \rho_k} \begin{cases} \pi_{(it)j} + \rho_j'(\delta_g - \pi_{(i,t-1)}) & \text{for } j = 1, \ldots, J-1 \\ 1 - \sum_{h=1}^{J-1} \left[\pi_{(it)h} + \rho_h'(\delta_g - \pi_{(i,t-1)})\right] & \text{for } j = J, \end{cases}$$

$$= \begin{cases} (\delta_g - \pi_{(i,t-1)}) & \text{for } j = 1, \ldots, J-1;\ k = j \\ 0 & \text{for } j = 1, \ldots, J-1;\ k \neq j \\ -(\delta_g - \pi_{(i,t-1)}) & \text{for } j = J;\ k = 1, \ldots, J-1. \end{cases} \tag{4.57}$$

It then follows from (4.49) that the likelihood estimating equation for ρ_k, $k = 1, \ldots, J-1$, is given by

$$\frac{\partial Log\ L(\beta, \rho_M)}{\partial \rho_k} = \sum_{i=1}^{K} \sum_{t=2}^{T} \sum_{g=1}^{J} \left[\sum_{j=1}^{J-1} \frac{y_{itj}}{\lambda^{(j)}_{it|t-1}(g)} I_{j|k}(\delta_g - \pi_{(i,t-1)}) - \frac{y_{itJ}}{\lambda^{(J)}_{it|t-1}(g)}(\delta_g - \pi_{(i,t-1)}) \right] = 0, \tag{4.58}$$

where, for a selected value of k, $I_{j|k}$ is an indicator variable such that

$$I_{j|k} = \begin{cases} 1 \text{ for } j = k \\ 0 \text{ for } j \neq k, \end{cases}$$

leading to the estimating equations for the elements of $\rho^* = (\rho_1', \ldots, \rho_j', \ldots, \rho_{J-1}')'$ as

$$\frac{\partial Log\, L(\beta, \rho_M)}{\partial \rho^*} = \begin{pmatrix} \frac{\partial Log\, L(\beta, \rho_M)}{\partial \rho_1} \\ \vdots \\ \frac{\partial Log\, L(\beta, \rho_M)}{\partial \rho_k} \\ \vdots \\ \frac{\partial Log\, L(\beta, \rho_M)}{\partial \rho_{J-1}} \end{pmatrix} = 0 : (J-1)^2 \times 1. \tag{4.59}$$

Similar to Chap. 3 (see (3.201)), one may solve these likelihood equations in (4.59) for ρ^* by using the iterative equation

$$\hat{\rho}^*(r+1) = \hat{\rho}^*(r) - \left[\left\{ \frac{\partial^2 \text{Log}\, L(\beta, \rho_M)}{\partial \rho^* \partial \rho^{*\prime}} \right\}^{-1} \frac{\partial \text{Log}\, L(\beta, \rho_M)}{\partial \rho^*} \right]_{|\rho^* = \hat{\rho}^*(r)}, \tag{4.60}$$

where the $(J-1)^2 \times (J-1)^2$ second derivative matrix is computed by using the formulas

$$\frac{\partial^2 \text{Log}\, L(\beta, \rho_M)}{\partial \rho_k \partial \rho_k'} = -\sum_{i=1}^{K} \sum_{t=2}^{T} \sum_{g=1}^{J} \left[\sum_{j=1}^{J-1} \frac{y_{itj}}{\{\lambda_{it|t-1}^{(j)}(g)\}^2} I_{j|k} (\delta_g - \pi_{(i,t-1)})(\delta_g - \pi_{(i,t-1)})' \right.$$
$$\left. + \frac{y_{itJ}}{\{\lambda_{it|t-1}^{(J)}(g)\}^2} (\delta_g - \pi_{(i,t-1)})(\delta_g - \pi_{(i,t-1)})' \right], \tag{4.61}$$

for all $k = 1, \ldots, J-1$, and

$$\frac{\partial^2 \text{Log}\, L(\beta, \rho_M)}{\partial \rho_h \partial \rho_k'} = -\sum_{i=1}^{K} \sum_{t=2}^{T} \sum_{g=1}^{J} \left[\frac{y_{itJ}}{\{\lambda_{it|t-1}^{(J)}(g)\}^2} (\delta_g - \pi_{(i,t-1)})(\delta_g - \pi_{(i,t-1)})' \right], \tag{4.62}$$

for all $h \neq k; h, k = 1, \ldots, J-1$.

4.4 NSMDL Model

The MDL models with time independent covariates were discussed in Chap. 3, more specifically in Sect. 3.5.2. In this section we deal with a general MDL model where covariates can be time dependent. As far as the marginal probabilities at time $t = 1$

are concerned, they remain the same as in (4.1), see also (4.35) under the LDCMP model. For convenience we rewrite these probabilities from (4.35) as

$$P[y_{i1} = y_{i1}^{(j)} = \delta_{i1j}] = \pi_{(i1)j} = \begin{cases} \frac{\exp(w_{i1}^{*'}\beta_j^*)}{1+\sum_{g=1}^{J-1}\exp(w_{i1}^{*'}\beta_g^*)} & \text{for } j = 1,\ldots,J-1 \\ \frac{1}{1+\sum_{g=1}^{J-1}\exp(w_{i1}^{*'}\beta_g^*)} & \text{for } j = J, \end{cases} \quad (4.63)$$

where $w_{i1}^* = \left(1 \ w_{i1}'\right)'$, w_{i1} being the p-dimensional covariate vector recorded at time $t = 1$, and $\beta_j^* = (\beta_{j0}, \beta_j')'$ is the effect of w_{i1}^*, leading to the regression parameters set as

$$\beta \equiv (\beta_1^{*'}, \ldots, \beta_j^{*'}, \ldots, \beta_{J-1}^{*}{}')' : (J-1)(p+1) \times 1.$$

However, unlike the LDCMP model (4.20), at times $t = 2, \ldots, T$, we now use the logit type non-linear conditional probabilities given by

$$\eta_{it|t-1}^{(j)}(g) = P\left(Y_{it} = y_{it}^{(j)} \,\middle|\, Y_{i,t-1} = y_{i,t-1}^{(g)}\right) = \begin{cases} \frac{\exp\left[w_{it}^{*'}\beta_j^* + \gamma_j' y_{i,t-1}^{(g)}\right]}{1+\sum_{v=1}^{J-1}\exp\left[w_{it}^{*'}\beta_v^* + \gamma_v' y_{i,t-1}^{(g)}\right]}, & \text{for } j = 1,\ldots,J-1 \\ \frac{1}{1+\sum_{v=1}^{J-1}\exp\left[w_{it}^{*'}\beta_v^* + \gamma_v' y_{i,t-1}^{(g)}\right]}, & \text{for } j = J, \end{cases} \quad (4.64)$$

where $\gamma_j = (\gamma_{j1}, \ldots, \gamma_{jv}, \ldots, \gamma_{j,J-1})'$ denotes the dynamic dependence parameters, which may be referred to as the correlation index or a particular type of odds ratio parameters. More specifically, the correlations of the repeated multinomial responses will be functions of these γ parameters. Furthermore, the marginal probabilities (4.63) at time $t = 1$ and conditional probabilities (4.64) for $t = 2, \ldots, T$, yield the marginal probabilities at time $t(t = 2, \ldots)$ as function of $w_{it}^{*'}$ and they are also influenced by γ parameters. Suppose that unlike in the LDCMP model, we use $\tilde{\pi}_{(it)j}$ for the marginal probabilities under the present MDL model for all time $t = 1, \ldots, T$. When marginal probabilities under the MDL model are computed recursively by using (4.63) and (4.64), it becomes clear that even though

$$\tilde{\pi}_{(i1)j} = P[y_{i1} = y_{i1}^{(j)}] = \pi_{(i1)j} = \begin{cases} \frac{\exp(w_{i1}^{*'}\beta_j^*)}{1+\sum_{g=1}^{J-1}\exp(w_{i1}^{*'}\beta_g^*)} & \text{for } j = 1,\ldots,J-1 \\ \frac{1}{1+\sum_{g=1}^{J-1}\exp(w_{i1}^{*'}\beta_g^*)} & \text{for } j = J, \end{cases} \quad (4.65)$$

$$\tilde{\pi}_{(it)j} = P[y_{it} = y_{it}^{(j)}] \neq \pi_{(it)j} = \begin{cases} \frac{\exp(w_{it}^{*'}\beta_j^*)}{1+\sum_{g=1}^{J-1}\exp(w_{it}^{*'}\beta_g^*)} & \text{for } j = 1,\ldots,J-1;\ t = 2,\ldots,T \\ \frac{1}{1+\sum_{g=1}^{J-1}\exp(w_{it}^{*'}\beta_g^*)} & \text{for } j = J;\ t = 2,\ldots,T. \end{cases} \quad (4.66)$$

The formulas for the marginal probabilities $\tilde{\pi}_{(it)j}$ are given below under the basic properties of the model (4.63)–(4.64).

4.4.1 Basic Moment Properties of the MDL Model

4.4.1.1 Marginal Expectation Vector and Covariance Matrix at $t = 1$

For $t = 1$, the expectation and covariance matrix of the response vector y_{i1} are the same as in (4.21) and (4.29) under the LDCMP model. That is,

$$\begin{aligned} E[Y_{i1}] &= \sum_{g=1}^{J} y_{i1}^{(g)} P[Y_{i1} = y_{i1}^{(g)}] = \sum_{g=1}^{J} y_{i1}^{(g)} \pi_{(i1)g} \\ &= [\pi_{(i1)1}, \ldots, \pi_{(i1)j}, \ldots, \pi_{(i1)(J-1)}]' = \pi_{(i1)} \\ &\equiv [\tilde{\pi}_{(i1)1}, \ldots, \tilde{\pi}_{(i1)j}, \ldots, \tilde{\pi}_{(i1)(J-1)}]' \\ &= \tilde{\pi}_{(i1)} : (J-1) \times 1, \end{aligned} \tag{4.67}$$

and

$$\begin{aligned} \mathrm{var}[Y_{i1}] &= \mathrm{diag}[\pi_{(i1)1}, \ldots, \pi_{(i1)j}, \ldots, \pi_{(i1),J-1}] - \pi_{(i1)}\pi'_{(i1)} = \Sigma_{(i,11)}(\beta) \\ &\equiv \mathrm{diag}[\tilde{\pi}_{(i1)1}, \ldots, \tilde{\pi}_{(i1)j}, \ldots, \tilde{\pi}_{(i1),J-1}] - \tilde{\pi}_{(i1)}\tilde{\pi}'_{(i1)} \\ &= \tilde{\Sigma}_{(i,11)}(\beta), \text{ (say).} \end{aligned} \tag{4.68}$$

4.4.1.2 Marginal Expectation Vectors and Covariance Matrices for $t = 2, \ldots, T$

For $t = 2, \ldots, T$, by using the initial marginal model (4.63) for $t = 1$ and the conditional probability model (4.64) for $t = 2, \ldots, T$, one may derive the recursive relationships for the unconditional means, variance and covariance matrices (see also Loredo-Osti and Sutradhar 2012, unpublished Ph.D. thesis by Chowdhury 2011) as

$$\begin{aligned} E[Y_{it}] &= \tilde{\pi}_{(it)}(\beta, \gamma) = \eta_{(it|t-1)}(J) + \left[\eta_{(it|t-1),M} - \eta_{(it|t-1)}(J)1'_{J-1}\right] \tilde{\pi}_{(i,t-1)} \\ &= (\tilde{\pi}_{(it)1}, \ldots, \tilde{\pi}_{(it)j}, \ldots, \tilde{\pi}_{(it)(J-1)})' : (J-1) \times 1 \end{aligned} \tag{4.69}$$

$$\begin{aligned} \mathrm{var}[Y_{it}] &= \mathrm{diag}[\tilde{\pi}_{(it)1}, \ldots, \tilde{\pi}_{(it)j}, \ldots, \tilde{\pi}_{(it)(J-1)}] - \tilde{\pi}_{(it)}\tilde{\pi}'_{(it)} \\ &= (\mathrm{cov}(Y_{itj}, Y_{itk})) = (\tilde{\sigma}_{(i,tt)jk}), \; j,k = 1, \ldots, J-1 \\ &= \tilde{\Sigma}_{(i,tt)}(\beta, \gamma) \end{aligned} \tag{4.70}$$

$$\begin{aligned} \mathrm{cov}[Y_{iu}, Y_{it}] &= \Pi_{s=u+1}^{t} \left[\eta_{(is|s-1),M} - \eta_{(is|s-1)}(J)1'_{J-1}\right] \mathrm{var}[Y_{iu}], \text{ for } u < t \\ &= (\mathrm{cov}(Y_{iuj}, Y_{itk})) = (\tilde{\sigma}_{(i,ut)jk}), \; j,k = 1, \ldots, J-1 \\ &= \tilde{\Sigma}_{(i,ut)}(\beta, \gamma), \end{aligned} \tag{4.71}$$

where

$$\eta_{(is|s-1)}(J) = [\eta^{(1)}_{is|s-1}(J), \ldots, \eta^{(j)}_{is|s-1}(J) \ldots, \eta^{(J-1)}_{is|s-1}(J)]' = \pi_{(is)} : (J-1) \times 1, \text{ by (4.64) and (4.66);}$$

$$\eta_{(is|s-1),M} = \begin{pmatrix} \eta^{(1)}_{is|s-1}(1) & \cdots & \eta^{(1)}_{is|s-1}(g) & \cdots & \eta^{(1)}_{is|s-1}(J-1) \\ \vdots & \vdots & \vdots & \vdots & \vdots \\ \eta^{(j)}_{is|s-1}(1) & \cdots & \eta^{(j)}_{is|s-1}(g) & \cdots & \eta^{(j)}_{is|s-1}(J-1) \\ \vdots & \vdots & \vdots & \vdots & \vdots \\ \eta^{(J-1)}_{is|s-1}(1) & \cdots & \eta^{(J-1)}_{is|s-1}(g) & \cdots & \eta^{(J-1)}_{is|s-1}(J-1) \end{pmatrix} : (J-1) \times (J-1),$$

with

$$\eta^{(j)}_{is|s-1}(g) = \begin{cases} \frac{\exp\left[w^{*'}_{is}\beta^*_j + \gamma_{jg}\right]}{1+\sum_{v=1}^{J-1}\exp\left[w^{*'}_{is}\beta^*_v + \gamma_{vg}\right]}, & \text{for } j = 1,\ldots,J-1;\ g = 1,\ldots,J-1 \\ \frac{\exp\left[w^{*'}_{is}\beta^*_j\right]}{1+\sum_{v=1}^{J-1}\exp\left[w^{*'}_{is}\beta^*_v\right]}, & \text{for } j = 1,\ldots,J-1;\ g = J, \end{cases} \tag{4.72}$$

by (4.64).

4.4.1.3 Illustration

We illustrate the computation of the marginal means, variance and covariances for the case with $T = 2$.

For $t = 1$, the formulas for the mean $E[Y_{i1}]$, variance–covariance matrix $\text{var}[Y_{i1}]$ are derived in (4.67) and (4.68), respectively.

For $t = 2$, the formula for $E[Y_{i2}]$ given in (4.69) can be derived, for example, as follows:

Computation of $E[Y_{i2}]$:

$$\begin{aligned} E[Y_{i2}] &= E_{Y_{i1}} E[Y_{i2}|y_{i1}] \\ &= E_{Y_{i1}}[\sum_{j=1}^{J} y^{(j)}_{i2}\eta^{(j)}_{i2|1}(y_{i1})] \end{aligned} \tag{4.73}$$

$$\begin{aligned} &= E_{Y_{i1}} \begin{pmatrix} \eta^{(1)}_{i2|1}(y_{i1}) \\ \vdots \\ \eta^{(j)}_{i2|1}(y_{i1}) \\ \vdots \\ \eta^{(J-1)}_{i2|1}(y_{i1}) \end{pmatrix} \\ &= E_{Y_{i1}}[\eta_{i2|1}(y_{i1})], \end{aligned} \tag{4.74}$$

where $\eta^{(j)}_{it|t-1}(y^{(g)}_{i1})$ is given by (4.64). Next because

$$Y_{i1} = y^{(g)}_{i1} = \begin{cases} (y^{(g)}_{i11}, \ldots, y^{(g)}_{i1g}, \ldots, y^{(g)}_{i1,J-1})' = (01'_{g-1}, 1, 01'_{J-1-g})' & \text{for } g = 1, \ldots, J-1; \\ (01_{J-1}) & \text{for } g = J, \end{cases} \tag{4.75}$$

with

$$P[Y_{i1} = y^{(g)}_{i1}] = \pi_{(i1)g} \equiv \tilde{\pi}_{(i1)g},$$

where

$$\tilde{\pi}_{(i1)J} = 1 - \sum_{g=1}^{J-1} \tilde{\pi}_{(i1)g},$$

it then follows that

$$\begin{aligned} E_{Y_{i1}}[\eta_{i2|1}(y_{i1})] &= \sum_{g=1}^{J} [\eta_{i2|1}(y^{(g)}_{i1})]\tilde{\pi}_{(i1)g} \\ &= \sum_{g=1}^{J} \begin{pmatrix} \eta^{(1)}_{i2|1}(g) \\ \vdots \\ \eta^{(j)}_{i2|1}(g) \\ \vdots \\ \eta^{(J-1)}_{i2|1}(g) \end{pmatrix} \tilde{\pi}_{(i1)g} \\ &= \sum_{g=1}^{J-1} \begin{pmatrix} \eta^{(1)}_{i2|1}(g) \\ \vdots \\ \eta^{(j)}_{i2|1}(g) \\ \vdots \\ \eta^{(J-1)}_{i2|1}(g) \end{pmatrix} \tilde{\pi}_{(i1)g} + \begin{pmatrix} \eta^{(1)}_{i2|1}(J) \\ \vdots \\ \eta^{(j)}_{i2|1}(J) \\ \vdots \\ \eta^{(J-1)}_{i2|1}(J) \end{pmatrix} [1 - \sum_{g=1}^{J-1} \tilde{\pi}_{(i1)g}] \\ &= \begin{pmatrix} \eta^{(1)}_{i2|1}(J) \\ \vdots \\ \eta^{(j)}_{i2|1}(J) \\ \vdots \\ \eta^{(J-1)}_{i2|1}(J) \end{pmatrix} + \sum_{g=1}^{J-1} \left[\begin{pmatrix} \eta^{(1)}_{i2|1}(g) \\ \vdots \\ \eta^{(j)}_{i2|1}(g) \\ \vdots \\ \eta^{(J-1)}_{i2|1}(g) \end{pmatrix} - \begin{pmatrix} \eta^{(1)}_{i2|1}(J) \\ \vdots \\ \eta^{(j)}_{i2|1}(J) \\ \vdots \\ \eta^{(J-1)}_{i2|1}(J) \end{pmatrix} \right] \tilde{\pi}_{(i1)g} \end{aligned}$$

$$
= \begin{pmatrix} \eta_{i2|1}^{(1)}(J) \\ \vdots \\ \eta_{i2|1}^{(j)}(J) \\ \vdots \\ \eta_{i2|1}^{(J-1)}(J) \end{pmatrix} + \left[\begin{pmatrix} \eta_{i2|1}^{(1)}(1) & \cdots & \eta_{i2|1}^{(1)}(g) & \cdots & \eta_{i2|1}^{(1)}(J-1) \\ \vdots & \vdots & \vdots & \vdots & \vdots \\ \eta_{i2|1}^{(j)}(1) & \cdots & \eta_{i2|1}^{(j)}(g) & \cdots & \eta_{i2|1}^{(j)}(J-1) \\ \vdots & \vdots & \vdots & \vdots & \vdots \\ \eta_{i2|1}^{(J-1)}(1) & \cdots & \eta_{i2|1}^{(J-1)}(g) & \cdots & \eta_{i2|1}^{(J-1)}(J-1) \end{pmatrix} \right.
$$

$$
\left. - \begin{pmatrix} \eta_{i2|1}^{(1)}(J) \\ \vdots \\ \eta_{i2|1}^{(j)}(J) \\ \vdots \\ \eta_{i2|1}^{(J-1)}(J) \end{pmatrix} 1'_{J-1} \right] \tilde{\pi}_{(i1)}
$$

$$
\begin{aligned}
&= \eta_{(i2|1)}(J) + \left[\eta_{(i2|1),M} - \eta_{(i2|1)}(J) 1'_{J-1} \right] \tilde{\pi}_{(i1)} \\
&= \tilde{\pi}_{(i2)} = [\tilde{\pi}_{(i2)1}, \ldots, \tilde{\pi}_{(i2)j}, \ldots, \tilde{\pi}_{(i2)(J-1)}]'. \qquad (4.76)
\end{aligned}
$$

Computation of var$[Y_{i2}]$:

$$
\begin{aligned}
\text{var}[Y_{i2}] &= E[Y_{i2} - \tilde{\pi}_{(i2)}][Y_{i2} - \tilde{\pi}_{(i2)}]' \\
&= E[Y_{i2}Y'_{i2}] - \tilde{\pi}_{(i2)}\tilde{\pi}'_{(i2)}. \qquad (4.77)
\end{aligned}
$$

Notice from (4.64) that

$$
\eta_{i2|1}^{(j)}(g) = P\left(Y_{i2} = y_{i2}^{(j)} \,\middle|\, Y_{i1} = y_{i1}^{(g)}\right)
$$

for all j with $\eta_{i2|1}^{(J)}(g) = 1 - \sum_{j=1}^{J-1} \eta_{i2|1}^{(j)}(g)$, yielding the conditional multinomial covariance matrix

$$
\text{var}[Y_{i2}|y_{i1}^{(g)}] = \text{diag}[\eta_{i2|1}^{(1)}(g), \ldots, \eta_{i2|1}^{(j)}(g), \ldots, \eta_{i2|1}^{(J-1)}(g)] - \eta_{i2|1}(g)\eta'_{i2|1}(g), \qquad (4.78)
$$

where

$$
\eta_{i2|1}(g) = [\eta_{i2|1}^{(1)}(g), \ldots, \eta_{i2|1}^{(j)}(g), \ldots, \eta_{i2|1}^{(J-1)}(g)]'.
$$

By (4.78), it then follows from (4.77) that

$$
\begin{aligned}
\text{var}[Y_{i2}] &= E_{Y_{i1}} E[Y_{i2}Y'_{i2}|y_{i1}] - \tilde{\pi}_{(i2)}\tilde{\pi}'_{(i2)} \\
&= E_{Y_{i1}} \text{diag}[\eta_{i2|1}^{(1)}(y_{i1}), \ldots, \eta_{i2|1}^{(j)}(y_{i1}), \ldots, \eta_{i2|1}^{(J-1)}(y_{i1})] - \tilde{\pi}_{(i2)}\tilde{\pi}'_{(i2)} \\
&= \text{diag}[\tilde{\pi}_{(i2)1}, \ldots, \tilde{\pi}_{(i2)j}, \ldots, \tilde{\pi}_{(i2)(J-1)}] - \tilde{\pi}_{(i2)}\tilde{\pi}'_{(i2)}, \qquad (4.79)
\end{aligned}
$$

by (4.76).

Computation of cov$[Y_{i2}, Y_{i1}]$:

$$
\begin{aligned}
\mathrm{cov}[Y_{i2},Y_{i1}] &= E_{Y_{i1}} Y_{i1} E[Y'_{i2}|y_{i1}] - \tilde{\pi}_{(i1)}\tilde{\pi}'_{(i2)} \\
&= E_{Y_{i1}} Y_{i1}[\eta^{(1)}_{i2|1}(y_{i1}),\ldots,\eta^{(j)}_{i2|1}(y_{i1}),\ldots,\eta^{(J-1)}_{i2|1}(y_{i1})] - \tilde{\pi}_{(i1)}\tilde{\pi}'_{(i2)} \\
&= \sum_{g=1}^{J}\left[y^{(g)}_{i1}\left\{\eta^{(1)}_{i2|1}(y^{(g)}_{i1}),\ldots,\eta^{(j)}_{i2|1}(y^{(g)}_{i1}),\ldots,\eta^{(J-1)}_{i2|1}(y^{(g)}_{i1})\right\}\right]\tilde{\pi}_{(i1)g} - \tilde{\pi}_{(i1)}\tilde{\pi}'_{(i2)} \\
&= \mathrm{diag}[\tilde{\pi}_{(i1)1},\ldots,\tilde{\pi}_{(i1)j},\ldots,\tilde{\pi}_{(i1)(J-1)}] \\
&\times \begin{pmatrix}
\eta^{(1)}_{i2|1}(1) & \cdots & \eta^{(j)}_{i2|1}(1) & \cdots & \eta^{(J-1)}_{i2|1}(1) \\
\vdots & \vdots & \vdots & \vdots & \vdots \\
\eta^{(1)}_{i2|1}(j) & \cdots & \eta^{(j)}_{i2|1}(j) & \cdots & \eta^{(J-1)}_{i2|1}(j) \\
\vdots & \vdots & \vdots & \vdots & \vdots \\
\eta^{(1)}_{i2|1}(J-1) & \cdots & \eta^{j}_{i2|1}(J-1) & \cdots & \eta^{(J-1)}_{i2|1}(J-1)
\end{pmatrix} - \tilde{\pi}_{(i1)}\tilde{\pi}'_{(i2)} \\
&= \mathrm{diag}[\tilde{\pi}_{(i1)1},\ldots,\tilde{\pi}_{(i1)j},\ldots,\tilde{\pi}_{(i1)(J-1)}]\eta'_{(i2|1),M} - \tilde{\pi}_{(i1)}\tilde{\pi}'_{(i2)} \\
&= \mathrm{diag}[\tilde{\pi}_{(i1)1},\ldots,\tilde{\pi}_{(i1)j},\ldots,\tilde{\pi}_{(i1)(J-1)}]\eta'_{(i2|1),M} \\
&- \tilde{\pi}_{(i1)}\left[\eta_{(i2|1)}(J) + \left[\eta_{(i2|1),M} - \eta_{(i2|1)}(J)1'_{J-1}\right]\tilde{\pi}_{(i1)}\right]' \\
&= \mathrm{diag}[\tilde{\pi}_{(i1)1},\ldots,\tilde{\pi}_{(i1)j},\ldots,\tilde{\pi}_{(i1)(J-1)}]\eta'_{(i2|1),M} \\
&- \tilde{\pi}_{(i1)}\eta'_{(i2|1)}(J) - \tilde{\pi}_{(i1)}\tilde{\pi}'_{(i1)}\eta'_{(i2|1),M} + \tilde{\pi}_{(i1)}\tilde{\pi}'_{(i1)}1_{J-1}\eta'_{(i2|1)}(J) \\
&= \mathrm{diag}[\tilde{\pi}_{(i1)1},\ldots,\tilde{\pi}_{(i1)j},\ldots,\tilde{\pi}_{(i1)(J-1)}]\eta'_{(i2|1),M} \\
&- \mathrm{diag}[\tilde{\pi}_{(i1)1},\ldots,\tilde{\pi}_{(i1)j},\ldots,\tilde{\pi}_{(i1)(J-1)}]1_{J-1}\eta'_{(i2|1)}(J) - \tilde{\pi}_{(i1)}\tilde{\pi}'_{(i1)}\eta'_{(i2|1),M} \\
&+ \tilde{\pi}_{(i1)}\tilde{\pi}'_{(i1)}1_{J-1}\eta'_{(i2|1)}(J) \\
&= \mathrm{var}[Y_{i1}]\left[\eta'_{(i2|1),M} - 1_{J-1}\eta'_{(i2|1)}(J)\right] \\
&= \left[\eta_{(i2|1),M} - \eta_{(i2|1)}(J)1'_{J-1}\right]\mathrm{var}[Y_{i1}].
\end{aligned}
\tag{4.80}
$$

4.4.2 Existing Models for Dynamic Dependence Parameters and Drawbacks

Recall from (4.6) that odds ratios are, in general, defined based on joint probabilities or joint cell frequencies from an associated contingency table. However by defining odds ratios based on a transitional or conditional (on previous time) contingency table, such as Table 3.24 from Chap. 3, one may verify that the dynamic dependence parameters $\{\gamma_{jg}\}$ parameters in the conditional probabilities (4.64) (see also (4.72)) have interpretation of such odds ratio parameters. To be specific, irrespective of time $t = 2, \ldots, T$, the lag 1 dynamic dependence parameter may be expressed as

$$\begin{aligned}\gamma_{jg} &\equiv \gamma_{jg}(t|t-1) \\ &= log \frac{\eta^{(j)}_{it|t-1}(g)\eta^{(J)}_{it|t-1}(J)}{\eta^{(J)}_{it|t-1}(g)\eta^{(j)}_{it|t-1}(J)}. \end{aligned} \quad (4.81)$$

To illustrate this odds ratio, consider $J = 3$, for example. By (4.72) one writes

$$\begin{aligned}
\eta^{(1)}_{it|t-1}(1) &= \frac{\exp\left[w^{*'}_{it}\beta^*_1 + \gamma_{11}\right]}{1 + \sum_{v=1}^2 \exp\left[w^{*'}_{it}\beta^*_v + \gamma_{v1}\right]};\ \eta^{(2)}_{it|t-1}(1) = \frac{\exp\left[w^{*'}_{it}\beta^*_2 + \gamma_{21}\right]}{1 + \sum_{v=1}^2 \exp\left[w^{*'}_{it}\beta^*_v + \gamma_{v1}\right]}; \\
\eta^{(3)}_{it|t-1}(1) &= \frac{1}{1 + \sum_{v=1}^2 \exp\left[w^{*'}_{it}\beta^*_v + \gamma_{v1}\right]};\ \eta^{(1)}_{it|t-1}(2) = \frac{\exp\left[w^{*'}_{it}\beta^*_1 + \gamma_{12}\right]}{1 + \sum_{v=1}^2 \exp\left[w^{*'}_{it}\beta^*_v + \gamma_{v2}\right]}; \\
\eta^{(2)}_{it|t-1}(2) &= \frac{\exp\left[w^{*'}_{it}\beta^*_2 + \gamma_{22}\right]}{1 + \sum_{v=1}^2 \exp\left[w^{*'}_{it}\beta^*_v + \gamma_{v2}\right]};\ \eta^{(3)}_{it|t-1}(2) = \frac{1}{1 + \sum_{v=1}^2 \exp\left[w^{*'}_{it}\beta^*_v + \gamma_{v2}\right]}; \\
\eta^{(1)}_{it|t-1}(3) &= \frac{\exp\left[w^{*'}_{it}\beta^*_1\right]}{1 + \sum_{v=1}^2 \exp\left[w^{*'}_{it}\beta^*_v\right]};\ \eta^{(2)}_{it|t-1}(3) = \frac{\exp\left[w^{*'}_{it}\beta^*_2\right]}{1 + \sum_{v=1}^2 \exp\left[w^{*'}_{it}\beta^*_v\right]}; \\
\eta^{(3)}_{it|t-1}(3) &= \frac{1}{1 + \sum_{v=1}^2 \exp\left[w^{*'}_{it}\beta^*_v\right]}.
\end{aligned} \quad (4.82)$$

It is clear, for example, that

$$\frac{\eta^{(1)}_{it|t-1}(2)\eta^{(3)}_{it|t-1}(3)}{\eta^{(3)}_{it|t-1}(2)\eta^{(1)}_{it|t-1}(3)} = \frac{\exp\left[w^{*'}_{it}\beta^*_1 + \gamma_{12}\right]}{\exp\left[w^{*'}_{it}\beta^*_1\right]}, \quad (4.83)$$

yielding

$$\gamma_{12} = log \frac{\eta^{(1)}_{it|t-1}(2)\eta^{(3)}_{it|t-1}(3)}{\eta^{(3)}_{it|t-1}(2)\eta^{(1)}_{it|t-1}(3)}. \quad (4.84)$$

Note that these dynamic dependence parameters $\{\gamma_{jg}(t|t-1),\ j,g = 1,\ldots,J-1\}$ in conditional probabilities also get involved in the joint and marginal probabilities. For example, by (4.69),

$$\begin{aligned}P[Y_{it} = y^{(j)}_{it}] &= \tilde{\pi}_{(it)j} = E[Y^{(j)}_{it}] \\ &= \eta^{(j)}_{it|t-1}(J) + \sum_{g=1}^{J-1}[\{\eta^{(j)}_{it|t-1}(g) - \eta^{(j)}_{it|t-1}(J)\}\tilde{\pi}_{(i,t-1)j}], \end{aligned} \quad (4.85)$$

showing that $\{\gamma_{jg}(t|t-1),\ j,g=1,\ldots,J-1\}$ are involved in the marginal probability in a complicated way. Some authors such as Chen et al. (2009, Eq. (4), see also Sect. 3.1) determine the values of these dynamic dependence parameters by equating $\tilde{\pi}_{(it)j}$ in (4.85) to a LDCM (4.20) type marginal probability

$$\pi_{(it)j} = \begin{cases} \frac{\exp(w_{it}^{*'}\beta_j^*)}{1+\sum_{g=1}^{J-1}\exp(w_{it}^{*'}\beta_g^*)} & \text{for } j=1,\ldots,J-1;\ t=2,\ldots,T \\ \frac{1}{1+\sum_{g=1}^{J-1}\exp(w_{it}^{*'}\beta_g^*)} & \text{for } j=J;\ t=2,\ldots,T. \end{cases}$$

But as shown in (4.66), under the present MDL model, marginal probabilities except for initial time $t=1$, do not have the form as $\pi_{(it)j}$. That is,

$$\tilde{\pi}_{(it)j} = P[y_{it} = y_{it}^{(j)}] \neq \pi_{(it)j}. \tag{4.86}$$

Thus, the restriction, that is, $\tilde{\pi}_{(it)j} = P[y_{it} = y_{it}^{(j)}] = \pi_{(it)j}$, used in Chen et al. (2009, Eq. (4), see also Section 3.1) to understand the odds ratio parameters, is not justified.

In fact, as we demonstrate in the next section, under the present MDL model (4.63)–(4.64), the dynamic dependence parameters $\{\gamma_{jg}(t|t-1),\ j,g=1,\ldots,J-1\}$ along with regression parameters (β), can be estimated easily by using the traditional likelihood estimation method, without any additional restrictions.

4.5 Likelihood Estimation for NSMDL Model Parameters

The likelihood estimation for a similar MDL model was discussed in Chap. 3, more specifically in Sect. 3.4.2 for an MDL model involving no covariates (see Eqs. (3.206)–(3.207)) and in Sect. 3.5.2 for an MDL model involving a categorical covariate with $p+1$ levels (see Eqs. (3.275)–(3.276)). In this section, we construct the likelihood function and develop estimating equations for the parameters of the general NSMDL model (see Eqs. (4.63)–(4.64)), where covariates involved are general, that is, they can vary from individual to individual and they can be time dependent as well. These general covariates are denoted by $w_{it}^* = \left(1\ w_{it}'\right)'$, w_{it} being the p-dimensional covariate vector recorded from the ith individual at time $t=1,\ldots,T$.

4.5.1 Likelihood Function

Note that y_{it} is a J category based multinomial variable at any time point $t=1,\ldots,T$. At $t=1$, y_{i1} has the marginal distribution as

$$f(y_{i1}) = \frac{1!}{y_{i11}!\ldots y_{i1j}!\ldots y_{i1,J-1}!y_{i1J}!}\Pi_{j=1}^{J}\left[\pi_{(i1)j}\right]^{y_{i1j}}, \tag{4.87}$$

where by (4.63),

$$\pi_{(i1)j} = \begin{cases} \frac{\exp(w_{i1}^{*'}\beta_j^*)}{1+\sum_{g=1}^{J-1}\exp(w_{i1}^{*'}\beta_g^*)} & \text{for } j=1,\ldots,J-1 \\ \frac{1}{1+\sum_{g=1}^{J-1}\exp(w_{i1}^{*'}\beta_g^*)} & \text{for } j=J. \end{cases}$$

Next, at time $t = 2,\ldots,T$, conditional on $Y_{i,t-1} = y_{i,t-1}^{(g)}$, one may write the conditional distribution of y_{it} as

$$f(y_{it}|y_{i,t-1}^{(g)}) = \frac{1!}{y_{it1}!\ldots y_{itj}!\ldots y_{it,J-1}!y_{itJ}!}\Pi_{j=1}^J\left[\eta_{it|t-1}^{(j)}(g)\right]^{y_{itj}}, \ g=1,\ldots,J \tag{4.88}$$

where $\eta_{it|t-1}^{(j)}(g)$ for $j=1,\ldots,J$, by (4.64), have the formulas

$$\eta_{it|t-1}^{(j)}(g) = P\left(Y_{it}=y_{it}^{(j)}\Big|Y_{i,t-1}=y_{i,t-1}^{(g)}\right) = \begin{cases} \frac{\exp\left[w_{it}^{*'}\beta_j^*+\gamma_j'y_{i,t-1}^{(g)}\right]}{1+\sum_{v=1}^{J-1}\exp\left[w_{it}^{*'}\beta_v^*+\gamma_v'y_{i,t-1}^{(g)}\right]}, & \text{for } j=1,\ldots,J-1 \\ \frac{1}{1+\sum_{v=1}^{J-1}\exp\left[w_{it}^{*'}\beta_v^*+\gamma_v'y_{i,t-1}^{(g)}\right]}, & \text{for } j=J, \end{cases}$$

where $\gamma_j = (\gamma_{j1},\ldots,\gamma_{jv},\ldots,\gamma_{j,J-1})'$ denotes the dynamic dependence parameters. Similar to (4.1)–(4.3), we use

$$\beta \equiv (\beta_1^{*'},\ldots,\beta_j^{*'},\ldots,\beta_{J-1}^{*'})' : (J-1)(p+1)\times 1,$$

where $\beta_j^* = (\beta_{j0},\beta_j')'$, with $\beta_j = [\beta_{j1},\ldots,\beta_{js},\ldots,\beta_{jp}]'$. Also, the dynamic dependence parameters are conveniently denoted by γ_M with

$$\gamma_M = \begin{pmatrix} \gamma_1' \\ \vdots \\ \gamma_j' \\ \vdots \\ \gamma_{J-1}' \end{pmatrix} : (J-1)\times(J-1). \tag{4.89}$$

One may then write the likelihood function for β and γ_M, under the present MDL model, as

$$\begin{aligned} L(\beta,\gamma_M) &= \Pi_{i=1}^K\left[f(y_{i1})\Pi_{t=2}^T f(y_{it}|y_{i,t-1})\right] \\ &= \left[\Pi_{i=1}^K f(y_{i1})\right] \\ &\times \Pi_{i=1}^K\Pi_{t=2}^T\Pi_{g=1}^J\left[f(y_{it}|y_{i,t-1}^{(g)})\right] \\ &= c_0^*\left[\Pi_{i=1}^K\Pi_{j=1}^J\pi_{(i1)j}^{y_{i1j}}\right] \\ &\times \Pi_{i=1}^K\Pi_{t=2}^T\Pi_{j=1}^J\Pi_{g=1}^J\left\{\eta_{it|t-1}^{(j)}(y_{i,t-1}^{(g)})\right\}^{y_{itj}}, \end{aligned} \tag{4.90}$$

where c_0^* is the normalizing constant free from any parameters. This yields the log likelihood function as

$$Log\ L(\beta, \gamma_M) = log\ c_0^* + \sum_{i=1}^{K}\sum_{j=1}^{J} y_{i1j} log\ \pi_{(i1)j} + \sum_{i=1}^{K}\sum_{t=2}^{T}\sum_{j=1}^{J}\sum_{g=1}^{J}\left[y_{itj} log\ \eta_{it|t-1}^{(j)}(g)\right]. \quad (4.91)$$

For further notational convenience, we re-express the conditional probabilities in (4.91) as

$$\eta_{it|t-1}^{(j)}(g) = \begin{cases} \frac{\exp\left[w_{it}^{*'}\beta_j^* + \gamma_j'\delta_{(i,t-1)g}\right]}{1+\sum_{v=1}^{J-1}\exp\left[w_{it}^{*'}\beta_v^* + \gamma_v'\delta_{(i,t-1)g}\right]}, & \text{for } j = 1,\ldots,J-1 \\ \frac{1}{1+\sum_{v=1}^{J-1}\exp\left[w_{it}^{*'}\beta_v^* + \gamma_v'\delta_{(i,t-1)g}\right]}, & \text{for } j = J, \end{cases}$$

where for all $i = 1,\ldots,K$, and $t = 2,\ldots,T$, $\delta_{(i,t-1)g}$ is defined as

$$\delta_{(i,t-1)g} = \begin{cases} [01_{g-1}', 1, 01_{J-1-g}']' & \text{for } g = 1,\ldots,J-1 \\ 01_{J-1} & \text{for } g = J. \end{cases}$$

4.5.1.1 Likelihood Estimating Equation for β

It follows from the log likelihood function in (4.91) that the likelihood estimating equations for β has the form

$$\frac{\partial Log\ L(\beta, \gamma_M)}{\partial \beta} = \sum_{i=1}^{K}\sum_{j=1}^{J}\frac{y_{i1j}}{\pi_{(i1)j}}\frac{\partial \pi_{(i1)j}}{\partial \beta} + \sum_{i=1}^{K}\sum_{t=2}^{T}\sum_{j=1}^{J}\sum_{g=1}^{J}\left[\frac{y_{itj}}{\eta_{it|t-1}^{(j)}(g)}\frac{\partial \eta_{it|t-1}^{(j)}(g)}{\partial \beta}\right] = 0, \quad (4.92)$$

where by (4.37)–(4.38),

$$\frac{\partial \pi_{(i1)j}}{\partial \beta_j^*} = \pi_{(i1)j}[1 - \pi_{(i1)j}]w_{i1}^*$$

$$\frac{\partial \pi_{(i1)j}}{\partial \beta_k^*} = -[\pi_{(i1)j}\pi_{(i1)k}]w_{i1}^*, \quad (4.93)$$

yielding

$$\frac{\partial \pi_{(i1)j}}{\partial \beta} = \begin{pmatrix} -\pi_{(i1)1}\pi_{(i1)j} \\ \vdots \\ \pi_{(i1)j}[1-\pi_{(i1)j}] \\ \vdots \\ -\pi_{(i1)(J-1)}\pi_{(i1)j} \end{pmatrix} \otimes w^*_{i1} : (J-1)(p+1) \times 1$$
$$= \left[\pi_{(i1)j}(\delta_{(i1)j} - \pi_{(i1)})\right] \otimes w^*_{i1}, \tag{4.94}$$

with

$$\delta_{(i1)j} = \begin{cases} [01'_{j-1}, 1, 01'_{J-1-j}]' & \text{for } j = 1,\ldots,J-1;\ i = 1,\ldots,K \\ 01_{J-1} & \text{for } j = J;\ i = 1,\ldots,K. \end{cases}$$

Similarly, for $t = 2,\ldots,T$, it follows from (4.91) that

$$\frac{\partial \eta^{(j)}_{it|t-1}(g)}{\partial \beta^*_j} = \eta^{(j)}_{it|t-1}(g)[1-\eta^{(j)}_{it|t-1}(g)]w^*_{it}$$
$$\frac{\partial \eta^{(j)}_{it|t-1}(g)}{\partial \beta^*_k} = -[\eta^{(j)}_{it|t-1}(g)\eta^{(k)}_{it|t-1}(g)]w^*_{it}, \tag{4.95}$$

yielding

$$\frac{\partial \eta^{(j)}_{it|t-1}(g)}{\partial \beta} = \begin{pmatrix} -\eta^{(1)}_{it|t-1}(g)\eta^{(j)}_{it|t-1}(g) \\ \vdots \\ \eta^{(j)}_{it|t-1}(g)[1-\eta^{(j)}_{it|t-1}(g)] \\ \vdots \\ -\eta^{(J-1)}_{it|t-1}(g)\eta^{(j)}_{it|t-1}(g) \end{pmatrix} \otimes w^*_{it} : (J-1)(p+1) \times 1$$
$$= \left[\eta^{(j)}_{it|t-1}(g)(\delta_{(i,t-1)j} - \eta_{it|t-1}(g))\right] \otimes w^*_{it}, \tag{4.96}$$

where

$$\eta_{it|t-1}(g) = [\eta^{(1)}_{it|t-1}(g),\ldots,\eta^{(j)}_{it|t-1}(g),\ldots,\eta^{(J-1)}_{it|t-1}(g)]'.$$

Thus, the likelihood equation in (4.92) has the computational formula

$$\frac{\partial Log\, L(\beta,\gamma_M)}{\partial \beta} = \sum_{i=1}^{K}\sum_{j=1}^{J} \frac{y_{i1j}}{\pi_{(i1)j}} \left[\{\pi_{(i1)j}(\delta_{(i1)j}-\pi_{(i1)})\} \otimes w^*_{i1}\right]$$

$$+ \sum_{i=1}^{K}\sum_{t=2}^{T}\sum_{j=1}^{J}\sum_{g=1}^{J} \frac{y_{itj}}{\eta^{(j)}_{it|t-1}(g)} \left[\left\{\eta^{(j)}_{it|t-1}(g)(\delta_{(i,t-1)j}-\eta_{it|t-1}(g))\right\} \otimes w^*_{it}\right] = 0, \quad (4.97)$$

For given γ_M (4.89), the likelihood equations in (4.97) may be solved iteratively by using the iterative equations for β given by

$$\hat{\beta}(r+1) = \hat{\beta}(r) - \left[\left\{\frac{\partial^2 \mathrm{Log}\, L(\beta,\gamma_M)}{\partial \beta' \partial \beta}\right\}^{-1} \frac{\partial \mathrm{Log}\, L(\beta,\gamma_M)}{\partial \beta}\right]_{|\beta=\hat{\beta}(r)} ; \; (J-1)(p+1)\times 1, \quad (4.98)$$

where the formula for the second order derivative matrix $\frac{\partial^2 Log\, L(\beta,\gamma_M)}{\partial \beta' \partial \beta}$ may be derived by taking the derivative of the $(J-1)(p+1)\times 1$ vector with respect to β'. The exact derivative has a complicated formula. We provide an approximation first and then give the exact formula for the sake of completeness.

An approximation for $\frac{\partial^2 Log\, L(\beta,\gamma_M)}{\partial \beta' \partial \beta}$ based on iteration principle:
In this approach, one assumes that β in the derivatives in (4.92), that is, β involved in $\frac{\partial \pi_{(i1)j}}{\partial \beta}$ and $\frac{\partial \eta^{(j)}_{it|t-1}(g)}{\partial \beta}$ are known from a previous iteration, and then take the derivative of $\frac{\partial Log\, L(\beta,\gamma_M)}{\partial \beta}$ in (4.92) or (4.97), with respect to β'. This provides a simpler formula for the second order derivative as

$$\frac{\partial^2 Log\, L(\beta,\gamma_M)}{\partial \beta' \partial \beta} = -\sum_{i=1}^{K}\sum_{j=1}^{J} \frac{y_{i1j}}{[\pi_{(i1)j}]^2} \left[\{\pi_{(i1)j}(\delta_{(i1)j}-\pi_{(i1)})\} \otimes w^*_{i1}\right] \left[\{\pi_{(i1)j}(\delta_{(i1)j}-\pi_{(i1)})\} \otimes w^*_{i1}\right]'$$

$$- \sum_{i=1}^{K}\sum_{t=2}^{T}\sum_{j=1}^{J}\sum_{g=1}^{J} \left[\frac{y_{itj}}{[\eta^{(j)}_{it|t-1}(g)]^2} \left[\left\{\eta^{(j)}_{it|t-1}(g)(\delta_{(i,t-1)j}-\eta_{it|t-1}(g))\right\} \otimes w^*_{it}\right]\right.$$

$$\times \left.\left[\left\{\eta^{(j)}_{it|t-1}(g)(\delta_{(i,t-1)j}-\eta_{it|t-1}(g))\right\} \otimes w^*_{it}\right]'\right] : (J-1)(p+1)\times (J-1)(p+1). \quad (4.99)$$

Exact formula for $\frac{\partial^2 Log\, L(\beta,\gamma_M)}{\partial \beta' \partial \beta}$:

Here it is assumed that β in the derivatives in (4.92), that is, β involved in $\frac{\partial \pi_{(i1)j}}{\partial \beta}$ and $\frac{\partial \eta^{(j)}_{it|t-1}(g)}{\partial \beta}$ are unknown, implying that the second order derivatives of these quantities cannot be zero. Hence, instead of (4.99), one obtains

$$\frac{\partial^2 Log\, L(\beta,\gamma_M)}{\partial \beta' \partial \beta} = -\sum_{i=1}^{K}\sum_{j=1}^{J} \frac{y_{i1j}}{[\pi_{(i1)j}]^2} \left[\{\pi_{(i1)j}(\delta_{(i1)j}-\pi_{(i1)})\} \otimes w^*_{i1}\right] \left[\{\pi_{(i1)j}(\delta_{(i1)j}-\pi_{(i1)})\} \otimes w^*_{i1}\right]'$$

$$+ \sum_{i=1}^{K}\sum_{j=1}^{J} \frac{y_{i1j}}{\pi_{(i1)j}} \frac{\partial}{\partial \beta'} \left[\{\pi_{(i1)j}(\delta_{(i1)j}-\pi_{(i1)})\} \otimes w^*_{i1}\right]$$

$$- \sum_{i=1}^{K}\sum_{t=2}^{T}\sum_{j=1}^{J}\sum_{g=1}^{J}\left[\frac{y_{itj}}{[\eta^{(j)}_{it|t-1}(g)]^2}\left[\left\{\eta^{(j)}_{it|t-1}(g)(\delta_{(i,t-1)j}-\eta_{it|t-1}(g))\right\}\otimes w^*_{it}\right]\right.$$
$$\left.\times\left[\left\{\eta^{(j)}_{it|t-1}(g)(\delta_{(i,t-1)j}-\eta_{it|t-1}(g))\right\}\otimes w^*_{it}\right]'\right]$$
$$+ \sum_{i=1}^{K}\sum_{t=2}^{T}\sum_{j=1}^{J}\sum_{g=1}^{J}\frac{y_{itj}}{\eta^{(j)}_{it|t-1}(g)}\frac{\partial}{\partial\beta'}\left[\left\{\eta^{(j)}_{it|t-1}(g)(\delta_{(i,t-1)j}-\eta_{it|t-1}(g))\right\}\otimes w^*_{it}\right], \tag{4.100}$$

where $\frac{\partial}{\partial\beta'}\left[\{\pi_{(i1)j}(\delta_{(i1)j}-\pi_{(i1)})\}\otimes w^*_{i1}\right]$ and $\frac{\partial}{\partial\beta'}\left[\left\{\eta^{(j)}_{it|t-1}(g)(\delta_{(i,t-1)j}-\eta_{it|t-1}(g))\right\}\right.$ $\left.\otimes w^*_{it}\right]$ are computed as follows.

Computation of $\frac{\partial}{\partial\beta'}\left[\{\pi_{(i1)j}(\delta_{(i1)j}-\pi_{(i1)})\}\otimes w^*_{i1}\right]$:

By (4.94),

$$\frac{\partial}{\partial\beta'}\left[\{\pi_{(i1)j}(\delta_{(i1)j}-\pi_{(i1)})\}\otimes w^*_{i1}\right]$$
$$= \frac{\partial}{\partial\beta'}\left[\begin{pmatrix} -\pi_{(i1)1}\pi_{(i1)j} \\ \vdots \\ \pi_{(i1)j}[1-\pi_{(i1)j}] \\ \vdots \\ -\pi_{(i1)(J-1)}\pi_{(i1)j}\end{pmatrix}\otimes w^*_{i1}\right]$$
$$= \begin{pmatrix} \left[-\pi_{(i1)1}\pi_{(i1)j}\left\{\left(\delta_{(i1)j}+\delta_{(i1)1}-2\pi_{(i1)}\right)'\otimes w^{*'}_{i1}\right\}\right]\otimes w^*_{i1} \\ \left[-\pi_{(i1)2}\pi_{(i1)j}\left\{\left(\delta_{(i1)j}+\delta_{(i1)2}-2\pi_{(i1)}\right)'\otimes w^{*'}_{i1}\right\}\right]\otimes w^*_{i1} \\ \vdots \\ \left[\pi_{(i1)j}(1-2\pi_{(i1)j})\left\{\left(\delta_{(i1)j}-\pi_{(i1)}\right)'\otimes w^{*'}_{i1}\right\}\right]\otimes w^*_{i1} \\ \vdots \\ \left[-\pi_{(i1)(J-1)}\pi_{(i1)j}\left\{\left(\delta_{(i1)j}+\delta_{(i1)(J-1)}-2\pi_{(i1)}\right)'\otimes w^{*'}_{i1}\right\}\right]\otimes w^*_{i1}\end{pmatrix}. \tag{4.101}$$

Computation of $\frac{\partial}{\partial\beta'}\left[\left\{\eta^{(j)}_{it|t-1}(g)(\delta_{(i,t-1)j}-\eta_{it|t-1}(g))\right\}\otimes w^*_{it}\right]$:

By (4.96),

$$\frac{\partial}{\partial\beta'}\left[\left\{\eta^{(j)}_{it|t-1}(g)(\delta_{(i,t-1)j}-\eta_{it|t-1}(g))\right\}\otimes w^*_{it}\right]$$

$$= \frac{\partial}{\partial \beta'} \left[\begin{pmatrix} -\eta^{(1)}_{it|t-1}(g)\eta^{(j)}_{it|t-1}(g) \\ \vdots \\ \eta^{(j)}_{it|t-1}(g)[1-\eta^{(j)}_{it|t-1}(g)] \\ \vdots \\ -\eta^{(J-1)}_{it|t-1}(g)\eta^{(j)}_{it|t-1}(g) \end{pmatrix} \otimes w^*_{it} \right]$$

$$= \begin{pmatrix} \left[-\eta^{(1)}_{it|t-1}(g)\eta^{(j)}_{it|t-1}(g)\left\{\left(\delta_{(i,t-1)j}+\delta_{(i,t-1)1}-2\eta_{it|t-1}(g)\right)' \otimes w^{*'}_{it}\right\}\right] \otimes w^*_{it} \\ \left[-\eta^{(2)}_{it|t-1}(g)\eta^{(j)}_{it|t-1}(g)\left\{\left(\delta_{(i,t-1)j}+\delta_{(i,t-1)2}-2\eta_{it|t-1}(g)\right)' \otimes w^{*'}_{it}\right\}\right] \otimes w^*_{it} \\ \vdots \\ \left[\eta^{(j)}_{it|t-1}(g)(1-2\eta^{(j)}_{it|t-1}(g))\left\{\left(\delta_{(i,t-1)j}-\eta_{it|t-1}(g)\right)' \otimes w^{*'}_{it}\right\}\right] \otimes w^*_{it} \\ \vdots \\ \left[-\eta^{(J-1)}_{it|t-1}(g)\eta^{(j)}_{it|t-1}(g)\left\{\left(\delta_{(i,t-1)j}+\delta_{(i,t-1)(J-1)}-2\eta_{it|t-1}(g)\right)' \otimes w^{*'}_{it}\right\}\right] \otimes w^*_{it} \end{pmatrix}. \tag{4.102}$$

4.5.1.2 Likelihood Estimating Equation for γ_M

Consider γ^* equivalent to γ_M (4.89), where

$$\gamma^* = (\gamma'_1,\ldots,\gamma'_j,\ldots,\gamma'_{J-1})' : (J-1)^2 \times 1; \text{ with } \gamma_j = (\gamma_{j1},\ldots,\gamma_{jh},\ldots,\gamma_{j,J-1})' \tag{4.103}$$

as the $(J-1)\times 1$ vector of dynamic dependence parameters involved in the conditional multinomial logit function in (4.64). See also (4.91) for an equivalent but simpler expression for these conditional logit functions. Using this latter form (4.91), one obtains

$$\frac{\partial \eta^{(h)}_{it|t-1}(g)}{\partial \gamma_j} = \begin{cases} \delta_{(i,t-1)g}\eta^{(j)}_{it|t-1}(g)[1-\eta^{(j)}_{it|t-1}(g)] & \text{for } h=j; h,j=1,\ldots,J-1 \\ -\delta_{(i,t-1)g}\eta^{(j)}_{it|t-1}(g)\eta^{(h)}_{it|t-1}(g) & \text{for } h \neq j; h,j=1,\ldots,J-1 \\ -\delta_{(i,t-1)g}\eta^{(j)}_{it|t-1}(g)\eta^{(J)}_{it|t-1}(g) & \text{for } h=J;\ j=1,\ldots,J-1, \end{cases} \tag{4.104}$$

for all $g = 1,\ldots,J$. Using these derivatives, it follows from the likelihood function (4.91) that

$$\frac{\partial Log\, L(\beta,\gamma_M)}{\partial \gamma_j} = \sum_{i=1}^{K}\sum_{t=2}^{T}\sum_{h=1}^{J}\sum_{g=1}^{J}\left[\frac{y_{ith}}{\eta^{(h)}_{it|t-1}(g)}\frac{\partial \eta^{(h)}_{it|t-1}(g)}{\partial \gamma_j}\right]$$
$$= \sum_{i=1}^{K}\sum_{t=2}^{T}\sum_{g=1}^{J} y_{itj}\delta_{(i,t-1)g}[1-\eta^{(j)}_{it|t-1}(g)]$$
$$- \sum_{i=1}^{K}\sum_{t=2}^{T}\sum_{g=1}^{J}\sum_{h\neq j}^{J}\frac{y_{ith}}{\eta^{(h)}_{it|t-1}(g)}\delta_{(i,t-1)g}\left(\eta^{(j)}_{it|t-1}(g)\eta^{(h)}_{it|t-1}(g)\right)$$
$$= \sum_{i=1}^{K}\sum_{t=2}^{T}\sum_{g=1}^{J} y_{itj}\delta_{(i,t-1)g}$$
$$- \sum_{i=1}^{K}\sum_{t=2}^{T}\sum_{g=1}^{J}\sum_{h=1}^{J} y_{ith}\delta_{(i,t-1)g}\left(\eta^{(j)}_{it|t-1}(g)\right)$$
$$= 0, \tag{4.105}$$

for $j = 1,\ldots,J-1$, leading to the estimating equations for the elements of $\gamma^* = (\gamma_1',\ldots,\gamma_j',\ldots,\gamma_{J-1}')'$ as

$$\frac{\partial Log\, L(\beta,\gamma_M)}{\partial \gamma^*} = \begin{pmatrix} \frac{\partial Log\, L(\beta,\gamma_M)}{\partial \gamma_1} \\ \vdots \\ \frac{\partial Log\, L(\beta,\gamma_M)}{\partial \gamma_j} \\ \vdots \\ \frac{\partial Log\, L(\beta,\gamma_M)}{\partial \gamma_{J-1}} \end{pmatrix} = 0 : (J-1)^2 \times 1. \tag{4.106}$$

One may solve this likelihood equation (4.106) for γ^* by using the iterative equation

$$\hat{\gamma}^*(r+1) = \hat{\gamma}^*(r) - \left[\left\{\frac{\partial^2 \text{Log}\, L(\beta,\gamma_M)}{\partial \gamma^* \partial \gamma^{*\prime}}\right\}^{-1}\frac{\partial \text{Log}\, L(\beta,\gamma_M)}{\partial \gamma^*}\right]_{|\gamma^*=\hat{\gamma}^*(r)}, \tag{4.107}$$

where the $(J-1)^2 \times (J-1)^2$ second derivative matrix is computed by using the formulas

$$\frac{\partial^2 \text{Log}\, L(\beta,\gamma_M)}{\partial \gamma_j \partial \gamma_j'} = -\sum_{i=1}^{K}\sum_{t=2}^{T}\sum_{g=1}^{J}\sum_{h=1}^{J} y_{ith}\left[\eta^{(j)}_{it|t-1}(g)\left(1-\eta^{(j)}_{it|t-1}(g)\right)\delta_{(i,t-1)g}\delta'_{(i,t-1)g}\right] \tag{4.108}$$

for all $j = 1,\ldots,J-1$, and

$$\frac{\partial^2 \text{Log } L(\beta, \gamma_M)}{\partial \gamma_j \partial \gamma_k'} = \sum_{i=1}^{K}\sum_{t=2}^{T}\sum_{g=1}^{J}\sum_{h=1}^{J}\left[y_{ith}\left(\eta_{it|t-1}^{(j)}(g)\eta_{it|t-1}^{(k)}(g)\right)\delta_{(i,t-1)g}\delta_{(i,t-1)g}'\right], \tag{4.109}$$

for all $j \neq k; j,k = 1,\ldots,J-1$.

References

Chen, B., Yi, G. Y., & Cook, R. (2009). Likelihood analysis of joint marginal and conditional models for longitudinal categorical data. *The Canadian Journal of Statistics*, *37*, 182–205.

Chen, B., Yi, G. Y., & Cook, R. (2010). Weighted generalized estimating functions for longitudinal response and covariate data that are missing at random. *Journal of the American Statistical Association*, *105*, 336–353.

Chowdhury, R. I. (2011). *Inferences in Longitudinal Multinomial Fixed and Mixed Models*. Unpublished Ph.D. thesis, Memorial University, Canada.

Crowder, M. (1995). On the use of a working correlation matrix in using generalized linear models for repeated measures. *Biometrika*, *82*, 407–410.

Fitzmaurice, G.M. & Laird, N. M. (1993). A likelihood-based method for analysing longitudinal binary responses. *Biometrika*, **80**, 141–151.

Liang, K-Y. & Zeger, S. L. (1986). Longitudinal data analysis using generalized linear models. *Biometrika*, *73*, 13–22.

Lipsitz, S. R., Kim, K., & Zhao, L. (1994). Analysis of repeated categorical data using generalized estimating equations. *Statistics in Medicine*, *13*, 1149–1163.

Lipsitz, S. R., Laird, N. M., & Harrington, D. P. (1991). Generalized estimating equations for correlated binary data: Using the odds ratio as a measure of association. *Biometrika*, *78*, 53–160.

Loredo-Osti, J. C. & Sutradhar, B. C. (2012). Estimation of regression and dynamic dependence parameters for non-stationary multinomial time series. *Journal of Time Series Analysis*, *33*, 458–467.

Sutradhar, B.C. (2003). An overview on regression models for discrete longitudinal responses. *Statistical Science*, *18*, 377–393.

Sutradhar, B.C. (2011). *Dynamic Mixed Models for Familial Longitudinal Data*. Springer: New York.

Sutradhar, B. C. & Das, K. (1999). On the efficiency of regression estimators in generalized linear models for longitudinal data. *Biometrika*, *86*, 459–465.

Williamson, J. M., Kim, K., & Lipsitz, S. R. (1995). Analyzing bivariate ordinal data using a global odds ratio. *Journal of American Statistical Association*, *90*, 1432–1437.

Yi, G. Y. & Cook, R. (2002). Marginal methods for incomplete longitudinal data arising in clusters. *Journal of the American Statistical Association*, *97*, 1071–1080.

Chapter 5
Multinomial Models for Cross-Sectional Bivariate Categorical Data

Let Y_i and Z_i denote the two multinomial response variables. Suppose that Y_i from the ith ($i = 1,\ldots,K$) individual belongs to one of J categories, and Z_i belongs to one of R categories (J≥2, R≥2). For example, in a diabetic retinopathy (DR) study, when left and right eyes retinopathy status of a patient, say in three categories such as absence of DR, non-severe DR, and severe DR, are studied, Y_i with $J = 3$, and Z_i with $R = 3$, may be used to represent the three status of the left and right eyes, respectively. In general, we express these two responses as $y_i = (y_{i1},\ldots,y_{ij},\ldots,y_{i,J-1})'$ and $z_i = (z_{i1},\ldots,z_{ir},\ldots,z_{i,R-1})'$. Further if y_i falls into the jth category, then we denote this by $y_i = y_i^{(j)} = (y_{i1}^{(j)},\ldots,y_{ij}^{(j)},\ldots,y_{i,J-1}^{(j)})' = (\mathbf{0}'_{j-1},1,\mathbf{0}'_{J-1-j})'$. Similarly, if z_i falls into the rth category, we denote this by writing $z_i = z_i^{(r)} = (z_{i1}^{(r)},\ldots,z_{ir}^{(r)},\ldots,z_{i,R-1}^{(r)})' = (\mathbf{0}'_{r-1},1,\mathbf{0}'_{R-1-r})'$.

5.1 Familial Correlation Models for Bivariate Data with No Covariates

5.1.1 Marginal Probabilities

Before writing the marginal probabilities for each of y and z variables, it is important to note that because y_i and z_i are two categorical responses for the same ith individual, it is quite likely that these responses, on top of category prune effect, will also be influenced by certain common effect, say ξ_i^*, shared by both variables. This common effect is usually treated to be random and will cause correlation between y_i and z_i. Suppose that

$$\xi_i^* \overset{iid}{\sim} N(0,\sigma_\xi^2), \text{ or equivalently } \xi_i = \frac{\xi_i^*}{\sigma_\xi} \overset{iid}{\sim} N(0,1). \tag{5.1}$$

B.C. Sutradhar, *Longitudinal Categorical Data Analysis*, Springer Series in Statistics, DOI 10.1007/978-1-4939-2137-9_5

Now as an extension of the univariate multinomial model from Chap. 2, more specifically from (2.1)–(2.2), it is sensible to condition on ξ_i and write the marginal probabilities for y_i and z_i, as

$$P[y_i = y_i^{(j)}|\xi_i^*] = \pi^*_{(i)j\cdot}(\xi_i) = \begin{cases} \frac{\exp(\beta_{j0}+\sigma_\xi \xi_i)}{1+\sum_{u=1}^{J-1}\exp(\beta_{u0}+\sigma_\xi \xi_i)} & \text{for } j = 1,\ldots,J-1 \\ \frac{1}{1+\sum_{h=1}^{J-1}\exp(\beta_{h0}+\sigma_\xi \xi_i)} & \text{for } j = J, \end{cases} \tag{5.2}$$

and

$$P[z_i = z_i^{(r)}|\xi_i^*] = \pi^*_{(i)\cdot r}(\xi_i) = \begin{cases} \frac{\exp(\alpha_{r0}+\sigma_\xi \xi_i)}{1+\sum_{h=1}^{R-1}\exp(\alpha_{h0}+\sigma_\xi \xi_i)} & \text{for } r = 1,\ldots,R-1 \\ \frac{1}{1+\sum_{h=1}^{R-1}\exp(\alpha_{h0}+\sigma_\xi \xi_i)} & \text{for } r = R, \end{cases} \tag{5.3}$$

respectively. By (5.1), it follows from (5.2) and (5.3) that the unconditional marginal probabilities have the forms

$$\begin{aligned} \pi_{(i)j\cdot} &= P(y_i = y_i^{(j)}) = E_{\xi_i}E[Y_{ij}|\xi_i] = E_{\xi_i}[\pi^*_{(i)j\cdot}(\xi_i)|\xi_i]. \\ &= \int_{-\infty}^{\infty} \pi^*_{(i)j\cdot}(\xi_i) f_N(\xi_i) d\xi_i, \end{aligned} \tag{5.4}$$

and

$$\begin{aligned} \pi_{(i)\cdot r} &= P(z_i = z_i^{(r)}) = E_{\xi_i}E[Z_{ir}|\xi_i] = E_{\xi_i}[\pi^*_{(i)\cdot r}(\xi_i)|\xi_i] \\ &= \int_{-\infty}^{\infty} \pi^*_{(i)\cdot r}(\xi_i) f_N(\xi_i) d\xi_i, \end{aligned} \tag{5.5}$$

with $f_N(\xi_i) = \frac{\exp(\frac{-\xi_i^2}{2})}{\sqrt{2\pi}}$.

Note that there is no closed form expressions for these expectations. However, as shown in Sect. 5.3, they can be computed empirically.

5.1.2 *Joint Probabilities and Correlations*

As far as the computation of the joint probabilities is concerned, two variables y_i and z_i are independent conditional on the common random effect ξ_i. Thus,

$$\begin{aligned} P[\{y_i = y_i^{(j)}, z_i = z_i^{(r)}\}|\xi_i] &= \pi^*_{(i)j\cdot}(\xi_i)\pi^*_{(i)\cdot r}(\xi_i) \\ &= \pi^*_{(i)jr}(\xi_i), \text{ (say)}, \end{aligned} \tag{5.6}$$

yielding the unconditional joint probabilities as

$$\begin{aligned} P[y_i = y_i^{(j)}, z_i = z_i^{(r)}] &= \int_{-\infty}^{\infty} \pi^*_{(i)jr}(\xi_i) f_N(\xi_i) d\xi_i \\ &= \pi_{(i)jr}. \end{aligned} \tag{5.7}$$

This further produces the correlations between y_{ij} and z_{ir} as

$$\begin{aligned} \text{corr}[Y_{ij}, Z_{ir}] &= \frac{\text{cov}[Y_{ij}, Z_{ir}]}{[\text{var}(Y_{ij})\text{var}(Z_{ir})]^{\frac{1}{2}}} \\ &= \frac{P[y_i = y_i^{(j)}, z_i = z_i^{(r)}] - P(y_i = y_i^{(j)})P(z_i = z_i^{(r)})}{[\text{var}(Y_{ij})\text{var}(Z_{ir})]^{\frac{1}{2}}} \\ &= \frac{\pi_{(i)jr} - \pi_{(i)j\cdot}\pi_{(i)\cdot r}}{[\{\pi_{(i)j\cdot}(1-\pi_{(i)j\cdot})\}\{\pi_{(i)\cdot r}(1-\pi_{(i)\cdot r})\}]^{\frac{1}{2}}}, \end{aligned} \tag{5.8}$$

where the unconditional marginal and joint probabilities are given in (5.4), (5.5), and (5.7).

It is clear from (5.4) and (5.5) that the computation of the marginal probabilities requires the estimation of $\beta = (\beta_{10}, \ldots, \beta_{j0}, \ldots, \beta_{(J-1)0})'$, $\alpha = (\alpha_{10}, \ldots, \alpha_{r0}, \ldots, \alpha_{(R-1)0})'$, and σ^2_ξ. This inference problem will be discussed in Sect. 5.3 in detail. In Sect. 5.2, we consider an existing approach of modeling the joint probabilities by using a two-way ANOVA concept.

5.1.3 Remarks on Similar Random Effects Based Models

For familial data modeling, it is standard to use a common random effect shared by family members which causes correlations among the responses of the same family. For this type binary data modeling, we, for example, refer to Sutradhar (2011, Chapter 5). The bivariate multinomial model introduced in (5.1)–(5.3) may be treated as a generalization of familial binary model with a family consisting of two members. The ith individual in (5.1)–(5.3) is compared to ith family with two (bivariate) responses which are equivalent to responses from two members of the family. Some other authors such as MacDonald (1994) used individual random effects to construct correlation models for longitudinal binary data. Various scenarios for the distribution of the random effects are considered. This approach, however, appears to be more suitable in the present bivariate multinomial setup as opposed to the univariate longitudinal setup. As far as the distribution of the random effects is concerned, in (5.2)–(5.3), we have used normal random effects similar to Breslow and Clayton (1993), for example, and develop the familial correlation model through such random effects. In a familial longitudinal setup, Ten Have and

Morabia (1999) used a mixed model similar to (5.2)–(5.3) to model the binary data. More specifically, they have used two different random effects for two binary responses to represent possible overdispersion only, which however do not cause any familial or structural correlations between the bivariate binary responses at a given time. The bivariate association between the two binary responses was modeled through certain additional random effects based odds ratios, but the estimation of the odds ratios requires an extra regression modeling (equivalent to 'working' correlation approach) as pointed out in Chap. 4, specifically in Sect. 4.2.1, which is a limitation to this approach.

5.2 Two-Way ANOVA Type Covariates Free Joint Probability Model

Let K_{rj} and m_{rj} denote the observed and expected counts in the (r, j)-th cell of a two-way ANOVA type table, where $K = \sum_{r=1}^{R}\sum_{j=1}^{J} K_{rj}$ is the total number of individuals. Suppose that $m = \sum_{r=1}^{R}\sum_{j=1}^{J} m_{rj}$. When K individuals are distributed to the RJ cells following a Poisson distribution, one writes

$$K_{rj} \sim Poi(\mu_{rj}),\; r = 1,\ldots,R;\; j = 1,\ldots,J,$$

where $Poi(\mu_{rj})$ denotes the Poisson distribution with mean μ_{rj}, that is,

$$P(K_{rj}|\mu_{rj}) = \frac{\exp(-\mu_{rj})\mu_{rj}^{K_{rj}}}{K_{rj}!},\; K_{rj} = 0,1,2,\ldots \tag{5.9}$$

Also suppose that K_{rj}'s are independent for all $r = 1,\ldots,R;\; j = 1,\ldots,J$. It then follows that

$$K = \sum_{r=1}^{R}\sum_{j=1}^{J} K_{rj} \sim Poi(\mu = \sum_{r=1}^{R}\sum_{j=1}^{J} \mu_{rj}),$$

and conditional on total K, the joint distribution of the counts $\{K_{rj}, r \neq R \cap j \neq J\}$ has the form

$$P[\{K_{rj}, r \neq R \cap j \neq J\}|K] = \frac{\Pi_{r=1}^{R}\Pi_{j=1}^{J}[\frac{\exp(-\mu_{rj})\mu_{rj}^{K_{rj}}}{K_{rj}!}]}{\frac{\exp(-\mu)\mu^{K}}{K!}},$$

where now $K_{RJ} = K - \sum_{r \neq R \cap j \neq J} K_{rj}$ is known. Now by using $\pi_{rj} = \frac{\mu_{rj}}{\mu}$, one obtains the multinomial distribution

$$P[\{K_{rj}, r \neq R \cap j \neq J\}] = \frac{K!}{\Pi_{r=1}^{R} \Pi_{j=1}^{J} K_{rj}!} \Pi_{r=1}^{R} \Pi_{j=1}^{J} \pi_{rj}^{\sum_{i=1}^{K} y_{ij} z_{ir}}$$
$$= \frac{K!}{K_{11}! \cdots K_{rj}! \cdots K_{RJ}!} \Pi_{r=1}^{R} \Pi_{j=1}^{J} \pi_{rj}{}^{K_{rj}}. \quad (5.10)$$

where $\pi_{RJ} = 1 - \sum_{r \neq R \cap j \neq J} \pi_{rj}$ is known. In (5.10), y_{ij} and z_{ir} are the jth and rth component of the multinomial response vector y_i and z_i, respectively, as in the last section. Further, when $K = 1$, one obtains the desired multinomial distribution from (5.10) by using $K_{rj} = y_{ij} z_{ir}$ as a special case.

Note that in Poisson case, one models the means $\{\mu_{rj}, r = 1, \ldots, R; j = 1, \ldots, J\}$ or $\{\log(\mu_{rj}), r = 1, \ldots, R; j = 1, \ldots, J\}$, and in the multinomial case one models the probabilities $\{\pi_{rj}, r = 1, \ldots, R; j = 1, \ldots, J\}$. However, as opposed to the random effects approach discussed in the last section, many studies over the last two decades modeled these joint probabilities directly by using the so-called two-way ANOVA type relationship

$$\pi_{irj} = Pr(y_i = y_i^{(j)}, z_i = z_i^{(r)})$$
$$= \frac{\exp(\alpha_r + \beta_j + \gamma_{rj})}{\sum_{r=1}^{R} \sum_{j=1}^{J} \exp(\alpha_r + \beta_j + \gamma_{rj})} = \frac{\mu_{rj}}{\mu},$$
$$\equiv \pi_{rj}, \ r = 1, \ldots, R, \ j = 1, \ldots, J, \quad (5.11)$$

(e.g., Agresti 2002, Eqn. (8.4); Fienberg 2007, Eqn. (2.19)) for all $i = 1, \ldots, K$. In (5.11), for a constant effect m_0, the two-way ANOVA type relationship is observed for $\log(\mu_{rj})$ as

$$\log(\mu_{rj}) = m_{rj} = m_0 + \alpha_r + \beta_j + \gamma_{rj}. \quad (5.12)$$

These parameters α_r and β_j are treated to be rth row and jth column effect, and γ_{rj} are so-called interaction effects, satisfying the restrictions

$$\sum_{r=1}^{R} \alpha_r = 0; \ \sum_{j=1}^{J} \beta_j = 0; \ \sum_{r=1}^{R} \gamma_{rj} = \sum_{j=1}^{J} \gamma_{rj} = 0. \quad (5.13)$$

Thus, when the bivariate cell counts follow a Poisson model, that is, K is random, one would estimate the model parameters in the right-hand side of (5.12) to compute the mean (or log of the mean) rate for an individual to be in that cell. Because, by using (5.13), it follows from (5.12) that

$$m_0 = \frac{\sum_{r=1}^{R} \sum_{j=1}^{J} m_{rj}}{RJ} = m_{++}$$

$$\alpha_r = \frac{\sum_{j=1}^{J} m_{rj}}{J} - m_0 = m_{r+} - m_{++}$$

$$\beta_j = \frac{\sum_{r=1}^{R} m_{rj}}{R} - m_0 = m_{+j} - m_{++}$$

$$\gamma_{rj} = [m_{rj} - m_{r+} - m_{+j} + m_{++}], \tag{5.14}$$

as indicated above, α_r and β_j may be interpreted as the marginal effects and γ_{rj} as the interaction effect, in the two-way table for the log of the cell counts.

5.2.1 *Marginal Probabilities and Parameter Interpretation Difficulties*

As opposed to (5.14), the interpretation of the parameters α_r, β_j, and γ_{rj} to understand their role in marginal probabilities in multinomial setup (5.11) is not easy. This is because, using a simple logit transformation to (5.11) does not separate α_r from β_j. That is, one cannot understand the role of α_r in row effect probabilities $\pi_{r\cdot} = \sum_{j=1}^{J} \pi_{rj}$ without knowing β_j. To be more clear, by a direct calculation, one writes the marginal probabilities from (5.11) as

$$\pi_{\cdot j} = \sum_{r=1}^{R} \pi_{rj} = \frac{\sum_{r=1}^{R} \exp(\alpha_r + \beta_j + \gamma_{rj})}{\sum_{r=1}^{R} \sum_{j=1}^{J} \exp(\alpha_r + \beta_j + \gamma_{rj})}$$

$$\pi_{r\cdot} = \sum_{j=1}^{J} \pi_{rj} = \frac{\sum_{j=1}^{J} \exp(\alpha_r + \beta_j + \gamma_{rj})}{\sum_{r=1}^{R} \sum_{j=1}^{J} \exp(\alpha_r + \beta_j + \gamma_{rj})}. \tag{5.15}$$

These formulas show that the marginal probabilities for one variable are complicated functions of marginal and association parameters for both variables, making the interpretation of parameter effects on marginal probabilities unnecessary difficult. But, as opposed to the two-way ANOVA type model, the marginal probabilities under the familial model, for example, $\pi_{(i)j\cdot}$ in (5.4) is a function of β_{j0} but not of α_{r0}.

However, the estimation of the parameters in the ANOVA type model (5.11) may be achieved relatively easily, for example, by using the likelihood approach, and subsequently one can compute the joint and marginal probabilities by using such estimates. We demonstrate this in the following section.

5.2.2 *Parameter Estimation in Two-Way ANOVA Type Multinomial Probability Model*

5.2.2.1 Likelihood Estimating Equations

For π_{rj} in (5.11), it follows from (5.10) that the log likelihood function is given by

$$\begin{aligned} \log L(\cdot) &= \text{const.} + \sum_{r=1}^{R} \sum_{j=1}^{J} K_{rj} \log \pi_{rj} \\ &= \text{const.} + \sum_{r=1}^{R} \sum_{j=1}^{J} K_{rj} \log \left(\frac{\mu_{rj}}{\mu}\right) \\ &= \text{const.} + \sum_{r=1}^{R} \sum_{j=1}^{J} K_{rj} \log \mu_{rj} - K \log \mu, \end{aligned} \tag{5.16}$$

with

$$\mu_{rj} = \exp(\alpha_r + \beta_j + \gamma_{rj}),\ \mu = \sum_{r=1}^{R} \sum_{j=1}^{J} \exp(\alpha_r + \beta_j + \gamma_{rj}).$$

Parameter Constraints *(C)*:
As far as the parameter constraints are concerned, in the multinomial case as opposed to the Poisson case, it is convenient to use the constraints
$C: \alpha_R = \beta_J = 0;\ \gamma_{Rj} = 0$ for $j = 1, \ldots, J$; and $\gamma_{rJ} = 0$ for $r = 1, \ldots, R$.

Likelihood estimating equations under the constraint *C*:
Note that because of the constraint on the parameters, there are $(R-1) + (J-1) + \{RJ - (R+J-1)\} = RJ - 1$ parameters to estimate under the present two-way table based multinomial model. When the restriction **C** is used, the formulas for μ_{rj} and μ can be conveniently expressed as

$$\mu_{rj}|_C = \begin{cases} \exp(\alpha_r + \beta_j + \gamma_{rj}) & \text{for } r = 1, \ldots, R-1;\ j = 1, \ldots, J-1 \\ \exp(\alpha_r) & \text{for } r = 1, \ldots, R-1, \text{ and } j = J \\ \exp(\beta_j) & \text{for } r = R, \text{ and } j = 1, \ldots, J-1 \\ 1 & \text{for } r = R \text{ and } j = J, \end{cases} \tag{5.17}$$

and

$$\mu|_C = 1 + \sum_{r=1}^{R-1} \exp(\alpha_r) + \sum_{j=1}^{J-1} \exp(\beta_j) + \sum_{r=1}^{R-1} \sum_{j=1}^{J-1} \exp(\alpha_r + \beta_j + \gamma_{rj}), \tag{5.18}$$

respectively. One may then write the likelihood function under the constraints as

$$\log L(\cdot)|_C = \text{const.} + \sum_{r=1}^{R}\sum_{j=1}^{J} K_{rj} \log \mu_{rj}|_C - K \log \mu|_C$$
$$= \text{const.} + \left[K_{RJ} + \sum_{r=1}^{R-1} K_{rJ}\alpha_r + \sum_{j=1}^{J-1} K_{Rj}\beta_j + \sum_{r=1}^{R-1}\sum_{j=1}^{J-1} K_{rj}\{\alpha_r + \beta_j + \gamma_{rj}\}\right]$$
$$-K \log\left[1 + \sum_{r=1}^{R-1} \exp(\alpha_r) + \sum_{j=1}^{J-1} \exp(\beta_j) + \sum_{r=1}^{R-1}\sum_{j=1}^{J-1} \exp(\alpha_r + \beta_j + \gamma_{rj})\right]. \quad (5.19)$$

It then follows that

$$\frac{\partial log\, L(\cdot)|_C}{\partial \alpha_r} = \left[K_{rJ} + \sum_{j=1}^{J-1} K_{rj}\right] - K\frac{1}{\mu|_C}\left[\exp(\alpha_r) + \sum_{j=1}^{J-1} \exp(\alpha_r + \beta_j + \gamma_{rj})\right]$$
$$\frac{\partial log\, L(\cdot)|_C}{\partial \beta_j} = \left[K_{Rj} + \sum_{r=1}^{R-1} K_{rj}\right] - K\frac{1}{\mu|_C}\left[\exp(\beta_j) + \sum_{r=1}^{R-1} \exp(\alpha_r + \beta_j + \gamma_{rj})\right]$$
$$\frac{\partial log\, L(\cdot)|_C}{\partial \gamma_{rj}} = [K_{rj}] - K\frac{1}{\mu|_C}\left[\exp(\alpha_r + \beta_j + \gamma_{rj})\right], \quad (5.20)$$

and the likelihood equations are given by

$$\frac{\partial log\, L(\cdot)|_C}{\partial \alpha_r} = 0$$
$$\frac{\partial log\, L(\cdot)|_C}{\partial \beta_j} = 0$$
$$\frac{\partial log\, L(\cdot)|_C}{\partial \gamma_{rj}} = 0. \quad (5.21)$$

Let

$$\theta = [\alpha_1, \ldots, \alpha_{R-1}, \beta_1, \ldots, \beta_{J-1}, \lambda_{11}, \ldots, \lambda_{1,J-1}, \ldots, \lambda_{R-1,1}, \ldots, \lambda_{R-1,J-1}]'$$
$$= [\alpha', \beta', \gamma']', \quad (5.22)$$

be the $(RJ-1) \times 1$ vector of regression parameters. One may then solve the likelihood equations in (5.21) by using the iterative equations

$$\hat{\theta}(q+1) = \hat{\theta}(q) + \left(\left[\frac{\partial^2 log\, L|_C}{\partial \theta'}\right]^{-1}\left[\frac{\partial log\, L|_C}{\partial \theta}\right]\right)|_{\theta=\hat{\theta}(q)}, \quad (5.23)$$

where, by (5.20), one writes

$$\frac{\partial log\ L|_C}{\partial\theta} = \begin{pmatrix} \frac{\partial log\ L(\cdot)|_C}{\partial\alpha} \\ \frac{\partial log\ L(\cdot)|_C}{\partial\beta} \\ \frac{\partial log\ L(\cdot)|_C}{\partial\gamma} \end{pmatrix} : (RJ-1)\times 1. \tag{5.24}$$

Now to compute the second order derivatives in (5.23), it is sufficient to compute the following elements-wise derivatives:

$$\begin{aligned}
\frac{\partial^2 log\ L(\cdot)|_C}{\partial\alpha_r^2} &= -K\left[\frac{\exp(\alpha_r)+\Sigma_{j=1}^{J-1}\exp(\alpha_r+\beta_j+\gamma_{rj})}{\mu|_C}\left\{1-\frac{\exp(\alpha_r)+\Sigma_{j=1}^{J-1}\exp(\alpha_r+\beta_j+\gamma_{rj})}{\mu|_C}\right\}\right] \\
\frac{\partial^2 log\ L(\cdot)|_C}{\partial\alpha_r\partial\alpha_s} &= K\left[\frac{\exp(\alpha_r)+\Sigma_{j=1}^{J-1}\exp(\alpha_r+\beta_j+\gamma_{rj})}{\mu|_C}\left\{\frac{\exp(\alpha_s)+\Sigma_{j=1}^{J-1}\exp(\alpha_s+\beta_j+\gamma_{sj})}{\mu|_C}\right\}\right], \text{ for } r\neq s \\
\frac{\partial^2 log\ L(\cdot)|_C}{\partial\alpha_r\partial\beta_j} &= -K\left[\frac{\exp(\alpha_r+\beta_j+\gamma_{rj})}{\mu|_C}\right. \\
&\quad \left. -\left\{\frac{\exp(\alpha_r)+\Sigma_{j=1}^{J-1}\exp(\alpha_r+\beta_j+\gamma_{rj})}{\mu|_C}\right\}\left\{\frac{\exp(\beta_j)+\Sigma_{r=1}^{R-1}\exp(\alpha_r+\beta_j+\gamma_{rj})}{\mu|_C}\right\}\right] \\
\frac{\partial^2 log\ L(\cdot)|_C}{\partial\alpha_r\partial\gamma_{rj}} &= -K\left[\frac{\exp(\alpha_r+\beta_j+\gamma_{rj})}{\mu|_C}\left\{1-\frac{\exp(\alpha_r)+\Sigma_{j=1}^{J-1}\exp(\alpha_r+\beta_j+\gamma_{rj})}{\mu|_C}\right\}\right] \\
\frac{\partial^2 log\ L(\cdot)|_C}{\partial\alpha_r\partial\gamma_{sj}} &= -K\left[\frac{\exp(\alpha_s+\beta_j+\gamma_{sj})}{\mu|_C}\left\{1-\frac{\exp(\alpha_r)+\Sigma_{j=1}^{J-1}\exp(\alpha_r+\beta_j+\gamma_{rj})}{\mu|_C}\right\}\right] \\
\frac{\partial^2 log\ L(\cdot)|_C}{\partial\beta_j^2} &= -K\left[\frac{\exp(\beta_j)+\Sigma_{r=1}^{R-1}\exp(\alpha_r+\beta_j+\gamma_{rj})}{\mu|_C}\left\{1-\frac{\exp(\beta_j)+\Sigma_{r=1}^{R-1}\exp(\alpha_r+\beta_j+\gamma_{rj})}{\mu|_C}\right\}\right] \\
\frac{\partial^2 log\ L(\cdot)|_C}{\partial\beta_j\partial\beta_s} &= K\left[\frac{\exp(\beta_j)+\Sigma_{r=1}^{R-1}\exp(\alpha_r+\beta_j+\gamma_{rj})}{\mu|_C}\left\{\frac{\exp(\beta_s)+\Sigma_{r=1}^{R-1}\exp(\alpha_r+\beta_s+\gamma_{rs})}{\mu|_C}\right\}\right], \text{ for } r\neq s \\
\frac{\partial^2 log\ L(\cdot)|_C}{\partial\beta_j\partial\gamma_{rj}} &= -K\left[\frac{\exp(\alpha_r+\beta_j+\gamma_{rj})}{\mu|_C}\left\{1-\frac{\exp(\beta_j)+\Sigma_{r=1}^{R-1}\exp(\alpha_r+\beta_j+\gamma_{rj})}{\mu|_C}\right\}\right] \\
\frac{\partial^2 log\ L(\cdot)|_C}{\partial\beta_j\partial\gamma_{rs}} &= -K\left[\frac{\exp(\alpha_r+\beta_s+\gamma_{rs})}{\mu|_C}\left\{1-\frac{\exp(\beta_j)+\Sigma_{r=1}^{R-1}\exp(\alpha_r+\beta_j+\gamma_{rj})}{\mu|_C}\right\}\right] \\
\frac{\partial log\ L(\cdot)|_C}{\partial\gamma_{rj}^2} &= -K\left[\frac{\exp(\alpha_r+\beta_j+\gamma_{rj})}{\mu|_C}\left\{1-\frac{\exp(\alpha_r+\beta_j+\gamma_{rj})}{\mu|_C}\right\}\right]. \\
\frac{\partial log\ L(\cdot)|_C}{\partial\gamma_{rj}\partial\gamma_{sk}} &= K\left[\left\{\frac{\exp(\alpha_r+\beta_j+\gamma_{rj})}{\mu|_C}\right\}\left\{\frac{\exp(\alpha_s+\beta_k+\gamma_{sk})}{\mu|_C}\right\}\right].
\end{aligned} \tag{5.25}$$

5.2.2.2 (Alternative) Likelihood Estimation Using Regression Form

Let c denote the cth cell of the two-way table with RJ cells. Suppose that the RJ cells are read across the R rows of the table as follows:

$$c \equiv \begin{cases} (J-1)(r-1)+j & \text{for } r=1,\ldots,R-1;\ j=1,\ldots,J-1 \\ (R-1)(J-1)+r & \text{for } r=1,\ldots,R-1, \text{ and } j=J \\ (R-1)J+j & \text{for } r=R, \text{ and } j=1,\ldots,J-1 \\ RJ & \text{for } r=R \text{ and } j=J. \end{cases} \tag{5.26}$$

Notice that following this layout in (5.26), $log\ \mu_{rj}|C$ in (5.17) can be expressed as

$$log\ \mu_c = x_c'\theta, \quad (5.27)$$

where

$$\theta = [\alpha_1, \ldots, \alpha_{R-1}, \beta_1, \ldots, \beta_{J-1}, \lambda_{11}, \ldots, \lambda_{1,J-1}, \ldots, \lambda_{R-1,1}, \ldots, \lambda_{R-1,J-1}]' : (RJ-1) \times 1,$$

and $x_c' = [x_{c1}, \ldots, x_{cd}, \ldots, x_{c,RJ-1}]$ be the cth row of the $RJ \times (RJ-1)$ covariate matrix $X = (x_{cd})$ involving $RJ-1$ dummy covariates. To be specific, for $c = 1, \ldots, RJ$, $x_c' :\ 1 \times (RJ-1)$ are defined as

$$\begin{aligned}
x'_{(J-1)(r-1)+j} &= [\delta'_{1,r}, \delta'_{2,j}, \delta'_{3,(r,j)}] \text{ for } r = 1, \ldots, R-1;\ j = 1, \ldots, J-1 \\
x'_{(R-1)(J-1)+r} &= [\delta'_{1,r}, 01'_{J-1}, 01'_{(R-1)(J-1)}] \text{ for } r = 1, \ldots, R-1, \text{ and } j = J \\
x'_{(R-1)J+j} &= [01'_{R-1}, \delta'_{2,j}, 01'_{(R-1)(J-1)}] \text{ for } r = R, \text{ and } j = 1, \ldots, J-1 \\
x'_{RJ} &= [01'_{RJ-1}] \text{ for } r = R \text{ and } j = J,
\end{aligned} \quad (5.28)$$

where $\delta'_{1,r}$ is a $1 \times (R-1)$ row vector with all elements except the rth element as zero, the rth element being 1; similarly $\delta'_{2,j}$ is a $1 \times (J-1)$ row vector with all elements except the jth element as zero, the jth element being 1; and $\delta'_{3,(r,j)}$ is a $1 \times (R-1)(J-1)$ stacked row vector constructed by stacking the elements of a matrix with all elements except the (r,j)th element as zero, the (r,j)th element being 1. Furthermore, in (5.28), $1'_b$, for example, is the $1 \times b$ row vector with all elements as 1. Consequently, the multinomial log likelihood function (5.19) reduces to

$$\begin{aligned}
log\ L(\cdot)|C &= \text{const.} + \sum_{r=1}^{R}\sum_{j=1}^{J} K_{rj}\ log\ (\frac{\mu_{rj}|C}{\mu|C}) \\
&= \sum_{c=1}^{RJ} K_c log\ \frac{\mu_c}{\mu|C},
\end{aligned} \quad (5.29)$$

where $\mu|C = \sum_{c=1}^{RJ} \mu_c|C$.

By using (5.27), this log likelihood function may be re-written as

$$log\ L(\cdot)|C = \text{const.} + \sum_{c=1}^{RJ} K_c x_c'\theta - K log\left[\sum_{c=1}^{RJ} \exp(x_c'\theta)\right]. \quad (5.30)$$

Thus, the likelihood equation for θ is given by

$$\begin{aligned}
\frac{\partial log\ L(\cdot)|C}{\partial\theta} &= \sum_{c=1}^{RJ} K_c x_c - K\frac{1}{\sum_{c=1}^{RJ} \exp(x_c'\theta)} \sum_{c=1}^{RJ} \mu_c x_c \\
&= X'y - KX'\pi = 0,
\end{aligned} \quad (5.31)$$

where $X' = [x_1,\ldots,x_c,\ldots,x_{RJ}]$ is the $(RJ-1)\times RJ$ covariate matrix, $y = [K_1,\ldots,K_c,\ldots,K_{RJ}]'$ is the $RJ\times 1$ response vector of counts, and $\pi = [\pi_1,\ldots,\pi_c,\ldots,\pi_{RJ}]'$ is the corresponding multinomial probability vector, with $\pi_c = \frac{\mu_c}{\mu}$.

Now to solve the likelihood estimating equation (5.31), we use the iterative equation

$$\hat{\theta}(q+1) = \hat{\theta}(q) + \left(\left[\frac{\partial^2 log\, L}{\partial\theta'}\right]^{-1}[X'y - KX'\pi]\right)_{\hat{\theta}(q)}, \tag{5.32}$$

with

$$\begin{aligned}\frac{\partial^2 log\, L}{\partial\theta'} &= -KX'\frac{\partial\pi}{\partial\theta'}\\ &= -KX'[\mathrm{diag}(\pi) - \pi\pi']X,\end{aligned} \tag{5.33}$$

because $\pi_c = \frac{\mu_c}{\mu} = \exp(x_c'\theta)/\sum_{c=1}^{RJ}\exp(x_c'\theta)$, and

$$\begin{aligned}\frac{\partial\pi_c}{\partial\theta_d} &= \frac{\mu\,\mu_c x_{cd} - \mu_c\sum_{c=1}^{RJ}\mu_c x_{cd}}{\mu^2}\\ &= \pi_c x_{cd} - \pi_c\sum_{k=1}^{RJ}\pi_k x_{kd},\end{aligned} \tag{5.34}$$

yielding

$$\frac{\partial\pi}{\partial\theta'} = [\mathrm{diag}(\pi) - \pi\pi']X. \tag{5.35}$$

5.2.2.2.1 Cov($\hat{\theta}$) and its Estimate

Note that $\hat{\theta}$, the likelihood estimator of θ, is computed from (5.31)–(5.32). It then follows that Cov($\hat{\theta}$) has the formula given by

$$\begin{aligned}\mathrm{Cov}(\hat{\theta}) &= -\left[E\frac{\partial^2 log\, L}{\partial\theta'}\right]^{-1}\\ &= \frac{1}{K}\left[X'\left\{\mathrm{diag}(\pi) - \pi\pi'\right\}X\right]^{-1},\end{aligned} \tag{5.36}$$

by (5.33). Next, this covariance may be estimated by replacing π with its estimate $\hat{\pi}$.

5.2.2.2.2 Estimation of π and the Covariance Matrix of its Estimate

Because π represents the cell probabilities, that is,

$$\pi = [\pi_1, \ldots, \pi_i, \ldots, \pi_{RJ}]'$$

with

$$\pi_c = \frac{\mu_c}{\mu} = \exp(x_c'\theta) / \sum_{c=1}^{RJ} \exp(x_c'\theta),$$

one may obtain the likelihood estimate of π by using $\hat{\theta}$ (likelihood estimate of θ) from (5.31)–(5.32), for θ in π_c, that is,

$$\hat{\pi}_c = \exp(x_c'\hat{\theta}) / \sum_{k=1}^{RJ} \exp(x_k'\hat{\theta}), \tag{5.37}$$

for all $c = 1, \ldots, RJ$.

Computation of Cov$(\hat{\pi})$:
Write

$$\hat{\pi}_c = \exp(x_c'\hat{\theta}) / \sum_{k=1}^{RJ} \exp(x_k'\hat{\theta}) = g_c(\hat{\theta}),$$

so that

$$\hat{\pi} = [g_1(\hat{\theta}), \ldots, g_c(\hat{\theta}), \ldots, g_{RJ}(\hat{\theta})]'.$$

Because by first order Taylor's expansion, one can write

$$\begin{aligned} g_c(\hat{\theta}) &= g_c(\theta + \hat{\theta} - \theta) \\ &\approx g_c(\theta) + \sum_{k=1}^{RJ-1} (\hat{\theta}_k - \theta_k) g_c'(\theta_k), \end{aligned} \tag{5.38}$$

with $g_c'(\theta_k) = \frac{\partial g_c(\theta)}{\partial \theta_k}$, it then follows that

$$\begin{aligned} E[g_c(\hat{\theta})] &= g_c(\theta) \\ \text{var}(g_c(\hat{\theta})) &= \sum_{k=1}^{RJ-1} \text{var}(\hat{\theta}_k)[g_c'(\theta_k)]^2 + \sum_{k \neq \ell}^{RJ-1} \text{cov}(\hat{\theta}_k, \widehat{\theta_\ell}) g_c'(\theta_k) g_c'(\theta_\ell) \\ &= [g_c'(\theta_1), \ldots, g_c'(\theta_k), \ldots, g_c'(\theta_{RJ-1})] \text{cov}(\hat{\theta}) [g_c'(\theta_1), \ldots, g_c'(\theta_k), \ldots, g_c'(\theta_{RJ-1})]' \\ \text{cov}(g_c(\hat{\theta}), g_m(\hat{\theta})) &= [g_c'(\theta_1), \ldots, g_c'(\theta_k), \ldots, g_c'(\theta_{RJ-1})] \text{cov}(\hat{\theta}) \end{aligned}$$

$$\times\ [g'_m(\theta_1),\ldots,g'_m(\theta_k),\ldots,g'_m(\theta_{RJ-1})]'. \tag{5.39}$$

Because $g'_c(\theta_k) = \frac{\partial g_c(\theta)}{\partial \theta_k} = \frac{\partial \pi_c}{\partial \theta_k}$, $\mathrm{cov}(\hat{\pi})$ has the formula

$$\mathrm{cov}(\hat{\pi}) = [\frac{\partial \pi}{\partial \theta'}]\mathrm{cov}(\hat{\theta})[\frac{\partial \pi'}{\partial \theta}] \tag{5.40}$$

Furthermore, as $\frac{\partial \pi}{\partial \theta'} = [\mathrm{diag}(\pi) - \pi\pi']X$ by (5.35), the covariance matrix in (5.40) may be expressed as

$$\begin{aligned}\mathrm{cov}(\hat{\pi}) &= [\mathrm{diag}(\pi) - \pi\pi']X\mathrm{cov}(\hat{\theta})X'[\mathrm{diag}(\pi) - \pi\pi'] \\ &= [\mathrm{diag}(\pi) - \pi\pi']X\frac{1}{K}\left[X'\left\{\mathrm{diag}(\pi) - \pi\pi'\right\}X\right]^{-1}X'[\mathrm{diag}(\pi) - \pi\pi'],\end{aligned} \tag{5.41}$$

by (5.36).

Remark that the likelihood estimating equation (5.31) for θ, the formula for $\mathrm{Cov}(\hat{\theta})$ given by (5.36), and the formula for $\mathrm{Cov}(\hat{\pi})$ given by (5.41) are also available in the standard textbooks. See, for example, Agresti (2002, Sections 8.6.6–8.6.8).

5.3 Estimation of Parameters for Covariates Free Familial Bivariate Model (5.4)–(5.7)

Remark that for a situation when binary responses are collected from the members of a family, these responses become correlated as they share a common family effect (equivalent to a random effect). For the estimation of the effects of the covariates of the individual members as well as the random effects variance parameter for the underlying familial binary model (equivalent to binary mixed model), one may refer to the simulated GQL and simulated MLE approaches discussed in Sutradhar (2011, Sections 5.2.3 and 5.2.4). Because the present familial bivariate multinomial model may be treated as a generalization of the familial binary model for families with two members with a difference that now each of the two members is providing multinomial instead of binary responses, similar to the familial binary model, one may develop GQL and MLE approaches for the estimation of the parameters of the present multinomial mixed model.

To be specific, similar to Sutradhar (2011, Section 5.2.3) we first develop both marginal GQL (MGQL) and joint GQL (JGQL) estimating equations for the parameters of the bivariate mixed model (5.4)–(5.7) in the next section. These parameters are

$$\{\beta_{j0},\ j = 1,\ldots,J-1\}; \{\alpha_{r0},\ r = 1,\ldots,R-1\}; \text{and } \sigma^2_\xi. \tag{5.42}$$

We then discuss the ML estimation of the parameters in Sect. 5.3.2. Note however that instead of simulation (of random effects) approach, we will use the so-called binomial approximation to construct the MGQL, JGQL, and ML estimating equations.

5.3.1 Binomial Approximation Based GQL Estimation

5.3.1.1 Binomial Approximation Based MGQL Estimation

As far as the marginal properties of $y_i = (y_{i1}, \ldots, y_{ij}, \ldots, y_{i,J-1})'$ and $z_i = (z_{i1}, \ldots, z_{ir}, \ldots, z_{i,R-1})'$ are concerned, it follows, for example, from Chap. 3 [see Eqs. (3.148) and (3.150)] that the mean, variance, and structural covariance of these two multinomial variables are given by:

$$E(Y_{ij}) = \pi_{(i)j\cdot}, \ \mathrm{var}(Y_{ij}) = \pi_{(i)j\cdot}(1-\pi_{(i)j\cdot}), \ \mathrm{cov}(Y_{ij}, Y_{i\ell}) = -\pi_{(i)j\cdot}\pi_{(i)\ell\cdot};$$
$$\text{and } E(Z_{ir}) = \pi_{(i)\cdot r}, \ \mathrm{var}(Z_{ir}) = \pi_{(i)\cdot r}(1-\pi_{(i)\cdot r}), \ \mathrm{cov}(Z_{ir}, Z_{iq}) = -\pi_{(i)\cdot r}\pi_{(i)\cdot q}. \quad (5.43)$$

One may then write the covariance matrices for y_i and z_i as

$$\begin{aligned} \mathrm{var}(Y_i) &= \mathrm{diag}[\pi_{(i)1\cdot}, \ldots, \pi_{(i)j\cdot}, \ldots, \pi_{(i)(J-1)\cdot}] - \pi_{(i)y}(\beta, \sigma_\xi)\pi'_{(i)y}(\beta, \sigma_\xi) \\ &= \Sigma_{(i)yy}; \\ \mathrm{var}(Z_i) &= \mathrm{diag}[\pi_{(i)\cdot 1}, \ldots, \pi_{(i)\cdot r}, \ldots, \pi_{(i)\cdot(R-1)}] - \pi_{(i)z}(\alpha, \sigma_\xi)\pi'_{(i)z}(\alpha, \sigma_\xi) \\ &= \Sigma_{(i)zz}, \end{aligned} \quad (5.44)$$

where

$$\pi_{(i)y}(\beta, \sigma_\xi) = E[Y_i] = [\pi_{(i)1\cdot}, \ldots, \pi_{(i)j\cdot}, \ldots, \pi_{(i)(J-1)\cdot}]',$$
$$\pi_{(i)z}(\alpha, \sigma_\xi) = E[Z_i] = [\pi_{(i)\cdot 1}, \ldots, \pi_{(i)\cdot r}, \ldots, \pi_{(i)\cdot(R-1)}]',$$

with $\beta = (\beta_{10}, \ldots, \beta_{j0}, \ldots, \beta_{(J-1)0})'$ and $\alpha = (\alpha_{10}, \ldots, \alpha_{r0}, \ldots, \alpha_{(R-1)0})'$ from Sect. 5.1.2.

5.3.1.1.1 MGQL Estimation for $\psi = (\beta', \alpha')'$

Next by using the notation $\psi = (\beta', \alpha')'$, for known σ_ξ^2, we write the MGQL estimating equation for ψ as

$$f(\psi) = \sum_{i=1}^{K} \frac{\partial(\pi'_{(i)y}(\beta,\sigma_\xi), \pi'_{(i)z}(\alpha,\sigma_\xi))}{\partial \psi} \Sigma^{-1}_{(i)11}(\psi,\sigma_\xi) \begin{pmatrix} y_i - \pi_{(i)y}(\beta,\sigma_\xi) \\ z_i - \pi_{(i)z}(\alpha,\sigma_\xi) \end{pmatrix} = 0, \tag{5.45}$$

(Sutradhar 2011) where $\Sigma_{(i)11}(\psi,\sigma_\xi)$ has the formula given by

$$\Sigma_{(i)11}(\psi,\sigma_\xi) = \begin{pmatrix} \Sigma_{(i)yy} & \Sigma_{(i)yz} \\ \Sigma'_{(i)yz} & \Sigma_{(i)zz} \end{pmatrix} \tag{5.46}$$

with

$$\Sigma_{(i)yz} = \text{cov}(Y_i, Z'_i) = (\pi_{(i)jr}) - \pi_{(i)y}\pi'_{(i)z}, \tag{5.47}$$

where $\pi_{(i)jr}$ is the joint probability with its formula given as in (5.7).

Computation of the mean vectors and covariance matrix:
To compute the mean vectors $\pi_{(i)y}(\beta,\sigma_\xi)$ and $\pi_{(i)z}(\alpha,\sigma_\xi)$, and the covariance matrix $\Sigma_{(i)11}(\psi,\sigma_\xi)$ involved in (5.45), it is sufficient to compute

$$\pi_{(i)j\cdot},\ \pi_{(i)\cdot r},\ \pi_{(i)jr}$$

for $j = 1,\ldots,J-1$; $r = 1,\ldots,R-1$. Exact computation for these probabilities by (5.4), (5.5), and (5.7), respectively, is however not possible because of the difficulty of the evaluation of the integral involved in these probabilities. As a remedy to this integration problem, we, therefore, use a Binomial approximation (Sutradhar 2011, eqns. (5.24)–(5.27); Ten Have and Morabia 1999, eqn. (7)) and compute these probabilities as

$$\pi_{(i)j\cdot} = \int_{-\infty}^{\infty} \pi^*_{(i)j\cdot}(\xi_i) f_N(\xi_i) d\xi_i$$

$$\equiv \begin{cases} \sum_{v_i=0}^{V} [\frac{\exp(\beta_{j0}+\sigma_\xi \xi_i(v_i))}{1+\sum_{u=1}^{J-1}\exp(\beta_{u0}+\sigma_\xi \xi_i(v_i))}] \binom{V}{v_i} (1/2)^{v_i}(1/2)^{V-v_i} & \text{for } j = 1,\ldots,J-1 \\ \sum_{v_i=0}^{V} [\frac{1}{1+\sum_{h=1}^{J-1}\exp(\beta_{h0}+\sigma_\xi \xi_i(v_i))}] \binom{V}{v_i} (1/2)^{v_i}(1/2)^{V-v_i} & \text{for } j = J, \end{cases} \tag{5.48}$$

$$\pi_{(i)\cdot r} = \int_{-\infty}^{\infty} \pi^*_{(i)\cdot r}(\xi_i) f_N(\xi_i) d\xi_i$$

$$\equiv \begin{cases} \sum_{v_i=0}^{V} [\frac{\exp(\alpha_{r0}+\sigma_\xi \xi_i(v_i))}{1+\sum_{h=1}^{R-1}\exp(\alpha_{h0}+\sigma_\xi \xi_i(v_i))}] \binom{V}{v_i} (1/2)^{v_i}(1/2)^{V-v_i} & \text{for } r = 1,\ldots,R-1 \\ \sum_{v_i=0}^{V} [\frac{1}{1+\sum_{h=1}^{R-1}\exp(\alpha_{h0}+\sigma_\xi \xi_i(v_i))}] \binom{V}{v_i} (1/2)^{v_i}(1/2)^{V-v_i} & \text{for } r = R, \end{cases} \tag{5.49}$$

and

$$\pi_{(i)jr} = \int_{-\infty}^{\infty} \pi^*_{(i)j\cdot}(\xi_i)\pi^*_{(i)\cdot r}(\xi_i) f_N(\xi_i) d\xi_i$$

$$\equiv \begin{cases} \Sigma_{v_i=0}^{V}[\{\frac{\exp(\beta_{j0}+\sigma_\xi \xi_i(v_i))}{1+\Sigma_{u=1}^{J-1}\exp(\beta_{u0}+\sigma_\xi \xi_i(v_i))}\}\{\frac{\exp(\alpha_{r0}+\sigma_\xi \xi_i(v_i))}{1+\Sigma_{h=1}^{R-1}\exp(\alpha_{h0}+\sigma_\xi \xi_i(v_i))}\}] \\ \times \binom{V}{v_i}(1/2)^{v_i}(1/2)^{V-v_i} & \text{for } j=1,\ldots,J-1;\ r=1,\ldots,R-1 \\ \Sigma_{v_i=0}^{V}[\{\frac{\exp(\beta_{j0}+\sigma_\xi \xi_i(v_i))}{1+\Sigma_{u=1}^{J-1}\exp(\beta_{u0}+\sigma_\xi \xi_i(v_i))}\}\{\frac{1}{1+\Sigma_{h=1}^{R-1}\exp(\alpha_{h0}+\sigma_\xi \xi_i(v_i))}\}] \\ \times \binom{V}{v_i}(1/2)^{v_i}(1/2)^{V-v_i} & \text{for } j=1,\ldots,J-1;\ r=R \\ \Sigma_{v_i=0}^{V}[\{\frac{1}{1+\Sigma_{u=1}^{J-1}\exp(\beta_{u0}+\sigma_\xi \xi_i(v_i))}\}\{\frac{\exp(\alpha_{r0}+\sigma_\xi \xi_i(v_i))}{1+\Sigma_{h=1}^{R-1}\exp(\alpha_{h0}+\sigma_\xi \xi_i(v_i))}\}] \\ \times \binom{V}{v_i}(1/2)^{v_i}(1/2)^{V-v_i} & \text{for } j=J;\ r=1,\ldots,R-1 \\ \Sigma_{v_i=0}^{V}[\{\frac{1}{1+\Sigma_{u=1}^{J-1}\exp(\beta_{u0}+\sigma_\xi \xi_i(v_i))}\}\{\frac{1}{1+\Sigma_{h=1}^{R-1}\exp(\alpha_{h0}+\sigma_\xi \xi_i(v_i))}\}] \\ \times \binom{V}{v_i}(1/2)^{v_i}(1/2)^{V-v_i} & \text{for } j=J;\ r=R, \end{cases} \tag{5.50}$$

respectively, where, for $v_i \sim \text{binomial}(V, 1/2)$ with a suitable V such as $V = 10$, one writes

$$\xi_i(v_i) = \frac{v_i - V(1/2)}{\sqrt{V(1/2)(1/2)}}.$$

Computation of the Derivative $\frac{\partial(\pi'_{(i)y}(\beta,\sigma_\xi),\pi'_{(i)z}(\alpha,\sigma_\xi))}{\partial\psi}$: $(J+R-2)\times(J+R-2)$

Because $\psi = (\beta', \alpha')'$, this derivative matrix may be computed as follows:

$$\frac{\partial \pi'_{(i)y}(\beta,\sigma_\xi)}{\partial \beta} = \left[\frac{\partial \pi_{(i)1\cdot}}{\partial \beta}, \ldots, \frac{\partial \pi_{(i)j\cdot}}{\partial \beta}, \ldots, \frac{\partial \pi_{(i)(J-1)\cdot}}{\partial \beta}\right], \tag{5.51}$$

where, for $j = 1, \ldots, J-1$,

$$\begin{aligned} \frac{\partial \pi_{(i)j\cdot}}{\partial \beta} &= \int_{-\infty}^{\infty} \frac{\partial \pi^*_{(i)j\cdot}(\xi_i)}{\partial \beta} f_N(\xi_i) d\xi_i \\ &= \int_{-\infty}^{\infty} [\pi^*_{(i)j\cdot}(\xi_i)x_j - \pi^*_{(i)j\cdot}(\xi_i)\sum_{g=1}^{J-1} x_g \pi^*_{(i)g\cdot}(\xi_i)] f_N(\xi_i) d\xi_i, \end{aligned} \tag{5.52}$$

where $x'_j = [01'_{j-1}, 1, 01'_{(J-1)-j}]$ is the $1 \times J-1$ row vector with jth element as 1 and others 0. By using (5.52) in (5.51), we obtain

$$\frac{\partial \pi'_{(i)y}(\beta,\sigma_\xi)}{\partial \beta} = \int_{-\infty}^{\infty} [\Sigma^*_{(i)yy}(\xi_i)] f_N(\xi_i) d\xi_i, \tag{5.53}$$

where

$$\Sigma^*_{(i)yy}(\xi_i) = \text{diag}[\pi^*_{(i)1\cdot}(\xi_i), \ldots, \pi^*_{(i)j\cdot}(\xi_i), \ldots, \pi^*_{(i)(J-1)\cdot}(\xi_i)] - \pi^*_{(i)y}(\xi_i)\pi^{*\prime}_{(i)y}(\xi_i),$$

with

$$\pi^*_{(i)y}(\xi_i) = [\pi^*_{(i)1\cdot}(\xi_i), \ldots, \pi^*_{(i)j\cdot}(\xi_i), \ldots, \pi^*_{(i)(J-1)\cdot}(\xi_i)]',$$

and

$$\pi^*_{(i)j\cdot}(\xi_i) = \frac{\exp(\beta_{j0} + \sigma_\xi \xi_i)}{1 + \sum_{u=1}^{J-1} \exp(\beta_{u0} + \sigma_\xi \xi_i)}.$$

By calculations similar to that of (5.53), one obtains

$$\frac{\partial \pi'_{(i)z}(\alpha, \sigma_\xi)}{\partial \alpha} = \int_{-\infty}^{\infty} [\Sigma^*_{(i)zz}(\xi_i)] f_N(\xi_i) d\xi_i, \tag{5.54}$$

where

$$\Sigma^*_{(i)zz}(\xi_i) = \text{diag}[\pi^*_{(i)\cdot 1}(\xi_i), \ldots, \pi^*_{(i)\cdot r}(\xi_i), \ldots, \pi^*_{(i)\cdot(R-1)}(\xi_i)] - \pi^*_{(i)z}(\xi_i)\pi^{*\prime}_{(i)z}(\xi_i),$$

with

$$\pi^*_{(i)z}(\xi_i) = [\pi^*_{(i)\cdot 1}(\xi_i), \ldots, \pi^*_{(i)\cdot r}(\xi_i), \ldots, \pi^*_{(i)\cdot(R-1)}(\xi_i)]',$$

and

$$\pi^*_{(i)\cdot r}(\xi_i) = \frac{\exp(\alpha_{r0} + \sigma_\xi \xi_i)}{1 + \sum_{h=1}^{R-1} \exp(\alpha_{h0} + \sigma_\xi \xi_i)}.$$

Consequently, we obtain

$$\frac{\partial(\pi'_{(i)y}(\beta, \sigma_\xi), \pi'_{(i)z}(\alpha, \sigma_\xi))}{\partial \psi} = \int_{-\infty}^{\infty} \begin{pmatrix} \Sigma^*_{(i)yy}(\xi_i) & 0 \\ 0 & \Sigma^*_{(i)zz}(\xi_i) \end{pmatrix} f_N(\xi_i) d\xi_i. \tag{5.55}$$

Remark that applying the aforementioned formulas for the mean vectors, associated covariance matrix, and the derivative matrix, one may now solve the MGQL estimating equation (5.45) for $\psi = (\beta', \alpha,)'$ by using the iterative equation

$$\begin{aligned} \hat{\psi}(q+1) = \hat{\psi}(q) + & \left[\left\{ \sum_{i=1}^{K} \frac{\partial(\pi'_{(i)y}(\beta, \sigma_\xi), \pi'_{(i)z}(\alpha, \sigma_\xi))}{\partial \psi} \Sigma^{-1}_{(i)11}(\psi, \sigma_\xi) \frac{\partial(\pi'_{(i)y}(\beta, \sigma_\xi), \pi'_{(i)z}(\alpha, \sigma_\xi))'}{\partial \psi'} \right\}^{-1} \right. \\ & \left. \times \left\{ \sum_{i=1}^{K} \frac{\partial(\pi'_{(i)y}(\beta, \sigma_\xi), \pi'_{(i)z}(\alpha, \sigma_\xi))}{\partial \psi} \Sigma^{-1}_{(i)11}(\psi, \sigma_\xi) \begin{pmatrix} y_i - \pi_{(i)y}(\beta, \sigma_\xi) \\ z_i - \pi_{(i)z}(\alpha, \sigma_\xi) \end{pmatrix} \right\} \right] |_{\psi = \hat{\psi}(q)}. \end{aligned} \tag{5.56}$$

5.3.1.1.2 MGQL Estimation for σ_ξ^2

We exploit the pair-wise products of the bivariate responses to estimate this random effects variance component parameter σ_ξ^2. Let

$$g_i = (y_{i1}z_{i1}, \ldots, y_{ij}z_{ir}, \ldots, y_{i,J-1}z_{i,R-1})' \tag{5.57}$$

which has the mean

$$\begin{aligned} E[G_i] &= (\pi_{(i)11}, \ldots, \pi_{(i)jr}, \ldots, \pi_{(i),J-1,R-1})' \\ &= \pi_{(i)yz}(\psi, \sigma_\xi), \end{aligned} \tag{5.58}$$

where, for $j = 1, \ldots, J-1; r = 1, \ldots, R-1$,

$$\pi_{(i)jr} = \int_{-\infty}^{\infty} \pi^*_{(i)j\cdot}(\xi_i)\pi^*_{(i)\cdot r}(\xi_i) f_N(\xi_i) d\xi_i$$

is computed by (5.50). Notice that by using the joint cell probabilities $\pi_{(i)jr}$, the likelihood function for the parameters involved in $\phi = (\psi', \sigma_\xi^2)'$ may be written as

$$L(\phi) = \prod_{i=1}^{K} \pi_{(i)11}^{y_{i1}z_{i1}} \ldots \pi_{(i)jr}^{y_{ij}z_{ir}} \ldots \pi_{(i)JR}^{y_{iJ}z_{iR}}. \tag{5.59}$$

This multinomial probability function for the bivariate cells also implies that

$$\begin{aligned} \mathrm{cov}(G_i) &= \mathrm{diag}(\pi_{(i)yz}(\psi, \sigma_\xi)) - \pi_{(i)yz}(\psi, \sigma_\xi)\pi'_{(i)yz}(\psi, \sigma_\xi) \\ &= \mathrm{diag}[\pi_{(i)11}, \ldots, \pi_{(i)jr}, \ldots, \pi_{(i)J-1,R-1}] - \pi_{(i)yz}(\psi, \sigma_\xi)\pi'_{(i)yz}(\psi, \sigma_\xi) \\ &= \Sigma_{(i)22}(\psi, \sigma_\xi), \text{ (say)}, \end{aligned} \tag{5.60}$$

where $\pi_{(i)jr}$ is given in (5.58). Next we compute the gradient function, that is, the derivative of $E[G_i]$ with respect to σ_ξ^2 as

$$\begin{aligned} \frac{\partial E[G_i]}{\partial \sigma_\xi^2} &= \frac{\partial \pi_{(i)yz}(\psi, \sigma_\xi)}{\partial \sigma_\xi^2} \\ &= (\frac{\partial \pi_{(i)11}}{\partial \sigma_\xi^2}, \ldots, \frac{\partial \pi_{(i)jr}}{\partial \sigma_\xi^2}, \ldots, \frac{\partial \pi_{(i)J-1,R-1}}{\partial \sigma_\xi^2})', \end{aligned} \tag{5.61}$$

where, for example,

$$\frac{\partial \pi_{(i)jr}}{\partial \sigma_\xi^2} = \int_{-\infty}^{\infty} \frac{\partial \left[\pi^*_{(i)j\cdot}(\xi_i)\pi^*_{(i)\cdot r}(\xi_i)\right]}{\partial \sigma_\xi^2} f_N(\xi_i)d\xi_i$$
$$= \frac{1}{2\sigma_\xi}\int_{-\infty}^{\infty} \xi_i \left[\pi^*_{(i)j\cdot}(\xi_i)\pi^*_{(i)\cdot r}(\xi_i)\right]$$
$$\times \left[\frac{1}{1+\Sigma_{u=1}^{J-1}\exp(\beta_{u0}+\sigma_\xi\xi_i)} + \frac{1}{1+\Sigma_{h=1}^{R-1}\exp(\alpha_{h0}+\sigma_\xi\xi_i)}\right] f_N(\xi_i)d\xi_i, \tag{5.62}$$

for all $j = 1,\ldots,J-1;\ r = 1,\ldots,R-1$.

By using (5.57)–(5.58), (5.60), and (5.61)–(5.62), one may construct the MGQL estimating equation for σ_ξ^2 as

$$\sum_{i=1}^{K} \frac{\partial \pi'_{(i)yz}(\psi,\sigma_\xi)}{\partial \sigma_\xi^2} \Sigma^{-1}_{(i)22}(\psi,\sigma_\xi)[g_i - \pi_{(i)yz}(\psi,\sigma_\xi)] = 0, \tag{5.63}$$

which for known $\psi = (\beta',\alpha')'$ may be solved iteratively by using the formula

$$\hat{\sigma}_\xi^2(q+1) = \hat{\sigma}_\xi^2(q) + \left[\left\{\sum_{i=1}^{K} \frac{\partial \pi'_{(i)yz}(\psi,\sigma_\xi)}{\partial \sigma_\xi^2} \Sigma^{-1}_{(i)22}(\psi,\sigma_\xi)\frac{\partial \pi_{(i)yz}(\psi,\sigma_\xi)}{\partial \sigma_\xi^2}\right\}^{-1} \times \left\{\sum_{i=1}^{K} \frac{\partial \pi'_{(i)yz}(\psi,\sigma_\xi)}{\partial \sigma_\xi^2} \Sigma^{-1}_{(i)22}(\psi,\sigma_\xi)[g_i - \pi_{(i)yz}(\psi,\sigma_\xi)]\right\}\right]_{|\sigma_\xi^2=\hat{\sigma}_\xi^2(q)}. \tag{5.64}$$

5.3.1.2 Binomial Approximation Based JGQL Estimation

In the MGQL approach, we have estimated the intercept parameters $\psi = (\beta',\alpha')'$ and the variance component parameter σ_ξ^2, by solving two separate, i.e., MGQL estimating equations (5.45) and (5.63). As opposed to this MGQL approach, we now estimate these parameters jointly by using a single GQL estimating equation which is constructed by combining (5.45) and (5.63) as follows.

Notice from (5.59) that ϕ denotes a stacked vector of parameters ψ and σ_ξ^2. A JGQL estimating equation for ϕ by combining (5.45) and (5.63) has the form given by

$$f(\phi) = \sum_{i=1}^{K} \frac{\partial(\pi'_{(i)y}(\beta,\sigma_\xi), \pi'_{(i)z}(\alpha,\sigma_\xi), \pi'_{(i)yz}(\psi,\sigma_\xi))}{\partial \phi} \Sigma_{(i)}^{-1}(\psi,\sigma_\xi) \begin{pmatrix} y_i - \pi_{(i)y}(\beta,\sigma_\xi) \\ z_i - \pi_{(i)z}(\alpha,\sigma_\xi) \\ g_i - \pi_{(i)yz}(\psi,\sigma_\xi) \end{pmatrix} = 0, \tag{5.65}$$

where

$$\Sigma_{(i)}(\psi,\sigma_\xi) = \begin{pmatrix} \Sigma_{(i)11}(\psi,\sigma_\xi) & \Sigma_{(i)12}(\psi,\sigma_\xi) \\ \Sigma'_{(i)12}(\psi,\sigma_\xi) & \Sigma_{(i)22}(\psi,\sigma_\xi) \end{pmatrix}, \tag{5.66}$$

with $\Sigma_{(i)11}(\psi,\sigma_\xi)$ and $\Sigma_{(i)22}(\psi,\sigma_\xi)$ are as in (5.46) and (5.60), respectively, and $\Sigma_{(i)12}(\psi,\sigma_\xi)$ has the form

$$\begin{aligned} \Sigma_{(i)12}(\psi,\sigma_\xi) &= \text{cov}\left[\begin{pmatrix} Y_i \\ Z_i \end{pmatrix}, G'_i\right] \\ &= \begin{pmatrix} \text{cov}(Y_i, G'_i) \\ \text{cov}(Z_i, G'_i) \end{pmatrix}, \end{aligned} \tag{5.67}$$

where

$$\text{cov}(Y_i, G'_i) = [\text{cov}(y_{ik}, y_{ij}z_{ir})]_{(J-1)\times(J-1)(R-1)} \tag{5.68}$$

with

$$\text{cov}(y_{ik}, y_{ij}z_{ir}) = \begin{cases} \pi_{(i)jr}(1-\pi_{(i)j\cdot}) & j = k, \\ -\pi_{(i)k\cdot}\pi_{(i)jr} & j \neq k, \end{cases} \tag{5.69}$$

and similarly

$$\text{cov}(Z_i, G'_i) = [\text{cov}(z_{iq}, y_{ij}z_{ir})]_{(R-1)\times(J-1)(R-1)} \tag{5.70}$$

with

$$\text{cov}(z_{iq}, y_{ij}z_{ir}) = \begin{cases} \pi_{(i)jr}(1-\pi_{(i)\cdot r}) & r = q, \\ -\pi_{(i)\cdot q}\pi_{(i)jr} & r \neq q. \end{cases} \tag{5.71}$$

Furthermore, in (5.65), the gradient function may be computed as

$$\frac{\partial(\pi'_{(i)y}(\beta,\sigma_\xi), \pi'_{(i)z}(\alpha,\sigma_\xi), \pi'_{(i)yz}(\psi,\sigma_\xi))}{\partial \phi} = \begin{pmatrix} \frac{\partial(\pi'_{(i)y}(\beta,\sigma_\xi),\pi'_{(i)z}(\alpha,\sigma_\xi))}{\partial \psi} & \frac{\partial \pi'_{(i)yz}(\psi,\sigma_\xi)}{\partial \psi} \\ \frac{\partial(\pi'_{(i)y}(\beta,\sigma_\xi),\pi'_{(i)z}(\alpha,\sigma_\xi))}{\partial \sigma_\xi^2} & \frac{\partial \pi'_{(i)yz}(\psi,\sigma_\xi)}{\partial \sigma_\xi^2} \end{pmatrix}, \tag{5.72}$$

where the formulas for

$$\frac{\partial(\pi'_{(i)y}(\beta,\sigma_\xi),\pi'_{(i)z}(\alpha,\sigma_\xi))}{\partial\psi} \text{ and } \frac{\partial\pi'_{(i)yz}(\psi,\sigma_\xi)}{\partial\sigma^2_\xi},$$

are given by (5.55) and (5.61), respectively. The formulas for remaining two derivatives are derived as follows.

Computation of $\frac{\partial\pi'_{(i)yz}(\psi,\sigma_\xi)}{\partial\psi}$ **:**
Similar to (5.61), we write

$$\frac{\partial\pi'_{(i)yz}(\psi,\sigma_\xi)}{\partial\psi} = \left(\frac{\partial\pi_{(i)11}}{\partial\psi},\ldots,\frac{\partial\pi_{(i)jr}}{\partial\psi},\ldots,\frac{\partial\pi_{(i)J-1,R-1}}{\partial\psi}\right), \tag{5.73}$$

where

$$\frac{\partial\pi_{(i)jr}}{\partial\psi} = \begin{pmatrix}\frac{\partial\pi_{(i)jr}}{\partial\beta}\\ \frac{\partial\pi_{(i)jr}}{\partial\alpha}\end{pmatrix}, \tag{5.74}$$

with

$$\begin{aligned}\frac{\partial\pi_{(i)jr}}{\partial\beta} &= \int_{-\infty}^{\infty}\frac{\partial\left[\pi^*_{(i)j\cdot}(\xi_i)\pi^*_{(i)\cdot r}(\xi_i)\right]}{\partial\beta}f_N(\xi_i)d\xi_i\\ &= \int_{-\infty}^{\infty}\pi^*_{(i)\cdot r}(\xi_i)\frac{\partial\left[\pi^*_{(i)j\cdot}(\xi_i)\right]}{\partial\beta}f_N(\xi_i)d\xi_i,\end{aligned} \tag{5.75}$$

for all $j = 1,\ldots,J-1$; $r = 1,\ldots,R-1$, the formula for $\frac{\partial\left[\pi^*_{(i)j\cdot}(\xi_i)\right]}{\partial\beta}$ is being given by (5.52). Now for convenience of applying the result from (5.75) to (5.73), we first re-express (5.73) as

$$\begin{aligned}\frac{\partial\pi'_{(i)yz}(\psi,\sigma_\xi)}{\partial\psi} = \Bigg[&\frac{\partial\pi_{(i)11}}{\partial\psi},\ldots,\frac{\partial\pi_{(i)j1}}{\partial\psi},\ldots,\frac{\partial\pi_{(i)J-1,1}}{\partial\psi},\\ &\ldots\ldots\ldots\ldots\ldots\\ &\frac{\partial\pi_{(i)1r}}{\partial\psi},\ldots,\frac{\partial\pi_{(i)jr}}{\partial\psi},\ldots,\frac{\partial\pi_{(i)J-1,r}}{\partial\psi},\\ &\ldots\ldots\ldots\ldots\ldots\\ &\frac{\partial\pi_{(i)1,R-1}}{\partial\psi},\ldots,\frac{\partial\pi_{(i)j,R-1}}{\partial\psi},\ldots,\frac{\partial\pi_{(i)J-1,R-1}}{\partial\psi}\Bigg].\end{aligned} \tag{5.76}$$

Next by using (5.53) and (5.75), we obtain

$$\frac{\partial \pi'_{(i)yz}(\psi,\sigma_\xi)}{\partial \beta} = \left[\frac{\partial \pi_{(i)11}}{\partial \beta},\ldots,\frac{\partial \pi_{(i)j1}}{\partial \beta},\ldots,\frac{\partial \pi_{(i)J-1,1}}{\partial \beta},\right.$$
$$\ldots\ldots\ldots\ldots\ldots$$
$$\frac{\partial \pi_{(i)1r}}{\partial \beta},\ldots,\frac{\partial \pi_{(i)jr}}{\partial \beta},\ldots,\frac{\partial \pi_{(i)J-1,r}}{\partial \beta},$$
$$\ldots\ldots\ldots\ldots\ldots$$
$$\left.\frac{\partial \pi_{(i)1,R-1}}{\partial \beta},\ldots,\frac{\partial \pi_{(i)j,R-1}}{\partial \beta},\ldots,\frac{\partial \pi_{(i)J-1,R-1}}{\partial \beta}\right]$$
$$= \int_{-\infty}^{\infty}\left(\pi^*_{(i)\cdot 1}(\xi_i)\Sigma^*_{(i)yy}(\xi_i)\ \ldots\ \pi^*_{(i)\cdot r}(\xi_i)\Sigma^*_{(i)yy}(\xi_i)\ \ldots\ \pi^*_{(i)\cdot,R-1}(\xi_i)\Sigma^*_{(i)yy}(\xi_i)\right)$$
$$\times f_N(\xi_i)d\xi_i. \tag{5.77}$$

Similarly, one obtains

$$\frac{\partial \pi'_{(i)yz}(\psi,\sigma_\xi)}{\partial \alpha} = \left[\frac{\partial \pi_{(i)11}}{\partial \alpha},\ldots,\frac{\partial \pi_{(i)j1}}{\partial \alpha},\ldots,\frac{\partial \pi_{(i)J-1,1}}{\partial \alpha},\right.$$
$$\ldots\ldots\ldots\ldots\ldots$$
$$\frac{\partial \pi_{(i)1r}}{\partial \alpha},\ldots,\frac{\partial \pi_{(i)jr}}{\partial \alpha},\ldots,\frac{\partial \pi_{(i)J-1,r}}{\partial \alpha},$$
$$\ldots\ldots\ldots\ldots\ldots$$
$$\left.\frac{\partial \pi_{(i)1,R-1}}{\partial \alpha},\ldots,\frac{\partial \pi_{(i)j,R-1}}{\partial \alpha},\ldots,\frac{\partial \pi_{(i)J-1,R-1}}{\partial \alpha}\right]$$
$$= \int_{-\infty}^{\infty}\left[\pi^*_{(i)1\cdot}\{\pi^*_{(i)\cdot 1}(x_1-\pi^*_{(i)z})\},\ldots,\pi^*_{(i)j\cdot}\{\pi^*_{(i)\cdot 1}(x_1-\pi^*_{(i)z})\},\ldots,\pi^*_{(i),J-1\cdot}\{\pi^*_{(i)\cdot 1}(x_1-\pi^*_{(i)z})\},\right.$$
$$\ldots\ldots\ldots\ldots\ldots$$
$$\pi^*_{(i)1\cdot}\{\pi^*_{(i)\cdot r}(x_r-\pi^*_{(i)z})\},\ldots,\pi^*_{(i)j\cdot}\{\pi^*_{(i)\cdot r}(x_r-\pi^*_{(i)z})\},\ldots,\pi^*_{(i),J-1\cdot}\{\pi^*_{(i)\cdot r}(x_r-\pi^*_{(i)z})\},$$
$$\ldots\ldots\ldots\ldots\ldots$$
$$\pi^*_{(i)1\cdot}\{\pi^*_{(i)\cdot,R-1}(x_{R-1}-\pi^*_{(i)z})\},\ldots,\pi^*_{(i)j\cdot}\{\pi^*_{(i)\cdot,R-1}(x_{R-1}-\pi^*_{(i)z})\},\ldots,$$
$$\left.\pi^*_{(i),J-1\cdot}\{\pi^*_{(i)\cdot,R-1}(x_{R-1}-\pi^*_{(i)z})\}\right] f_N(\xi_i)d\xi_i$$
$$= \int_{-\infty}^{\infty}\left[{\pi^*}'_{(i)y}\otimes\{\pi^*_{(i)\cdot 1}(x_1-\pi^*_{(i)z})\},\ldots,{\pi^*}'_{(i)y}\otimes\{\pi^*_{(i)\cdot r}(x_r-\pi^*_{(i)z})\},\ldots,\right.$$
$$\left.{\pi^*}'_{(i)y}\otimes\{\pi^*_{(i)\cdot,R-1}(x_{R-1}-\pi^*_{(i)z})\}\right] f_N(\xi_i)d\xi_i, \tag{5.78}$$

where similar to (5.52), $x'_r = [01'_{r-1}, 1, 01'_{(R-1)-R}]$ is the $1 \times R-1$ row vector with rth element as 1 and others 0; $\otimes$ denotes the Kronecker or direct product, and

$$\pi^*_{(i)y} = [\pi^*_{(i)1\cdot}(\xi),\ldots,\pi^*_{(i)j\cdot}(\xi),\ldots,\pi^*_{(i)(J-1)\cdot}(\xi)]',$$
$$\pi^*_{(i)z} = [\pi^*_{(i)\cdot 1}(\xi),\ldots,\pi^*_{(i)\cdot r}(\xi),\ldots,\pi^*_{(i)\cdot,R-1}(\xi)]'.$$

Computation of $\frac{\partial(\pi'_{(i)y}(\beta,\sigma_\xi),\pi'_{(i)z}(\alpha,\sigma_\xi))}{\partial\sigma^2_\xi}$:

To compute these derivatives, we compute, for example, the formula for $\frac{\partial\pi'_{(i)y}(\beta,\sigma_\xi)}{\partial\sigma^2_\xi}$. One may then write a similar formula for the other derivative. Note that

$$\frac{\partial\pi'_{(i)y}(\beta,\sigma_\xi)}{\partial\sigma^2_\xi} = \left[\frac{\partial\pi_{(i)1\cdot}}{\partial\sigma^2_\xi},\ldots,\frac{\partial\pi_{(i)j\cdot}}{\partial\sigma^2_\xi},\ldots,\frac{\partial\pi_{(i)(J-1)\cdot}}{\partial\sigma^2_\xi}\right], \tag{5.79}$$

where, for $j = 1,\ldots,J-1$,

$$\begin{aligned}\frac{\partial\pi_{(i)j\cdot}}{\partial\sigma^2_\xi} &= \int_{-\infty}^{\infty}\frac{\pi^*_{(i)j\cdot}(\xi_i)}{\partial\sigma^2_\xi}f_N(\xi_i)d\xi_i \\ &= \frac{1}{2\sigma_\xi}\int_{-\infty}^{\infty}\xi_i\pi^*_{(i)j\cdot}\left[\frac{1}{1+\sum_{u=1}^{J-1}\exp(\beta_{u0}+\sigma_\xi\xi_i)}\right]f_N(\xi_i)d\xi_i. \end{aligned} \tag{5.80}$$

Similarly, one computes

$$\frac{\partial\pi'_{(i)z}(\alpha,\sigma_\xi)}{\partial\sigma^2_\xi} = \left[\frac{\partial\pi_{(i)\cdot 1}}{\partial\sigma^2_\xi},\ldots,\frac{\partial\pi_{(i)\cdot r}}{\partial\sigma^2_\xi},\ldots,\frac{\partial\pi_{(i)\cdot(R-1)}}{\partial\sigma^2_\xi}\right], \tag{5.81}$$

where, for $r = 1,\ldots,R-1$,

$$\begin{aligned}\frac{\partial\pi_{(i)\cdot r}}{\partial\sigma^2_\xi} &= \int_{-\infty}^{\infty}\frac{\pi^*_{(i)\cdot r}(\xi_i)}{\partial\sigma^2_\xi}f_N(\xi_i)d\xi_i \\ &= \frac{1}{2\sigma_\xi}\int_{-\infty}^{\infty}\xi_i\pi^*_{(i)\cdot r}\left[\frac{1}{1+\sum_{u=1}^{R-1}\exp(\alpha_{u0}+\sigma_\xi\xi_i)}\right]f_N(\xi_i)d\xi_i. \end{aligned} \tag{5.82}$$

Because the formulas for the derivatives and the covariance matrix involved in the JGQL estimating equation (5.65) are obtained, one may now solve this equation by applying the iterative equation given by

$$\begin{aligned}\hat{\phi}(m+1) &= \hat{\phi}(m) + \left[\left\{\sum_{i=1}^{K}\frac{\partial(\pi'_{(i)y}(\beta,\sigma_\xi),\pi'_{(i)z}(\alpha,\sigma_\xi),\pi'_{(i)yz}(\psi,\sigma_\xi))}{\partial\phi}\right.\right. \\ &\times\left.\Sigma^{-1}_{(i)}(\psi,\sigma_\xi)\frac{\partial(\pi'_{(i)y}(\beta,\sigma_\xi),\pi'_{(i)z}(\alpha,\sigma_\xi),\pi'_{(i)yz}(\psi,\sigma_\xi))'}{\partial\phi'}\right\}^{-1} \\ &\times\left.\sum_{i=1}^{K}\frac{\partial(\pi'_{(i)y}(\beta,\sigma_\xi),\pi'_{(i)z}(\alpha,\sigma_\xi),\pi'_{(i)yz}(\psi,\sigma_\xi))}{\partial\phi}\Sigma^{-1}_{(i)}(\psi,\sigma_\xi)\begin{pmatrix}y_i-\pi_{(i)y}(\beta,\sigma_\xi)\\ z_i-\pi_{(i)z}(\alpha,\sigma_\xi)\\ g_i-\pi_{(i)yz}(\psi,\sigma_\xi)\end{pmatrix}\right]_{|\phi=\hat{\phi}(m)}. \end{aligned} \tag{5.83}$$

5.3.2 Binomial Approximation Based ML Estimation

In this section we demonstrate how one can compute the maximum likelihood (ML) estimate of

$$\phi = (\psi', \sigma_\xi^2)' = (\beta', \alpha', \sigma_\xi^2)'$$

by exploiting likelihood function given in (5.59). For the purpose, write the log likelihood function as

$$Log\ L(\phi) = \sum_{i=1}^{K} \left[\sum_{j=1}^{J} \sum_{r=1}^{R} y_{ij} z_{ir} log\ \pi_{(i)jr} \right], \tag{5.84}$$

where

$$\pi_{(i)jr} = \int_{-\infty}^{\infty} [\pi^*_{(i)j\cdot} \pi^*_{(i)\cdot r}] f_N(\xi_i) d\xi_i,$$

with

$$\pi^*_{(i)j\cdot}(\xi_i) = \begin{cases} \frac{\exp(\beta_{j0} + \sigma_\xi \xi_i)}{1 + \sum_{u=1}^{J-1} \exp(\beta_{u0} + \sigma_\xi \xi_i)} & \text{for } j = 1, \ldots, J-1 \\ \frac{1}{1 + \sum_{h=1}^{J-1} \exp(\beta_{h0} + \sigma_\xi \xi_i)} & \text{for } j = J, \end{cases}$$

as in (5.2), and

$$\pi^*_{(i)\cdot r}(\xi_i) = \begin{cases} \frac{\exp(\alpha_{r0} + \sigma_\xi \xi_i)}{1 + \sum_{h=1}^{R-1} \exp(\alpha_{h0} + \sigma_\xi \xi_i)} & \text{for } r = 1, \ldots, R-1 \\ \frac{1}{1 + \sum_{h=1}^{R-1} \exp(\alpha_{h0} + \sigma_\xi \xi_i)} & \text{for } r = R, \end{cases}$$

as in (5.3). One may then write the likelihood estimating equation for ϕ as

$$\frac{\partial Log\ L(\phi)}{\partial \phi} = \sum_{i=1}^{K} \left[\sum_{j=1}^{J} \sum_{r=1}^{R} y_{ij} z_{ir} \frac{1}{\pi_{(i)jr}} \frac{\partial \pi_{(i)jr}}{\partial \phi} \right] = 0, \tag{5.85}$$

where for all $j = 1, \ldots, J$; $r = 1, \ldots, R$, the cell probabilities $\pi_{(i)jr}$ are computed by the binomial approximation based formulas given by (5.50). Because $\phi = (\beta', \alpha', \sigma_\xi^2)'$, for convenience, we express the first order derivatives in (5.85) as

$$\frac{\partial \pi_{(i)jr}}{\partial \phi} = \begin{pmatrix} \frac{\partial \pi_{(i)jr}}{\partial \beta} \\ \frac{\partial \pi_{(i)jr}}{\partial \alpha} \\ \frac{\partial \pi_{(i)jr}}{\partial \sigma_\xi^2} \end{pmatrix}, \tag{5.86}$$

and compute the components as follows.

In (5.86), for all $j = 1, \ldots, J;\ r = 1, \ldots, R$,

$$\frac{\partial \pi_{(i)jr}}{\partial \beta} = \int_{-\infty}^{\infty} \frac{\partial [\pi^*_{(i)j\cdot} \pi^*_{(i)\cdot r}]}{\partial \beta} f_N(\xi_i) d\xi_i$$

$$= \int_{-\infty}^{\infty} \pi^*_{(i)\cdot r} \frac{\partial [\pi^*_{(i)j\cdot}]}{\partial \beta} f_N(\xi_i) d\xi_i; \tag{5.87}$$

$$\frac{\partial \pi_{(i)jr}}{\partial \alpha} = \int_{-\infty}^{\infty} \frac{\partial [\pi^*_{(i)j\cdot} \pi^*_{(i)\cdot r}]}{\partial \alpha} f_N(\xi_i) d\xi_i$$

$$= \int_{-\infty}^{\infty} \pi^*_{(i)j\cdot} \frac{\partial [\pi^*_{(i)\cdot r}]}{\partial \alpha} f_N(\xi_i) d\xi_i; \tag{5.88}$$

$$\frac{\partial \pi_{(i)jr}}{\partial \sigma^2_\xi} = \int_{-\infty}^{\infty} \frac{\partial [\pi^*_{(i)j\cdot} \pi^*_{(i)\cdot r}]}{\partial \sigma^2_\xi} f_N(\xi_i) d\xi_i. \tag{5.89}$$

where, by (5.52),

$$\frac{\partial \pi_{(i)j\cdot}}{\partial \beta} = \int_{-\infty}^{\infty} \frac{\partial \pi^*_{(i)j\cdot}(\xi_i)}{\partial \beta} f_N(\xi_i) d\xi_i$$

$$= \begin{cases} \int_{-\infty}^{\infty} \pi^*_{(i)j\cdot}(\xi_i)[x_j - \pi^*_{(i)y}] f_N(\xi_i) d\xi_i & \text{for } j = 1, \ldots, J-1 \\ -\int_{-\infty}^{\infty} \pi^*_{(i)J\cdot}(\xi_i) \pi^*_{(i)y} f_N(\xi_i) d\xi_i & \text{for } j = J \end{cases}$$

$$= \int_{-\infty}^{\infty} \pi^*_{(i)j\cdot}(\xi_i)[x_j - \pi^*_{(i)y}] f_N(\xi_i) d\xi_i, \tag{5.90}$$

for all $j = 1, \ldots, J$, with

$$x_j = \begin{cases} [01'_{j-1}, 1, 01'_{(J-1)-j}] & \text{for } j = 1, \ldots, J-1 \\ 01'_{J-1} & \text{for } j = J, \end{cases}$$

and

$$\pi^*_{(i)y} = [\pi^*_{(i)1\cdot}(\xi), \ldots, \pi^*_{(i)j\cdot}(\xi), \ldots, \pi^*_{(i)(J-1)\cdot}(\xi)]';$$

and similarly

$$\frac{\partial \pi_{(i)\cdot r}}{\partial \alpha} = \int_{-\infty}^{\infty} \frac{\partial \pi^*_{(i)\cdot r}(\xi_i)}{\partial \alpha} f_N(\xi_i) d\xi_i$$

$$= \begin{cases} \int_{-\infty}^{\infty} \pi^*_{(i)\cdot r}(\xi_i)[x_r - \pi^*_{(i)z}] f_N(\xi_i) d\xi_i & \text{for } r = 1, \ldots, R-1 \\ -\int_{-\infty}^{\infty} \pi^*_{(i)\cdot R}(\xi_i) \pi^*_{(i)z} f_N(\xi_i) d\xi_i & \text{for } r = R \end{cases}$$

$$= \int_{-\infty}^{\infty} \pi^*_{(i)\cdot r}(\xi_i)[x_r - \pi^*_{(i)z}] f_N(\xi_i) d\xi_i, \tag{5.91}$$

for all $r = 1, \ldots, R$, with

$$x_r = \begin{cases} [01'_{r-1}, 1, 01'_{(R-1)-r}] & \text{for } r = 1, \ldots, R-1 \\ 01'_{R-1} & \text{for } r = R, \end{cases}$$

and

$$\pi^*_{(i)z} = [\pi^*_{(i)\cdot 1}(\xi), \ldots, \pi^*_{(i)\cdot r}(\xi), \ldots, \pi^*_{(i)\cdot, R-1}(\xi)]'.$$

This completes the computation for the derivatives in (5.87) and (5.88). The remaining derivatives, that is, the derivatives in (5.89) may be computed as follows for all $j = 1, \ldots, J$; $r = 1, \ldots, R$. More specifically, by using (5.62), (5.80), and (5.82), one obtains

$$\frac{\partial \pi_{(i)jr}}{\partial \sigma^2_\xi} = \begin{cases} \frac{1}{2\sigma_\xi} \int_{-\infty}^{\infty} \xi_i \left[\pi^*_{(i)j\cdot}\pi^*_{(i)\cdot r}\right] \left[\pi^*_{(i)J\cdot} + \pi^*_{(i)\cdot R}\right] f_N(\xi_i) d\xi_i & \text{for } j = 1, \ldots, J-1; r = 1, \ldots, R-1 \\ \frac{1}{2\sigma_\xi} \int_{-\infty}^{\infty} \xi_i \left[\pi^*_{(i)j\cdot}\pi^*_{(i)\cdot R}\right] [\pi^*_{(i)J\cdot} + \pi^*_{(i)\cdot R} - 1] f_N(\xi_i) d\xi_i & \text{for } j = 1, \ldots, J-1; r = R \\ \frac{1}{2\sigma_\xi} \int_{-\infty}^{\infty} \xi_i \left[\pi^*_{(i)J\cdot}\pi^*_{(i)\cdot r}\right] [\pi^*_{(i)J\cdot} + \pi^*_{(i)\cdot R} - 1] f_N(\xi_i) d\xi_i & \text{for } j = J; r = 1, \ldots, R-1 \\ \frac{1}{2\sigma_\xi} \int_{-\infty}^{\infty} \xi_i \left[\pi^*_{(i)J\cdot}\pi^*_{(i)\cdot R}\right] [\pi^*_{(i)J\cdot} + \pi^*_{(i)\cdot R} - 2] f_N(\xi_i) d\xi_i & \text{for } j = J; r = R. \end{cases} \quad (5.92)$$

Notice that by (5.90) and (5.91), for the sake of completeness, we write

$$\frac{\partial \pi_{(i)jr}}{\partial \beta} = \int_{-\infty}^{\infty} \pi^*_{(i)\cdot r}\pi^*_{(i)j\cdot}[x_j - \pi^*_{(i)y}] f_N(\xi_i) d\xi_i \quad (5.93)$$

$$\frac{\partial \pi_{(i)jr}}{\partial \alpha} = \int_{-\infty}^{\infty} \pi^*_{(i)j\cdot}\pi^*_{(i)\cdot r}[x_r - \pi^*_{(i)z}] f_N(\xi_i) d\xi_i, \quad (5.94)$$

for all $j = 1, \ldots, J$; $r = 1, \ldots, R$.

Thus, the derivatives in (5.86) required for the computation of the likelihood equation (5.85) are computed by (5.93), (5.94), and (5.92). One may now solve the likelihood estimating equation (5.85) for ϕ by applying the iterative equation given by

$$\hat{\phi}(m+1) = \hat{\phi}(m) + \left[\left\{\frac{\partial^2 Log\, L(\phi)}{\partial \phi \partial \phi'}\right\}^{-1} \frac{\partial Log\, L(\phi)}{\partial \phi}\right]_{|\phi = \hat{\phi}(m)}, \quad (5.95)$$

where the second order derivative matrix $\frac{\partial^2 Log\, L(\phi)}{\partial \phi \partial \phi'}$ is computed as follows.

5.3.2.1 An Approximation for $\frac{\partial^2 Log\, L(\phi)}{\partial\phi\partial\phi'}$

In the spirit of iteration, suppose that the parameters in the derivatives, that is, in $\frac{\partial\pi_{(i)jr}}{\partial\phi}$, of the likelihood estimating function

$$\frac{\partial Log\, L(\phi)}{\partial\phi} = \sum_{i=1}^{K}\left[\sum_{j=1}^{J}\sum_{r=1}^{R} y_{ij}z_{ir}\frac{1}{\pi_{(i)jr}}\frac{\partial\pi_{(i)jr}}{\partial\phi}\right],$$

are known from the previous iteration. One may then obtain an approximate formula for the second derivative of this likelihood estimating function as

$$\frac{\partial^2 Log\, L(\phi)}{\partial\phi\partial\phi'} = -\sum_{i=1}^{K}\left[\sum_{j=1}^{J}\sum_{r=1}^{R} y_{ij}z_{ir}\frac{1}{\pi^2_{(i)jr}}\left\{\frac{\partial\pi_{(i)jr}}{\partial\phi}\frac{\partial\pi_{(i)jr}}{\partial\phi'}\right\}\right] : (J+R-1)\times(J+R-1), \tag{5.96}$$

where $\frac{\partial\pi_{(i)jr}}{\partial\phi'}$ is the transpose of the $(J+R-1)\times 1$ column vector $\frac{\partial\pi_{(i)jr}}{\partial\phi}$ already computed by (5.92)–(5.94).

5.3.2.2 Exact Computational Formula for $\frac{\partial^2 Log\, L(\phi)}{\partial\phi\partial\phi'}$

The first order derivatives involved in the likelihood estimating function (5.85) contain unknown ϕ parameter. Therefore, as opposed to the approximation used in (5.96), the exact second order derivatives of the log likelihood function $Log\, L(\phi)$ are given by

$$\begin{aligned}\frac{\partial^2 Log\, L(\phi)}{\partial\phi\partial\phi'} = &-\sum_{i=1}^{K}\left[\sum_{j=1}^{J}\sum_{r=1}^{R} y_{ij}z_{ir}\frac{1}{\pi^2_{(i)jr}}\left\{\frac{\partial\pi_{(i)jr}}{\partial\phi}\frac{\partial\pi_{(i)jr}}{\partial\phi'}\right\}\right]\\ &+\sum_{i=1}^{K}\left[\sum_{j=1}^{J}\sum_{r=1}^{R} y_{ij}z_{ir}\frac{1}{\pi_{(i)jr}}\left\{\frac{\partial^2\pi_{(i)jr}}{\partial\phi\partial\phi'}\right\}\right],\end{aligned} \tag{5.97}$$

where the first term is computed as in (5.96), and the computation of the second term requires the formula for $\frac{\partial^2\pi_{(i)jr}}{\partial\phi\partial\phi'}$ which may be computed as follows.

By (5.93), we obtain

$$\frac{\partial^2 \pi_{(i)jr}}{\partial\beta\partial\beta'} = \int_{-\infty}^{\infty} \pi^*_{(i)\cdot r}\pi^*_{(i)j\cdot}\left[(x_j - \pi^*_{(i)y})(x_j - \pi^*_{(i)y})' - \begin{pmatrix} \pi^*_{(i)1\cdot}(x_1 - \pi^*_{(i)y})' \\ \vdots \\ \pi^*_{(i)j\cdot}(\xi_i)(x_j - \pi^*_{(i)y})' \\ \vdots \\ \pi^*_{(i)(J-1)\cdot}(x_{J-1} - \pi^*_{(i)y})' \end{pmatrix}\right] f_N(\xi_i)d\xi_i. \tag{5.98}$$

Similarly, by (5.93) and (5.94), we obtain

$$\frac{\partial^2 \pi_{(i)jr}}{\partial\beta\partial\alpha'} = \int_{-\infty}^{\infty} \pi^*_{(i)\cdot r}\pi^*_{(i)j\cdot}\left[(x_j - \pi^*_{(i)y})(x_r - \pi^*_{(i)z})'\right] f_N(\xi_i)d\xi_i, \tag{5.99}$$

and by (5.92) and (5.93), one computes

$$\frac{\partial^2 \pi_{(i)jr}}{\partial\beta\partial\sigma^2_\xi} = \begin{cases} \frac{1}{2\sigma_\xi}\int_{-\infty}^{\infty}\xi_i\pi^*_{(i)j\cdot}\pi^*_{(i)\cdot r} \\ \left[(\pi^*_{(i)J\cdot} + \pi^*_{(i)\cdot R})(x_j - \pi^*_{(i)y}) - \pi^*_{(i)J\cdot}\pi^*_{(i)y}\right] f_N(\xi_i)d\xi_i & \text{for } j = 1,\ldots,J-1; r = 1,\ldots,R-1 \\ \frac{1}{2\sigma_\xi}\int_{-\infty}^{\infty}\xi_i\pi^*_{(i)j\cdot}\pi^*_{(i)\cdot R} \\ \left[(\pi^*_{(i)J\cdot} + \pi^*_{(i)\cdot R} - 1)(x_j - \pi^*_{(i)y}) - \pi^*_{(i)J\cdot}\pi^*_{(i)y}\right] f_N(\xi_i)d\xi_i & \text{for } j = 1,\ldots,J-1; r = R \\ \frac{1}{2\sigma_\xi}\int_{-\infty}^{\infty}\xi_i\pi^*_{(i)J\cdot}\pi^*_{(i)\cdot r} \\ \left[(\pi^*_{(i)J\cdot} + \pi^*_{(i)\cdot R} - 1)(x_j - \pi^*_{(i)y}) - \pi^*_{(i)J\cdot}\pi^*_{(i)y}\right] f_N(\xi_i)d\xi_i & \text{for } j = J; r = 1,\ldots,R-1 \\ \frac{1}{2\sigma_\xi}\int_{-\infty}^{\infty}\xi_i\pi^*_{(i)J\cdot}\pi^*_{(i)\cdot R} \\ \left[(\pi^*_{(i)J\cdot} + \pi^*_{(i)\cdot R} - 2)(x_j - \pi^*_{(i)y}) - \pi^*_{(i)J\cdot}\pi^*_{(i)y}\right] f_N(\xi_i)d\xi_i & \text{for } j = J; r = R. \end{cases} \tag{5.100}$$

Next by similar operation as in (5.98) and (5.100), it follows from (5.94) that

$$\frac{\partial^2 \pi_{(i)jr}}{\partial\alpha\partial\alpha'} = \int_{-\infty}^{\infty} \pi^*_{(i)\cdot r}\pi^*_{(i)j\cdot}\left[(x_r - \pi^*_{(i)z})(x_r - \pi^*_{(i)z})' - \begin{pmatrix} \pi^*_{(i)\cdot 1}(x_1 - \pi^*_{(i)z})' \\ \vdots \\ \pi^*_{(i)\cdot r}(\xi_i)(x_r - \pi^*_{(i)z})' \\ \vdots \\ \pi^*_{(i)\cdot(R-1)}(x_{R-1} - \pi^*_{(i)z})' \end{pmatrix}\right] f_N(\xi_i)d\xi_i, \tag{5.101}$$

and by (5.94) and (5.92), one writes

$$\frac{\partial^2 \pi_{(i)jr}}{\partial\alpha\partial\sigma_\xi^2} = \begin{cases} \frac{1}{2\sigma_\xi}\int_{-\infty}^{\infty}\xi_i\pi^*_{(i)j\cdot}\pi^*_{(i)\cdot r} \\ \left[(\pi^*_{(i)J\cdot}+\pi^*_{(i)\cdot R})(x_r-\pi^*_{(i)z})-\pi^*_{(i)\cdot R}\pi^*_{(i)z}\right] f_N(\xi_i)d\xi_i & \text{for } j=1,\ldots,J-1; r=1,\ldots,R-1 \\ \frac{1}{2\sigma_\xi}\int_{-\infty}^{\infty}\xi_i\pi^*_{(i)\cdot r}\pi^*_{(i)J\cdot} \\ \left[(\pi^*_{(i)J\cdot}+\pi^*_{(i)\cdot R}-1)(x_r-\pi^*_{(i)z})-\pi^*_{(i)\cdot R}\pi^*_{(i)z}\right] f_N(\xi_i)d\xi_i & \text{for } j=J; r=1,\ldots,R-1 \\ \frac{1}{2\sigma_\xi}\int_{-\infty}^{\infty}\xi_i\pi^*_{(i)\cdot R}\pi^*_{(i)j\cdot} \\ \left[(\pi^*_{(i)J\cdot}+\pi^*_{(i)\cdot R}-1)(x_r-\pi^*_{(i)z})-\pi^*_{(i)\cdot R}\pi^*_{(i)z}\right] f_N(\xi_i)d\xi_i & \text{for } j=1,\ldots,J-1; r=R \\ \frac{1}{2\sigma_\xi}\int_{-\infty}^{\infty}\xi_i\pi^*_{(i)J\cdot}\pi^*_{(i)\cdot R} \\ \left[(\pi^*_{(i)J\cdot}+\pi^*_{(i)\cdot R}-2)(x_r-\pi^*_{(i)z})-\pi^*_{(i)\cdot R}\pi^*_{(i)z}\right] f_N(\xi_i)d\xi_i & \text{for } j=J; r=R. \end{cases} \tag{5.102}$$

The remaining second order derivative, that is, $\frac{\partial^2 \pi_{(i)jr}}{\partial\sigma_\xi^4}$ is computed by (5.92) as

$$\frac{\partial^2 \pi_{(i)jr}}{\partial\sigma_\xi^4} = \begin{cases} \int_{-\infty}^{\infty}\frac{\xi_i(\pi^*_{(i)j\cdot}\pi^*_{(i)\cdot r})}{4\sigma_\xi^2}\left[\xi_i\left\{\pi^*_{(i)J\cdot}+\pi^*_{(i)\cdot R}\right\}^2\right. \\ -\xi_i[\pi^*_{(i)J\cdot}(1-\pi^*_{(i)J\cdot})+\pi^*_{(i)\cdot R}(1-\pi^*_{(i)\cdot R})] \\ \left.-\frac{1}{\sigma_\xi}\left\{\pi^*_{(i)J\cdot}+\pi^*_{(i)\cdot R}\right\}\right] f_N(\xi_i)d\xi_i & \text{for } j=1,\ldots,J-1; r=1,\ldots,R-1 \\ \int_{-\infty}^{\infty}\frac{\xi_i(\pi^*_{(i)j\cdot}\pi^*_{(i)\cdot R})}{4\sigma_\xi^2}\left[\xi_i\left\{\pi^*_{(i)J\cdot}+\pi^*_{(i)\cdot R}-1\right\}^2\right. \\ -\xi_i[\pi^*_{(i)J\cdot}(1-\pi^*_{(i)J\cdot})+\pi^*_{(i)\cdot R}(1-\pi^*_{(i)\cdot R})] \\ \left.-\frac{1}{\sigma_\xi}\left\{\pi^*_{(i)J\cdot}+\pi^*_{(i)\cdot R}-1\right\}\right] f_N(\xi_i)d\xi_i & \text{for } j=1,\ldots,J-1; r=R \\ \int_{-\infty}^{\infty}\frac{\xi_i(\pi^*_{(i)J\cdot}\pi^*_{(i)\cdot r})}{4\sigma_\xi^2}\left[\xi_i\left\{\pi^*_{(i)J\cdot}+\pi^*_{(i)\cdot R}-1\right\}^2\right. \\ -\xi_i[\pi^*_{(i)J\cdot}(1-\pi^*_{(i)J\cdot})+\pi^*_{(i)\cdot R}(1-\pi^*_{(i)\cdot R})] \\ \left.-\frac{1}{\sigma_\xi}\left\{\pi^*_{(i)J\cdot}+\pi^*_{(i)\cdot R}-1\right\}\right] f_N(\xi_i)d\xi_i & \text{for } j=J; r=1,\ldots,R-1 \\ \int_{-\infty}^{\infty}\frac{\xi_i(\pi^*_{(i)J\cdot}\pi^*_{(i)\cdot R})}{4\sigma_\xi^2}\left[\xi_i\left\{\pi^*_{(i)J\cdot}+\pi^*_{(i)\cdot R}-2\right\}^2\right. \\ -\xi_i[\pi^*_{(i)J\cdot}(1-\pi^*_{(i)J\cdot})+\pi^*_{(i)\cdot R}(1-\pi^*_{(i)\cdot R})] \\ \left.-\frac{1}{\sigma_\xi}\left\{\pi^*_{(i)J\cdot}+\pi^*_{(i)\cdot R}-2\right\}\right] f_N(\xi_i)d\xi_i & \text{for } j=J; r=R. \end{cases} \tag{5.103}$$

5.4 Familial (Random Effects Based) Bivariate Multinomial Regression Model

For the univariate case, a multinomial regression model was discussed in Chap. 2, more specifically in Sect. 2.2. However, the covariates were considered to be categorical. In this and next sections, also in the next chapter, we consider general covariates which can be continuous, categorical or both. Note that in the absence of covariates, this model to be discussed in this section reduces to the covariates free bivariate multinomial model studied in the last three Sects. 5.1–5.3.

We use similar notations for covariates as in Sect. 2.2. In the present bivariate case, suppose that w_{i1} and w_{i2} are covariate vectors corresponding to y_i and z_i. More specifically, we write

$$w_{i1} = (w'_{iy} : 1 \times p_1, w'_{ic} : 1 \times p_2)' : p \times 1, \; w_{i2} = (w'_{iz} : 1 \times q_1, w'_{ic} : 1 \times p_2)' : q \times 1, \tag{5.104}$$

where w_{iy} and w_{iz} are individual response specific covariates and w_{ic} is a common covariate vector influencing both responses of the ith individual. For example, the so-called WESDR (Wisconsin Epidemiologic Study of Diabetic Retinopathy) data set (see Williamson et al. 1995, for example) contains diabetic categorical retinopathy status of left and right eyes (two response variables) of $K = 996$ individuals along with their associated covariates. This data set did not have any individual response variable specific covariates, but there were seven important common covariates, namely: (1) duration of diabetes (DD), (2) glycosylated hemoglobin level (GHL), (3) diastolic blood pressure (DBP), (4) gender, (5) proteinuria (Pr), (6) dose of insulin per day (DI), and (7) macular edema (ME). Thus, in notation of (5.104), $p_1 = q_1 = 0$, and $p_2 = 7$. Note that these covariates w_{i1} and w_{i2} are considered to be fixed and known. However, as the bivariate categorical responses Y_i and Z_i are collected from the same ith individual, they are likely to be correlated, and it may be reasonable to assume that this bivariate correlation is caused by a common individual latent effect shared by both responses. Thus, conditional on such latent/random effects, we may modify the marginal probabilities given in (5.1) and (5.2) to incorporate the covariates and write these new marginal probabilities conditional on the random effects as

$$P[y_i = y_i^{(j)} | \xi_i^*, w_{i1}] = \pi^*_{(i)j\cdot}(\xi_i, w_{i1}) = \begin{cases} \frac{\exp(\beta_{j0} + \beta'_j w_{i1} + \sigma_\xi \xi_i)}{1 + \sum_{u=1}^{J-1} \exp(\beta_{u0} + \beta'_u w_{i1} + \sigma_\xi \xi_i)} & \text{for } j = 1, \ldots, J-1 \\ \frac{1}{1 + \sum_{u=1}^{J-1} \exp(\beta_{u0} + \beta'_u w_{i1} + \sigma_\xi \xi_i)} & \text{for } j = J, \end{cases} \tag{5.105}$$

and

$$P[z_i = z_i^{(r)} | \xi_i^*, w_{i2}] = \pi^*_{(i)\cdot r}(\xi_i, w_{i2}) = \begin{cases} \frac{\exp(\alpha_{r0} + \alpha'_r w_{i2} + \sigma_\xi \xi_i)}{1 + \sum_{h=1}^{R-1} \exp(\alpha_{h0} + \alpha'_h w_{i2} + \sigma_\xi \xi_i)} & \text{for } r = 1, \ldots, R-1 \\ \frac{1}{1 + \sum_{h=1}^{R-1} \exp(\alpha_{h0} + \alpha'_h w_{i2} + \sigma_\xi \xi_i)} & \text{for } r = R, \end{cases} \tag{5.106}$$

where

$$\beta_j = (\beta_{j1}, \ldots, \beta_{j\ell}, \ldots, \beta_{jp})', \text{and } \alpha_r = (\alpha_{r1}, \ldots, \alpha_{rm}, \ldots, \alpha_{rq})',$$

for $j = 1, \ldots, J-1$, and $r = 1, \ldots, R-1$.

Similar to Sect. 2.1 (from Chap. 2), define

$$\begin{aligned} \beta_j^* &= [\beta_{j0}, \beta'_j]' \\ \theta_1^* &= [\beta_1^{*'}, \ldots, \beta_j^{*'}, \ldots, \beta_{J-1}^{*'}]'; \\ \alpha_r^* &= [\alpha_{r0}, \alpha'_r]' \\ \theta_2^* &= [\alpha_1^{*'}, \ldots, \alpha_r^{*'}, \ldots, \alpha_{R-1}^{*'}]'. \end{aligned} \tag{5.107}$$

Also define

$$\begin{aligned} w^*_{i1} &= [1, w'_{i1}]' \\ w^*_{i2} &= [1, w'_{i2}]'. \end{aligned} \tag{5.108}$$

Using the notations from (5.107) and (5.108), re-express the marginal probabilities conditional on the random effects from (5.105)–(5.106) as

$$P[y_i = y_i^{(j)} | \xi_i^*, w^*_{i1}] = \pi^*_{(i)j\cdot}(\xi_i, w^*_{i1}) = \begin{cases} \frac{\exp(\beta_j^{*\prime} w^*_{i1} + \sigma_\xi \xi_i)}{1+\sum_{u=1}^{J-1}\exp(\beta_u^{*\prime} w^*_{i1} + \sigma_\xi \xi_i)} & \text{for } j = 1, \ldots, J-1 \\ \frac{1}{1+\sum_{u=1}^{J-1}\exp(\beta_u^{*\prime} w^*_{i1} + \sigma_\xi \xi_i)} & \text{for } j = J, \end{cases} \tag{5.109}$$

and

$$P[z_i = z_i^{(r)} | \xi_i^*, w^*_{i2}] = \pi^*_{(i)\cdot r}(\xi_i, w^*_{i2}) = \begin{cases} \frac{\exp(\alpha_r^{*\prime} w^*_{i2} + \sigma_\xi \xi_i)}{1+\sum_{h=1}^{R-1}\exp(\alpha_h^{*\prime} w^*_{i2} + \sigma_\xi \xi_i)} & \text{for } r = 1, \ldots, R-1 \\ \frac{1}{1+\sum_{h=1}^{R-1}\exp(\alpha_h^{*\prime} w^*_{i2} + \sigma_\xi \xi_i)} & \text{for } r = R, \end{cases} \tag{5.110}$$

where w^*_{i1} and w^*_{i2} are fixed and known covariates, whereas $\xi_i \overset{iid}{\sim} N(0,1)$ as in (5.1).

Hence, the (unconditional) marginal and joint probabilities have the formulas

$$\pi_{(i)j\cdot}(w^*_{i1}) = P(y_i = y_i^{(j)}) = \int_{-\infty}^{\infty} \pi^*_{(i)j\cdot}(\xi_i, w^*_{i1}) f_N(\xi_i) d\xi_i; \tag{5.111}$$

$$\pi_{(i)\cdot r}(w^*_{i2}) = P(z_i = z_i^{(r)}) == \int_{-\infty}^{\infty} \pi^*_{(i)\cdot r}(\xi_i, w^*_{i2}) f_N(\xi_i) d\xi_i; \tag{5.112}$$

$$\begin{aligned} \pi_{(i)jr}(w^*_{i1}, w^*_{i2}) &= P[y_i = y_i^{(j)}, z_i = z_i^{(r)}] \\ &= \int_{-\infty}^{\infty} [\pi^*_{(i)j\cdot}(\xi_i, w^*_{i1}) \pi^*_{(i)\cdot r}(\xi_i, w^*_{i2})] f_N(\xi_i) d\xi_i, \end{aligned} \tag{5.113}$$

where $f_N(\xi_i) = \frac{\exp(\frac{-\xi_i^2}{2})}{\sqrt{2\pi}}$. Notice that the integrations in (5.111)–(5.113) for the computation of marginal and joint probabilities may be computed by using the binomial approximation similar to that of (5.48)–(5.50). For example,

$$\begin{aligned} \pi_{(i)j\cdot}(w^*_{i1}) &= \int_{-\infty}^{\infty} \pi^*_{(i)j\cdot}(\xi_i, w^*_{i1}) f_N(\xi_i) d\xi_i \\ &\equiv \begin{cases} \sum_{v_i=0}^{V} [\frac{\exp(\beta_j^{*\prime} w^*_{i1} + \sigma_\xi \xi_i(v_i))}{1+\sum_{u=1}^{J-1}\exp(\beta_u^{*\prime} w^*_{i1} + \sigma_\xi \xi_i(v_i))}] \binom{V}{v_i} (1/2)^{v_i} (1/2)^{V-v_i} & \text{for } j = 1, \ldots, J-1 \\ \sum_{v_i=0}^{V} [\frac{1}{1+\sum_{h=1}^{J-1}\exp(\beta_j^{*\prime} w^*_{i1} + \sigma_\xi \xi_i(v_i))}] \binom{V}{v_i} (1/2)^{v_i} (1/2)^{V-v_i} & \text{for } j = J, \end{cases} \end{aligned} \tag{5.114}$$

where, for $v_i \sim \text{binomial}(V, 1/2)$ with a user's choice large V,

$$\xi_i(v_i) = \frac{v_i - V(1/2)}{\sqrt{V(1/2)(1/2)}}.$$

The parameters of the model (5.111)–(5.113), namely

$$\theta_1^* = (\beta_1^{*\prime}, \ldots, \beta_j^{*\prime}, \ldots, \beta_{J-1}^{*}{}')'; \theta_2^* = (\alpha_1^{*\prime}, \ldots, \alpha_r^{*\prime}, \ldots, \alpha_{R-1}^{*}{}')'; \text{and } \sigma_\xi^2,$$

may be estimated by using the MGQL, JGQL, or ML approach discussed in the last section. In the next section, we, however, demonstrate how one can construct the MGQL estimating equations for these parameters. The formulas for the estimating equations under other two approaches may be obtained similarly.

5.4.1 MGQL Estimation for the Parameters

Using the marginal probabilities from (5.111) and (5.112) we first write

$$\pi_{(i)y}(\theta_1^*, \sigma_\xi, w_{i1}^*) = E[Y_i] = [\pi_{(i)1\cdot}(w_{i1}^*), \ldots, \pi_{(i)j\cdot}(w_{i1}^*), \ldots, \pi_{(i)(J-1)\cdot}(w_{i1}^*)]', \quad (5.115)$$

$$\pi_{(i)z}(\theta_2^*, \sigma_\xi, w_{i2}^*) = E[Z_i] = [\pi_{(i)\cdot 1}(w_{i2}^*), \ldots, \pi_{(i)\cdot r}(w_{i2}^*), \ldots, \pi_{(i)\cdot(R-1)}(w_{i2}^*)]', \quad (5.116)$$

$$\begin{aligned}\text{var}(Y_i) &= \text{diag}[\pi_{(i)1\cdot}(w_{i1}^*), \ldots, \pi_{(i)j\cdot}(w_{i1}^*), \ldots, \pi_{(i)(J-1)\cdot}(w_{i1}^*)] - \pi_{(i)y}(\theta_1^*, \sigma_\xi, w_{i1}^*)\pi_{(i)y}'(\theta_1^*, \sigma_\xi, w_{i1}^*) \\ &= \Sigma_{(i)yy}(\theta_1^*, \sigma_\xi, w_{i1}^*); \quad (5.117) \\ \text{var}(Z_i) &= \text{diag}[\pi_{(i)\cdot 1}(w_{i2}^*), \ldots, \pi_{(i)\cdot r}(w_{i2}^*), \ldots, \pi_{(i)\cdot(R-1)}(w_{i2}^*)] - \pi_{(i)z}(\theta_2^*, \sigma_\xi, w_{i2}^*)\pi_{(i)z}'(\theta_2^*, \sigma_\xi, w_{i2}^*) \\ &= \Sigma_{(i)zz}(\theta_2^*, \sigma_\xi, w_{i2}^*), \quad (5.118)\end{aligned}$$

and

$$\begin{aligned}\text{cov}(Y_i, Z_i') &= \Sigma_{(i)yz}(\theta_1^*, \theta_2^*, \sigma_\xi, w_{i1}^*, w_{i2}^*) \\ &= (\pi_{(i)jr}(\theta_1^*, \theta_2^*, w_{i1}^*, w_{i2}^*)) - \pi_{(i)y}(\theta_1^*, \sigma_\xi, w_{i1}^*)\pi_{(i)z}'(\theta_2^*, \sigma_\xi, w_{i2}^*), \quad (5.119)\end{aligned}$$

where

$$\pi_{(i)jr}(\theta_1^*, \theta_2^*, w_{i1}^*, w_{i2}^*) \equiv \pi_{(i)jr}(w_{i1}^*, w_{i2}^*)$$

is the joint probability with its formula given in (5.113).

Next, use $\psi^* = (\theta_1^{*\prime}, \theta_2^{*\prime})'$ and construct the MGQL for this vector parameter as in the next section.

5.4.1.1 MGQL Estimation for $\psi^* = (\theta_1^{*\prime}, \theta_2^{*\prime})'$

For known σ_ξ^2, we write the MGQL estimating equation for ψ^* as

$$f(\psi^*) = \sum_{i=1}^{K} \frac{\partial(\pi'_{(i)y}(\theta_1^*, \sigma_\xi, w_{i1}^*), \pi'_{(i)z}(\theta_2^*, \sigma_\xi, w_{i2}^*))}{\partial \psi^*}$$

$$\times \Sigma_{(i)11}^{-1}(\psi^*, \sigma_\xi, w_{i1}^*, w_{i2}^*) \begin{pmatrix} y_i - \pi_{(i)y}(\theta_1^*, \sigma_\xi, w_{i1}^*) \\ z_i - \pi_{(i)z}(\theta_2^*, \sigma_\xi, w_{i2}^*) \end{pmatrix} = 0, \quad (5.120)$$

(Sutradhar 2004) where $\Sigma_{(i)11}(\psi^*, \sigma_\xi, w_{i1}^*, w_{i2}^*)$ has the formula given by

$$\Sigma_{(i)11}(\psi^*, \sigma_\xi, w_{i1}^*, w_{i2}^*) = \begin{pmatrix} \Sigma_{(i)yy}(\theta_1^*, \sigma_\xi, w_{i1}^*) & \Sigma_{(i)yz}(\theta_1^*, \theta_2^*, \sigma_\xi, w_{i1}^*, w_{i2}^*) \\ \Sigma'_{(i)yz}(\theta_1^*, \theta_2^*, \sigma_\xi, w_{i1}^*, w_{i2}^*) & \Sigma_{(i)zz}(\theta_2^*, \sigma_\xi, w_{i2}^*) \end{pmatrix}. \quad (5.121)$$

In (5.120), the first order derivative matrix is computed as follows.

Computation of the derivative $\frac{\partial(\pi'_{(i)y}(\theta_1^*, \sigma_\xi, w_{i1}^*), \pi'_{(i)z}(\theta_2^*, \sigma_\xi, w_{i2}^*))}{\partial \psi^*}$: $((J-1)(p+1) + (R-1)(q+1)) \times (J+R-2)$

For the purpose, we first re-express the marginal probabilities in (5.109)–(5.110) as functions of $\theta_1^*, \theta_2^*, \sigma_\xi$, as follows.

$$\pi_{(i)j\cdot}^*(\xi_i, w_{i1}^*) = \begin{cases} \frac{\exp(\theta_1^{*\prime} x_{ij}^* + \sigma_\xi \xi_i)}{1 + \sum_{u=1}^{J-1} \exp(\theta_1^{*\prime} x_{iu}^* + \sigma_\xi \xi_i)} & \text{for } j = 1, \ldots, J-1 \\ \frac{1}{1 + \sum_{u=1}^{J-1} \exp(\theta_1^{*\prime} x_{iu}^* + \sigma_\xi \xi_i)} & \text{for } j = J, \end{cases} \quad (5.122)$$

with

$$x_{ij}^* = \begin{pmatrix} 01_{(j-1)(p+1)} \\ w_{i1}^* \\ 01_{(J-1-j)(p+1)} \end{pmatrix},$$

for $j = 1, \ldots, J-1$; and

$$\pi_{(i)\cdot r}^*(\xi_i, w_{i2}^*) = \begin{cases} \frac{\exp(\theta_2^{*\prime} \tilde{x}_{ir} + \sigma_\xi \xi_i)}{1 + \sum_{h=1}^{R-1} \exp(\theta_2^{*\prime} \tilde{x}_{ih} + \sigma_\xi \xi_i)} & \text{for } r = 1, \ldots, R-1 \\ \frac{1}{1 + \sum_{h=1}^{R-1} \exp(\theta_2^{*\prime} \tilde{x}_{ih} + \sigma_\xi \xi_i)} & \text{for } r = R, \end{cases} \quad (5.123)$$

with

$$\tilde{x}_{ir} = \begin{pmatrix} 01_{(r-1)(q+1)} \\ w_{i2}^* \\ 01_{(R-1-r)(q+1)} \end{pmatrix},$$

for $r = 1, \ldots, R-1$.

Because $\psi^* = (\theta_1^{*\prime}, \theta_2^{*\prime})'$, the desired derivative matrix may be computed as follows:

$$\frac{\partial \pi'_{(i)y}(\theta_1^*, \sigma_\xi, w_{i1}^*)}{\partial \theta_1^*} = \left[\frac{\partial \pi_{(i)1\cdot}}{\partial \theta_1^*}, \ldots, \frac{\partial \pi_{(i)j\cdot}}{\partial \theta_1^*}, \ldots, \frac{\partial \pi_{(i)(J-1)\cdot}}{\partial \theta_1^*}\right], \tag{5.124}$$

where, for $j = 1, \ldots, J-1$,

$$\begin{aligned} \frac{\partial \pi_{(i)j\cdot}}{\partial \theta_1^*} &= \int_{-\infty}^{\infty} \frac{\partial \pi^*_{(i)j\cdot}(\xi_i, w_{i1}^*)}{\partial \theta_1^*} f_N(\xi_i) d\xi_i \\ &= \int_{-\infty}^{\infty} \pi^*_{(i)j\cdot}(\xi_i, w_{i1}^*)[x_{ij}^* - \sum_{g=1}^{J-1} x_{ig}^* \pi^*_{(i)g\cdot}(\xi_i, w_{i1}^*)] f_N(\xi_i) d\xi_i, \end{aligned} \tag{5.125}$$

where $x_{ij}^{*\prime} = [01'_{(j-1)(p+1)}, w_{i1}^{*\prime}, 01'_{(J-1-j)(p+1)}]$ is the $1 \times (J-1)(p+1)$ row vector as defined in (5.122). For convenience, we re-express the $(J-1)(p+1) \times 1$ vector in (5.125) as

$$\begin{aligned} \frac{\partial \pi_{(i)j\cdot}}{\partial \theta_1^*} &= \int_{-\infty}^{\infty} \begin{pmatrix} -\pi^*_{(i)j\cdot}(\xi_i, w_{i1}^*)\pi^*_{(i)1\cdot}(\xi_i, w_{i1}^*) w_{i1}^* \\ \vdots \\ -\pi^*_{(i)j\cdot}(\xi_i, w_{i1}^*)\pi^*_{(i)(j-1)\cdot}(\xi_i, w_{i1}^*) w_{i1}^* \\ [\pi^*_{(i)j\cdot}(\xi_i, w_{i1}^*)(1 - \pi^*_{(i)j\cdot}(\xi_i, w_{i1}^*))] w_{i1}^* \\ -\pi^*_{(i)j\cdot}(\xi_i, w_{i1}^*)\pi^*_{(i)(j+1)\cdot}(\xi_i, w_{i1}^*) w_{i1}^* \\ \vdots \\ -\pi^*_{(i)j\cdot}(\xi_i, w_{i1}^*)\pi^*_{(i)(J-1)\cdot}(\xi_i, w_{i1}^*) w_{i1}^* \end{pmatrix} f_N(\xi_i) d\xi_i \\ &= \int_{-\infty}^{\infty} \left[\{\pi^*_{(i)j\cdot}(\xi_i, w_{i1}^*) 1_{J-1} - \pi^*_{(i)j\cdot}(\xi_i, w_{i1}^*) \pi_{(i)y}(\theta_1^*, \sigma_\xi, w_{i1}^*)\}\right. \\ &\qquad \left. \otimes w_{i1}^*\right] f_N(\xi_i) d\xi_i, \end{aligned} \tag{5.126}$$

and write the formula for the derivative as

$$\frac{\partial \pi'_{(i)y}(\theta_1^*, \sigma_\xi, w_{i1}^*)}{\partial \theta_1^*} = \int_{-\infty}^{\infty} [\Sigma_{(i)yy}(\theta_1^*, \sigma_\xi, w_{i1}^*) \otimes w_{i1}^*] f_N(\xi_i) d\xi_i, \tag{5.127}$$

where $\Sigma_{(i)yy}(\theta_1^*, \sigma_\xi, w_{i1}^*)$ is the $(J-1) \times (J-1)$ covariance matrix of y_i as given by (5.117). By calculations similar to that of (5.127), one obtains

$$\frac{\partial \pi'_{(i)z}(\theta_2^*, \sigma_\xi, w_{i2}^*)}{\partial \theta_2^*} = \int_{-\infty}^{\infty} [\Sigma_{(i)zz}(\theta_2^*, \sigma_\xi, w_{i2}^*) \otimes w_{i2}^*] f_N(\xi_i) d\xi_i, \tag{5.128}$$

where $\Sigma_{(i)zz}(\theta_2^*, \sigma_\xi, w_{i2}^*)$ is the $(R-1) \times (R-1)$ covariance matrix of z_i as given by (5.118). Consequently, we obtain

$$\frac{\partial(\pi'_{(i)y}(\theta_1^*, \sigma_\xi, w_{i1}^*), \pi'_{(i)z}(\theta_2^*, \sigma_\xi, w_{i2}^*))}{\partial \psi^*}$$
$$= \int_{-\infty}^{\infty} \begin{pmatrix} \Sigma_{(i)yy}(\theta_1^*, \sigma_\xi, w_{i1}^*) \otimes w_{i1}^* & 0 \\ 0 & \Sigma_{(i)zz}(\theta_2^*, \sigma_\xi, w_{i2}^*) \otimes w_{i2}^* \end{pmatrix} f_N(\xi_i) d\xi_i. \quad (5.129)$$

Remark that applying the aforementioned formulas for the mean vectors [(5.115)–(5.116)], associated covariance matrix (5.121), and the derivative matrix (5.129), one may now solve the MGQL estimating equation (5.120) for $\psi^* = (\theta_1^{*\prime}, \theta_2^{*\prime})'$ by using the iterative equation

$$\hat{\psi}^*(m+1) = \hat{\psi}^*(m) + \left[\left\{ \sum_{i=1}^{K} \frac{\partial(\pi'_{(i)y}(\theta_1^*, \sigma_\xi, w_{i1}^*), \pi'_{(i)z}(\theta_2^*, \sigma_\xi, w_{i2}^*))}{\partial \psi^*} \Sigma_{(i)11}^{-1}(\psi^*, \sigma_\xi, w_{i1}^*, w_{i2}^*) \right.\right.$$
$$\left. \times \frac{\partial(\pi'_{(i)y}(\theta_1^*, \sigma_\xi, w_{i1}^*), \pi'_{(i)z}(\theta_2^*, \sigma_\xi, w_{i2}^*))'}{\partial \psi^{*\prime}} \right\}^{-1} \left\{ \sum_{i=1}^{K} \frac{\partial(\pi'_{(i)y}(\theta_1^*, \sigma_\xi, w_{i1}^*), \pi'_{(i)z}(\theta_2^*, \sigma_\xi, w_{i2}^*))}{\partial \psi^*} \right.$$
$$\left.\left. \times\ \Sigma_{(i)11}^{-1}(\psi^*, \sigma_\xi, w_{i1}^*, w_{i2}^*) \begin{pmatrix} y_i - \pi_{(i)y}(\theta_1^*, \sigma_\xi, w_{i1}^*) \\ z_i - \pi_{(i)z}(\theta_2^*, \sigma_\xi, w_{i2}^*) \end{pmatrix} \right\} \right] |_{\psi^* = \hat{\psi}^*(m)}. \quad (5.130)$$

5.4.1.2 MGQL Estimation for σ_ξ^2

Similar to Sect. 5.3.1.1.2, we exploit the pair-wise products of the bivariate responses to estimate this random effects variance component parameter σ_ξ^2. Let

$$g_i = (y_{i1}z_{i1}, \ldots, y_{ij}z_{ir}, \ldots, y_{i,J-1}z_{i,R-1})' \quad (5.131)$$

which has the mean

$$E[G_i] = (\pi_{(i)11}(w_{i1}^*, w_{i2}^*), \ldots, \pi_{(i)jr}(w_{i1}^*, w_{i2}^*), \ldots, \pi_{(i),J-1,R-1}(w_{i1}^*, w_{i2}^*))'$$
$$= \pi_{(i)yz}(\psi^*, \sigma_\xi, w_{i1}^*, w_{i2}^*), \quad (5.132)$$

where, by (5.113),

$$\pi_{(i)jr}(w_{i1}^*, w_{i2}^*) = \int_{-\infty}^{\infty} [\pi_{(i)j\cdot}^*(\xi_i, w_{i1}^*) \pi_{(i)\cdot r}^*(\xi_i, w_{i2}^*)] f_N(\xi_i) d\xi_i,$$

for $j = 1, \ldots, J; r = 1, \ldots, R$.

Next following (5.60), one writes

$$\begin{aligned}\mathrm{cov}(G_i) &= \mathrm{diag}[\pi_{(i)11}(w^*_{i1},w^*_{i2}),\ldots,\pi_{(i)jr}(w^*_{i1},w^*_{i2}),\ldots,\pi_{(i)J-1,R-1}(w^*_{i1},w^*_{i2})] \\ &- \pi_{(i)yz}(\psi^*,\sigma_\xi,w^*_{i1},w^*_{i2})\pi'_{(i)yz}(\psi^*,\sigma_\xi,w^*_{i1},w^*_{i2}) \\ &= \Sigma_{(i)22}(\psi^*,\sigma_\xi,w^*_{i1},w^*_{i2}), \text{ (say)}. \end{aligned} \tag{5.133}$$

Furthermore, we compute the gradient function, that is, the derivative of $E[G_i]$ with respect to σ^2_ξ as

$$\begin{aligned}\frac{\partial E[G_i]}{\partial \sigma^2_\xi} &= \frac{\partial \pi_{(i)yz}(\psi^*,\sigma_\xi,w^*_{i1},w^*_{i2})}{\partial \sigma^2_\xi} \\ &= (\frac{\partial \pi_{(i)11}(w^*_{i1},w^*_{i2})}{\partial \sigma^2_\xi},\ldots,\frac{\partial \pi_{(i)jr}(w^*_{i1},w^*_{i2})}{\partial \sigma^2_\xi},\ldots,\frac{\partial \pi_{(i)J-1,R-1}(w^*_{i1},w^*_{i2})}{\partial \sigma^2_\xi})', \end{aligned} \tag{5.134}$$

where, for example,

$$\begin{aligned}\frac{\partial \pi_{(i)jr}(w^*_{i1},w^*_{i2})}{\partial \sigma^2_\xi} &= \int_{-\infty}^{\infty} \frac{\partial\left[\pi^*_{(i)j\cdot}(\xi_i,w^*_{i1})\pi^*_{(i)\cdot r}(\xi_i,w^*_{i2})\right]}{\partial \sigma^2_\xi} f_N(\xi_i)d\xi_i \\ &= \frac{1}{2\sigma_\xi}\int_{-\infty}^{\infty} \xi_i\left[\pi^*_{(i)j\cdot}(\xi_i,w^*_{i1})\pi^*_{(i)\cdot r}(\xi_i,w^*_{i2})\right] \\ &\times \left[\pi^*_{(i)J\cdot}(\xi_i,w^*_{i1})+\pi^*_{(i)\cdot R}(\xi_i,w^*_{i2})\right] f_N(\xi_i)d\xi_i, \end{aligned} \tag{5.135}$$

for all $j=1,\ldots,J-1;\ r=1,\ldots,R-1$.

By using (5.131)–(5.134), one may now construct the MGQL estimating equation for σ^2_ξ as

$$\sum_{i=1}^{K}\frac{\partial \pi'_{(i)yz}(\psi^*,\sigma_\xi,w^*_{i1},w^*_{i2})}{\partial \sigma^2_\xi}\Sigma^{-1}_{(i)22}(\psi^*,\sigma_\xi,w^*_{i1},w^*_{i2})[g_i-\pi_{(i)yz}(\psi^*,\sigma_\xi,w^*_{i1},w^*_{i2})]=0, \tag{5.136}$$

which, for known $\psi^*=(\theta^{*\prime}_1,\theta^{*\prime}_2)'$ may be solved iteratively by using the formula

$$\begin{aligned}&\hat{\sigma}^2_\xi(m+1)=\hat{\sigma}^2_\xi(m) \\ &+\left[\left\{\sum_{i=1}^{K}\frac{\partial \pi'_{(i)yz}(\psi^*,\sigma_\xi,w^*_{i1},w^*_{i2})}{\partial \sigma^2_\xi}\Sigma^{-1}_{(i)22}(\psi^*,\sigma_\xi,w^*_{i1},w^*_{i2})\frac{\partial \pi_{(i)yz}(\psi^*,\sigma_\xi,w^*_{i1},w^*_{i2})}{\partial \sigma^2_\xi}\right\}^{-1}\right. \\ &\times\left.\left\{\sum_{i=1}^{K}\frac{\partial \pi'_{(i)yz}(\psi^*,\sigma_\xi,w^*_{i1},w^*_{i2})}{\partial \sigma^2_\xi}\Sigma^{-1}_{(i)22}(\psi^*,\sigma_\xi,w^*_{i1},w^*_{i2})[g_i-\pi_{(i)yz}(\psi^*,\sigma_\xi,w^*_{i1},w^*_{i2})]\right\}\right]_{|\sigma^2_\xi=\hat{\sigma}^2_\xi(m)}. \end{aligned} \tag{5.137}$$

5.5 Bivariate Normal Linear Conditional Multinomial Probability Model

In Sect. 5.4, the correlation between two multinomial variables is modeled in a natural way through a random effect shared by these variables. Recently in an unpublished Ph.D. thesis, Sun (2013) (see also Sun and Sutradhar 2014) has used a bivariate normal type linear conditional multinomial probability (BNLCMP) model to explain the correlations between two multinomial variables. This model is simpler than the random effects based model discussed in the last section. However, the ranges for the correlations under such a linear conditional probability model may be narrow because of the restriction that the conditional probability of one variable is linear in other variable. We discuss this simpler model in the following section.

5.5.1 *Bivariate Normal Type Model and its Properties*

In this approach, unlike in random effects approach (5.105)–(5.110), we assume that Y_i and Z_i marginally follow the multinomial distributions with marginal probabilities as

$$P[y_i = y_i^{(j)}|w_{i1}] = \pi_{(i)j\cdot}(w_{i1}) = \begin{cases} \frac{\exp(\beta_{j0}+\beta_j' w_{i1})}{1+\sum_{u=1}^{J-1}\exp(\beta_{u0}+\beta_u' w_{i1})} & \text{for } j = 1,\ldots,J-1 \\ \frac{1}{1+\sum_{u=1}^{J-1}\exp(\beta_{u0}+\beta_u' w_{i1})} & \text{for } j = J, \end{cases} \tag{5.138}$$

and

$$P[z_i = z_i^{(r)}|w_{i2}] = \pi_{(i)\cdot r}(w_{i2}) = \begin{cases} \frac{\exp(\alpha_{r0}+\alpha_r' w_{i2})}{1+\sum_{h=1}^{R-1}\exp(\alpha_{h0}+\alpha_h' w_{i2})} & \text{for } r = 1,\ldots,R-1 \\ \frac{1}{1+\sum_{h=1}^{R-1}\exp(\alpha_{h0}+\alpha_h' w_{i2})} & \text{for } r = R, \end{cases} \tag{5.139}$$

where

$$\beta_j = (\beta_{j1},\ldots,\beta_{j\ell},\ldots,\beta_{jp})', \text{and } \alpha_r = (\alpha_{r1},\ldots,\alpha_{rm},\ldots,\alpha_{rq})',$$

for $j = 1,\ldots,J-1$, and $r = 1,\ldots,R-1$. Equivalently, writing

$$\begin{aligned} \beta_j^* &= [\beta_{j0},\beta_j']',\ w_{i1}^* = [1,w_{i1}']' \\ \alpha_r^* &= [\alpha_{r0},\alpha_r']',\ w_{i2}^* = [1,w_{i2}']', \end{aligned} \tag{5.140}$$

these marginal probabilities in (5.138)–(5.139) may be re-expressed as

$$P[y_i = y_i^{(j)}|w_{i1}^*] = \pi_{(i)j\cdot}(w_{i1}^*) = \begin{cases} \frac{\exp(\beta_j^{*\prime} w_{i1}^*)}{1+\sum_{u=1}^{J-1}\exp(\beta_u^{*\prime} w_{i1}^*)} & \text{for } j = 1,\ldots,J-1 \\ \frac{1}{1+\sum_{u=1}^{J-1}\exp(\beta_u^{*\prime} w_{i1}^*)} & \text{for } j = J, \end{cases} \quad (5.141)$$

and

$$P[z_i = z_i^{(r)}|w_{i2}^*] = \pi_{(i)\cdot r}(w_{i2}^*) = \begin{cases} \frac{\exp(\alpha_r^{*\prime} w_{i2}^*)}{1+\sum_{h=1}^{R-1}\exp(\alpha_h^{*\prime} w_{i2}^*)} & \text{for } r = 1,\ldots,R-1 \\ \frac{1}{1+\sum_{h=1}^{R-1}\exp(\alpha_h^{*\prime} w_{i2}^*)} & \text{for } r = R, \end{cases} \quad (5.142)$$

respectively. Note that these marginal probabilities in (5.140)–(5.141) are quite different and simpler than those random effects based marginal (unconditional) probabilities given in (5.111)–(5.112).

Now to develop a correlation model for $\{y_i, z_i\}$, Sun and Sutradhar (2014) have used a conditional regression approach. More specifically, to write a conditional regression function of y_i given z_i, these authors have used the aforementioned simpler marginal probabilities but assume a bivariate normal type correlation structure between y_i and z_i. Note that if y_i and z_i were bivariate normal responses, one would then relate them using the conditional mean of y_i given z_i, that is, through

$$E[Y_i|Z_i = z_i] = \mu_y + \Sigma_{y|z}^{-1}(z_i - \mu_z), \quad (5.143)$$

where μ_y and μ_z are the marginal mean vectors corresponding to y_i and z_i and $\Sigma_{y|z}$ is the conditional covariance matrix of y_i given z_i. However, as y_i and z_i in the present setup are two multinomial responses, we follow the linear form (4.20) [see Sect. 4.3] used in Chap. 4, for example, to model the conditional probabilities, i.e., $Pr(y_i|z_i)$, and write

$$\lambda_{iy|z}^{(j)}(r; w_{i1}^*, w_{i2}^*) = Pr(y_i = y_i^{(j)}|z_i = z_i^{(r)})$$
$$= \begin{cases} \pi_{(i)j\cdot}(w_{i1}^*) + \sum_{h=1}^{R-1}\rho_{jh}(z_{ih}^{(r)} - \pi_{(i)\cdot h}(w_{i2}^*)), & j = 1,\ldots,J-1;\ r = 1,\ldots,R, \\ 1 - \sum_{j=1}^{J-1}\lambda_{iy|z}^{(j)}(r), & j = J; r = 1,\ldots,R, \end{cases} \quad (5.144)$$

where $z_{ih}^{(r)}$ is the hth ($h = 1,\ldots,R-1$) component of $z_i^{(r)}$, with $z_{ih}^{(r)} = 1$ if $h = r$, and 0 otherwise; ρ_{jh} is referred to as the dependence parameter relating $y_i^{(j)}$ with $z_i^{(h)}$. Note that this conditional model (5.144) may not be symmetric especially when $J \neq R$. However, this does not cause any problems in inferences as we will use all unconditional product responses (see also Sect. 5.5.2.2) to estimate the dependence parameters.

5.5.1.1 Means, Variance, and Covariances of Marginal Variables

Using the marginal probabilities from (5.141) and (5.142), the mean vectors and covariance matrices for each of y_i and z_i are written as

$$\pi_{(i)y}(\theta_1^*, w_{i1}^*) = E[Y_i] = [\pi_{(i)1\cdot}(w_{i1}^*), \ldots, \pi_{(i)j\cdot}(w_{i1}^*), \ldots, \pi_{(i)(J-1)\cdot}(w_{i1}^*)]', \quad (5.145)$$

$$\pi_{(i)z}(\theta_2^*, w_{i2}^*) = E[Z_i] = [\pi_{(i)\cdot 1}(w_{i2}^*), \ldots, \pi_{(i)\cdot r}(w_{i2}^*), \ldots, \pi_{(i)\cdot (R-1)}(w_{i2}^*)]', \quad (5.146)$$

$$\begin{aligned} \mathrm{var}(Y_i) &= \mathrm{diag}[\pi_{(i)1\cdot}(w_{i1}^*), \ldots, \pi_{(i)j\cdot}(w_{i1}^*), \ldots, \pi_{(i)(J-1)\cdot}(w_{i1}^*)] - \pi_{(i)y}(\theta_1^*, w_{i1}^*)\pi'_{(i)y}(\theta_1^*, w_{i1}^*) \\ &= \Sigma_{(i)yy}(\theta_1^*, w_{i1}^*); \quad (5.147) \\ \mathrm{var}(Z_i) &= \mathrm{diag}[\pi_{(i)\cdot 1}(w_{i2}^*), \ldots, \pi_{(i)\cdot r}(w_{i2}^*), \ldots, \pi_{(i)\cdot (R-1)}(w_{i2}^*)] - \pi_{(i)z}(\theta_2^*, w_{i2}^*)\pi'_{(i)z}(\theta_2^*, w_{i2}^*) \\ &= \Sigma_{(i)zz}(\theta_2^*, w_{i2}^*), \quad (5.148) \end{aligned}$$

where

$$\theta_1^* = [\beta_1^{*\prime}, \ldots, \beta_j^{*\prime}, \ldots, \beta_{J-1}^{*\prime}]', \; \theta_2^* = [\alpha_1^{*\prime}, \ldots, \alpha_r^{*\prime}, \ldots, \alpha_{R-1}^{*\prime}]'.$$

Note that these formulas appear to be the same as in (5.111)–(5.118), except that the marginal probabilities, that is,

$$\pi_{(i)j\cdot}(w_{i1}^*), \text{ and } \pi_{(i)\cdot r}(w_{i2}^*),$$

are now given by (5.141) and (5.142), and they are free of σ_ξ.

5.5.1.2 Covariances and Correlations Between y_i and z_i

Using the proposed conditional probability from (5.144), one may write the joint probability $\pi_{(i)jr}(w_{i1}^*, w_{i2}^*)$ as

$$\begin{aligned} \pi_{(i)jr}(w_{i1}^*, w_{i2}^*) &= Pr[y_i = y_i^{(j)}, z_i = z_i^{(r)}] \\ &= Pr(y_i = y_i^{(j)} | z_i = z_i^{(r)}) Pr(z_i = z_i^{(r)}) = \lambda_{iy|z}^{(j)}(r; w_{i1}^*, w_{i2}^*)\pi_{(i)\cdot r}(w_{i2}^*) \\ &= \left[\pi_{(i)j\cdot}(w_{i1}^*) + \sum_{h=1}^{R-1} \rho_{jh}(z_{ih}^{(r)} - \pi_{(i)\cdot h}(w_{i2}^*))\right] \pi_{(i)\cdot r}(w_{i2}^*), \quad (5.149) \end{aligned}$$

yielding the covariance between Y_{ij} and Z_{ir} as

$$\begin{aligned} cov(Y_{ij}, Z_{ir}) &= E(Y_{ij}Z_{ir}) - E(Y_{ij})E(Z_{ir}) = \pi_{(i)jr}(w_{i1}^*, w_{i2}^*) - \pi_{(i)j\cdot}(w_{i1}^*)\pi_{(i)\cdot r}(w_{i2}^*) \\ &= \pi_{(i)\cdot r}(w_{i2}^*) \left[\sum_{h=1}^{R-1} \rho_{jh}(z_{ih}^{(r)} - \pi_{(i)\cdot h}(w_{i2}^*))\right]. \quad (5.150) \end{aligned}$$

Following (5.150), after some algebras, we can write the $R-1$ covariance quantities in

$$\mathrm{cov}(Z_i, Y_{ij}) = [\mathrm{cov}(Y_{ij}, Z_{i1}), \ldots, \mathrm{cov}(Y_{ij}, Z_{ir}), \ldots, \mathrm{cov}(Y_{ij}, Z_{i,R-1})]'$$

in a matrix form as

$$\begin{aligned}
\mathrm{cov}(Z_i, Y_{ij}) &= \begin{pmatrix} \pi_{(i)\cdot 1}(w_{i2}^*)\left[\sum_{h=1}^{R-1} \rho_{jh}(z_{ih}^{(1)} - \pi_{(i)\cdot h}(w_{i2}^*))\right] \\ \vdots \\ \pi_{(i)\cdot r}(w_{i2}^*)\left[\sum_{h=1}^{R-1} \rho_{jh}(z_{ih}^{(r)} - \pi_{(i)\cdot h}(w_{i2}^*))\right] \\ \vdots \\ \pi_{(i)\cdot (R-1)}(w_{i2}^*)\left[\sum_{h=1}^{R-1} \rho_{jh}(z_{ih}^{(R-1)} - \pi_{(i)\cdot h}(w_{i2}^*))\right] \end{pmatrix} \\
&= \begin{pmatrix} \pi_{(i)\cdot 1}(w_{i2}^*)\left[(1, 0'_{R-2}) - \pi'_{(i)z}(\theta_2^*, w_{i2}^*)\right]\rho_j \\ \vdots \\ \pi_{(i)\cdot r}(w_{i2}^*)\left[(0'_{r-1}, 1, 0'_{R-1-r}) - \pi'_{(i)z}(\theta_2^*, w_{i2}^*)\right]\rho_j \\ \vdots \\ \pi_{(i)\cdot r}(w_{i2}^*)\left[(0'_{R-2}, 1) - \pi'_{(i)z}(\theta_2^*, w_{i2}^*)\right]\rho_j \end{pmatrix} \\
&= \mathrm{var}(Z_i)\rho_j, \qquad (5.151)
\end{aligned}$$

where

$$\begin{aligned}
\rho_j &= [\rho_{j1}, \ldots, \rho_{jh}, \ldots, \rho_{j,R-1}]', \text{ and} \\
\pi_{(i)z}(\theta_2^*, w_{i2}^*) &= [\pi_{(i)\cdot 1}(w_{i2}^*), \ldots, \pi_{(i)\cdot r}(w_{i2}^*), \ldots, \pi_{(i)\cdot (R-1)}(w_{i2}^*)]',
\end{aligned}$$

by (5.146), and the $(R-1) \times (R-1)$ covariance matrix $\mathrm{var}(Z_i)$ is given in (5.148). Consequently, for every $j = 1, \ldots, J-1$, one obtains

$$\begin{aligned}
\mathrm{cov}(Z_i, Y_i') &= [\mathrm{var}(Z_i)\rho_1, \ldots, \mathrm{var}(Z_i)\rho_j, \ldots, \mathrm{var}(Z_i)\rho_{J-1}] \\
&= \mathrm{var}(Z_i)\rho_M \\
&= \Sigma_{(i)yz}(\theta_2^*, w_{i2}^*, \rho_M), \qquad (5.152)
\end{aligned}$$

where $\rho_M = [\rho_1, \ldots, \rho_j, \ldots, \rho_{J-1}]$ is the $(R-1) \times (J-1)$ matrix of dependence parameters. Next, by (5.152), one may compute the correlation matrix between the pair-wise components of y_i and z_i, as

$$\begin{aligned}\text{corr}(Z_i, Y_i') &= [\text{var}(Z_i)]^{-\frac{1}{2}} \text{var}(Z_i)\rho_M[\text{var}(Y_i)]^{-\frac{1}{2}} \\ &= [\text{var}(Z_i)]^{\frac{1}{2}} \rho_M[\text{var}(Y_i)]^{-\frac{1}{2}} \\ &= C_{iM}, \text{ (say).}\end{aligned} \tag{5.153}$$

Note however that these correlations given by (5.153) among the components of Z_i and Y_i for the ith individual may not have full range from -1 to 1, because of the fact that ρ_{jh} parameters in (5.144) are restricted by the constraint that $\lambda^{(j)}_{iy|z}(r; w^*_{i1}, w^*_{i2})$ has to lie between 0 and 1. This is however not a major problem as this type of linear conditional model was demonstrated to accommodate wider ranges for correlation index parameters for the binary data as compared to other competitive models (see Sutradhar 2011, Table 7.1). But it would be important to estimate these index parameters ρ_{jr} in ρ_M matrix in (5.152) consistently, so that regression parameters can be estimated consistently and as efficiently as possible. This estimation issue is discussed in the next section.

5.5.2 *Estimation of Parameters of the Proposed Correlation Model*

Recall that

$$\theta^*_1 = [\beta^{*\prime}_1, \ldots, \beta^{*\prime}_j, \ldots, \beta^{*}_{J-1}{}']', \; \theta^*_2 = [\alpha^{*\prime}_1, \ldots, \alpha^{*\prime}_r, \ldots, \alpha^{*}_{R-1}{}']'$$

are referred to as the regression parameters involved in the marginal probabilities (5.141)–(5.142), that is,

$$\begin{aligned}P[y_i = y_i^{(j)}|w^*_{i1}] = \pi_{(i)j\cdot}(w^*_{i1}) &= \begin{cases}\frac{\exp(\beta^{*\prime}_j w^*_{i1})}{1+\sum_{u=1}^{J-1}\exp(\beta^{*\prime}_u w^*_{i1})} & \text{for } j = 1, \ldots, J-1 \\ \frac{1}{1+\sum_{u=1}^{J-1}\exp(\beta^{*\prime}_u w^*_{i1})} & \text{for } j = J\end{cases} \\ &= \begin{cases}\frac{\exp(\theta^{*\prime}_1 x^*_{ij})}{1+\sum_{u=1}^{J-1}\exp(\theta^{*\prime}_1 x^*_{iu})} & \text{for } j = 1, \ldots, J-1 \\ \frac{1}{1+\sum_{u=1}^{J-1}\exp(\theta^{*\prime}_1 x^*_{iu})} & \text{for } j = J,\end{cases}\end{aligned} \tag{5.154}$$

with

$$x^*_{ij} = \begin{pmatrix} 01_{(j-1)(p+1)} \\ w^*_{i1} \\ 01_{(J-1-j)(p+1)} \end{pmatrix},$$

for $j = 1, \ldots, J-1$; and

$$P[z_i = z_i^{(r)}|w_{i2}^*] = \pi_{(i)\cdot r}(w_{i2}^*) = \begin{cases} \frac{\exp(\alpha_r^{*\prime} w_{i2}^*)}{1+\sum_{h=1}^{R-1}\exp(\alpha_h^{*\prime} w_{i2}^*)} & \text{for } r = 1,\ldots,R-1 \\ \frac{1}{1+\sum_{h=1}^{R-1}\exp(\alpha_h^{*\prime} w_{i2}^*)} & \text{for } r = R \end{cases}$$

$$= \begin{cases} \frac{\exp(\theta_2^{*\prime}\tilde{x}_{ir})}{1+\sum_{h=1}^{R-1}\exp(\theta_2^{*\prime}\tilde{x}_{ih})} & \text{for } r = 1,\ldots,R-1 \\ \frac{1}{1+\sum_{h=1}^{R-1}\exp(\theta_2^{*\prime}\tilde{x}_{ih})} & \text{for } r = R, \end{cases} \quad (5.155)$$

with

$$\tilde{x}_{ir} = \begin{pmatrix} 01_{(r-1)(q+1)} \\ w_{i2}^* \\ 01_{(R-1-r)(q+1)} \end{pmatrix},$$

for $r = 1,\ldots,R-1$, and the components in

$$\rho^* = (\rho_{11}, \rho_{12}, \ldots, \rho_{jr}, \ldots, \rho_{J-1,R-1})',$$

are variables dependence parameters involved in the conditional probabilities (5.144), or equivalently in the joint probabilities (5.149), that is,

$$\pi_{(i)jr}(w_{i1}^*, w_{i2}^*) = Pr[y_i = y_i^{(j)}, z_i = z_i^{(r)}]$$

$$= \left[\pi_{(i)j\cdot}(w_{i1}^*) + \sum_{h=1}^{R-1}\rho_{jh}(z_{ih}^{(r)} - \pi_{(i)\cdot h}(w_{i2}^*))\right]\pi_{(i)\cdot r}(w_{i2}^*)$$

$$= \left[\pi_{(i)j\cdot}(w_{i1}^*) + \left\{(0'_{r-1}, 1, 0'_{R-1-r}) - \pi'_{(i)z}(\theta_2^*, w_{i2}^*)\right\}\rho_j\right]\pi_{(i)\cdot r}(w_{i2}^*). \quad (5.156)$$

For convenience, we write

$$\psi = (\theta_1^{*\prime}, \theta_2^{*\prime})', \text{ and}$$
$$\phi = (\psi', \rho^{*\prime})', \quad (5.157)$$

and estimate the parameters in ϕ by using the so-called GQL estimation approach. More specifically, we use two GQL approaches, first, an MGQL (marginal GQL) approach, and then a joint GQL (JGQL) approach.

5.5.2.1 MGQL Approach

In this approach, for known $\rho_M \equiv \rho^*$, we exploit the first order moments to estimate $\psi = (\theta_1^{*\prime}, \theta_2^{*\prime})'$ parameter at the first stage. This we do by using the GQL approach. Once an estimate of $\psi = (\theta_1^{*\prime}, \theta_2^{*\prime})'$ is available, we use it as a known value of ψ in the moment estimating equation for ρ_M which is developed exploiting both first and second order moments.

5.5.2.1.1 MGQL Estimation for ψ

The MGQL estimating equation for $\psi = (\theta_1^{*\prime}, \theta_2^{*\prime})'$ is given by

$$f(\psi) = \sum_{i=1}^{K} \frac{\partial(\pi'_{(i)y}(\theta_1^*, w_{i1}^*), \pi'_{(i)z}(\theta_2^*, w_{i2}^*))}{\partial \psi} \Sigma_{i11}^{-1}(\psi, \rho_M) \begin{pmatrix} y_i - \pi_{(i)y}(\theta_1^*, w_{i1}^*) \\ z_i - \pi_{(i)z}(\theta_2^*, w_{i2}^*) \end{pmatrix} = 0, \tag{5.158}$$

where, by (5.147)–(5.148) and (5.152), $\Sigma_{i11}(\psi, \rho_M)$ has the form

$$\begin{aligned} \Sigma_{i11}(\psi, \rho_M) &= \mathrm{cov}\begin{pmatrix} Y_i \\ Z_i \end{pmatrix} \\ &= \begin{pmatrix} \mathrm{var}(Y_i) & \mathrm{cov}(Y_i, Z_i') \\ \mathrm{cov}(Z_i, Y_i') & \mathrm{var}(Z_i) \end{pmatrix} \\ &= \begin{pmatrix} \Sigma_{(i)yy}(\theta_1^*, w_{i1}^*) & \Sigma'_{(i)yz}(\theta_2^*, w_{i2}^*, \rho_M) \\ \Sigma_{(i)yz}(\theta_2^*, w_{i2}^*, \rho_M) & \Sigma_{(i)zz}(\theta_2^*, w_{i2}^*) \end{pmatrix}. \end{aligned} \tag{5.159}$$

Computation of the Derivative $\frac{\partial(\pi'_{(i)y}(\theta_1^*, w_{i1}^*), \pi'_{(i)z}(\theta_2^*, w_{i2}^*))}{\partial \psi}$**:**
Because $\psi = (\theta_1^{*\prime}, \theta_2^{*\prime})'$, the desired derivative matrix may be computed as follows:

$$\frac{\partial \pi'_{(i)y}(\theta_1^*, w_{i1}^*)}{\partial \theta_1^*} = \left[\frac{\partial \pi_{(i)1\cdot}}{\partial \theta_1^*}, \ldots, \frac{\partial \pi_{(i)j\cdot}}{\partial \theta_1^*}, \ldots, \frac{\partial \pi_{(i)(J-1)\cdot}}{\partial \theta_1^*}\right], \tag{5.160}$$

where, for $j = 1, \ldots, J-1$, by (5.154),

$$\frac{\partial \pi_{(i)j\cdot}}{\partial \theta_1^*} = \pi_{(i)j\cdot}(w_{i1}^*)[x_{ij}^* - \sum_{g=1}^{J-1} x_{ig}^* \pi_{(i)g\cdot}(w_{i1}^*)], \tag{5.161}$$

where $x_{ij}^{*\prime} = [01'_{(j-1)(p+1)}, w_{i1}^{*\prime}, 01'_{(J-1-j)(p+1)}]$ is the $1 \times (J-1)(p+1)$ row vector as defined in (5.154). For convenience, we re-express the $(J-1)(p+1) \times 1$ vector in (5.161) as

$$\begin{aligned} \frac{\partial \pi_{(i)j\cdot}}{\partial \theta_1^*} &= \begin{pmatrix} -\pi_{(i)j\cdot}(w_{i1}^*)\pi_{(i)1\cdot}(w_{i1}^*)w_{i1}^* \\ \vdots \\ -\pi_{(i)j\cdot}(w_{i1}^*)\pi_{(i)(j-1)\cdot}(w_{i1}^*)w_{i1}^* \\ [\pi_{(i)j\cdot}(w_{i1}^*)(1 - \pi_{(i)j\cdot}(w_{i1}^*))]w_{i1}^* \\ -\pi_{(i)j\cdot}(w_{i1}^*)\pi_{(i)(j+1)\cdot}(w_{i1}^*)w_{i1}^* \\ \vdots \\ -\pi_{(i)j\cdot}(w_{i1}^*)\pi_{(i)(J-1)\cdot}(w_{i1}^*)w_{i1}^* \end{pmatrix} \\ &= [\{\pi_{(i)j\cdot}(w_{i1}^*)1_{J-1} - \pi_{(i)j\cdot}(w_{i1}^*)\pi_{(i)y}(\theta_1^*, w_{i1}^*)\} \\ &\quad \otimes w_{i1}^*], \end{aligned} \tag{5.162}$$

and write the formula for the derivative as

$$\frac{\partial \pi'_{(i)y}(\theta_1^*, w_{i1}^*)}{\partial \theta_1^*} = [\Sigma_{(i)yy}(\theta_1^*, w_{i1}^*) \otimes w_{i1}^*], \tag{5.163}$$

where $\Sigma_{(i)yy}(\theta_1^*, w_{i1}^*)$ is the $(J-1) \times (J-1)$ covariance matrix of y_i as given by (5.147). By calculations similar to that of (5.163), one obtains

$$\frac{\partial \pi'_{(i)z}(\theta_2^*, w_{i2}^*)}{\partial \theta_2^*} = [\Sigma_{(i)zz}(\theta_2^*, w_{i2}^*) \otimes w_{i2}^*], \tag{5.164}$$

where $\Sigma_{(i)zz}(\theta_2^*, w_{i2}^*)$ is the $(R-1) \times (R-1)$ covariance matrix of z_i as given by (5.148). Consequently, we obtain

$$\frac{\partial(\pi'_{(i)y}(\theta_1^*, w_{i1}^*), \pi'_{(i)z}(\theta_2^*, w_{i2}^*))}{\partial \psi} = \begin{pmatrix} \Sigma_{(i)yy}(\theta_1^*, w_{i1}^*) \otimes w_{i1}^* & 0 \\ 0 & \Sigma_{(i)zz}(\theta_2^*, w_{i2}^*) \otimes w_{i2}^* \end{pmatrix}. \tag{5.165}$$

For known ρ_M, one may then solve the MGQL estimating equation (5.158) for ψ by applying the iterative equation

$$\hat{\psi}(m+1) = \hat{\psi}(m) + \left[\left\{ \sum_{i=1}^{K} \frac{\partial(\pi'_{(i)y}(\theta_1^*, w_{i1}^*), \pi'_{(i)z}(\theta_2^*, w_{i2}^*))}{\partial \psi} \Sigma_{(i)11}^{-1}(\psi, w_{i1}^*, w_{i2}^*) \right.\right.$$
$$\left. \times \frac{\partial(\pi'_{(i)y}(\theta_1^*, w_{i1}^*), \pi'_{(i)z}(\theta_2^*, w_{i2}^*))'}{\partial \psi'} \right\}^{-1} \left\{ \sum_{i=1}^{K} \frac{\partial(\pi'_{(i)y}(\theta_1^*, w_{i1}^*), \pi'_{(i)z}(\theta_2^*, w_{i2}^*))}{\partial \psi} \right.$$
$$\left.\left. \times \Sigma_{(i)11}^{-1}(\psi, w_{i1}^*, w_{i2}^*) \begin{pmatrix} y_i - \pi_{(i)y}(\theta_1^*, w_{i1}^*) \\ z_i - \pi_{(i)z}(\theta_2^*, w_{i2}^*) \end{pmatrix} \right\} \right] \Big|_{\psi = \hat{\psi}(m)}. \tag{5.166}$$

Furthermore, it follows that the MGQL estimator, say $\hat{\psi}_{MGQL}$, obtained from (5.166) has the asymptotic variance given by

$$\text{limit}_{K \to \infty} \text{var}[\hat{\psi}_{MGQL}] = \left\{ \sum_{i=1}^{K} \frac{\partial(\pi'_{(i)y}(\theta_1^*, w_{i1}^*), \pi'_{(i)z}(\theta_2^*, w_{i2}^*))}{\partial \psi} \Sigma_{(i)11}^{-1}(\psi, w_{i1}^*, w_{i2}^*) \right.$$
$$\left. \times \frac{\partial(\pi'_{(i)y}(\theta_1^*, w_{i1}^*), \pi'_{(i)z}(\theta_2^*, w_{i2}^*))'}{\partial \psi'} \right\}^{-1}. \tag{5.167}$$

5.5.2.1.2 MM Estimation for ρ_M

At the second stage we estimate ρ^* or equivalently ρ_M by using the well-known method of moments (MM). Because

$$\mathrm{cov}(Z_i, Y_i') = [\mathrm{var}(Z_i)]\,\rho_M. \tag{5.168}$$

by (5.152), and because this relationship holds for all $i = 1,\ldots,K$, by taking averages on both sides, we obtain the method of moments (MM) estimator of ρ_M as

$$\hat{\rho}_{M,MM} = \left[\frac{1}{K}\sum_{i=1}^{K}\hat{\mathrm{var}}(Z_i)\right]^{-1}\left[\frac{1}{K}\sum_{i=1}^{K}\hat{\mathrm{cov}}(Z_i, Y_i')\right], \tag{5.169}$$

where $\hat{\mathrm{cov}}(Z_{ir}, Y_{ij})$ in $\hat{\mathrm{cov}}(Z_i, Y_i')$, for example, has the formula, $\hat{\mathrm{cov}}(Z_{ir}, Y_{ij}) = (z_{ir} - \hat{\pi}_{(i)\cdot r})(y_{ij} - \hat{\pi}_{(i)j\cdot})$.

5.5.2.2 JGQL Approach

In the last section, the regression effects $\psi = (\theta_1^{*\prime}, \theta_2^{*\prime})'$ were estimated by using the GQL approach, whereas the bivariate response dependence parameters in ρ_M were estimated by the method of moments. In this section we estimate all these parameters jointly by using the GQL approach only. Thus, the JGQL estimating equation for

$$\phi = (\psi', \rho^{*\prime})'$$

will be a generalization of the GQL estimating equation for ψ given by (5.158). For the purpose, because the joint cell probabilities $\pi_{(i)jr}(w_{i1}^*, w_{i2}^*)$ given in (5.156), i.e.,

$$\begin{aligned}
\pi_{(i)jr}(w_{i1}^*, w_{i2}^*) &= Pr[y_i = y_i^{(j)}, z_i = z_i^{(r)}] \\
&= \left[\pi_{(i)j\cdot}(w_{i1}^*) + \sum_{h=1}^{R-1}\rho_{jh}(z_{ih}^{(r)} - \pi_{(i)\cdot h}(w_{i2}^*))\right]\pi_{(i)\cdot r}(w_{i2}^*) \\
&= \left[\pi_{(i)j\cdot}(w_{i1}^*) + \left\{(0_{r-1}', 1, 0_{R-1-r}') - \pi_{(i)z}'(\theta_2^*, w_{i2}^*)\right\}\rho_j\right]\pi_{(i)\cdot r}(w_{i2}^*),
\end{aligned}$$

contain the parameters $\psi = (\theta_1^{*\prime}, \theta_2^{*\prime})'$ as well as

$$\begin{aligned}
\rho^* &= (\rho_1', \ldots, \rho_j', \ldots, \rho_{J-1}')' \\
&= (\rho_{11}, \ldots, \rho_{j1}, \ldots, \rho_{jr}, \ldots, \rho_{j,R-1}, \ldots, \rho_{J-1,R-1})',
\end{aligned}$$

we consider a statistic g_i with joint cell observations, namely

$$g_i = (y_{i1}z_{i1}, \ldots, y_{ij}z_{ir}, \ldots, y_{i,J-1}z_{i,R-1})', \tag{5.170}$$

for the estimation of ρ^*. This statistic g_i has the mean

$$E[G_i] = (\pi_{(i)11}, \ldots, \pi_{(i)jr}, \ldots, \pi_{(i)(J-1)(R-1)})' = \pi_{(i)yz}(\psi, \rho^*), \text{ (say).} \qquad (5.171)$$

As an extension of (5.158), one may now construct the JGQL estimating equation for $\phi = (\psi', \rho^{*\prime})'$ as

$$f(\phi) = \sum_{i=1}^{K} \frac{\partial(\pi'_{(i)y}(\theta_1^*, w_{i1}^*), \pi'_{(i)z}(\theta_2^*, w_{i2}^*), \pi'_{iyz}(\psi, \rho^*))}{\partial \phi}$$
$$\times \left[\text{cov}\begin{pmatrix} Y_i \\ Z_i \\ G_i \end{pmatrix}\right]^{-1} \begin{pmatrix} y_i - \pi_{(i)y}(\theta_1^*, w_{i1}^*) \\ z_i - \pi_{(i)z}(\theta_2^*, w_{i2}^*) \\ g_i - \pi_{iyz}(\psi, \rho^*) \end{pmatrix} = 0, \qquad (5.172)$$

which may be solved iteratively to obtain the JGQL estimates for all elements in ϕ, including ρ^*. The construction of the covariance matrix of $(Y_i', Z_i', G_i')'$ is outlined below.

5.5.2.2.1 Construction of the Covariance Matrix of $(Y_i', Z_i', G_i')'$ for the JGQL Approach

In (5.172), the covariance matrix of $(Y_i', Z_i', G_i')'$ has the form

$$\text{cov}\begin{pmatrix} Y_i \\ Z_i \\ G_i \end{pmatrix} = \begin{pmatrix} \Sigma_{i11}(\psi, \rho^*) & \Sigma_{i12}(\psi, \rho^*) \\ & \Sigma_{i22}(\psi, \rho^*) \end{pmatrix} = \Sigma_i(\psi, \rho^*) \ (say), \qquad (5.173)$$

where

$$\Sigma_{i11}(\psi, \rho^*) = \text{cov}\begin{pmatrix} Y_i \\ Z_i \end{pmatrix},$$

is already computed in (5.159), ρ^* being equivalent to ρ_M, with ρ_M as the $(R-1) \times (J-1)$ matrix given by $\rho_M = (\rho_1, \ldots, \rho_j, \ldots, \rho_{J-1})$, where $\rho_j = (\rho_{j1}, \ldots, \rho_{jr}, \ldots, \rho_{j,R-1})'$.

The computation for the remaining covariance matrices in (5.173) is done as follows. More specifically,

$$\begin{aligned} \Sigma_{i22}(\psi, \rho^*) &= \text{cov}(G_i) = \text{diag}(\pi_{iyz}(\psi, \rho^*)) - \pi_{iyz}(\psi, \rho^*)\pi'_{iyz}(\psi, \rho^*) \\ &= \text{diag}[\pi_{(i)11}, \ldots, \pi_{(i)jr}, \ldots, \pi_{(i)(J-1)(R-1)}] - \pi_{iyz}(\psi, \rho^*)\pi'_{iyz}(\psi, \rho^*), \end{aligned}$$

where $\pi_{iyz}(\psi,\rho^*) = [\pi_{(i)11},\ldots,\pi_{(i)jr},\ldots,\pi_{(i)(J-1)(R-1)}]'$ as in (5.171), with $\pi_{(i)jr}$ as given in (5.156). Next,

$$\Sigma_{i12}(\psi,\rho^*) = \begin{pmatrix} \mathrm{cov}(Y_i,G_i') \\ \mathrm{cov}(Z_i,G_i') \end{pmatrix}, \tag{5.174}$$

where

$$\mathrm{cov}(Y_i,G_i') = [\mathrm{cov}(y_{ih},y_{ij}z_{ir})] : (J-1)\times(J-1)(R-1) \tag{5.175}$$

with

$$\mathrm{cov}(y_{ih},y_{ij}z_{ir}) = \begin{cases} \pi_{(i)jr}(1-\pi_{(i)j\cdot}) & h=j, \\ -\pi_{(i)jr}\pi_{(i)j\cdot} & h\neq j, \end{cases} \tag{5.176}$$

and

$$\mathrm{cov}(Z_i,G_i') = [\mathrm{cov}(z_{iq},y_{ij}z_{ir})] : (R-1)\times(R-1)(J-1) \tag{5.177}$$

with

$$\mathrm{cov}(z_{iq},y_{ij}z_{ir}) = \begin{cases} \pi_{(i)jr}(1-\pi_{(i)\cdot r}) & q=r, \\ -\pi_{(i)jr}\pi_{(i)\cdot r} & q\neq r. \end{cases} \tag{5.178}$$

5.5.2.2.2 Computation of the Derivative Matrix $\frac{\partial(\pi'_{(i)y}(\theta_1^*,w_{i1}^*),\pi'_{(i)z}(\theta_2^*,w_{i2}^*),\pi'_{iyz}(\psi,\rho^*))}{\partial\phi}$

Because $\phi = (\psi',\rho^{*\prime})'$ with $\psi = (\theta_1^{*\prime},\theta_2^{*\prime})'$, and the derivative

$$\frac{\partial(\pi'_{(i)y}(\theta_1^*,w_{i1}^*),\pi'_{(i)z}(\theta_2^*,w_{i2}^*))}{\partial\psi}$$

was computed in (5.165), it is convenient to re-express the desired derivative matrix as

$$\frac{\partial(\pi'_{(i)y}(\theta_1^*,w_{i1}^*),\pi'_{(i)z}(\theta_2^*,w_{i2}^*),\pi'_{iyz}(\psi,\rho^*))}{\partial\phi}$$
$$= \begin{pmatrix} \frac{\partial(\pi'_{(i)y}(\theta_1^*,w_{i1}^*),\pi'_{(i)z}(\theta_2^*,w_{i2}^*))}{\partial\psi} & \frac{\partial(\pi'_{iyz}(\psi,\rho^*))}{\partial\psi} \\ \frac{\partial(\pi'_{(i)y}(\theta_1^*,w_{i1}^*),\pi'_{(i)z}(\theta_2^*,w_{i2}^*))}{\partial\rho^*} & \frac{\partial(\pi'_{iyz}(\psi,\rho^*))}{\partial\rho^*} \end{pmatrix}, \tag{5.179}$$

where

$$\frac{\partial(\pi'_{(i)y}(\theta_1^*, w_{i1}^*), \pi'_{(i)z}(\theta_2^*, w_{i2}^*))}{\partial \rho^*} = 0 : (J-1)(R-1) \times \{(J-1)+(R-1)\}$$

because the components in $\pi'_{(i)y}(\theta_1^*, w_{i1}^*)$ and $\pi'_{(i)z}(\theta_2^*, w_{i2}^*)$, that is, the marginal probabilities are free from ρ^*. The remaining two derivatives in (5.179) are computed as follows:

$$\frac{\partial(\pi'_{iyz}(\psi, \rho^*))}{\partial \psi} = \left(\frac{\partial \pi_{(i)11}}{\partial \psi} \cdots \frac{\partial \pi_{(i)jr}}{\partial \psi} \cdots \frac{\partial \pi_{(i)(J-1)(R-1)}}{\partial \psi} \right), \tag{5.180}$$

where by (5.156), for all $j = 1, \ldots, J-1$; $r = 1, \ldots, R-1$, one writes

$$\begin{aligned} \frac{\partial \pi_{(i)jr}}{\partial \psi} &= \frac{\partial \left[\left(\pi_{(i)j\cdot}(w_{i1}^*) + \left\{ (0'_{r-1}, 1, 0'_{R-1-r}) - \pi'_{(i)z}(\theta_2^*, w_{i2}^*) \right\} \rho_j \right) \pi_{(i)\cdot r}(w_{i2}^*) \right]}{\partial \psi} \\ &= \left[\left(\frac{\partial \pi_{(i)j\cdot}(w_{i1}^*)}{\partial \psi} + \left\{ (0'_{r-1}, 1, 0'_{R-1-r}) - \frac{\partial \pi'_{(i)z}(\theta_2^*, w_{i2}^*)}{\partial \psi} \right\} \rho_j \right) \pi_{(i)\cdot r}(w_{i2}^*) \right] \\ &+ \left[\left(\pi_{(i)j\cdot}(w_{i1}^*) + \left\{ (0'_{r-1}, 1, 0'_{R-1-r}) - \pi'_{(i)z}(\theta_2^*, w_{i2}^*) \right\} \rho_j \right) \frac{\partial \pi_{(i)\cdot r}(w_{i2}^*)}{\partial \psi} \right], \end{aligned} \tag{5.181}$$

with

$$\frac{\partial \pi_{(i)j\cdot}}{\partial \psi} = \begin{pmatrix} [\{\pi_{(i)j\cdot}(w_{i1}^*) 1_{J-1} - \pi_{(i)j\cdot}(w_{i1}^*) \pi_{(i)y}(\theta_1^*, w_{i1}^*)\} \otimes w_{i1}^*] \\ 0 \end{pmatrix} \tag{5.182}$$

$$\frac{\partial \pi_{(i)\cdot r}}{\partial \psi} = \begin{pmatrix} 0 \\ [\{\pi_{(i)\cdot r}(w_{i2}^*) 1_{R-1} - \pi_{(i)\cdot r}(w_{i2}^*) \pi_{(i)z}(\theta_2^*, w_{i2}^*)\} \otimes w_{i2}^*] \end{pmatrix} \tag{5.183}$$

$$\frac{\partial \pi'_{(i)z}(\theta_2^*, w_{i2}^*)}{\partial \psi} = \begin{pmatrix} 0 \\ \Sigma_{(i)zz}(\theta_2^*, w_{i2}^*) \otimes w_{i2}^* \end{pmatrix}, \tag{5.184}$$

by (5.162) and (5.165).

Next

$$\frac{\partial(\pi'_{iyz}(\psi, \rho^*))}{\partial \rho^*} = \left(\frac{\partial \pi_{(i)11}}{\partial \rho^*} \cdots \frac{\partial \pi_{(i)jr}}{\partial \rho^*} \cdots \frac{\partial \pi_{(i)(J-1)(R-1)}}{\partial \rho^*} \right), \tag{5.185}$$

where

$$\frac{\partial \pi_{(i)jr}}{\partial \rho^*} = \frac{\partial \left[\left(\pi_{(i)j\cdot}(w_{i1}^*) + \left\{ (0'_{r-1}, 1, 0'_{R-1-r}) - \pi'_{(i)z}(\theta_2^*, w_{i2}^*) \right\} \rho_j \right) \pi_{(i)\cdot r}(w_{i2}^*) \right]}{\partial \rho^*}. \tag{5.186}$$

Now because

$$\rho^* = [\rho_1', \ldots, \rho_j', \ldots, \rho_{J-1}']',$$

the derivative in (5.186) has the formula

$$\frac{\partial \pi_{(i)jr}}{\partial \rho^*} = \begin{pmatrix} 01_{(R-1)(j-1)} \\ -\pi_{(i)\cdot r}(w_{i2}^*)\pi_{(i)z}(\theta_2^*, w_{i2}^*) \\ 01_{(R-1)(J-1-j)} \end{pmatrix}, \tag{5.187}$$

for all $j = 1, \ldots, J-1$; $r = 1, \ldots, R-1$.

5.5.2.2.3 JGQL Estimate and Variance

By using the formulas for the covariance matrix given by (5.173) and the derivative matrix from the last section, one then solves the JGQL estimating equation (5.172) for ϕ by applying the iterative equation

$$\begin{aligned}
\hat{\phi}(m+1) &= \hat{\phi}(m) + \left[\left[\sum_{i=1}^{K} \left\{\frac{\partial(\pi_{(i)y}'(\theta_1^*, w_{i1}^*), \pi_{(i)z}'(\theta_2^*, w_{i2}^*), \pi_{iyz}'(\psi, \rho^*))}{\partial \phi}\right\} \Sigma_i^{-1}(\psi, \rho^*)\right.\right. \\
&\times \left.\left\{\frac{\partial(\pi_{(i)y}'(\theta_1^*, w_{i1}^*), \pi_{(i)z}'(\theta_2^*, w_{i2}^*), \pi_{iyz}'(\psi, \rho^*))'}{\partial \phi'}\right\}\right]^{-1} \\
&\times \left[\sum_{i=1}^{K} \frac{\partial(\pi_{(i)y}'(\theta_1^*, w_{i1}^*), \pi_{(i)z}'(\theta_2^*, w_{i2}^*), \pi_{iyz}'(\psi, \rho^*))}{\partial \phi} \Sigma_i^{-1}(\psi, \rho^*)\right. \\
&\times \left.\left.\begin{pmatrix} y_i - \pi_{(i)y}(\theta_1^*, w_{i1}^*) \\ z_i - \pi_{(i)z}(\theta_2^*, w_{i2}^*) \\ g_i - \pi_{iyz}(\psi, \rho^*) \end{pmatrix}\right]\right]_{\phi = \hat{\phi}(m)}.
\end{aligned} \tag{5.188}$$

Let $\text{var}[\hat{\phi}_{JGQL}]$ be the estimate obtained from (5.188). It then follows that this estimate has the asymptotic variance given by

$$\begin{aligned}
\text{limit}_{K\to\infty}\text{var}[\hat{\phi}_{JGQL}] &= \left[\sum_{i=1}^{K} \left\{\frac{\partial(\pi_{(i)y}'(\theta_1^*, w_{i1}^*), \pi_{(i)z}'(\theta_2^*, w_{i2}^*), \pi_{iyz}'(\psi, \rho^*))}{\partial \phi}\right\} \Sigma_i^{-1}(\psi, \rho^*)\right. \\
&\times \left.\left\{\frac{\partial(\pi_{(i)y}'(\theta_1^*, w_{i1}^*), \pi_{(i)z}'(\theta_2^*, w_{i2}^*), \pi_{iyz}'(\psi, \rho^*))'}{\partial \phi'}\right\}\right]^{-1}.
\end{aligned} \tag{5.189}$$

5.5.3 Fitting BNLCMP Model to a Diabetic Retinopathy Data: An Illustration

In this section, we illustrate an application of the bivariate multinomial model described by (5.138)–(5.139) and (5.144), under Sect. 5.5.1, by reanalyzing the so-called WESDR data, which was analyzed earlier by Williamson et al. (1995), for example. As far as the inference techniques are concerned, we apply both MGQL and JGQL approaches discussed in Sects. 5.5.2.1 and 5.5.2.2, respectively. Note that this illustration is also available in Sun and Sutradhar (2014). We now explain the WESDR data set in brief as follows. This data set contains diabetic retinopathy status on a ten-point interval scale for left and right eyes of 996 independent patients, along with information on various associated covariates. Williamson et al. (1995) have considered four categories, namely None, Mild, Moderate, and Proliferative, for the DR status for each eye. There were 743 subjects with complete response and covariate data. Some of the important covariates are: (1) duration of diabetes (DD), (2) glycosylated hemoglobin level (GHL), (3) diastolic blood pressure (DBP), (4) gender, (5) proteinuria (Pr), (6) dose of insulin per day (DI), and (7) macular edema (ME). Note that these covariates are not eye specific. That is, these covariates are common for both left and right eyes. Let $w_i = (w_{i1}, \ldots, w_{ip})'$ be the $p-$dimensional common (to both eyes) covariate for the ith individual. Also, in this example, the number of categories for DR status of two eyes would be the same. That is, $J = R$. Thus, one has to adjust the marginal probabilities in (5.138) and (5.139) as

$$P[y_i = y_i^{(j)}|w_i] = \pi_{(i)j\cdot}(w_i) = \begin{cases} \frac{\exp(\beta_{j0}+\theta_j' w_i)}{1+\sum_{u=1}^{J-1}\exp(\beta_{u0}+\theta_u' w_i)} & \text{for } j = 1,\ldots,J-1 \\ \frac{1}{1+\sum_{u=1}^{J-1}\exp(\beta_{u0}+\theta_u' w_i)} & \text{for } j = J, \end{cases} \tag{5.190}$$

and

$$P[z_i = z_i^{(r)}|w_i] = \pi_{(i)\cdot r}(w_i) = \begin{cases} \frac{\exp(\alpha_{r0}+\theta_r' w_i)}{1+\sum_{h=1}^{R-1}\exp(\alpha_{h0}+\theta_h' w_i)} & \text{for } r = 1,\ldots,R-1 \\ \frac{1}{1+\sum_{h=1}^{R-1}\exp(\alpha_{h0}+\theta_h' w_i)} & \text{for } r = R, \end{cases} \tag{5.191}$$

where for $j = r$ under $J = R$,

$$\theta_j = (\theta_{j1}, \ldots, \theta_{j\ell}, \ldots, \theta_{jp})',$$

which is the same for both y and z. Equivalently, writing

$$\begin{aligned} \beta_j^* &= [\beta_{j0}, \theta_j']', \\ \alpha_r^* &= [\alpha_{r0}, \theta_r']', \\ w_i^* &= [1, w_i']', \end{aligned} \tag{5.192}$$

one still can use the notation

$$\theta_1^* = [\beta_1^{*\prime}, \ldots, \beta_j^{*\prime}, \ldots, \beta_{J-1}^{*\prime}]', \; \theta_2^* = [\alpha_1^{*\prime}, \ldots, \alpha_r^{*\prime}, \ldots, \alpha_{R-1}^{*\prime}]'$$

as in the last section (see (5.147)–(5.148)), but there are fewer parameters now because $\theta_j : p \times 1$ is common to both β_j^* and α_r^* for all $j = r = 1, \ldots, J-1$. This common covariate situation would make the conditional probability (5.144) simpler, which now is given by

$$\lambda_{iy|z}^{(j)}(r; w_i^*) = Pr(y_i = y_i^{(j)} | z_i = z_i^{(r)})$$

$$= \begin{cases} \pi_{(i)j\cdot}(w_i^*) + \Sigma_{h=1}^{R-1} \rho_{jh}(z_{ih}^{(r)} - \pi_{(i)\cdot h}(w_i^*)), \; j = 1, \ldots, J-1; \; r = 1, \ldots, R, \\ 1 - \Sigma_{j=1}^{J-1} \lambda_{iy|z}^{(j)}(r), j = J; r = 1, \ldots, R. \end{cases} \quad (5.193)$$

To better understand the data, in Sect. 5.5.3.1, for simplicity, we first use two categories for each variable and fit such a bivariate binary model by computing the correlation index and regression parameters. This bivariate binary analysis is followed by a bivariate trinomial model fitting in Sect. 5.5.3.2.

As far as the dependence parameters $\{\rho_{jr}\}$ are concerned, for the binary case there is one parameter, namely ρ_{11}. For the trinomial case, because $J = K = 3$, there will be four dependence parameters, namely $\{\rho_{jr}\}$ for $j = 1, 2$ and $r = 1, 2$. These are interpreted as the left eye category j (for y) versus right eye category r (for z) dependence parameter.

5.5.3.1 Diabetic Retinopathy Data Analysis Using Bivariate Binary ($J = 2$, $R = 2$) Model

In this section, for simplicity, we collapsed the four categories of left and eye diabetic retinopathy (DR) status in Williamson et al. (1995) into two categories for each of the bivariate responses. More specifically, these two categories are 'presence' and 'absence' of DR. The DR responses in the bivariate binary format is shown in Table 5.1.

Table 5.1 Bivariate binary model based counts for left and right eyes diabetic retinopathy status

right eye \ left eye	Y=1 (presence of DR)	Y=0 (absence of DR)	Total
Z=1 (presence of DR)	424	31	455
Z=0 (absence of DR)	39	249	288
Total	463	280	743

As far as the covariates are concerned, we denote the seven covariates as follows. First, we categorize duration of diabetes (DD) into three categories, to do so we use two dummy covariates w_{i11} and w_{i12} defined as follows:

$$(w_{i11}, w_{i12}) = \begin{cases} (1,0), \ DD \ < 5 \ years \\ (0,0), \ DD \ between \ 5 \ and \ 10 \ years \\ (0,1), \ DD \ > 10 \ years. \end{cases}$$

The other six covariates are denoted as:

$$w_{i2} = \frac{GHL_i - \overline{GHL}}{se(GHL)}, \ w_{i3} = \begin{cases} 0, \ DBP \ < 80 \\ 1, \ DBP \geq 80, \end{cases} \ w_{i4} = \begin{cases} 0, \ male \\ 1, \ female, \end{cases}$$

$$. \ w_{i5} = \begin{cases} 0, \ Pr \ absence \\ 1, \ Pr \ presence, \end{cases} \ w_{i6} = \begin{cases} 0, \ DI \leq 1 \\ 1, \ DI \equiv 2, \end{cases} \ w_{i7} = \begin{cases} 0, \ ME \ absence \\ 1, \ ME \ presence. \end{cases}$$

The effects of the above seven covariates are denoted by

$$\theta_1 \equiv \theta = (\theta_{11}, \theta_{12}, \theta_2, \theta_3, \theta_4, \theta_5, \theta_6, \theta_7)'$$

on the binary response variables y_i and z_i.

The bivariate binary response counts from Table 5.1 and the above covariates are now used to fit the following marginal and correlation models:

$$\pi_{(i)y} = Pr(y_i = 1) = \frac{\exp(\beta_{10} + w_i'\theta)}{1 + \exp(\beta_{10} + w_i'\theta)},$$

$$\pi_{(i)z} = Pr(z_i = 1) = \frac{\exp(\alpha_{10} + w_i'\theta)}{1 + \exp(\alpha_{10} + w_i'\theta)},$$

$$\text{and } \lambda^{(1)}_{iy|z} = Pr(y_i = 1|z_i, w_i) = \pi_{(i)y} + \rho_{11}(z_i - \pi_{(i)z}). \tag{5.194}$$

These models are special cases of the marginal multinomial models (5.190)–(5.191) and the multinomial correlation model (5.193), where β_{10} $(\beta_{20} = 0)$ represents the category effect for the left eye and similarly, α_{10} $(\alpha_{20} = 0)$ represents the category effect for the right eye, and ρ_{11} represents the dependence of left eye DR on the right eye DR. Note that the bivariate binary model produces the correlation between left and right eye DR as

$$\rho_{(i)yz} = corr(y_i, z_i) = \frac{\pi_{(i)11} - \pi_{(i)z}\pi_{(i)y}}{\sqrt{\pi_{(i)y}(1 - \pi_{(i)y})\pi_{(i)z}(1 - \pi_{(i)z})}}$$

$$= \rho_{11}\sqrt{\frac{\pi_{(i)z}(1 - \pi_{(i)z})}{\pi_{(i)y}(1 - \pi_{(i)y})}}, \tag{5.195}$$

Table 5.2 The joint GQL (JGQL) and MGQL estimates for the regression effects and the left eye category $j = 1$ (for y) versus right eye category $k = 1$ (for z) dependence $(C11D)$ parameter $\{\rho_{kj}, j = 1; k = 1\}$, along with their estimated standard errors (ESE), under the normal linear conditional bivariate binary probability model for the diabetic retinopathy data

Approach	JGQL		MGQL	
Parameter (Effect of)	Estimate	ESE	Estimate	ESE
α_{10}	−0.317	0.197	−0.320	0.201
β_{10}	−0.215	0.197	−0.238	0.200
θ_{11} (DD low)	−2.040	0.274	−2.119	0.287
θ_{12} (DD high)	2.235	0.206	2.238	0.210
θ_2 (GHL)	0.387	0.093	0.417	0.095
θ_3 (DBP)	0.573	0.189	0.554	0.193
θ_4 (Gender)	−0.249	0.183	−0.230	0.187
θ_5 (Pr)	0.527	0.321	0.510	0.327
θ_6 (DI)	0.003	0.184	0.018	0.187
θ_7 (ME)	2.064	1.043	2.603	1.378
ρ_{11} (C11D)	0.637	0.039	0.636	–

where $\pi_{(i)11} = Pr(y_i = 1, z_i = 1) = Pr(z_i = 1)P(y_i = 1|z_i = 1) = \pi_{(i)z}\lambda^{(1)}_{iy|z} = \pi_{(i)z}[\pi_{(i)y} + \rho_{11}(1 - \pi_{(i)z})]$.

The MGQL estimates for the regression effects (θ) of the bivariate binary model (5.194) are computed by (5.166), along with their standard errors computed by (5.167). The MM estimate for ρ_{11} is computed by (5.169). Next, the JGQL estimates for both regression effects (θ) and dependence parameter (ρ) along with their standard errors are computed by using (5.188) and (5.189). These estimates for the parameters of bivariate binary model are given in Table 5.2.

Now by using the model parameter estimates given in Table 5.2, we can calculate the correlation ρ_{iyz} for each $i = 1, \ldots, 743$. This we do by using the MGQL estimates. As far as the correlation index parameter is concerned, it was found to be $\hat{\rho}_{11,JGQL} = 0.637$ $(\hat{\rho}_{11,MM} = 0.636)$ implying that right eye retinopathy status is highly dependent on the retinopathy status of left eye. This high dependence appears to reflect well the correlation indicated by the observations in Table 5.1. We also have computed the summary statistics for the distribution of $\rho_{(i)yz}$ (5.195) for $i = 1, \ldots, 743$. It was found that most correlations cluster around 0.61 which is far from zero correlation, whereas the correlations for some individuals may be larger than 0.61 and in some cases they can reach a high value such as 0.64. To be precise, the minimum of $\rho_{(i)yz}$ was found to be 0.611, and the maximum is 0.641, with average of $\rho_{(i)yz}$ given by $\bar{\rho}_{yz} = 0.617$. Thus, the present model helps to understand the correlation between the left and right eye retinopathy status.

The results from Table 5.2 show that the JGQL estimates are very close to the MGQL estimates. However, when ESEs (estimated standard errors) are compared, it is clear that the ESEs of the JGQL estimates are smaller than the corresponding MGQL estimates, which is expected because unlike the MGQL estimating equation, the JGQL estimating equation is fully standardized for all parameters. We now interpret the estimates. The results of the table show that the propensity of diabetic retinopathy (probability of having diabetic retinopathy problem) tends to increase with longer DD, higher GHL, higher DBP, male gender, presence of Pr, more DI per day, and presence of ME. Note that the estimates of effects of DD and ME are found to deviate from zero clearly, indicating that these two covariates are important risk factors of diabetic retinopathy problem. To be specific, (1) the marginal parameter estimates $\hat{\alpha}_{10,JGQL} = -0.317$ and $\hat{\beta}_{10,JGQL} = -0.215$ indicate that when other covariates are fixed, an individual has small probabilities to develop left and right eye retinopathy problem. Next, (2) because DD was coded as $(0,0)$ for duration between 5 and 10 years, the large positive value of $\hat{\theta}_{12,JGQL} = 2.235$ and negative value of $\hat{\theta}_{11,JGQL} = -2.040$ show that as DD increases, the probability of an individual to have retinopathy problem increases. (3) The positive values of $\hat{\theta}_{2,JGQL} = 0.387$ and $\hat{\theta}_{3,JGQL} = 0.573$ indicate that an individual with high GHL and DBP has greater probability to have retinopathy problem given the other covariates fixed, respectively. (4) The negative value of $\hat{\theta}_{4,JGQL} = -0.249$ indicates that males are more likely to develop retinopathy problem compared with females. Next, $\hat{\theta}_{5,JGQL} = 0.527$ show that presence of Pr (proteinuria) increases one's probability to develop retinopathy compared with those who don't have Pr problem. (6) The small values of $\hat{\theta}_6$ under both approaches, to be specific, $\hat{\theta}_{6,MGQL} = 0.018$, indicate that dose of insulin per day (DI) does not have much influence on one's propensity to have retinopathy problem. (7) The regression effect of ME (macular edema) on the probability of having diabetic retinopathy in left or right eye was found to be $\hat{\theta}_{7,MGQL} = 2.603$. Because ME was coded as $w_7 = 1$ in the presence of ME, this high positive value $\hat{\theta}_{7,MGQL} = 2.603$ indicates that ME has great effects on the retinopathy status.

5.5.3.2 Diabetic Retinopathy Data Analysis Using Trinomial ($K = 3$, $J = 3$) Model

Under the bivariate binary model fitted in the last section, dichotomous diabetic retinopathy status such as absence or presence of DR in both left and right eyes were considered. In this section we subdivide the presence of DR into two categories, i.e., non-severe DR and severe DR. Thus, for illustration of the proposed correlation model, altogether we consider three categories, namely none, non-severe, and severe, for both left (y) and right (z) eyes, whereas Williamson et al. (1995), for example, considered four categories, namely none, mild, moderate, and proliferative. This is done for simplicity only, whereas the proposed approach is quite general and is able to deal with any suitable finite number of categories for a response variable. In notation, we represent three categories of left eye diabetic retinopathy status by using two dummy variables y_{i1} and y_{i2} defined as follows:

$$(y_{i1}, y_{i2}) = \begin{cases} (1,0), \; non-severe\ DR\ (category\ 1) \\ (0,1), \; severe\ of\ DR\ (category\ 2) \\ (0,0), \; absence\ of\ DR\ (category\ 3). \end{cases}$$

Table 5.3 Trinomial model based counts of left and right eyes diabetic retinopathy status

right eye \ left eye	non-severe DR	severe DR	absence of DR	Total
non-severe DR	354	15	31	400
severe DR	12	43	0	55
absence of DR	39	0	249	288
Total	405	58	280	743

Similarly, we use two dummy variables z_{i1} and z_{i2} to represent the three categories of right eye diabetic retinopathy status as follows:

$$(z_{i1}, z_{i2}) = \begin{cases} (1,0), \ non-severe\ DR\ (category\ 1) \\ (0,1), \ severe\ DR\ (category\ 2) \\ (0,0), \ absence\ of\ DR\ (category\ 3). \end{cases}$$

The distribution of the 743 individuals under three categories of each of y and z are shown in Table 5.3.

As far as the covariates are concerned, in the bivariate binary analysis in the last section, we considered seven covariates. However, one of the covariates, namely dose of insulin per day (DI) was found to have no obvious effect on DR evident from the JGQL and MGQL estimates for this effect, which were found to be $\hat{\theta}_{6,JGQL} = 0.003$ and $\hat{\theta}_{6,MGQL} = 0.018$. Thus, we do not include DI in the present multinomial analysis. The rest of the covariates are: (1) duration of diabetes (DD), (2) glycosylated hemoglobin level (GHL), (3) diastolic blood pressure (DBP), (4) gender, (5) proteinuria (Pr), and (6) macular edema (ME); and it is of interest to find the effects of the six covariates on the trinomial status of DR. Furthermore, unlike in the previous section, in this section, we use standardized DD to estimate the effect of DD on DR. There are two obvious advantages of doing so, first the total number of model parameters can be reduced by two, yielding simpler calculations; second it is easier to interpret effects of DD on different categories of DR. We give the formula for standardizing DD as follows:

$$w_{i1} = \frac{DD_i - \overline{DD}}{se(DD)}. \tag{5.196}$$

Next, to specify the bivariate trinomial probabilities following (5.190)–(5.191), and (5.193), we use the notation $w_i = (w_{i1}, w_{i2}, w_{i3}, w_{i4}, w_{i5}, w_{i6})'$ to represent aforementioned 6 covariates, and use $\theta_1 = (\theta_{11}, \theta_{21}, \theta_{31}, \theta_{41}, \theta_{51}, \theta_{61})'$ to represent the effects of w_i on the response variables y_{i1} and z_{i1}, and $\theta_2 = (\theta_{12}, \theta_{22}, \theta_{32}, \theta_{42}, \theta_{52}, \theta_{62})'$ to represent the effects of w_i on the response variables y_{i2} and z_{i2}. For example, θ_{11} is the effect of DD on non-severe DR, and θ_{12} represent the effect of DD on severe retinopathy problem. Note that in addition to w_i, the probabilities for the response variables z_{i1} and z_{i2} are functions of marginal

Table 5.4 The marginal GQL (MGQL) estimates for the regression effects along with their estimated standard errors (ESE), and the estimates of the left eye category j (for y) versus right eye category r (for z) dependence ($CjrD$) parameters $\{\rho_{jr}, j = 1,2; r = 1,2\}$ under the normal linear conditional bivariate trinomial probability model for the diabetic retinopathy data

Parameter (Effect of)	Estimate	ESE
$(\alpha_{10}, \alpha_{20})$	(0.682,−2.528)	(0.147,0.312)
(β_{10}, β_{20})	(0.753,−2.388)	(0.148, 308)
θ_{11} (DD on non-severe DR)	2.177	0.141
θ_{12} (DD on severe DR)	2.591	0.177
θ_{21} (GHL on non-severe DR)	0.367	0.070
θ_{22} (GHL on severe DR)	0.391	0.132
θ_{31} (DBP on non-severe DR)	0.673	0.142
θ_{32} (DBP on severe DR)	1.146	0.287
θ_{41} (Gender on non-severe DR)	−0.190	0.138
θ_{42} (Gender on severe DR)	−0.374	0.261
θ_{51} (Pr on non-severe DR)	0.545	0.245
θ_{52} (Pr on severe DR)	1.741	0.335
θ_{61} (ME on non-severe DR)	2.077	1.035
θ_{62} (ME on severe DR)	4.154	1.050
ρ_{11} (C11D)	0.641	–
ρ_{21} (C12D)	0.017	–
ρ_{12} (C21D)	0.009	–
ρ_{22} (C22D)	0.674	–

parameters α_{10} and α_{20}, respectively; similarly, the probabilities for the response variables y_{i1} and y_{i2} are functions of marginal parameters β_{10} and β_{20}, respectively. These latter parameters are category effects.

Because there is no big difference between JGQL and MGQL estimation techniques, for simplicity, in this section we have used the MGQL approach only. The MGQL estimates of all model parameters and the estimated standard errors (ESE) of all regression parameters (α_{10}, α_{20}, β_{10}, β_{20}, θ_1 and θ_2) are reported in Table 5.4.

The results in Table 5.4 show that the propensity of diabetic retinopathy (probability of having diabetic retinopathy problem) tends to increase with longer DD, higher GHL, higher DBP, male gender, presence of proteinuria, and presence of ME. This observation agrees with the results in Table 5.2 under the bivariate binary analysis. To be specific, (1) the marginal parameter estimates $\hat{\alpha}_{10,MGQL} = 0.682$ and $\hat{\alpha}_{20,MGQL} = -2.528$, along with the marginal parameter estimates $\hat{\beta}_{10,MGQL} = 0.753$ and $\hat{\beta}_{10,MGQL} = -2.388$, indicate that when other covariates are fixed, a diabetic patient tends to develop retinopathy problem. However, the probability to have moderate (non-severe) retinopathy problem is larger as compared to the probability of having severe retinopathy problem. This observation agrees with the descriptive statistics in Table 5.3. (2) The large positive values of $\hat{\theta}_{11,MGQL} = 2.177$ and $\hat{\theta}_{12,MGQL} = 2.591$ show that as DD increases, the probability of an individual to have retinopathy problem increases, the longer DD, the severer retinopathy status will be. (3) The positive values of $\hat{\theta}_{31,MGQL} = 0.673$ and $\hat{\theta}_{32,MGQL} = 1.146$ indicate that an individual with higher DBP has greater probability to have retinopathy problem given the other covariates fixed. The positive values of $\hat{\theta}_{21}$ and $\hat{\theta}_{22}$ give similar interpretation of the effects of GHL on one's retinopathy status. (4) The negative values of $\hat{\theta}_{41,MGQL} = -0.190$ and $\hat{\theta}_{42,MGQL} = -0.374$ indicate that males are more likely to develop retinopathy problem as compared to females, and males are more likely to develop severe retinopathy problem than females. (5) The large positive values of $\hat{\theta}_{61} = 2.077$ and $\hat{\theta}_{62} = 4.154$ indicate that ME has a strong influence on one's propensity of diabetic retinopathy, and that presence of ME leads to severe DR more likely than moderate retinopathy problems.

Next, the large correlation index parameter values $\hat{\rho}_{11,MM} = 0.641$ and $\hat{\rho}_{22,MM} = 0.674$, and the small values of $\hat{\rho}_{21,MM} = 0.017$ and $\hat{\rho}_{12,MM} = 0.009$ imply that right eye retinopathy severity is highly correlated with the retinopathy severity of left eye. For example, for individuals whose left eye retinopathy status is non-severe, it is highly possible for them to have non-severe right eye retinopathy problem. Similarly, for those who have severe left eye retinopathy problem, it is greatly possible for them to have severe right eye retinopathy problem as well. This high correlation appears to reflect well the correlation indicated by the observations in Table 5.3.

Note that Williamson et al. (1995) also found similar but different (in magnitude) regression effect values as in Table 5.4, but the present estimation techniques provide more efficient estimates for the regression effects involved in the proposed normal linear conditional probability model. Furthermore, the correlation index parameters interpretation is quite appealing to understand the dependence of left eye retinopathy status on the right eye status and vice versa, whereas the odds ratio approach does not offer such correlation ideas but uses only one global odds ratio parameter to understand the dependence of multiple categories which appears to be inadequate.

References

Agresti, A. (2002). *Categorical data analysis* (2nd ed.) New York: Wiley.

Breslow, N. E., & Clayton, D. G. (1993). Approximate inference in generalized linear mixed models. *Journal of American Statistical Association, 88*, 9–25.

Fienberg, S. E. (2007). *The analysis of cross-classified categorical data.* New York: Springer.

MacDonald, B. W. (1994). Two random effects models for multivariate binary data. *Biometrics, 50*, 164–172.

Sun, B. (2013). *Bivariate multinomial models.* Unpublished Ph.D. thesis, Memorial University, Canada.

Sun, B., & Sutradhar, B. C. (2014). Bivariate categorical data analysis using normal linear conditional multinomial probability model. *Statistics in Medicine.* In Press.

Sutradhar, B. C. (2004). On exact quasilikelihood inference in generalized linear mixed models. *Sankhya, 66*, 261–289.
Sutradhar, B. C. (2011). *Dynamic mixed models for familial longitudinal data*. New York: Springer.
Ten Have, T. R., & Morabia, A. (1999). Mixed effects models with bivariate and univariate association parameters for longitudinal bivariate binary response data. *Biometrics, 55*, 85–93.
Williamson, J. M., Kim, K., & Lipsitz, S. R. (1995). Analyzing bivariate ordinal data using a global odds ratio. *Journal of American Statistical Association, 90*, 1432–1437.

Chapter 6
Multinomial Models for Longitudinal Bivariate Categorical Data

6.1 Preamble: Longitudinal Fixed Models for Two Multinomial Response Variables Ignoring Correlations

Recall from Chap. 4, specifically from Sect. 4.4 that the marginal probability at initial time ($t = 1$) and all possible lag 1 conditional probabilities for a multinomial response repeated over time were modeled as:

Marginal probability at $t = 1$ for y variable:

$$P[y_{i1} = y_{i1}^{(j)}] = \pi_{(i1)j}(y) = \begin{cases} \frac{\exp(w_{i1}^{*'}\beta_j^*)}{1+\sum_{g=1}^{J-1}\exp(w_{i1}^{*'}\beta_g^*)} & \text{for } j = 1,\ldots,J-1 \\ \frac{1}{1+\sum_{g=1}^{J-1}\exp(w_{i1}^{*'}\beta_g^*)} & \text{for } j = J, \end{cases} \quad (6.1)$$

where $w_{i1}^* = \left(1 \; w_{i1}'\right)'$, w_{i1} being the $p-$dimensional covariate vector recorded at time $t = 1$, and $\beta_j^* = (\beta_{j0}, \beta_j')'$ is the effect of w_{i1}^* influencing y_{i1} to be $y_{i1}^{(j)}$. Here $\beta_j = [\beta_{j1},\ldots,\beta_{ju},\ldots,\beta_{jp}]'$.

Lag 1 based conditional probabilities at $t = 2,\ldots,T$, for y variable:

$$\eta_{it|t-1}^{(j)}(g|y) = P\left(Y_{it} = y_{it}^{(j)} \middle| Y_{i,t-1} = y_{i,t-1}^{(g)}\right) = \begin{cases} \frac{\exp\left[w_{it}^{*'}\beta_j^*+\gamma_j' y_{i,t-1}^{(g)}\right]}{1+\sum_{v=1}^{J-1}\exp\left[w_{it}^{*'}\beta_v^*+\gamma_v' y_{i,t-1}^{(g)}\right]}, & \text{for } j = 1,\ldots,J-1 \\ \frac{1}{1+\sum_{v=1}^{J-1}\exp\left[w_{it}^{*'}\beta_v^*+\gamma_v' y_{i,t-1}^{(g)}\right]}, & \text{for } j = J, \end{cases} \quad (6.2)$$

where $g = 1,\ldots,J$, is a given (known) category, and $\gamma_j = (\gamma_{j1},\ldots,\gamma_{jv},\ldots,\gamma_{j,J-1})'$ denotes the dynamic dependence parameters.

Also recall from Chap. 5 that in the bivariate multinomial case in cross-sectional setup, one collects two multinomial responses y_i and z_i from the ith individual. In the longitudinal setup, both responses will be repeatedly collected over time

B.C. Sutradhar, *Longitudinal Categorical Data Analysis*, Springer Series in Statistics, DOI 10.1007/978-1-4939-2137-9_6

$t = 1,\ldots,T$. Using individual specific covariate (i.e., common covariate for both responses), a separate marginal and conditional probabilities model for z_{it}, similar to (6.1)–(6.2) may be written as

Marginal probability at $t = 1$ for z variable:

$$P[z_{i1} = z_{i1}^{(r)}] = \pi_{(i1)r}(z) = \begin{cases} \frac{\exp(w_{i1}^{*'}\alpha_r^*)}{1+\sum_{g=1}^{R-1}\exp(w_{i2}^{*'}\alpha_g^*)} & \text{for } r = 1,\ldots,R-1 \\ \frac{1}{1+\sum_{g=1}^{R-1}\exp(w_{i1}^{*'}\alpha_g^*)} & \text{for } r = R, \end{cases} \tag{6.3}$$

where $\alpha_r^* = (\alpha_{r0}, \alpha_r')'$ is the effect of w_{i1}^* influencing z_{i1} to be $z_{i1}^{(r)}$, where $r = 1,\ldots,R-1$. Here $\alpha_r = [\alpha_{r1},\ldots,\alpha_{ru},\ldots,\alpha_{rp}]'$.

Lag 1 based conditional probabilities at $t = 2,\ldots,T$, for z variable:

$$\eta_{it|t-1}^{(r)}(h|z) = P\left(Z_{it} = z_{it}^{(r)} \,\middle|\, Z_{i,t-1} = z_{i,t-1}^{(h)}\right) = \begin{cases} \frac{\exp\left[w_{it}^{*'}\alpha_r^* + \lambda_r' z_{i,t-1}^{(h)}\right]}{1+\sum_{v=1}^{R-1}\exp\left[w_{it}^{*'}\alpha_v^* + \lambda_v' z_{i,t-1}^{(h)}\right]}, & \text{for } r = 1,\ldots,R-1 \\ \frac{1}{1+\sum_{v=1}^{R-1}\exp\left[w_{it}^{*'}\alpha_v^* + \lambda_v' z_{i,t-1}^{(h)}\right]}, & \text{for } r = R, \end{cases} \tag{6.4}$$

where $h = 1,\ldots,R$ is a given (known) category, and $\lambda_r = (\lambda_{r1},\ldots,\lambda_{rv},\ldots,\lambda_{r,R-1})'$ denotes the dynamic dependence parameters.

6.2 Correlation Model for Two Longitudinal Multinomial Response Variables

Notice that $y_{it} = (y_{it1},\ldots,y_{itj},\ldots,y_{it,J-1})'$ and $z_{it} = (z_{it1},\ldots,z_{itr},\ldots,z_{it,R-1})'$ are two multinomial responses recorded at time t for the ith individual. Thus, two multinomial responses for the ith individual may be expressesd as

$$\begin{aligned} y_i &= [y_{i1}',\ldots,y_{it}',\ldots,y_{iT}']' : (J-1)T \times 1, \\ z_i &= [z_{i1}',\ldots,z_{it}',\ldots,z_{iT}']' : (R-1)T \times 1. \end{aligned} \tag{6.5}$$

Similar to Sect. 5.4 (specifically see (5.109)–(5.110)), it is quite reasonable to assume that these two responses are influenced by a common random or latent effect ξ_i^*. Conditional on this random effect ξ_i^*, one may then modify (6.1)–(6.2), and develop the marginal and conditional probabilities for the repeated responses $y_{i1},\ldots,y_{it},\ldots,y_{iT}$ as

$$P[y_{i1} = y_{i1}^{(j)}|\xi_i^*] = \pi_{(i1)j\cdot}^* = \begin{cases} \frac{\exp(w_{i1}^{*'}\beta_j^* + \xi_i^*)}{1+\sum_{g=1}^{J-1}\exp(w_{i1}^{*'}\beta_g^* + \xi_i^*)} & \text{for } j = 1,\ldots,J-1 \\ \frac{1}{1+\sum_{g=1}^{J-1}\exp(w_{i1}^{*'}\beta_g^* + \xi_i^*)} & \text{for } j = J, \end{cases} \tag{6.6}$$

and

$$\eta^{*(j\cdot)}_{it|t-1}(g) = P\Big(Y_{it} = y^{(j)}_{it} \Big| Y_{i,t-1} = y^{(g)}_{i,t-1}, \xi^*_i\Big)$$
$$= \begin{cases} \frac{\exp\left[w^{*'}_{it}\beta^*_j + \gamma'_j y^{(g)}_{i,t-1} + \xi^*_i\right]}{1+\sum_{v=1}^{J-1}\exp\left[w^{*'}_{it}\beta^*_v + \gamma'_v y^{(g)}_{i,t-1} + \xi^*_i\right]}, \text{ for } j = 1,\ldots,J-1 \\ \frac{1}{1+\sum_{v=1}^{J-1}\exp\left[w^{*'}_{it}\beta^*_v + \gamma'_v y^{(g)}_{i,t-1} + \xi^*_i\right]}, \text{ for } j = J, \end{cases} \tag{6.7}$$

for $t = 2,\ldots,T$. We will use

$$\beta = [\beta^{*'}_1,\ldots,\beta^{*'}_j,\ldots,\beta^{*'}_{J-1}]' : (J-1)(p+1)\times 1$$

to denote regression parameters under all categories, and

$$\gamma = [\gamma^{*'}_1,\ldots,\gamma^{*'}_j,\ldots,\gamma^{*'}_{J-1}]' : (J-1)(J-1)\times 1$$

to denote all dynamic dependence parameters.

Similarly, by modifying (6.3)–(6.4), one may develop the marginal and conditional probabilities for $z_{i1},\ldots,z_{it},\ldots,z_{iT}$ as

$$P[z_{i1} = z^{(r)}_{i1}|\xi^*_i] = \pi^*_{(i1)\cdot r} = \begin{cases} \frac{\exp(w^{*'}_{i1}\alpha^*_r + \xi^*_i)}{1+\sum_{g=1}^{R-1}\exp(w^{*'}_{i2}\alpha^*_g + \xi^*_i)} & \text{for } r = 1,\ldots,R-1 \\ \frac{1}{1+\sum_{g=1}^{R-1}\exp(w^{*'}_{i1}\alpha^*_g + \xi^*_i)} & \text{for } r = R, \end{cases} \tag{6.8}$$

and

$$\eta^{*(\cdot r)}_{it|t-1}(h) = P\Big(Z_{it} = z^{(r)}_{it} \Big| Z_{i,t-1} = z^{(h)}_{i,t-1}, \xi^*_i\Big)$$
$$= \begin{cases} \frac{\exp\left[w^{*'}_{it}\alpha^*_r + \lambda'_r z^{(h)}_{i,t-1} + \xi^*_i\right]}{1+\sum_{v=1}^{R-1}\exp\left[w^{*'}_{it}\alpha^*_v + \lambda'_v z^{(h)}_{i,t-1} + \xi^*_i\right]}, \text{ for } r = 1,\ldots,R-1 \\ \frac{1}{1+\sum_{v=1}^{R-1}\exp\left[w^{*'}_{it}\alpha^*_v + \lambda'_v z^{(h)}_{i,t-1} + \xi^*_i\right]}, \text{ for } r = R, \end{cases} \tag{6.9}$$

for $t = 2,\ldots,T$. All regression and dynamic dependence parameters corresponding to the z response variable will be denoted by

$$\alpha = [\alpha^{*'}_1,\ldots,\alpha^{*'}_r,\ldots,\alpha^{*'}_{R-1}]' : (R-1)(q+1)\times 1,$$

and

$$\lambda = [\lambda^{*'}_1,\ldots,\lambda^{*'}_r,\ldots,\lambda^{*'}_{R-1}]' : (R-1)(R-1)\times 1,$$

respectively.

6.2.1 Correlation Properties For Repeated Bivariate Responses

6.2.1.1 (a) Marginal Expectation Vector and Covariance Matrix for y Response Variable at Time t

Conditional on ξ_i^* or equivalently $\xi_i = \frac{\xi_i^*}{\sigma_\xi}$ (see (5.1)), these expectation vector and covariance matrix may be written following Chap. 4, specifically following Sect. 4.4.1. Thus these properties will be constructed as follows by combining the longitudinal properties of a variable from Sect. 4.4.1 and its possible common correlation property with another variable as discussed in Sect. 5.4.1. That is, in notation of (6.6)–(6.7), we write

$$E[Y_{it}|\xi_i] = \begin{cases} [\pi^*_{(i1)1\cdot},\ldots,\pi^*_{(i1)j\cdot},\ldots,\pi^*_{(i1)(J-1)\cdot}]' = \pi^*_{(i1)*\cdot} & \text{for } t=1, \\ \pi^{*(*\cdot)}_{(i1)}(\beta,\gamma,\sigma_\xi|\xi_i) = \pi^*_{(i1)*\cdot} & \text{for } t=1, \\ \pi^{*(*\cdot)}_{(it)}(\beta,\gamma,\sigma_\xi|\xi_i) = \eta^{*(*\cdot)}_{(it|t-1)}(J) & \\ +\left[\eta^{*(*\cdot)}_{(it|t-1),M} - \eta^{*(*\cdot)}_{(it|t-1)}(J)1'_{J-1}\right]\pi^{*(*\cdot)}_{(i,t-1)}(\beta,\gamma,\sigma_\xi|\xi_i) & \\ = [\pi^{*(1\cdot)}_{(it)},\ldots,\pi^{*(j\cdot)}_{(it)},\ldots,\pi^{*((J-1)\cdot)}_{(it)}]' & \text{for } t=2,\ldots,T, \end{cases} \tag{6.10}$$

and

$$\text{var}[Y_{it}|\xi_i] = \begin{cases} \text{diag}[\pi^*_{(i1)1\cdot},\ldots,\pi^*_{(i1)j\cdot},\ldots,\pi^*_{(i1)(J-1)\cdot}] - \pi^*_{(i1)*\cdot}\pi^{*\prime}_{(i1)*\cdot} & \text{for } t=1, \\ \text{diag}[\pi^{*(1\cdot)}_{(it)},\ldots,\pi^{*(j\cdot)}_{(it)},\ldots,\pi^{*((J-1)\cdot)}_{(it)}] - \pi^{*(*\cdot)}_{(it)}\pi^{*(*\cdot)\prime}_{(it)} & \text{for } t=2,\ldots,T. \end{cases} \tag{6.11}$$

$$= \Sigma^{*(*\cdot)}_{(i,tt)}(\beta,\gamma,\sigma_\xi|\xi_i) : (J-1)\times(J-1), \text{ (say), for } t=1,\ldots,T. \tag{6.12}$$

In (6.10)–(6.11),

$$\eta^{*(*\cdot)}_{(it|t-1)}(J) = [\eta^{*(1\cdot)}_{(it|t-1)}(J),\ldots,\eta^{*(j\cdot)}_{(it|t-1)}(J),\ldots,\eta^{*((J-1)\cdot)}_{(it|t-1)}(J)]'$$

$$= \pi^{*(*\cdot)}_{(i1)}(\beta,\gamma=0,\sigma_\xi|\xi_i) \tag{6.13}$$

$$\eta^{*(*\cdot)}_{(it|t-1),M}$$

$$= \begin{pmatrix} \eta^{*(1\cdot)}_{(it|t-1)}(1) & \cdots & \eta^{*(1\cdot)}_{(it|t-1)}(g) & \cdots & \eta^{*(1\cdot)}_{(it|t-1)}(J-1) \\ \vdots & \vdots & \vdots & \vdots & \vdots \\ \eta^{*(j\cdot)}_{(it|t-1)}(1) & \cdots & \eta^{*(j\cdot)}_{(it|t-1)}(g) & \cdots & \eta^{*(j\cdot)}_{(it|t-1)}(J-1) \\ \vdots & \vdots & \vdots & \vdots & \vdots \\ \eta^{*((J-1)\cdot)}_{(it|t-1)}(1) & \cdots & \eta^{*((J-1)\cdot)}_{(it|t-1)}(g) & \cdots & \eta^{*((J-1)\cdot)}_{(it|t-1)}(J-1) \end{pmatrix} : (J-1)\times(J-1), \tag{6.14}$$

with $\eta^{*(j\cdot)}_{(it|t-1)}(g)$ as in (6.7), for $j,g=1,\ldots,J-1$.

Now to obtain the unconditional mean vector and covariance matrix for y_{it}, similar to (5.1), we assume that the random effects are independent and they follow the standard normal distribution, i.e., $\xi_i = \frac{\xi_i^*}{\sigma_\xi} \overset{iid}{\sim} N(0,1)$. More specifically, after taking the average over the distribution of ξ_i, these unconditional moment properties are obtained from (6.10)–(6.11), as follows:

Unconditional mean vector at time $t = 1,\ldots,T$:

$$E[Y_{it}] = E_{\xi_i} E[Y_{it}|\xi_i] = \begin{cases} \int_{-\infty}^{\infty} \pi^*_{(i1)*\cdot}(\beta, \sigma_\xi|\xi_i) f_N(\xi_i) d\xi_i & \text{for } t = 1, \\ \int_{-\infty}^{\infty} \pi^{*(*\cdot)}_{(it)}(\beta, \gamma, \sigma_\xi|\xi_i) f_N(\xi_i) d\xi_i & \text{for } t = 2,\ldots,T, \end{cases} \tag{6.15}$$

$$= \pi^{(*\cdot)}_{(it)}(\beta, \gamma, \sigma_\xi) : (J-1) \times 1, \text{ (say), for } t = 1,\ldots,T, \tag{6.16}$$

where $f_N(\xi_i) = \frac{1}{\sqrt{2\pi}} \exp[-\frac{1}{2}\xi_i^2]$. Note that all integrations over the desired functions in normal random effects in this chapter including (6.16) may be computed by using the binomial approximation, for example, introduced in the last chapter, specifically in Sect. 5.3.

Unconditional covariance matrix at time $t = 1,\ldots,T$:

$$\begin{aligned} \text{var}[Y_{it}] &= E_{\xi_i}\text{var}[Y_{it}|\xi_i] + \text{var}_{\xi_i} E[Y_{it}|\xi_i] \\ &= \int_{-\infty}^{\infty} \Sigma^{*(*\cdot)}_{(i,tt)}(\beta, \gamma, \sigma_\xi|\xi_i) f_N(\xi_i) d\xi_i + \text{var}_{\xi_i}[\pi^{*(*\cdot)}_{(it)}(\beta, \gamma, \sigma_\xi|\xi_i)] \\ &= \int_{-\infty}^{\infty} \Sigma^{*(*\cdot)}_{(i,tt)}(\beta, \gamma, \sigma_\xi|\xi_i) f_N(\xi_i) d\xi_i + \int_{-\infty}^{\infty} [\{\pi^{*(*\cdot)}_{(it)}(\beta, \gamma, \sigma_\xi|\xi_i)\} \\ &\qquad \{\pi^{*(*\cdot)}_{(it)}(\beta, \gamma, \sigma_\xi|\xi_i)'\}] f_N(\xi_i) d\xi_i \\ &\quad - \pi^{(*\cdot)}_{(it)}(\beta, \gamma, \sigma_\xi) \pi^{(*\cdot)'}_{(it)}(\beta, \gamma, \sigma_\xi) \\ &= \Sigma^{(*\cdot)}_{(i,tt)}(\beta, \gamma, \sigma_\xi), \end{aligned} \tag{6.17}$$

where $\pi^{(*\cdot)}_{(it)}(\beta, \gamma, \sigma_\xi)$ is given in (6.16).

6.2.1.1 (b) Auto-Covariances Between Repeated Responses for y Variable Recorded at Times $u < t$

Conditional on ξ_i, following (4.71), the covariance matrix between the response vectors y_{iu} and y_{it} has the form

$$\text{cov}[\{Y_{iu}, Y_{it}\}|\xi_i] = \Pi_{s=u+1}^{t} \left[\eta^{*(*\cdot)}_{(is|s-1),M} - \eta^{*(*\cdot)}_{(is|s-1)}(J)1'_{J-1}\right] \text{var}[Y_{iu}|\xi_i], \text{ for } u < t$$

$$= (\mathrm{cov}(Y_{iuj}, Y_{itk})) = (\sigma^{*(*\cdot)}_{(i,ut)jk}),\ j,k = 1,\ldots,J-1$$

$$= \Sigma^{*(*\cdot)}_{(i,ut)}(\beta,\gamma,\sigma_\xi|\xi_i). \tag{6.18}$$

One then obtains the unconditional covariance matrix as follows by using the conditioning un-conditioning principle.

Unconditional covariance matrix between y_{iu} and y_{it} for $u < t$:

$$\begin{aligned}
\mathrm{cov}[Y_{iu}, Y'_{it}] &= E_{\xi_i}\mathrm{cov}[\{Y_{iu}, Y'_{it}\}|\xi_i] + \mathrm{cov}_{\xi_i}[E[Y_{iu}|\xi_i], E[Y'_{it}|\xi_i]] \\
&= \int_{-\infty}^{\infty} \Sigma^{*(*\cdot)}_{(i,ut)}(\beta,\gamma,\sigma_\xi|\xi_i) f_N(\xi_i) d\xi_i + \mathrm{cov}_{\xi_i}[\{\pi^{*(*\cdot)}_{(iu)}(\beta,\gamma,\sigma_\xi|\xi_i)\}, \{\pi^{*(*\cdot)'}_{(it)}(\beta,\gamma,\sigma_\xi|\xi_i)\}] \\
&= \int_{-\infty}^{\infty} \Sigma^{*(*\cdot)}_{(i,ut)}(\beta,\gamma,\sigma_\xi|\xi_i) f_N(\xi_i) d\xi_i + \int_{-\infty}^{\infty} [\{\pi^{*(*\cdot)}_{(iu)}(\beta,\gamma,\sigma_\xi|\xi_i)\}\{\pi^{*(*\cdot)}_{(it)}(\beta,\gamma,\sigma_\xi|\xi_i)'\}] f_N(\xi_i) d\xi_i \\
&- \pi^{(*\cdot)}_{(iu)}(\beta,\gamma,\sigma_\xi)\pi^{(*\cdot)'}_{(it)}(\beta,\gamma,\sigma_\xi) \\
&= \Sigma^{(*\cdot)}_{(i,ut)}(\beta,\gamma,\sigma_\xi),
\end{aligned} \tag{6.19}$$

where $\pi^{(*\cdot)}_{(it)}(\beta,\gamma,\sigma_\xi)$ is given in (6.16), and $\Sigma^{*(*\cdot)}_{(i,ut)}(\beta,\gamma,\sigma_\xi|\xi_i)$ for $u < t$ is given by (6.18).

6.2.1.2 (a) Marginal Expectation Vector and Covariance Matrix for z Response Variable at Time t

The computation for these moments is similar to those for the moments of y. More specifically, replacing the notations $\pi^*_{(i1)j\cdot}$, $\pi^{*(*\cdot)}_{(it)}(\beta,\gamma,\sigma_\xi|\xi_i)$, and $\eta^{*(j\cdot)}_{(it|t-1)}(g)$ in the formulas for the moments of y variable, with $\pi^*_{(i1)\cdot r}$ (6.8), $\pi^{*(\cdot *)}_{(it)}(\alpha,\lambda,\sigma_\xi|\xi_i)$, and $\eta^{*(\cdot r)}_{(it|t-1)}(h)$ (6.9), respectively, one may write the formulas for the moments for z variable. To be brief, we write the formulas only as follows, without giving any further explanation on computation.

$$E[Z_{it}|\xi_i] = \begin{cases}
[\pi^*_{(i1)\cdot 1},\ldots,\pi^*_{(i1)\cdot r},\ldots,\pi^*_{(i1)\cdot(R-1)}]' = \pi^*_{(i1)\cdot *} & \text{for } t = 1, \\
\pi^{*(\cdot *)}_{(i1)}(\alpha,\lambda,\sigma_\xi|\xi_i) = \pi^*_{(i1)\cdot *} & \text{for } t = 1, \\
\pi^{*(\cdot *)}_{(it)}(\alpha,\lambda,\sigma_\xi|\xi_i) = \eta^{*(\cdot *)}_{(it|t-1)}(R) & \\
+\left[\eta^{*(\cdot *)}_{(it|t-1),M} - \eta^{*(\cdot *)}_{(it|t-1)}(R)1'_{R-1}\right]\pi^{*(\cdot *)}_{(i,t-1)}(\alpha,\lambda,\sigma_\xi) & \\
= [\pi^{*(\cdot 1)}_{(it)},\ldots,\pi^{*(\cdot r)}_{(it)},\ldots,\pi^{*(\cdot(R-1))}_{(it)}]' & \text{for } t = 2,\ldots,T,
\end{cases} \tag{6.20}$$

using $\pi^{*(\cdot *)}_{(i1)}(\alpha, \lambda = 0, \sigma_\xi) = \pi^*_{(i1)\cdot *}$, and

$$\mathrm{var}[Z_{it}|\xi_i] = \begin{cases} \mathrm{diag}[\pi^*_{(i1)\cdot 1}, \ldots, \pi^*_{(i1)\cdot r}, \ldots, \pi^*_{(i1)\cdot (R-1)}] - \pi^*_{(i1)\cdot *}\pi^{*'}_{(i1)\cdot *} & \text{for } t = 1, \\ \mathrm{diag}[\pi^{*(\cdot 1)}_{(it)}, \ldots, \pi^{*(\cdot r)}_{(it)}, \ldots, \pi^{*(\cdot (R-1))}_{(it)}] - \pi^{*(\cdot *)}_{(it)}\pi^{*(\cdot *)'}_{(it)} & \text{for } t = 2, \ldots, T. \end{cases} \tag{6.21}$$

$$= \Sigma^{*(\cdot *)}_{(i,tt)}(\alpha, \lambda, \sigma_\xi|\xi_i) : (R-1) \times (R-1), \text{ (say), for } t = 1, \ldots, T. \tag{6.22}$$

In (6.20)–(6.21),

$$\eta^{*(\cdot *)}_{(it|t-1)}(R) = [\eta^{*(\cdot 1)}_{(it|t-1)}(R), \ldots, \eta^{*(\cdot r)}_{(it|t-1)}(R), \ldots, \eta^{*(\cdot (R-1))}_{(it|t-1)}(R)]'$$
$$= \pi^{*(\cdot *)}_{(i1)}(\alpha, \lambda, \sigma_\xi|\xi_i) \tag{6.23}$$

$$\eta^{*(\cdot *)}_{(it|t-1),M}$$
$$= \begin{pmatrix} \eta^{*(\cdot 1)}_{(it|t-1)}(1) & \cdots & \eta^{*(\cdot 1)}_{(it|t-1)}(g) & \cdots & \eta^{*(\cdot 1)}_{(it|t-1)}(R-1) \\ \vdots & \vdots & \vdots & \vdots & \vdots \\ \eta^{*(\cdot r)}_{(it|t-1)}(1) & \cdots & \eta^{*(\cdot r)}_{(it|t-1)}(g) & \cdots & \eta^{*(\cdot r)}_{(it|t-1)}(R-1) \\ \vdots & \vdots & \vdots & \vdots & \vdots \\ \eta^{*(\cdot (R-1))}_{(it|t-1)}(1) & \cdots & \eta^{*(\cdot (R-1))}_{(it|t-1)}(g) & \cdots & \eta^{*(\cdot (R-1))}_{(it|t-1)}(R-1) \end{pmatrix} : (R-1) \times (R-1), \tag{6.24}$$

with $\eta^{*(\cdot r)}_{(it|t-1)}(g)$ as in (6.9), for $r, g = 1, \ldots, R-1$.

Next the unconditional moments are obtained by taking the average of the desired quantities over the distribution of the random effects xi_i.:

Unconditional mean vector at time $t = 1, \ldots, T$:

$$E[Z_{it}] = E_{\xi_i}E[Z_{it}|\xi_i] = \begin{cases} \int_{-\infty}^{\infty} \pi^*_{(i1)\cdot *}(\alpha, \sigma_\xi|\xi_i)f_N(\xi_i)d\xi_i & \text{for } t = 1, \\ \int_{-\infty}^{\infty} \pi^{*(\cdot *)}_{(it)}(\alpha, \lambda, \sigma_\xi|\xi_i)f_N(\xi_i)d\xi_i & \text{for } t = 2, \ldots, T, \end{cases} \tag{6.25}$$

$$= \pi^{(\cdot *)}_{(it)}(\alpha, \lambda, \sigma_\xi) : (J-1) \times 1, \text{ (say), for } t = 1, \ldots, T, \tag{6.26}$$

where $f_N(\xi_i) = \frac{1}{\sqrt{2\pi}} \exp[-\frac{1}{2}\xi_i^2]$.

Unconditional covariance matrix at time $t = 1, \ldots, T$:

$$\begin{aligned} \mathrm{var}[Z_{it}] &= E_{\xi_i}\mathrm{var}[Z_{it}|\xi_i] + \mathrm{var}_{\xi_i}E[Z_{it}|\xi_i] \\ &= \int_{-\infty}^{\infty} \Sigma^{*(\cdot *)}_{(i,tt)}(\alpha, \lambda, \sigma_\xi|\xi_i)f_N(\xi_i)d\xi_i + \mathrm{var}_{\xi_i}[\pi^{*(\cdot *)}_{(it)}(\alpha, \lambda, \sigma_\xi|\xi_i)] \\ &= \int_{-\infty}^{\infty} \Sigma^{*(\cdot *)}_{(i,tt)}(\alpha, \lambda, \sigma_\xi|\xi_i)f_N(\xi_i)d\xi_i + \int_{-\infty}^{\infty} [\{\pi^{*(\cdot *)}_{(it)}(\alpha, \lambda, \sigma_\xi|\xi_i)\}\{\pi^{*(\cdot *)}_{(it)}(\alpha, \lambda, \sigma_\xi|\xi_i)'\}]f_N(\xi_i)d\xi_i \end{aligned}$$

$$- \pi^{(\cdot *)}_{(it)}(\alpha,\lambda,\sigma_\xi)\pi^{(\cdot *)'}_{(it)}(\alpha,\lambda,\sigma_\xi)$$
$$= \Sigma^{(\cdot *)}_{(i,tt)}(\alpha,\lambda,\sigma_\xi), \quad (6.27)$$

where $\pi^{(\cdot *)}_{(it)}(\alpha,\lambda,\sigma_\xi)$ is given in (6.26).

6.2.1.2 (b) Auto-Covariances Between Repeated Responses for z Variable Recorded at Times $u < t$

Similar to (6.18), the covariance matrix between the response vectors z_{iu} and z_{it} has the form

$$\begin{aligned}
\mathrm{cov}[\{Z_{iu},Z_{it}\}|\xi_i] &= \Pi^t_{s=u+1}\left[\eta^{*(\cdot *)}_{(is|s-1),M} - \eta^{*(\cdot *)}_{(is|s-1)}(R)1'_{R-1}\right]\mathrm{var}[Z_{iu}|\xi_i], \text{ for } u<t \\
&= (\mathrm{cov}(Z_{iuj},Z_{itk})) = (\sigma^{*(\cdot *)}_{(i,ut)r\ell}),\ r,\ell = 1,\ldots,R-1 \\
&= \Sigma^{*(\cdot *)}_{(i,ut)}(\alpha,\lambda,\sigma_\xi|\xi_i). \qquad (6.28)
\end{aligned}$$

One then obtains the unconditional covariance matrix as follows by using the conditioning un-conditioning principle.

Unconditional covariance matrix between z_{iu} and z_{it} for $u < t$:]

$$\begin{aligned}
\mathrm{cov}[Z_{iu},Z'_{it}] &= E_{\xi_i}\mathrm{cov}[\{Z_{iu},Z'_{it}\}|\xi_i] + \mathrm{cov}_{\xi_i}[E[Z_{iu}|\xi_i],E[Z'_{it}|\xi_i]] \\
&= \int_{-\infty}^{\infty}\Sigma^{*(\cdot *)}_{(i,ut)}(\alpha,\lambda,\sigma_\xi|\xi_i)f_N(\xi_i)d\xi_i + \mathrm{cov}_{\xi_i}[\{\pi^{*(\cdot *)}_{(iu)}(\alpha,\lambda,\sigma_\xi|\xi_i)\},\{\pi^{*(\cdot *)'}_{(it)}(\alpha,\lambda,\sigma_\xi|\xi_i)\}] \\
&= \int_{-\infty}^{\infty}\Sigma^{*(\cdot *)}_{(i,ut)}(\alpha,\lambda,\sigma_\xi|\xi_i)f_N(\xi_i)d\xi_i + \int_{-\infty}^{\infty}[\{\pi^{*(\cdot *)}_{(iu)}(\alpha,\lambda,\sigma_\xi|\xi_i)\}\{\pi^{*(\cdot *)}_{(it)}(\alpha,\lambda,\sigma_\xi|\xi_i)'\}]f_N(\xi_i)d\xi_i \\
&\quad - \pi^{(\cdot *)}_{(iu)}(\alpha,\lambda,\sigma_\xi)\pi^{(\cdot *)'}_{(it)}(\alpha,\lambda,\sigma_\xi) \\
&= \Sigma^{(\cdot *)}_{(i,ut)}(\alpha,\lambda,\sigma_\xi), \qquad (6.29)
\end{aligned}$$

where $\pi^{(\cdot *)}_{(it)}(\alpha,\lambda,\sigma_\xi)$ is given in (6.26), and $\Sigma^{*(\cdot *)}_{(i,ut)}(\alpha,\lambda,\sigma_\xi|\xi_i)$ for $u<t$ is given by (6.28).

6.2.1.3 (a) Covariance Matrix Between y_{it} and z_{it} of Dimension $(J-1)\times(R-1)$

Because y and z are uncorrelated conditional on ξ_i, the covariance matrix between these two multinomial response variables at a given time point may be computed as:

$$\mathrm{cov}[Y_{it},Z'_{it}] = E_{\xi_i}\mathrm{cov}[\{Y_{it},Z'_{it}\}|\xi_i] + \mathrm{cov}_{\xi_i}[E[Y_{it}|\xi_i],E[Z_{it}|\xi_i]]$$

$$= \text{cov}_{\xi_i}\left[E[Y_{it}|\xi_i], E[Z_{it}|\xi_i]\right]$$

$$= \begin{cases} \text{cov}_{\xi_i}\left[\pi^{*(*\cdot)}_{(i1)}(\beta,\gamma=0,\sigma_\xi|\xi_i), \pi^{*(\cdot *)'}_{(i1)}(\alpha,\lambda=0,\sigma_\xi|\xi_i)\right] & \text{for } t=1 \\ \text{cov}_{\xi_i}\left[\pi^{*(*\cdot)}_{(it)}(\beta,\gamma,\sigma_\xi|\xi_i), \pi^{*(\cdot *)'}_{(it)}(\alpha,\lambda,\sigma_\xi|\xi_i)\right] & \text{for } t=2,\ldots,T. \end{cases}$$

$$= \begin{cases} \int_{-\infty}^{\infty}\left[\pi^{*(*\cdot)}_{(i1)}(\beta,\gamma=0,\sigma_\xi|\xi_i)\pi^{*(\cdot *)'}_{(i1)}(\alpha,\lambda=0,\sigma_\xi|\xi_i)\right] f_N(\xi_i)d\xi_i & \\ -\pi^{(*\cdot)}_{(i1)}(\beta,\gamma=0,\sigma_\xi)\pi^{(\cdot *)'}_{(i1)}(\alpha,\lambda=0,\sigma_\xi) & \text{for } t=1 \\ \int_{-\infty}^{\infty}\left[\pi^{*(*\cdot)}_{(it)}(\beta,\gamma,\sigma_\xi|\xi_i)\pi^{*(\cdot *)'}_{(it)}(\alpha,\lambda,\sigma_\xi|\xi_i)\right] f_N(\xi_i)d\xi_i & \\ -\pi^{(*\cdot)}_{(it)}(\beta,\gamma,\sigma_\xi)\pi^{(\cdot *)'}_{(it)}(\alpha,\lambda,\sigma_\xi) & \text{for } t=2,\ldots,T. \end{cases}$$

$$= \Sigma^{(**)}_{(i,tt)}(\beta,\gamma,\alpha,\lambda,\sigma_\xi). \tag{6.30}$$

6.2.1.3 (b) Covariance Matrix Between y_{iu} and z_{it} of Dimension $(J-1)\times(R-1)$

For all u,t, this covariance matrix may be obtained as follows. Thus, the following formulas accommodate the $u=t$ case provided in Sect. 6.2.1.3(a). The general formula is given by

$$\begin{aligned} \text{cov}[Y_{iu}, Z'_{it}] &= E_{\xi_i}\text{cov}[\{Y_{iu}, Z'_{it}\}|\xi_i] + \text{cov}_{\xi_i}\left[E[Y_{iu}|\xi_i], E[Z_{it}|\xi_i]\right] \\ &= \text{cov}_{\xi_i}\left[E[Y_{iu}|\xi_i], E[Z_{it}|\xi_i]\right] \end{aligned}$$

$$= \begin{cases} \text{cov}_{\xi_i}\left[\pi^{*(*\cdot)}_{(i1)}(\beta,\gamma=0,\sigma_\xi|\xi_i), \pi^{*(\cdot *)'}_{(i1)}(\alpha,\lambda=0,\sigma_\xi|\xi_i)\right] & \text{for } u=1, t=1 \\ \text{cov}_{\xi_i}\left[\pi^{*(*\cdot)}_{(i1)}(\beta,\gamma=0,\sigma_\xi|\xi_i), \pi^{*(\cdot *)'}_{(it)}(\alpha,\lambda,\sigma_\xi|\xi_i)\right] & \text{for } u=1, t=2,\ldots,T \\ \text{cov}_{\xi_i}\left[\pi^{*(*\cdot)}_{(iu)}(\beta,\gamma,\sigma_\xi|\xi_i), \pi^{*(\cdot *)'}_{(i1)}(\alpha,\lambda=0,\sigma_\xi|\xi_i)\right] & \text{for } u=2,\ldots,T; t=1 \\ \text{cov}_{\xi_i}\left[\pi^{*(*\cdot)}_{(iu)}(\beta,\gamma,\sigma_\xi|\xi_i), \pi^{*(\cdot *)'}_{(it)}(\alpha,\lambda,\sigma_\xi|\xi_i)\right] & \text{for } u,t=2,\ldots,T. \end{cases}$$

$$= \begin{cases} \int_{-\infty}^{\infty}\left[\pi^{*(*\cdot)}_{(i1)}(\beta,\gamma=0,\sigma_\xi|\xi_i)\pi^{*(\cdot *)'}_{(i1)}(\alpha,\lambda=0,\sigma_\xi|\xi_i)\right] f_N(\xi_i)d\xi_i & \\ -\pi^{(*\cdot)}_{(i1)}(\beta,\gamma=0,\sigma_\xi)\pi^{(\cdot *)'}_{(i1)}(\alpha,\lambda=0,\sigma_\xi) & \text{for } u=t=1 \\ \int_{-\infty}^{\infty}\left[\pi^{*(*\cdot)}_{(i1)}(\beta,\gamma=0,\sigma_\xi|\xi_i)\pi^{*(\cdot *)'}_{(it)}(\alpha,\lambda,\sigma_\xi|\xi_i)\right] f_N(\xi_i)d\xi_i & \\ -\pi^{(*\cdot)}_{(i1)}(\beta,\gamma=0,\sigma_\xi)\pi^{(\cdot *)'}_{(it)}(\alpha,\lambda,\sigma_\xi) & \text{for } u=1; t=2,\ldots,T \\ \int_{-\infty}^{\infty}\left[\pi^{*(*\cdot)}_{(iu)}(\beta,\gamma,\sigma_\xi|\xi_i)\pi^{*(\cdot *)'}_{(i1)}(\alpha,\lambda=0,\sigma_\xi|\xi_i)\right] f_N(\xi_i)d\xi_i & \\ -\pi^{(*\cdot)}_{(iu)}(\beta,\gamma,\sigma_\xi)\pi^{(\cdot *)'}_{(i1)}(\alpha,\lambda=0,\sigma_\xi) & \text{for } u=2,\ldots,T; t=1 \\ \int_{-\infty}^{\infty}\left[\pi^{*(*\cdot)}_{(iu)}(\beta,\gamma,\sigma_\xi|\xi_i)\pi^{*(\cdot *)'}_{(it)}(\alpha,\lambda,\sigma_\xi|\xi_i)\right] f_N(\xi_i)d\xi_i & \\ -\pi^{(*\cdot)}_{(iu)}(\beta,\gamma,\sigma_\xi)\pi^{(\cdot *)'}_{(it)}(\alpha,\lambda,\sigma_\xi) & \text{for } u,t=2,\ldots,T. \end{cases}$$

$$= \Sigma^{(**)}_{(i,ut)}(\beta,\gamma,\alpha,\lambda,\sigma_\xi). \tag{6.31}$$

6.3 Estimation of Parameters

6.3.1 MGQL Estimation for Regression Parameters

Recall that the regression parameters involved in the marginal (6.6) and conditional (6.7) probabilities for the y variable with J categories are denoted by

$$\begin{aligned}\beta_j^* &= (\beta_{j0}, \beta_j')', \; j = 1, \ldots, J-1 \\ &= (\beta_{j0}, \beta_{j1}, \ldots, \beta_{jp})', \; j = 1, \ldots, J-1,\end{aligned}$$

and similarly the regression parameters involved in the marginal (6.8) and conditional (6.9) probabilities for the z variable with R categories are denoted by

$$\begin{aligned}\alpha_r^* &= (\alpha_{r0}, \alpha_r')', \; r = 1, \ldots, R-1 \\ &= (\alpha_{r0}, \alpha_{r1}, \ldots, \alpha_{rq})', \; r = 1, \ldots, R-1.\end{aligned}$$

Also recall that

$$\begin{aligned}\beta &= (\beta_1^{*\prime}, \ldots, \beta_j^{*\prime}, \ldots, \beta_{J-1}^{*}{}')' : (J-1)(p+1) \times 1 \\ \alpha &= (\alpha_1^{*\prime}, \ldots, \alpha_r^{*\prime}, \ldots, \alpha_{R-1}^{*}{}')' : (R-1)(q+1) \times 1,\end{aligned}$$

and by further stacking we write

$$\mu = [\beta', \alpha']' : \{(J-1)(p+1) + (R-1)(q+1)\} \times 1. \tag{6.32}$$

Next, for dynamic dependence parameters we use

$$\theta = (\gamma', \lambda')' : \{(J-1)^2 + (R-1)^2\} \times 1, \tag{6.33}$$

where

$$\begin{aligned}\gamma &= (\gamma_1', \ldots, \gamma_j', \ldots, \gamma_{J-1}')' : (J-1)^2 \times 1 \\ \lambda &= (\lambda_1', \ldots, \lambda_r', \ldots, \lambda_{R-1}')' : (R-1)^2 \times 1.\end{aligned}$$

In this section, it is of interest to estimate the regression (μ) parameters by exploiting the GQL estimation (Sutradhar et al. 2008; Sutradhar 2011, Chapter 11) approach. Note that this GQL approach was used in Chap. 5, specifically in Sect. 5.4, for the estimation of both regression and random effects variance parameters involved in the cross-sectional bivariate multinomial models, whereas in this chapter, more specifically in this section, the GQL approach is used only for the estimation of regression parameters involved in the longitudinal bivariate multinomial model. The application of the GQL approach for the estimation of dynamic dependence parameters as well as σ_ξ^2 would be complex for the present bivariate longitudinal model. For simplicity we estimate these latter parameters by using the traditional method of moments (MM) in the next two sections. Note that, similar to the GQL approach, the MM approach also produces consistent estimators but they will be less efficient than the corresponding GQL estimators.

We now turn back to the GQL estimation of the regression parameter $\mu = (\beta', \alpha')'$. This is also referred to as the marginal GQL (MGQL) approach as it is constructed for a marginal set of parameters. For known γ, λ, the MGQL estimating equation for $\mu = (\beta', \alpha')'$ is given by

$$f(\mu) = \sum_{i=1}^{K} \frac{\partial(\pi_{(i)}^{(*\cdot)'}(\beta,\gamma,\sigma_\xi), \pi_{(i)}^{(\cdot*)'}(\alpha,\lambda,\sigma_\xi))}{\partial\mu} \times \Sigma_{(i)}^{-1}(\mu,\gamma,\lambda,\sigma_\xi) \begin{pmatrix} y_i - \pi_{(i)}^{(*\cdot)}(\beta,\gamma,\sigma_\xi) \\ z_i - \pi_{(i)}^{(\cdot*)}(\alpha,\lambda,\sigma_\xi) \end{pmatrix} = 0, \quad (6.34)$$

where, for

$$y_i = [y'_{i1}, \ldots, y'_{it}, \ldots, y'_{iT}]' : (J-1)T \times 1, \text{ and}$$
$$z_i = [z'_{i1}, \ldots, z'_{it}, \ldots, z'_{iT}]' : (R-1)T \times 1,$$

$$E[Y_i] = \pi_{(i)}^{(*\cdot)}(\beta,\gamma,\sigma_\xi) = [\pi_{(i1)}^{(*\cdot)'}(\cdot), \ldots, \pi_{(it)}^{(*\cdot)'}(\cdot), \ldots, \pi_{(iT)}^{(*\cdot)'}(\cdot)]', \quad (6.35)$$

by (6.16). Similarly by (6.26), one writes

$$E[Z_i] = \pi_{(i)}^{(\cdot*)}(\alpha,\lambda,\sigma_\xi) = [\pi_{(i1)}^{(\cdot*)'}(\cdot), \ldots, \pi_{(it)}^{(\cdot*)'}(\cdot), \ldots, \pi_{(iT)}^{(\cdot*)'}(\cdot)]'. \quad (6.36)$$

Note that in (6.35),

$$\pi_{(it)}^{(*\cdot)}(\cdot) \equiv \pi_{(it)}^{(*\cdot)}(\beta,\gamma,\sigma_\xi) = [\pi_{(it)}^{(1\cdot)}(\beta,\gamma,\sigma_\xi), \ldots, \pi_{(it)}^{(j\cdot)}(\beta,\gamma,\sigma_\xi), \ldots, \pi_{(it)}^{((J-1)\cdot)}(\beta,\gamma,\sigma_\xi)]', \quad (6.37)$$

with

$$\pi_{(it)}^{(j\cdot)}(\beta,\gamma,\sigma_\xi) = \int_{-\infty}^{\infty} \pi_{(it)}^{*(j\cdot)}(\beta,\gamma,\sigma_\xi|\xi_i) f_N(\xi_i) d\xi_i,$$

as in (6.10) and (6.16). Similarly, in (6.36),

$$\pi^{(\cdot*)}_{(it)}(\cdot) \equiv \pi^{(\cdot*)}_{(it)}(\alpha,\lambda,\sigma_\xi)$$
$$= [\pi^{(\cdot 1)}_{(it)}(\alpha,\lambda,\sigma_\xi),\ldots,\pi^{(\cdot r)}_{(it)}(\alpha,\lambda,\sigma_\xi),\ldots,\pi^{(\cdot (R-1))}_{(it)}(\alpha,\lambda,\sigma_\xi)]', \quad (6.38)$$

with

$$\pi^{(\cdot r)}_{(it)}(\alpha,\lambda,\sigma_\xi) = \int_{-\infty}^{\infty} \pi^{*(\cdot r)}_{(it)}(\alpha,\lambda,\sigma_\xi|\xi_i) f_N(\xi_i) d\xi_i,$$

as in (6.20) and (6.26).

6.3.1.1 Construction of the Covariance Matrix $\Sigma_i(\mu,\gamma,\lambda,\sigma_\xi)$

In (6.34), the covariance matrix has the formula

$$\Sigma_i(\mu,\gamma,\lambda,\sigma_\xi) = \text{cov}\begin{pmatrix} Y_i \\ Z_i \end{pmatrix} : \{(J-1)+(R-1)\}T \times \{(J-1)+(R-1)\}T$$
$$= \begin{pmatrix} \text{var}(Y_i) : (J-1)T \times (J-1)T & \text{cov}(Y_i, Z_i') : (J-1)T \times (R-1)T \\ \text{cov}(Z_i, Y_i') : (R-1)T \times (J-1)T & \text{var}(Z_i) : (R-1)T \times (R-1)T \end{pmatrix}, \quad (6.39)$$

where

$$\text{var}(Y_i) = \text{var}\begin{pmatrix} Y_{i1} \\ \vdots \\ Y_{it} \\ \vdots \\ Y_{iT} \end{pmatrix} : (J-1)T \times (J-1)T$$
$$= \begin{pmatrix} \text{var}[Y_{i1}] & \cdots & \text{cov}[Y_{i1}, Y_{it}'] & \cdots & \text{cov}[Y_{i1}, Y_{iT}'] \\ \vdots & & \vdots & & \vdots \\ \text{cov}[Y_{it}, Y_{i1}'] & \cdots & \text{var}[Y_{it}] & \cdots & \text{cov}[Y_{it}, Y_{iT}'] \\ \vdots & & \vdots & & \vdots \\ \text{cov}[Y_{iT}, Y_{i1}'] & \cdots & \text{cov}[Y_{iT}, Y_{it}'] & \cdots & \text{var}[Y_{iT}] \end{pmatrix}$$
$$= \begin{pmatrix} \Sigma^{(*\cdot)}_{(i,11)}(\beta,\gamma,\sigma_\xi) & \cdots & \Sigma^{(*\cdot)}_{(i,1t)}(\beta,\gamma,\sigma_\xi) & \cdots & \Sigma^{(*\cdot)}_{(i,1T)}(\beta,\gamma,\sigma_\xi) \\ \vdots & & \vdots & & \vdots \\ \Sigma^{(*\cdot)}_{(i,t1)}(\beta,\gamma,\sigma_\xi) & \cdots & \Sigma^{(*\cdot)}_{(i,tt)}(\beta,\gamma,\sigma_\xi) & \cdots & \Sigma^{(*\cdot)}_{(i,tT)}(\beta,\gamma,\sigma_\xi) \\ \vdots & & \vdots & & \vdots \\ \Sigma^{(*\cdot)}_{(i,T1)}(\beta,\gamma,\sigma_\xi) & \cdots & \Sigma^{(*\cdot)}_{(i,Tt)}(\beta,\gamma,\sigma_\xi) & \cdots & \Sigma^{(*\cdot)}_{(i,TT)}(\beta,\gamma,\sigma_\xi) \end{pmatrix}, \quad (6.40)$$

with block diagonal variance matrices as in (6.17) and off-diagonal covariance matrices as in (6.19). Note that

$$\Sigma^{(*\cdot)}_{(i,tu)}(\beta,\gamma,\sigma_\xi) = \Sigma^{(*\cdot)'}_{(i,ut)}(\beta,\gamma,\sigma_\xi), \text{ for } u < t.$$

Similarly,

$$\mathrm{var}(Z_i) = \mathrm{var}\begin{pmatrix} Z_{i1} \\ \vdots \\ Z_{it} \\ \vdots \\ Z_{iT} \end{pmatrix} : (R-1)T \times (R-1)T$$

$$= \begin{pmatrix} \mathrm{var}[Z_{i1}] & \cdots & \mathrm{cov}[Z_{i1}, Z'_{it}] & \cdots & \mathrm{cov}[Z_{i1}, Z'_{iT}] \\ \vdots & & \vdots & & \vdots \\ \mathrm{cov}[Z_{it}, Z'_{i1}] & \cdots & \mathrm{var}[Z_{it}] & \cdots & \mathrm{cov}[Z_{it}, Z'_{iT}] \\ \vdots & & \vdots & & \vdots \\ \mathrm{cov}[Z_{iT}, Z'_{i1}] & \cdots & \mathrm{cov}[Z_{iT}, Z'_{it}] & \cdots & \mathrm{var}[Z_{iT}] \end{pmatrix}$$

$$= \begin{pmatrix} \Sigma^{(\cdot*)}_{(i,11)}(\alpha,\lambda,\sigma_\xi) & \cdots & \Sigma^{(\cdot*)}_{(i,1t)}(\alpha,\lambda,\sigma_\xi) & \cdots & \Sigma^{(\cdot*)}_{(i,1T)}(\alpha,\lambda,\sigma_\xi) \\ \vdots & & \vdots & & \vdots \\ \Sigma^{(\cdot*)}_{(i,t1)}(\alpha,\lambda,\sigma_\xi) & \cdots & \Sigma^{(\cdot*)}_{(i,tt)}(\alpha,\lambda,\sigma_\xi) & \cdots & \Sigma^{(\cdot*)}_{(i,tT)}(\alpha,\lambda,\sigma_\xi) \\ \vdots & & \vdots & & \vdots \\ \Sigma^{(\cdot*)}_{(i,T1)}(\alpha,\lambda,\sigma_\xi) & \cdots & \Sigma^{(\cdot*)}_{(i,Tt)}(\alpha,\lambda,\sigma_\xi) & \cdots & \Sigma^{(\cdot*)}_{(i,TT)}(\alpha,\lambda,\sigma_\xi) \end{pmatrix}, \quad (6.41)$$

with block diagonal variance matrices as in (6.27) and off-diagonal covariance matrices as in (6.29). Note that

$$\Sigma^{(\cdot*)}_{(i,tu)}(\alpha,\lambda,\sigma_\xi) = \Sigma^{(\cdot*)}_{(i,ut)}(\alpha,\lambda,\sigma_\xi), \text{ for } u < t.$$

We now compute the formula for $\mathrm{cov}[Y_i, Z'_i]$ as follows.

$$\mathrm{cov}(Y_i, Z'_i) = \mathrm{cov}\left[\begin{pmatrix} Y_{i1} \\ \vdots \\ Y_{iu} \\ \vdots \\ Y_{it} \\ \vdots \\ Y_{iT} \end{pmatrix}, \begin{pmatrix} Z'_{i1} & \cdots & Z'_{iu} & \cdots & Z'_{it} & \cdots & Z'_{iT} \end{pmatrix}\right] : (J-1)T \times (R-1)T$$

$$= \begin{pmatrix} \text{cov}[Y_{i1}, Z'_{i1}] & \cdots & \text{cov}[Y_{i1}, Z'_{iu}] & \cdots & \text{cov}[Y_{i1}, Z'_{it}] & \cdots & \text{cov}[Y_{i1}, Z'_{iT}] \\ \vdots & & \vdots & & \vdots & & \vdots \\ \text{cov}[Y_{iu}, Z'_{i1}] & \cdots & \text{cov}[Y_{iu}, Z'_{iu}] & \cdots & \text{cov}[Y_{iu}, Z'_{it}] & \cdots & \text{cov}[Y_{iu}, Z'_{iT}] \\ \vdots & & \vdots & & \vdots & & \vdots \\ \text{cov}[Y_{it}, Z'_{i1}] & \cdots & \text{cov}[Y_{it}, Z'_{iu}] & \cdots & \text{cov}[Y_{it}, Z'_{it}] & \cdots & \text{cov}[Y_{it}, Z'_{iT}] \\ \vdots & & \vdots & & \vdots & & \vdots \\ \text{cov}[Y_{iT}, Z'_{i1}] & \cdots & \text{cov}[Y_{iT}, Z'_{iu}] & \cdots & \text{cov}[Y_{iT}, Z'_{it}] & \cdots & \text{cov}[Y_{iT}, Z'_{iT}] \end{pmatrix}$$

$$= \begin{pmatrix} \Sigma^{(**)}_{(i,11)}(\mu,\gamma,\lambda,\sigma_\xi) & \cdots & \Sigma^{(**)}_{(i,1u)}(\mu,\gamma,\lambda,\sigma_\xi) & \cdots & \Sigma^{(**)}_{(i,1t)}(\mu,\gamma,\lambda,\sigma_\xi) & \cdots & \Sigma^{(**)}_{(i,1T)}(\mu,\gamma,\lambda,\sigma_\xi) \\ \vdots & & \vdots & & \vdots & & \vdots \\ \Sigma^{(**)}_{(i,u1)}(\mu,\gamma,\lambda,\sigma_\xi) & \cdots & \Sigma^{(**)}_{(i,uu)}(\mu,\gamma,\lambda,\sigma_\xi) & \cdots & \Sigma^{(**)}_{(i,ut)}(\mu,\gamma,\lambda,\sigma_\xi) & \cdots & \Sigma^{(**)}_{(i,uT)}(\mu,\gamma,\lambda,\sigma_\xi) \\ \vdots & & \vdots & & \vdots & & \vdots \\ \Sigma^{(**)}_{(i,t1)}(\mu,\gamma,\lambda,\sigma_\xi) & \cdots & \Sigma^{(**)}_{(i,tu)}(\mu,\gamma,\lambda,\sigma_\xi) & \cdots & \Sigma^{(**)}_{(i,tt)}(\mu,\gamma,\lambda,\sigma_\xi) & \cdots & \Sigma^{(**)}_{(i,tT)}(\mu,\gamma,\lambda,\sigma_\xi) \\ \vdots & & \vdots & & \vdots & & \vdots \\ \Sigma^{(**)}_{(i,T1)}(\mu,\gamma,\lambda,\sigma_\xi) & \cdots & \Sigma^{(**)}_{(i,Tu)}(\mu,\gamma,\lambda,\sigma_\xi) & \cdots & \Sigma^{(**)}_{(i,Tt)}(\mu,\gamma,\lambda,\sigma_\xi) & \cdots & \Sigma^{(**)}_{(i,TT)}(\mu,\gamma,\lambda,\sigma_\xi) \end{pmatrix}, \quad (6.42)$$

with formulas for $\Sigma^{(**)}_{(i,tt)}(\mu,\gamma,\lambda,\sigma_\xi)$ as given by (6.30) for $t = 1,\ldots,T$, and the formulas for $\Sigma^{(**)}_{(i,ut)}(\mu,\gamma,\lambda,\sigma_\xi)$ as given by (6.31) for $u \neq t$.

6.3.1.2 Computation of the Derivative Matrix $\frac{\partial(\pi^{(*\cdot)'}_{(i)}(\beta,\gamma,\sigma_\xi),\pi^{(\cdot*)'}_{(i)}(\alpha,\lambda,\sigma_\xi))}{\partial\mu}$: $\{(J-1)(p+1)+(R-1)(q+1)\} \times \{(J-1)+(R-1)\}T$

Because $\mu = (\beta', \alpha')'$, the desired derivative matrix may be expressed as follows:

$$\frac{\partial(\pi^{(*\cdot)'}_{(i)}(\beta,\gamma,\sigma_\xi),\pi^{(\cdot*)'}_{(i)}(\alpha,\lambda,\sigma_\xi))}{\partial\mu} = \begin{pmatrix} \frac{\partial\pi^{(*\cdot)'}_{(i)}(\beta,\gamma,\sigma_\xi)}{\partial\beta} & \frac{\partial\pi^{(\cdot*)'}_{(i)}(\alpha,\lambda,\sigma_\xi)}{\partial\beta} \\ \frac{\partial\pi^{(*\cdot)'}_{(i)}(\beta,\gamma,\sigma_\xi)}{\partial\alpha} & \frac{\partial\pi^{(\cdot*)'}_{(i)}(\alpha,\lambda,\sigma_\xi)}{\partial\alpha} \end{pmatrix} = \begin{pmatrix} \frac{\partial\pi^{(*\cdot)'}_{(i)}(\beta,\gamma,\sigma_\xi)}{\partial\beta} & 0 \\ 0 & \frac{\partial\pi^{(\cdot*)'}_{(i)}(\alpha,\lambda,\sigma_\xi)}{\partial\alpha} \end{pmatrix}. \quad (6.43)$$

6.3.1.2 (a) Computation of the Derivative Matrix $\frac{\partial(\pi^{(*\cdot)'}_{(i)}(\beta,\gamma,\sigma_\xi)}{\partial\beta}$: $\{(J-1)(p+1)\} \times (J-1)T$

By (6.35) and (6.37), one may write

$$\frac{\partial \pi^{(*\cdot)'}_{(i)}(\beta,\gamma,\sigma_\xi)}{\partial \beta}$$
$$= [\frac{\partial \pi^{(*\cdot)'}_{(i1)}(\cdot)}{\partial \beta},\ldots,\frac{\partial \pi^{(*\cdot)'}_{(it)}(\cdot)}{\partial \beta},\ldots,\frac{\partial \pi^{(*\cdot)'}_{(iT)}(\cdot)}{\partial \beta}] : (J-1)(p+1)\times(J-1)T, \quad (6.44)$$

with

$$\frac{\partial \pi^{(*\cdot)'}_{(it)}(\cdot)}{\partial \beta} = [\frac{\partial \pi^{(1\cdot)}_{(it)}(\beta,\gamma,\sigma_\xi)}{\partial \beta},\ldots,\frac{\partial \pi^{(j\cdot)}_{(it)}(\beta,\gamma,\sigma_\xi)}{\partial \beta},\ldots,\frac{\partial \pi^{((J-1)\cdot)}_{(it)}(\beta,\gamma,\sigma_\xi)}{\partial \beta}], \quad (6.45)$$

where

$$\frac{\partial \pi^{(j\cdot)}_{(it)}(\beta,\gamma,\sigma_\xi)}{\partial \beta} = \int_{-\infty}^{\infty} \frac{\partial \pi^{*(j\cdot)}_{(it)}(\beta,\gamma,\sigma_\xi|\xi_i)}{\partial \beta} f_N(\xi_i)d\xi_i.$$

However, by applying (6.15)–(6.16) and (6.10), one may directly compute the derivative matrix in (6.44) as

$$\frac{\partial \pi^{(*\cdot)}_{(it)}(\cdot)'}{\partial \beta} = \begin{cases} \int_{-\infty}^{\infty} \frac{\partial \pi^{*'}_{(i1)*\cdot}(\beta,\sigma_\xi|\xi_i)}{\partial\beta} f_N(\xi_i)d\xi_i & \text{for } t=1, \\ \int_{-\infty}^{\infty} \frac{\partial \pi^{*(*\cdot)'}_{(it)}(\beta,\gamma,\sigma_\xi|\xi_i)}{\partial\beta} f_N(\xi_i)d\xi_i & \text{for } t=2,\ldots,T, \end{cases}$$
$$= \begin{cases} \int_{-\infty}^{\infty} \frac{\partial[\pi^*_{(i1)1\cdot},\ldots,\pi^*_{(i1)j\cdot},\ldots,\pi^*_{(i1)(J-1)\cdot}]}{\partial\beta} f_N(\xi_i)d\xi_i & \text{for } t=1, \\ \int_{-\infty}^{\infty} \frac{\partial}{\partial\beta}\Big[\eta^{*(*\cdot)}_{(it|t-1)}(J) + [\eta^{*(*\cdot)}_{(it|t-1),M} - \eta^{*(*\cdot)}_{(it|t-1)}(J)1'_{J-1}] \\ \pi^{*(*\cdot)}_{(i,t-1)}(\beta,\gamma,\sigma_\xi|\xi_i)\Big]' f_N(\xi_i)d\xi_i & \text{for } t=2,\ldots,T, \end{cases}$$
$$= \begin{cases} \int_{-\infty}^{\infty} \frac{\partial[\pi^*_{(i1)1\cdot},\ldots,\pi^*_{(i1)j\cdot},\ldots,\pi^*_{(i1)(J-1)\cdot}]}{\partial\beta} f_N(\xi_i)d\xi_i & \text{for } t=1, \\ \int_{-\infty}^{\infty} \frac{\partial}{\partial\beta}\Big[\eta^{*(*\cdot)'}_{(it|t-1)}(J) + \pi^{*(*\cdot)'}_{(i,t-1)}(\beta,\gamma,\sigma_\xi|\xi_i) \\ [\eta^{*(*\cdot)'}_{(it|t-1),M} - 1_{J-1}\eta^{*(*\cdot)'}_{(it|t-1)}(J)]\Big] f_N(\xi_i)d\xi_i & \text{for } t=2,\ldots,T, \end{cases} \quad (6.46)$$

Now the computation of the derivative in (6.46) can be completed by computing

$$\frac{\partial \pi^{*'}_{(i1)*\cdot}(\beta,\sigma_\xi|\xi_i)}{\partial \beta} = \frac{\partial[\pi^*_{(i1)1\cdot},\ldots,\pi^*_{(i1)j\cdot},\ldots,\pi^*_{(i1)(J-1)\cdot}]}{\partial \beta}, \text{ and} \quad (6.47)$$

$$\frac{\partial \pi^{*(*\cdot)'}_{(it)}(\beta,\gamma,\sigma_\xi|\xi_i)}{\partial \beta} = \frac{\partial}{\partial \beta}\left[\eta^{*(*\cdot)'}_{(it|t-1)}(J) + \pi^{*(*\cdot)'}_{(i,t-1)}(\beta,\gamma,\sigma_\xi|\xi_i) \times \left[\eta^{*(*\cdot)'}_{(it|t-1),M} - 1_{J-1}\eta^{*(*\cdot)'}_{(it|t-1)}(J)\right]\right], \text{ for } t=2,\ldots,T, \quad (6.48)$$

where, in (6.48), we treat

$$\pi^{*(*\cdot)'}_{(i1)}(\beta,\gamma,\sigma_\xi|\xi_i) \equiv \pi^{*(*\cdot)'}_{(i1)}(\beta,\gamma=0,\sigma_\xi|\xi_i) \equiv \pi^{*'}_{(i1)*\cdot}(\beta,\sigma_\xi|\xi_i).$$

Notice that to compute the derivative in (6.47), it is sufficient to compute $\frac{\partial \pi^*_{(i1)j\cdot}}{\partial \beta}$ and using back the results for all $j=1,\ldots,J-1$, in (6.47). Because $\beta = [\beta_1^{*'},\ldots,\beta_j^{*'},\ldots,\beta_{J-1}^{*'}]'$, by similar calculations as in (6.38), this derivative is given by

$$\begin{aligned}
\frac{\partial \pi^*_{(i1)j\cdot}}{\partial \beta} &= \frac{\partial}{\partial \beta}\left[\frac{\exp(w^{*'}_{i1}\beta^*_j + \sigma_\xi \xi_i)}{1+\sum_{g=1}^{J-1}\exp(w^{*'}_{i1}\beta^*_g + \sigma_\xi\xi_i)}\right], \text{ for } j=1,\ldots,J-1 \\
&= \begin{pmatrix} -\pi^*_{(i1)1\cdot}\pi^*_{(i1)j\cdot} \\ \vdots \\ \pi^*_{(i1)j\cdot}[1-\pi^*_{(i1)j\cdot}] \\ \vdots \\ -\pi^*_{(i1)(J-1)\cdot}\pi^*_{(i1)j\cdot} \end{pmatrix} \otimes w^*_{i1} : (J-1)(p+1)\times 1 \\
&= \left[\pi^*_{(i1)j\cdot}(\delta_j - \pi^*_{(i1)*\cdot})\right] \otimes w^*_{i1},
\end{aligned} \quad (6.49)$$

with $\delta_j = [01'_{j-1}, 1, 01'_{J-1-j}]'$ for $j=1,\ldots,J-1$. Thus,

$$\frac{\partial \pi^{*'}_{(i1)*\cdot}(\beta,\sigma_\xi|\xi_i)}{\partial \beta} = \Sigma^{*(*\cdot)}_{(i,11)}(\beta,\gamma,\sigma_\xi|\xi_i) \otimes w^*_{i1} : (J-1)(p+1)\times(J-1), \quad (6.50)$$

where

$$\Sigma^{*(*\cdot)}_{(i,11)}(\beta,\sigma_\xi|\xi_i) = \text{diag}[\pi^*_{(i1)1\cdot},\ldots,\pi^*_{(i1)j\cdot},\ldots,\pi^*_{(i1)(J-1)\cdot}] - \pi^*_{(i1)*\cdot}\pi^{*'}_{(i1)*\cdot},$$

yielding the derivative in (6.47).

We now compute the derivative matrices in (6.48) for all other $t=2,\ldots,T$. First we simplify (6.48) as

$$\frac{\partial \pi^{*(*\cdot)'}_{(it)}(\beta,\gamma,\sigma_\xi|\xi_i)}{\partial \beta} = \frac{\partial}{\partial \beta}\left[\eta^{*(*\cdot)'}_{(it|t-1)}(J)\right] + \frac{\partial}{\partial \beta}\left[\pi^{*(*\cdot)'}_{(i,t-1)}(\beta,\gamma,\sigma_\xi|\xi_i)\right]\left\{\eta^{*(*\cdot)'}_{(it|t-1),M} - 1_{J-1}\eta^{*(*\cdot)'}_{(it|t-1)}(J)\right\}$$

$$+\ \pi^{*(*\cdot)'}_{(i,t-1)}(\beta,\gamma,\sigma_\xi|\xi_i)\frac{\partial}{\partial \beta}\left[\eta^{*(*\cdot)'}_{(it|t-1),M} - 1_{J-1}\eta^{*(*\cdot)'}_{(it|t-1)}(J)\right]. \tag{6.51}$$

Notice that $\frac{\partial}{\partial \beta}\left[\pi^{*(*\cdot)'}_{(i,t-1)}(\beta,\gamma,\sigma_\xi|\xi_i)\right]$ in the second term in (6.51) is available recursive way. For $t=2$, the formula for $\frac{\partial}{\partial \beta}\left[\pi^{*(*\cdot)'}_{(i1)}(\beta,\gamma=0,\sigma_\xi|\xi_i)\right]$ is the same as in (6.50). Thus, to compute the formula in (6.51), we compute the first term as

$$\frac{\partial}{\partial \beta}\left[\eta^{*(*\cdot)'}_{(it|t-1)}(J)\right] = \frac{\partial}{\partial \beta}[\eta^{*(1\cdot)}_{(it|t-1)}(J),\ldots,\eta^{*(j\cdot)}_{(it|t-1)}(J),\ldots,\eta^{*((J-1)\cdot)}_{(it|t-1)}(J)]$$

$$= [\frac{\partial \eta^{*(1\cdot)}_{(it|t-1)}(J)}{\partial \beta},\ldots,\frac{\partial \eta^{*(j\cdot)}_{(it|t-1)}(J)}{\partial \beta},\ldots,\frac{\partial \eta^{*((J-1)\cdot)}_{(it|t-1)}(J)}{\partial \beta}]. \tag{6.52}$$

Next because for known category $g(g=1,\ldots,J)$ from the past,

$$\eta^{*(j\cdot)}_{it|t-1}(g) = P\left(Y_{it}=y^{(j)}_{it}\,\Big|\,Y_{i,t-1}=y^{(g)}_{i,t-1},\xi_i\right)$$

$$= \begin{cases} \frac{\exp\left[w^{*'}_{it}\beta^*_j+\gamma'_j y^{(g)}_{i,t-1}+\sigma_\xi\xi_i\right]}{1+\sum_{v=1}^{J-1}\exp\left[w^{*'}_{it}\beta^*_v+\gamma'_v y^{(g)}_{i,t-1}+\sigma_\xi\xi_i\right]}, & \text{for } j=1,\ldots,J-1 \\ \frac{1}{1+\sum_{v=1}^{J-1}\exp\left[w^{*'}_{it}\beta^*_v+\gamma'_v y^{(g)}_{i,t-1}+\sigma_\xi\xi_i\right]}, & \text{for } j=J, \end{cases} \tag{6.53}$$

for $t=2,\ldots,T$, by (6.7), it then follows that

$$\frac{\partial \eta^{*(j\cdot)}_{(it|t-1)}(g)}{\partial \beta} = \begin{pmatrix} -\eta^{*(1\cdot)}_{it|t-1}(g)\eta^{*(j\cdot)}_{it|t-1}(g) \\ \vdots \\ \eta^{*(j\cdot)}_{it|t-1}(g)[1-\eta^{*(j\cdot)}_{it|t-1}(g)] \\ \vdots \\ -\eta^{*((J-1)\cdot)}_{it|t-1}(g)\eta^{*(j\cdot)}_{it|t-1}(g) \end{pmatrix} \otimes w^*_{it} : (J-1)(p+1)\times 1$$

$$= \left[\eta^{*(j\cdot)}_{it|t-1}(g)(\delta_{(i,t-1)j}-\eta^{*(*\cdot)}_{it|t-1}(g))\right]\otimes w^*_{it}, \tag{6.54}$$

where

$$\delta_{(i,t-1)j} = [01'_{j-1},1,01'_{J-1-j}]'$$

$$\eta^{*(*\cdot)}_{it|t-1}(g) = [\eta^{*(1\cdot)}_{it|t-1}(g),\ldots,\eta^{*(j\cdot)}_{it|t-1}(g),\ldots,\eta^{*((J-1)\cdot)}_{it|t-1}(g)]'.$$

Hence by using (6.54) into (6.52), one obtains

$$\frac{\partial}{\partial \beta}\left[\eta^{*(*\cdot)'}_{(it|t-1)}(J)\right]$$
$$= \begin{pmatrix} \eta^{*(1\cdot)}_{it|t-1}(J)[1-\eta^{*(1\cdot)}_{it|t-1}(J)] \cdots & -\eta^{*(1\cdot)}_{it|t-1}(J)\eta^{*(j\cdot)}_{it|t-1}(J) & \cdots & -\eta^{*(1\cdot)}_{it|t-1}(J)\eta^{*((J-1)\cdot)}_{it|t-1}(J) \\ \vdots & \cdots \quad \vdots & \cdots & \vdots \\ -\eta^{*(j\cdot)}_{it|t-1}(J)\eta^{*(1\cdot)}_{it|t-1}(J) & \cdots -\eta^{*(j\cdot)}_{it|t-1}(J)[1-\eta^{*(j\cdot)}_{it|t-1}(J)] & \cdots & -\eta^{*(j\cdot)}_{it|t-1}(J)\eta^{*((J-1)\cdot)}_{it|t-1}(J) \\ \vdots & \cdots \quad \vdots & \cdots & \vdots \\ -\eta^{*(1\cdot)}_{it|t-1}(J)\eta^{*((J-1)\cdot)}_{it|t-1}(J) \cdots & -\eta^{*((J-1)\cdot)}_{it|t-1}(J)\eta^{*(j\cdot)}_{it|t-1}(J) & \cdots & \eta^{*((J-1)\cdot)}_{it|t-1}(J)[1-\eta^{*((J-1)\cdot)}_{it|t-1}(J)] \end{pmatrix}$$
$$\otimes\, w^*_{it}. \tag{6.55}$$

Now compute the third term in (6.51) as follows. First, re-express $\eta^{*(*\cdot)'}_{(it|t-1),M}$ matrix as

$$\eta^{*(*\cdot)'}_{(it|t-1),M}$$
$$= \begin{pmatrix} \eta^{*(1\cdot)}_{(it|t-1)}(1) & \cdots & \eta^{*(1\cdot)}_{(it|t-1)}(g) & \cdots & \eta^{*(1\cdot)}_{(it|t-1)}(J-1) \\ \vdots & \vdots & \vdots & \vdots & \vdots \\ \eta^{*(j\cdot)}_{(it|t-1)}(1) & \cdots & \eta^{*(j\cdot)}_{(it|t-1)}(g) & \cdots & \eta^{*(j\cdot)}_{(it|t-1)}(J-1) \\ \vdots & \vdots & \vdots & \vdots & \vdots \\ \eta^{*((J-1)\cdot)}_{(it|t-1)}(1) & \cdots & \eta^{*((J-1)\cdot)}_{(it|t-1)}(g) & \cdots & \eta^{*((J-1)\cdot)}_{(it|t-1)}(J-1) \end{pmatrix}' : (J-1)\times(J-1)$$
$$= \left(b_1 \cdots b_j \cdots b_{J-1}\right), \tag{6.56}$$

and the $1_{J-1}\eta^{*(*\cdot)'}_{(it|t-1)}(J)$ matrix as

$$1_{J-1}\eta^{*(*\cdot)'}_{(it|t-1)}(J) = \left(1_{J-1}\eta^{*(1\cdot)}_{(it|t-1)}(J) \cdots 1_{J-1}\eta^{*(j\cdot)}_{(it|t-1)}(J) \cdots 1_{J-1}\eta^{*((J-1)\cdot)}_{(it|t-1)}(J)\right)$$
$$= \left(f_1 \cdots f_j \cdots f_{J-1}\right). \tag{6.57}$$

The third term in (6.51) may then be written as

$$\pi^{*(*\cdot)'}_{(i,t-1)}(\beta,\gamma,\sigma_\xi|\xi_i)\frac{\partial}{\partial\beta}\left[\eta^{*(*\cdot)'}_{(it|t-1),M} - 1_J\eta^{*(*\cdot)'}_{(it|t-1)}(J)\right]$$
$$= \left(\frac{\partial b'_1}{\partial\beta}\pi^{*(*\cdot)}_{(i,t-1)}(\beta,\gamma,\sigma_\xi|\xi_i) \cdots \frac{\partial b'_j}{\partial\beta}\pi^{*(*\cdot)}_{(i,t-1)}(\beta,\gamma,\sigma_\xi|\xi_i) \cdots \frac{\partial b'_{J-1}}{\partial\beta}\pi^{*(*\cdot)}_{(i,t-1)}(\beta,\gamma,\sigma_\xi|\xi_i)\right)$$
$$- \left(\frac{\partial f'_1}{\partial\beta}\pi^{*(*\cdot)}_{(i,t-1)}(\beta,\gamma,\sigma_\xi|\xi_i) \cdots \frac{\partial f'_j}{\partial\beta}\pi^{*(*\cdot)}_{(i,t-1)}(\beta,\gamma,\sigma_\xi|\xi_i) \cdots \frac{\partial f'_{J-1}}{\partial\beta}\pi^{*(*\cdot)}_{(i,t-1)}(\beta,\gamma,\sigma_\xi|\xi_i)\right)$$

$$= \left(\frac{\partial b_1'}{\partial \beta} \cdots \frac{\partial b_j'}{\partial \beta} \cdots \frac{\partial b_{J-1}'}{\partial \beta}\right)[I_{J-1} \otimes \pi^{*(*\cdot)}_{(i,t-1)}(\beta,\gamma,\sigma_\xi|\xi_i)]$$
$$- \left(\frac{\partial f_1'}{\partial \beta} \cdots \frac{\partial f_j'}{\partial \beta} \cdots \frac{\partial f_{J-1}'}{\partial \beta}\right)[I_{J-1} \otimes \pi^{*(*\cdot)}_{(i,t-1)}(\beta,\gamma,\sigma_\xi|\xi_i)], \quad (6.58)$$

where

$$\frac{\partial b_j'}{\partial \beta} = \frac{\partial}{\partial \beta}\left(\eta^{*(j\cdot)}_{(it|t-1)}(1) \cdots \eta^{*(j\cdot)}_{(it|t-1)}(g) \cdots \eta^{*(j\cdot)}_{(it|t-1)}(J-1)\right)$$
$$= \left[\left\{\eta^{*(j\cdot)}_{it|t-1}(1)(\delta_{(i,t-1)j} - \eta^{*(*\cdot)}_{it|t-1}(1))\right\} \otimes w^*_{it}, \ldots, \left\{\eta^{*(j\cdot)}_{it|t-1}(g)(\delta_{(i,t-1)j} - \eta^{*(*\cdot)}_{it|t-1}(g))\right\} \otimes w^*_{it},\right.$$
$$\left.\ldots, \left\{\eta^{*(j\cdot)}_{it|t-1}(J-1)(\delta_{(i,t-1)j} - \eta^{*(*\cdot)}_{it|t-1}(J-1))\right\} \otimes w^*_{it}\right] : (J-1)(p+1) \times (J-1), \quad (6.59)$$

and

$$\frac{\partial f_j'}{\partial \beta} = \frac{\partial}{\partial \beta}[1'_{J-1}\eta^{*(j\cdot)}_{(it|t-1)}(J)]$$
$$= 1'_{J-1} \otimes \left[\left\{\eta^{*(j\cdot)}_{it|t-1}(J)(\delta_{(i,t-1)j} - \eta^{*(*\cdot)}_{it|t-1}(J))\right\} \otimes w^*_{it}\right]. \quad (6.60)$$

6.3.1.2 (b) Computation of the Derivative Matrix $\frac{\partial \pi^{(\cdot *)'}_{(i)}(\alpha,\lambda,\sigma_\xi)}{\partial \alpha}$: $\{(R-1)(q+1)\} \times (R-1)T$

The computation of this derivative matrix corresponding to z response variable is quite similar to that of $\frac{\partial(\pi^{(*\cdot)'}_{(i)}(\beta,\gamma,\sigma_\xi)}{\partial \beta}$ given in Sect. 6.3.1.2(a) corresponding to the y variable. For simplicity, we provide the formulas only without showing background derivations. To be specific,

$$\frac{\partial \pi^{(\cdot *)'}_{(i)}(\alpha,\lambda,\sigma_\xi)}{\partial \alpha}$$
$$= [\frac{\partial \pi^{(\cdot *)'}_{(i1)}(\cdot)}{\partial \alpha}, \ldots, \frac{\partial \pi^{(\cdot *)'}_{(it)}(\cdot)}{\partial \alpha}, \ldots, \frac{\partial \pi^{(\cdot *)'}_{(iT)}(\cdot)}{\partial \alpha}] : (R-1)(q+1) \times (R-1)T, \quad (6.61)$$

with

$$\frac{\partial \pi^{(\cdot *)'}_{(it)}(\cdot)}{\partial \alpha} = \int_{-\infty}^{\infty} [\frac{\partial \pi^{(\cdot 1)}_{(it)}(\alpha,\lambda,\sigma_\xi|\xi_i)}{\partial \alpha}, \ldots, \frac{\partial \pi^{(\cdot r)}_{(it)}(\alpha,\lambda,\sigma_\xi|\xi_i)}{\partial \alpha},$$

$$\ldots, \frac{\partial \pi^{(\cdot(R-1))}_{(it)}(\alpha,\lambda,\sigma_\xi|\xi_i)}{\partial \alpha}] f_N(\xi_i)d\xi_i \tag{6.62}$$

$$= \begin{cases} \int_{-\infty}^{\infty} \frac{\partial [\pi^*_{(i1)\cdot 1},\ldots,\pi^*_{(i1)\cdot r},\ldots,\pi^*_{(i1)\cdot(R-1)}]}{\partial \alpha} f_N(\xi_i)d\xi_i & \text{for } t=1, \\ \int_{-\infty}^{\infty} \frac{\partial}{\partial \alpha}\Big[\eta^{*(\cdot *)'}_{(it|t-1)}(R) + \pi^{*(\cdot *)'}_{(i,t-1)}(\alpha,\lambda,\sigma_\xi|\xi_i) & \\ [\eta^{*(\cdot *)'}_{(it|t-1),M} - 1_{R-1}\eta^{*(\cdot *)'}_{(it|t-1)}(R)]\Big] f_N(\xi_i)d\xi_i & \text{for } t=2,\ldots,T \end{cases} \tag{6.63}$$

$$= \begin{cases} \int_{-\infty}^{\infty} [\Sigma^{*(\cdot *)}_{(i,11)}(\alpha,\lambda,\sigma_\xi|\xi_i)\otimes w^*_{i1}] f_N(\xi_i)d\xi_i & \text{for } t=1, \\ \int_{-\infty}^{\infty} \Big[\frac{\partial}{\partial \alpha}\Big\{\eta^{*(\cdot *)'}_{(it|t-1)}(R)\Big\} + \frac{\partial}{\partial \alpha}\Big\{\pi^{*(\cdot *)'}_{(i,t-1)}(\alpha,\lambda,\sigma_\xi|\xi_i)\Big\} & \\ \times\Big\{\eta^{*(\cdot *)'}_{(it|t-1),M} - 1_{R-1}\eta^{*(\cdot *)'}_{(it|t-1)}(R)\Big\} + \pi^{*(\cdot *)'}_{(i,t-1)}(\alpha,\lambda,\sigma_\xi|\xi_i) & \\ \times \frac{\partial}{\partial \alpha}\Big\{\eta^{*(\cdot *)'}_{(it|t-1),M} - 1_{R-1}\eta^{*(\cdot *)'}_{(it|t-1)}(R)\Big\}\Big] f_N(\xi_i)d\xi_i & \text{for } t=2,\ldots,T \end{cases} \tag{6.64}$$

$$= \begin{cases} \int_{-\infty}^{\infty} \frac{\partial}{\partial \alpha}\Big\{\pi^{*(\cdot *)'}_{(i1)}(\alpha,\lambda,\sigma_\xi|\xi_i)\Big\} f_N(\xi_i)d\xi_i \text{ for } t=1, \\ \int_{-\infty}^{\infty} \frac{\partial}{\partial \alpha}\Big\{\pi^{*(\cdot *)'}_{(it)}(\alpha,\lambda,\sigma_\xi|\xi_i)\Big\} f_N(\xi_i)d\xi_i \text{ for } t=2,\ldots,T. \end{cases} \tag{6.65}$$

In (6.64),

$\Sigma^{*(\cdot *)}_{(i,11)}(\alpha,\sigma_\xi|\xi_i) = \text{diag}[\pi^*_{(i1)\cdot 1},\ldots,\pi^*_{(i1)\cdot r},\ldots,\pi^*_{(i1)\cdot(R-1)}] - \pi^*_{(i1)\cdot *}\pi^{*'}_{(i1)\cdot *}$, and

$$\frac{\partial}{\partial \alpha}\Big[\eta^{*(\cdot *)'}_{(it|t-1)}(R)\Big]$$

$$= \begin{pmatrix} \eta^{*(\cdot 1)}_{it|t-1}(R)[1-\eta^{*(\cdot 1)}_{it|t-1}(R)] & \cdots & -\eta^{*(\cdot 1)}_{it|t-1}(R)\eta^{*(\cdot r)}_{it|t-1}(R) & \cdots & -\eta^{*(\cdot 1)}_{it|t-1}(R)\eta^{*(\cdot(R-1))}_{it|t-1}(R) \\ \vdots & \cdots & \vdots & \cdots & \vdots \\ -\eta^{*(\cdot r)}_{it|t-1}(R)\eta^{*(\cdot 1)}_{it|t-1}(R) & \cdots & -\eta^{*(\cdot r)}_{it|t-1}(R)[1-\eta^{*(\cdot r)}_{it|t-1}(R)] & \cdots & -\eta^{*(\cdot r)}_{it|t-1}(R)\eta^{*(\cdot(R-1))}_{it|t-1}(R) \\ \vdots & \cdots & \vdots & \cdots & \vdots \\ -\eta^{*(\cdot 1)}_{it|t-1}(r)\eta^{*(\cdot(R-1))}_{it|t-1}(R) & \cdots & -\eta^{*(\cdot(R-1))}_{it|t-1}(R)\eta^{*(\cdot r)}_{it|t-1}(R) & \cdots & \eta^{*(\cdot(R-1))}_{it|t-1}(R)[1-\eta^{*(\cdot(R-1))}_{it|t-1}(R)] \end{pmatrix}$$

$$\otimes w^*_{it}. \tag{6.66}$$

Notice that the first term in (6.64) is computed by (6.66). The second term in (6.64) is computed recursive way by comparing (6.64) with (6.65). It remains to compute the third term in (6.64) which is, similar to (6.58), given as

$$\pi^{*(\cdot *)'}_{(i,t-1)}(\alpha,\lambda,\sigma_\xi|\xi_i)\frac{\partial}{\partial \alpha}\Big[\eta^{*(\cdot *)'}_{(it|t-1),M} - 1_R\eta^{*(\cdot *)'}_{(it|t-1)}(R)\Big]$$
$$= \Big(\frac{\partial m'_1}{\partial \beta}\pi^{*(\cdot *)}_{(i,t-1)}(\alpha,\lambda,\sigma_\xi|\xi_i) \cdots \frac{\partial m'_r}{\partial \beta}\pi^{*(\cdot *)}_{(i,t-1)}(\alpha,\lambda,\sigma_\xi|\xi_i) \cdots \frac{\partial m'_{R-1}}{\partial \beta}\pi^{*(\cdot *)}_{(i,t-1)}(\alpha,\lambda,\sigma_\xi|\xi_i)\Big)$$
$$- \Big(\frac{\partial h'_1}{\partial \beta}\pi^{*(\cdot *)}_{(i,t-1)}(\alpha,\lambda,\sigma_\xi|\xi_i) \cdots \frac{\partial h'_r}{\partial \beta}\pi^{*(\cdot *)}_{(i,t-1)}(\alpha,\lambda,\sigma_\xi|\xi_i) \cdots \frac{\partial h'_{R-1}}{\partial \beta}\pi^{*(\cdot *)}_{(i,t-1)}(\alpha,\lambda,\sigma_\xi|\xi_i)\Big)$$

$$= \left(\frac{\partial m_1'}{\partial \alpha} \cdots \frac{\partial m_r'}{\partial \alpha} \cdots \frac{\partial m_{R-1}'}{\partial \alpha}\right) [I_{R-1} \otimes \pi^{*(\cdot *)}_{(i,t-1)}(\alpha, \lambda, \sigma_\xi|\xi_i)]$$
$$- \left(\frac{\partial h_1'}{\partial \alpha} \cdots \frac{\partial h_r'}{\partial \alpha} \cdots \frac{\partial h_{R-1}'}{\partial \alpha}\right) [I_{R-1} \otimes \pi^{*(\cdot *)}_{(i,t-1)}(\alpha, \lambda, \sigma_\xi|\xi_i)], \quad (6.67)$$

where

$$\frac{\partial m_r'}{\partial \alpha} = \frac{\partial}{\partial \alpha}\left(\eta^{*(\cdot r)}_{(it|t-1)}(1) \cdots \eta^{*(\cdot r)}_{(it|t-1)}(g) \cdots \eta^{*(\cdot r)}_{(it|t-1)}(R-1)\right)$$
$$= \left[\left\{\eta^{*(\cdot r)}_{it|t-1}(1)(\delta_{(i,t-1)r} - \eta^{*(\cdot *)}_{it|t-1}(1))\right\} \otimes w^*_{it}, \ldots, \left\{\eta^{*(\cdot r)}_{it|t-1}(g)(\delta_{(i,t-1)r} - \eta^{*(\cdot *)}_{it|t-1}(g))\right\} \otimes w^*_{it},\right.$$
$$\left.\ldots, \left\{\eta^{*(\cdot r)}_{it|t-1}(R-1)(\delta_{(i,t-1)r} - \eta^{*(\cdot *)}_{it|t-1}(R-1))\right\} \otimes w^*_{it}\right] : (R-1)(q+1) \times (R-1), \quad (6.68)$$

and

$$\frac{\partial h_r'}{\partial \alpha} = \frac{\partial}{\partial \alpha}[1'_{R-1}\eta^{*(\cdot r)}_{(it|t-1)}(R)]$$
$$= 1'_{R-1} \otimes \left[\left\{\eta^{*(\cdot r)}_{it|t-1}(R)(\delta_{(i,t-1)r} - \eta^{*(\cdot *)}_{it|t-1}(R))\right\} \otimes w^*_{it}\right]. \quad (6.69)$$

Thus the computation for the derivative matrix in the MGQL estimating equation (6.34) is completed.

6.3.1.3 MGQL Estimator and its Asymptotic Covariance Matrix

Because the covariance matrix $\Sigma_{(i)}(\cdot)$ and the derivative matrix $\frac{\partial}{\partial \mu}[\cdot]$ in (6.34) are known, for given values of $\gamma, \lambda, \sigma_\xi$, one may now solve the MGQL estimating equation (6.34) for the regression parameter μ. Let $\hat{\mu}_{MGQL}$ be the estimate, i.e., the solution of (6.34). This estimate may be obtained by using the iterative equation

$$\hat{\mu}(m+1) = \hat{\mu}(m) + \left[\left\{\sum_{i=1}^{K} \frac{\partial(\pi^{(*\cdot)'}_{(i)}(\beta, \gamma, \sigma_\xi), \pi^{(\cdot *)'}_{(i)}(\alpha, \lambda, \sigma_\xi))}{\partial \mu} \Sigma^{-1}_{(i)}(\mu, \gamma, \lambda, \sigma_\xi)\right.\right.$$
$$\left. \times \frac{\partial(\pi^{(*\cdot)}_{(i)}(\beta, \gamma, \sigma_\xi), \pi^{(\cdot *)}_{(i)}(\alpha, \lambda, \sigma_\xi)q)}{\partial \mu'}\right\}^{-1} \left\{\sum_{i=1}^{K} \frac{\partial(\pi^{(*\cdot)'}_{(i)}(\beta, \gamma, \sigma_\xi), \pi^{(\cdot *)'}_{(i)}(\alpha, \lambda, \sigma_\xi))}{\partial \mu}\right.$$
$$\left.\left. \times \Sigma^{-1}_{(i)}(\mu, \gamma, \lambda, \sigma_\xi)\begin{pmatrix} y_i - \pi^{(*\cdot)}_{(i)}(\beta, \gamma, \sigma_\xi) \\ z_i - \pi^{(\cdot *)}_{(i)}(\alpha, \lambda, \sigma_\xi)\end{pmatrix}\right\}\right]|_{\mu = \hat{\mu}(m)}. \quad (6.70)$$

Furthermore, it follows that the MGQL estimator, $\hat{\mu}_{MGQL}$, obtained from (6.70) has the asymptotic variance given by

$$\text{limit}_{K\to\infty}\text{var}[\hat{\mu}_{MGQL}] = \left\{\sum_{i=1}^{K}\frac{\partial(\pi_{(i)}^{(*\cdot)'}(\beta,\gamma,\sigma_\xi),\pi_{(i)}^{(\cdot *)'}(\alpha,\lambda,\sigma_\xi))}{\partial\mu}\Sigma_{(i)}^{-1}(\mu,\gamma,\lambda,\sigma_\xi)\right.$$
$$\left.\times\frac{\partial(\pi_{(i)}^{(*\cdot)}(\beta,\gamma,\sigma_\xi),\pi_{(i)}^{(\cdot *)}(\alpha,\lambda,\sigma_\xi)q)}{\partial\mu'}\right\}^{-1} \tag{6.71}$$

6.3.2 *Moment Estimation of Dynamic Dependence (Longitudinal Correlation Index) Parameters*

Estimation of γ:
Notice from (6.7) that $\gamma_j(j=1,\ldots,J-1)$ is the lag 1 dynamic dependence parameter relating $y_{it}^{(j)}$ and $y_{i,t-1}^{(g)}$ where g is a known category and ranges from 1 to J. Thus, it would be appropriate to exploit all lag 1 product responses to estimate this parameter. More specifically, for $t=2,\ldots,T$, following (6.19), we first write

$$\begin{aligned}E[Y_{i,t-1}Y_{it}'] &= \int_{-\infty}^{\infty}\left[\left\{\eta_{(it|t-1),M}^{*(*\cdot)}-\eta_{(it|t-1)}^{*(*\cdot)}(J)1_{J-1}'\right\}\text{var}[Y_{i,t-1}|\xi_i]\right]f_N(\xi_i)d\xi_i\\ &+\int_{-\infty}^{\infty}[\{\pi_{(i,t-1)}^{*(*\cdot)}(\beta,\gamma,\sigma_\xi|\xi_i)\}\{\pi_{(it)}^{*(*\cdot)}(\beta,\gamma,\sigma_\xi|\xi_i)'\}]f_N(\xi_i)d\xi_i\\ &=\int_{-\infty}^{\infty}[M_{i,(t-1)t}^{*}(\beta,\gamma,\sigma_\xi|\xi_i)]f_N(\xi_i)d\xi_i : (J-1)\times(J-1),\ \text{(say)}.\end{aligned} \tag{6.72}$$

One may then obtain the moment estimator of γ_j by solving the moment equation

$$\sum_{i=1}^{K}\sum_{t=2}^{T}\sum_{h=1}^{J-1}\sum_{k=1}^{J-1}\int_{-\infty}^{\infty}\left[\frac{\partial}{\partial\gamma_j}[m_{i,(t-1)t;h,k}^{*}(\beta,\gamma,\sigma_\xi|\xi_i)]\right.$$
$$\left.\times\ \{y_{i,t-1,h}y_{itk}-m_{i,(t-1)t;h,k}^{*}(\beta,\gamma,\sigma_\xi|\xi_i)\}\right]f_N(\xi_i)d\xi_i=0, \tag{6.73}$$

where $m_{i,(t-1)t;h,k}^{*}(\beta,\gamma,\sigma_\xi|\xi_i)$ is the (h,k)th element of the $M_{i,(t-1)t}^{*}(\beta,\gamma,\sigma_\xi|\xi_i)$ matrix of dimension $(J-1)\times(J-1)$, and $y_{i,t-1,h}$ and y_{itk} are, respectively, the hth and kth elements of the multinomial response vectors $y_{i,t-1}=(y_{i,t-1,1},\ldots,y_{i,t-1,h},\ldots,y_{i,t-1,J-1})'$ and $y_{it}=(y_{it1},\ldots,y_{itk},\ldots,y_{it,J-1})'$, of the ith individual. Next, in the spirit of iteration, by assuming that γ_j in $\frac{\partial}{\partial\gamma_j}[m_{i,(t-1)t;h,k}^{*}(\beta,\gamma,\sigma_\xi|\xi_i)$ is known from previous iteration, the moment equation (6.73) may be solved for γ_j by using the iterative equation

$$\hat{\gamma}_j(\ell+1) = \hat{\gamma}_j(\ell) + \left[\sum_{i=1}^{K}\sum_{t=2}^{T}\sum_{h=1}^{J-1}\sum_{k=1}^{J-1}\int_{-\infty}^{\infty}\left\{\frac{\partial}{\partial \gamma_j}[m^*_{i,(t-1)t;h,k}(\beta,\gamma,\sigma_\xi|\xi_i)]\right.\right.$$
$$\times \left.\left.\frac{\partial}{\partial \gamma'_j}[m^*_{i,(t-1)t;h,k}(\beta,\gamma,\sigma_\xi|\xi_i)]\right\} f_N(\xi_i)d\xi_i\right]^{-1} \sum_{i=1}^{K}\sum_{t=2}^{T}\sum_{h=1}^{J-1}\sum_{k=1}^{J-1}\int_{-\infty}^{\infty}\left[\frac{\partial}{\partial \gamma_j}[m^*_{i,(t-1)t;h,k}(\beta,\gamma,\sigma_\xi|\xi_i)]\right.$$
$$\times \left.\left.\{y_{i,t-1,h}y_{itk}-m^*_{i,(t-1)t;h,k}(\beta,\gamma,\sigma_\xi|\xi_i)\}\right] f_N(\xi_i)d\xi_i\right]_{\gamma_j=\hat{\gamma}_j(\ell)}. \quad (6.74)$$

Note that to compute the derivative of the elements of the matrix $M^*_{i,(t-1)t}(\beta,\gamma,\sigma_\xi|\xi_i)$ with respect to γ_j, i.e., to compute $\frac{\partial}{\partial \gamma'_j}[m^*_{i,(t-1)t;h,k}(\beta,\gamma,\sigma_\xi|\xi_i)]$ in (6.73)–(6.74), we provide the following derivatives as an aid:

$$\frac{\partial \pi^*_{(i1)h\cdot}}{\partial \gamma_j} = \frac{\partial}{\partial \gamma_j}\begin{cases}\frac{\exp(w^{*\prime}_{i1}\beta^*_h+\sigma_\xi\xi_i)}{1+\sum_{g=1}^{J-1}\exp(w^{*\prime}_{i1}\beta^*_g+\sigma_\xi\xi_i)} & \text{for } h=1,\ldots,J-1\\ \frac{1}{1+\sum_{g=1}^{J-1}\exp(w^{*\prime}_{i1}\beta^*_g+\sigma_\xi\xi_i)} & \text{for } h=J,\end{cases}$$
$$= \begin{cases}0 \text{ for } h=j; h,j=1,\ldots,J-1\\ 0 \text{ for } h\neq j; h,j=1,\ldots,J-1\\ 0 \text{ for } h=J; j=1,\ldots,J-1,\end{cases} \quad (6.75)$$

and

$$\frac{\partial}{\partial \gamma_j}[\eta^{*(h\cdot)}_{it|t-1}(g)] = \frac{\partial}{\partial \gamma_j}\begin{cases}\frac{\exp\left[w^{*\prime}_{it}\beta^*_h+\gamma'_h y^{(g)}_{i,t-1}+\sigma_\xi\xi_i\right]}{1+\sum_{v=1}^{J-1}\exp\left[w^{*\prime}_{it}\beta^*_v+\gamma'_v y^{(g)}_{i,t-1}+\sigma_\xi\xi_i\right]}, & \text{for } h=1,\ldots,J-1\\ \frac{1}{1+\sum_{v=1}^{J-1}\exp\left[w^{*\prime}_{it}\beta^*_v+\gamma'_v y^{(g)}_{i,t-1}+\sigma_\xi\xi_i\right]}, & \text{for } h=J,\end{cases}$$
$$= \begin{cases}\delta_{(i,t-1)g}\eta^{*(j\cdot)}_{it|t-1}(g)[1-\eta^{*(j\cdot)}_{it|t-1}(g)] & \text{for } h=j; h,j=1,\ldots,J-1\\ -\delta_{(i,t-1)g}\eta^{*(j\cdot)}_{it|t-1}(g)\eta^{*(h\cdot)}_{it|t-1}(g) & \text{for } h\neq j; h,j=1,\ldots,J-1\\ -\delta_{(i,t-1)g}\eta^{*(j\cdot)}_{it|t-1}(g)\eta^{*(J\cdot)}_{it|t-1}(g) & \text{for } h=J;\ j=1,\ldots,J-1,\end{cases} \quad (6.76)$$

where for all $i=1,\ldots,K$, and $t=2,\ldots,T$, one writes

$$\delta_{(i,t-1)g} = \begin{cases}[01'_{g-1},1,01'_{J-1-g}]' & \text{for; } g=1,\ldots,J-1\\ 01'_{J-1} & \text{for } g=J.\end{cases} \quad (6.77)$$

Estimation of λ:

Recall that $\lambda=[\lambda'_1,\ldots,\lambda'_r,\ldots,\lambda'_{R-1}]'$ and the moment estimation of λ_r is quite similar to that of γ_j. The difference between the two is that γ_j is a dynamic dependence parameter vector for y response variable, whereas λ_r is a similar parameter vector for z response variables. More specifically, $\lambda_r (r=1,\ldots,R-1)$ is the lag 1 dynamic dependence parameter relating $z_{it}^{(r)}$ and $z_{i,t-1}^{(g)}$ where g is a known category and ranges from 1 to R. Thus, it would be appropriate to exploit all lag 1 product responses corresponding to the z variable in order to estimate this parameter. More specifically, for $t = 2,\ldots,T$, following (6.29), we write

$$\begin{aligned} E[Z_{i,t-1}Z'_{it}] &= \int_{-\infty}^{\infty} \left[\left\{\eta^{*(\cdot*)}_{(it|t-1),M} - \eta^{*(\cdot*)}_{(it|t-1)}(R)1'_{R-1}\right\} \mathrm{var}[Z_{i,t-1}|\xi_i]\right] f_N(\xi_i)d\xi_i \\ &+ \int_{-\infty}^{\infty} [\{\pi^{*(\cdot*)}_{(i,t-1)}(\alpha,\lambda,\sigma_\xi|\xi_i)\}\{\pi^{*(\cdot*)}_{(it)}(\alpha,\lambda,\sigma_\xi|\xi_i)'\}]f_N(\xi_i)d\xi_i \\ &= \int_{-\infty}^{\infty} [\tilde{M}_{i,(t-1)t}(\alpha,\lambda,\sigma_\xi|\xi_i)]f_N(\xi_i)d\xi_i : (R-1)\times(R-1), \text{ (say)}. \end{aligned} \quad (6.78)$$

It then follows that the moment estimator of λ_r may be obtained by solving the moment equation

$$\begin{aligned} &\sum_{i=1}^{K}\sum_{t=2}^{T}\sum_{h=1}^{R-1}\sum_{k=1}^{R-1}\int_{-\infty}^{\infty}\left[\frac{\partial}{\partial\lambda_r}[\tilde{m}_{i,(t-1)t;h,k}(\alpha,\lambda,\sigma_\xi|\xi_i)]\right. \\ &\times \left.\{z_{i,t-1,h}z_{itk} - \tilde{m}_{i,(t-1)t;h,k}(\alpha,\lambda,\sigma_\xi|\xi_i)\}\right] f_N(\xi_i)d\xi_i = 0, \end{aligned} \quad (6.79)$$

where $\tilde{m}_{i,(t-1)t;h,k}(\alpha,\lambda,\sigma_\xi|\xi_i)$ is the (h,k)th element of the $\tilde{M}_{i,(t-1)t}(\alpha,\lambda,\sigma_\xi|\xi_i)$ matrix of dimension $(R-1)\times(R-1)$, and $z_{i,t-1,h}$ and z_{itk} are, respectively, the hth and kth elements of the multinomial response vectors $z_{i,t-1} = (z_{i,t-1,1},\ldots,z_{i,t-1,h},\ldots,z_{i,t-1,R-1})'$ and $z_{it} = (z_{it1},\ldots,z_{itk},\ldots,z_{it,R-1})'$, of the ith individual. Next, in the spirit of iteration, by assuming that λ_r in $\frac{\partial}{\partial\lambda_r}[\tilde{m}_{i,(t-1)t;h,k}(\alpha,\lambda,\sigma_\xi|\xi_i)$ is known from previous iteration, the moment equation (6.79) may be solved for λ_r by using the iterative equation

$$\begin{aligned} \hat{\lambda}_r(\ell+1) &= \hat{\lambda}_r(\ell) + \left[\sum_{i=1}^{K}\sum_{t=2}^{T}\sum_{h=1}^{R-1}\sum_{k=1}^{R-1}\int_{-\infty}^{\infty}\left\{\frac{\partial}{\partial\lambda_r}[\tilde{m}_{i,(t-1)t;h,k}(\alpha,\lambda,\sigma_\xi|\xi_i)]\right.\right. \\ &\times \left.\left.\frac{\partial}{\partial\lambda'_j}[\tilde{m}_{i,(t-1)t;h,k}(\alpha,\lambda,\sigma_\xi|\xi_i)]\right\} f_N(\xi_i)d\xi_i\right]^{-1} \sum_{i=1}^{K}\sum_{t=2}^{T}\sum_{h=1}^{R-1}\sum_{k=1}^{R-1}\int_{-\infty}^{\infty}\left[\frac{\partial}{\partial\lambda_r}[\tilde{m}_{i,(t-1)t;h,k}(\alpha,\lambda,\sigma_\xi|\xi_i)]\right. \\ &\times \left.\{z_{i,t-1,h}z_{itk} - \tilde{m}_{i,(t-1)t;h,k}(\alpha,\lambda,\sigma_\xi|\xi_i)\}\right] f_N(\xi_i)d\xi_i\Big]_{\lambda_r=\hat{\lambda}_r(\ell)}. \end{aligned} \quad (6.80)$$

Note that to compute the derivative of the elements of the matrix $\tilde{M}_{i,(t-1)t}(\alpha,\lambda,\sigma_\xi|\xi_i)$ with respect to λ_r, i.e., to compute $\frac{\partial}{\partial\lambda'_r}[\tilde{m}_{i,(t-1)t;h,k}(\alpha,\lambda,\sigma_\xi|\xi_i)]$ in (6.79)–(6.80), we provide the following derivatives as an aid:

$$\frac{\partial \pi^*_{(i1)\cdot h}}{\partial \lambda_r} = \frac{\partial}{\partial \lambda_r}\begin{cases} \frac{\exp(w^{*'}_{i1}\alpha^*_h+\sigma_\xi \xi_i)}{1+\sum_{g=1}^{R-1}\exp(w^{*'}_{i1}\alpha^*_g+\sigma_\xi \xi_i)} & \text{for } h=1,\ldots,R-1 \\ \frac{1}{1+\sum_{g=1}^{R-1}\exp(w^{*'}_{i1}\alpha^*_g+\sigma_\xi \xi_i)} & \text{for } h=R, \end{cases}$$

$$= \begin{cases} 0 \text{ for } h=r; h,r=1,\ldots,R-1 \\ 0 \text{ for } h\neq r; h,r=1,\ldots,R-1 \\ 0 \text{ for } h=R; r=1,\ldots,R-1, \end{cases} \quad (6.81)$$

and

$$\frac{\partial}{\partial \lambda_r}[\eta^{*(\cdot h)}_{it|t-1}(g)] = \frac{\partial}{\partial \lambda_r}\begin{cases} \frac{\exp\left[w^{*'}_{it}\alpha^*_h+\lambda'_h z^{(g)}_{i,t-1}+\sigma_\xi \xi_i\right]}{1+\sum_{v=1}^{R-1}\exp\left[w^{*'}_{it}\alpha^*_v+\lambda'_v z^{(g)}_{i,t-1}+\sigma_\xi \xi_i\right]}, & \text{for } h=1,\ldots,R-1 \\ \frac{1}{1+\sum_{v=1}^{R-1}\exp\left[w^{*'}_{it}\alpha^*_v+\lambda'_v z^{(g)}_{i,t-1}+\sigma_\xi \xi_i\right]}, & \text{for } h=R, \end{cases}$$

$$= \begin{cases} \delta^*_{(i,t-1)g}\eta^{*(\cdot r)}_{it|t-1}(g)[1-\eta^{*(\cdot r)}_{it|t-1}(g)] & \text{for } h=r; h,r=1,\ldots,R-1 \\ -\delta^*_{(i,t-1)g}\eta^{*(\cdot r)}_{it|t-1}(g)\eta^{*(\cdot h)}_{it|t-1}(g) & \text{for } h\neq r; h,r=1,\ldots,R-1 \\ -\delta^*_{(i,t-1)g}\eta^{*(\cdot r)}_{it|t-1}(g)\eta^{*(\cdot R)}_{it|t-1}(g) & \text{for } h=R;\ r=1,\ldots,R-1, \end{cases} \quad (6.82)$$

where for all $i=1,\ldots,K$, and $t=2,\ldots,T$, one writes

$$\delta^*_{(i,t-1)g} = \begin{cases} [01'_{g-1},1,01'_{R-1-g}]' & \text{for}; g=1,\ldots,R-1 \\ 01'_{R-1} & \text{for } g=R. \end{cases} \quad (6.83)$$

6.3.3 Moment Estimation for σ^2_ξ (Familial Correlation Index Parameter)

Because σ^2_ξ is involved in all pair-wise product moments for y and z variables, we exploit the corresponding observed products as follows to develop a moment estimating equation for this scalar parameter.

Recall from (6.19) that for $u<t$,

$$E[Y_{iu}Y'_{it}] = \int_{-\infty}^{\infty}\left[\Sigma^{*(*\cdot)}_{(i,ut)}(\beta,\gamma,\sigma_\xi|\xi_i)+[\{\pi^{*(*\cdot)}_{(iu)}(\beta,\gamma,\sigma_\xi|\xi_i)\}\{\pi^{*(*\cdot)}_{(it)}(\beta,\gamma,\sigma_\xi|\xi_i)'\}]\right]f_N(\xi_i)d\xi_i$$

$$= \int_{-\infty}^{\infty}[M^*_{i,ut}(\beta,\gamma,\sigma_\xi|\xi_i)]f_N(\xi_i)d\xi_i : (J-1)\times(J-1) \quad (6.84)$$

(6.72) being a special case. Similarly, for $u < t$, one writes from (6.29) that

$$E[Z_{iu}Z'_{it}] = \int_{-\infty}^{\infty} \left[\Sigma^{*(\cdot*)}_{(i,ut)}(\alpha,\lambda,\sigma_\xi|\xi_i) + [\{\pi^{*(\cdot*)}_{(iu)}(\alpha,\lambda,\sigma_\xi|\xi_i)\}\{\pi^{*(\cdot*)}_{(it)}(\alpha,\lambda,\sigma_\xi|\xi_i)'\}]'\right] f_N(\xi_i)d\xi_i$$
$$= \int_{-\infty}^{\infty} [\tilde{M}_{i,ut}(\alpha,\lambda,\sigma_\xi|\xi_i)] f_N(\xi_i)d\xi_i : (R-1)\times(R-1) \quad (6.85)$$

(6.78) being a special case. Next for all u,t, the pair-wise product moments for y and z variables may be written from (6.31), as

$$E[Y_{iu}Z'_{it}] = \begin{cases} \int_{-\infty}^{\infty} \left[\pi^{*(*\cdot)}_{(i1)}(\beta,\gamma=0,\sigma_\xi|\xi_i)\pi^{*(\cdot*)'}_{(i1)}(\alpha,\lambda=0,\sigma_\xi|\xi_i)\right] f_N(\xi_i)d\xi_i & \text{for } u=t=1 \\ \int_{-\infty}^{\infty} \left[\pi^{*(*\cdot)}_{(i1)}(\beta,\gamma=0,\sigma_\xi|\xi_i)\pi^{*(\cdot*)'}_{(it)}(\alpha,\lambda,\sigma_\xi|\xi_i)\right] f_N(\xi_i)d\xi_i & \text{for } u=1; t=2,\ldots,T \\ \int_{-\infty}^{\infty} \left[\pi^{*(*\cdot)}_{(iu)}(\beta,\gamma,\sigma_\xi|\xi_i)\pi^{*(\cdot*)'}_{(i1)}(\alpha,\lambda=0,\sigma_\xi|\xi_i)\right] f_N(\xi_i)d\xi_i & \text{for } u=2,\ldots,T; t=1 \\ \int_{-\infty}^{\infty} \left[\pi^{*(*\cdot)}_{(iu)}(\beta,\gamma,\sigma_\xi|\xi_i)\pi^{*(\cdot*)'}_{(it)}(\alpha,\lambda,\sigma_\xi|\xi_i)\right] f_N(\xi_i)d\xi_i & \text{for } u,t=2,\ldots,T. \end{cases}$$
$$= \int_{-\infty}^{\infty} [Q^*_{i,ut}(\beta,\gamma;\alpha,\lambda;\sigma_\xi|\xi_i)] f_N(\xi_i)d\xi_i : (J-1)\times(R-1), \text{ (say)}$$
$$= \int_{-\infty}^{\infty} (q^*_{i,ut;h,k}(\beta,\gamma;\alpha,\lambda;\sigma_\xi|\xi_i)) f_N(\xi_i)d\xi_i : (J-1)\times(R-1). \quad (6.86)$$

Now by exploiting the moments from (6.84)–(6.86), we develop a moment equation for σ^2_ξ as

$$\sum_{i=1}^{K}\sum_{u=1}^{T-1}\sum_{t=u+1}^{T}\sum_{h=1}^{J-1}\sum_{k=1}^{J-1}\int_{-\infty}^{\infty}\left[\frac{\partial}{\partial\sigma^2_\xi}[m^*_{i,ut;h,k}(\beta,\gamma,\sigma_\xi|\xi_i)]\{y_{iuh}y_{itk} - m^*_{i,ut;h,k}(\beta,\gamma,\sigma_\xi|\xi_i)\}\right] f_N(\xi_i)d\xi_i$$
$$+\sum_{i=1}^{K}\sum_{u=1}^{T-1}\sum_{t=u+1}^{T}\sum_{h=1}^{R-1}\sum_{k=1}^{R-1}\int_{-\infty}^{\infty}\left[\frac{\partial}{\partial\sigma^2_\xi}[\tilde{m}_{i,ut;h,k}(\alpha,\lambda,\sigma_\xi|\xi_i)]\{z_{iuh}z_{itk} - \tilde{m}_{i,ut;h,k}(\alpha,\lambda,\sigma_\xi|\xi_i)\}\right] f_N(\xi_i)d\xi_i$$
$$+\sum_{i=1}^{K}\sum_{u=1}^{T-1}\sum_{t=u+1}^{T}\sum_{h=1}^{J-1}\sum_{k=1}^{R-1}\int_{-\infty}^{\infty}\left[\frac{\partial}{\partial\sigma^2_\xi}[q^*_{i,ut;h,k}(\beta,\gamma;\alpha,\lambda;\sigma_\xi|\xi_i)]\right.$$
$$\left.\times\ \{y_{iuh}z_{itk} - q^*_{i,ut;h,k}(\alpha,\lambda,\sigma_\xi|\xi_i)\}\right] f_N(\xi_i)d\xi_i = 0. \quad (6.87)$$

This moment equation (6.87) may be solved by using the iterative equation

$$\hat{\sigma}^2_\xi(\ell+1) = \hat{\sigma}^2_\xi(\ell)$$
$$+\left[\left[\left\{\sum_{i=1}^{K}\sum_{u=1}^{T-1}\sum_{t=u+1}^{T}\sum_{h=1}^{J-1}\sum_{k=1}^{J-1}\int_{-\infty}^{\infty}\left[\frac{\partial}{\partial\sigma^2_\xi}[m^*_{i,ut;h,k}(\beta,\gamma,\sigma_\xi|\xi_i)]\right]^2 f_N(\xi_i)d\xi_i\right.\right.\right.$$
$$+\sum_{i=1}^{K}\sum_{u=1}^{T-1}\sum_{t=u+1}^{T}\sum_{h=1}^{R-1}\sum_{k=1}^{R-1}\int_{-\infty}^{\infty}\left[\frac{\partial}{\partial\sigma^2_\xi}[\tilde{m}_{i,ut;h,k}(\alpha,\lambda,\sigma_\xi|\xi_i)]\right]^2 f_N(\xi_i)d\xi_i$$
$$\left.+\sum_{i=1}^{K}\sum_{u=1}^{T-1}\sum_{t=u+1}^{T}\sum_{h=1}^{J-1}\sum_{k=1}^{R-1}\int_{-\infty}^{\infty}\left[\frac{\partial}{\partial\sigma^2_\xi}[q^*_{i,ut;h,k}(\beta,\gamma;\alpha,\lambda;\sigma_\xi|\xi_i)]\right]^2 f_N(\xi_i)d\xi_i\right\}^{-1}$$

$$\times \left\{ \sum_{i=1}^{K}\sum_{u=1}^{T-1}\sum_{t=u+1}^{T}\sum_{h=1}^{J-1}\sum_{k=1}^{J-1}\int_{-\infty}^{\infty}\left[\frac{\partial}{\partial\sigma_\xi^2}[m^*_{i,ut;h,k}(\beta,\gamma,\sigma_\xi|\xi_i)]\{y_{iuh}y_{itk}-m^*_{i,ut;h,k}(\beta,\gamma,\sigma_\xi|\xi_i)\}\right] f_N(\xi_i)d\xi_i\right.$$

$$+\sum_{i=1}^{K}\sum_{u=1}^{T-1}\sum_{t=u+1}^{T}\sum_{h=1}^{R-1}\sum_{k=1}^{R-1}\int_{-\infty}^{\infty}\left[\frac{\partial}{\partial\sigma_\xi^2}[\tilde{m}_{i,ut;h,k}(\alpha,\lambda,\sigma_\xi|\xi_i)]\{z_{iuh}z_{itk}-\tilde{m}_{i,ut;h,k}(\alpha,\lambda,\sigma_\xi|\xi_i)\}\right] f_N(\xi_i)d\xi_i$$

$$+\sum_{i=1}^{K}\sum_{u=1}^{T-1}\sum_{t=u+1}^{T}\sum_{h=1}^{J-1}\sum_{k=1}^{R-1}\int_{-\infty}^{\infty}\left[\frac{\partial}{\partial\sigma_\xi^2}[q^*_{i,ut;h,k}(\beta,\gamma;\alpha,\lambda;\sigma_\xi|\xi_i)]\right.$$

$$\times \left.\left.\{y_{iuh}z_{itk}-q^*_{i,ut;h,k}(\alpha,\lambda,\sigma_\xi|\xi_i)\}\right] f_N(\xi_i)d\xi_i\right\}\Big]_{\sigma_\xi^2=\hat{\sigma}_\xi^2(\ell)}. \quad (6.88)$$

Note that the computation of the derivatives for the elements of three matrices will require the following basic derivatives:

$$\frac{\partial\pi^*_{(i1)h\cdot}}{\partial\sigma_\xi^2}=\frac{\partial}{\partial\sigma_\xi^2}\begin{cases}\frac{\exp(w^{*\prime}_{i1}\beta^*_h+\sigma_\xi\xi_i)}{1+\sum_{g=1}^{J-1}\exp(w^{*\prime}_{i1}\beta^*_g+\sigma_\xi\xi_i)} & \text{for } h=1,\ldots,J-1\\ \frac{1}{1+\sum_{g=1}^{J-1}\exp(w^{*\prime}_{i1}\beta^*_g+\sigma_\xi\xi_i)} & \text{for } h=J,\end{cases}$$

$$=\begin{cases}\frac{\xi_i}{\sigma_\xi}\pi^*_{(i1)h\cdot}\pi^*_{(i1)J\cdot} & \text{for } h=1,\ldots,J-1\\ -\frac{\xi_i}{\sigma_\xi}\pi^*_{(i1)J\cdot}[1-\pi^*_{(i1)J\cdot}] & \text{for } h=J;\end{cases} \quad (6.89)$$

$$\frac{\partial}{\partial\sigma_\xi^2}[\eta^{*(h\cdot)}_{it|t-1}(g)]=\frac{\partial}{\partial\sigma_\xi^2}\begin{cases}\frac{\exp\left[w^{*\prime}_{it}\beta^*_h+\gamma'_h y^{(g)}_{i,t-1}+\sigma_\xi\xi_i\right]}{1+\sum_{v=1}^{J-1}\exp\left[w^{*\prime}_{it}\beta^*_v+\gamma'_v y^{(g)}_{i,t-1}+\sigma_\xi\xi_i\right]}, & \text{for } h=1,\ldots,J-1\\ \frac{1}{1+\sum_{v=1}^{J-1}\exp\left[w^{*\prime}_{it}\beta^*_v+\gamma'_v y^{(g)}_{i,t-1}+\sigma_\xi\xi_i\right]}, & \text{for } h=J,\end{cases}$$

$$=\begin{cases}\frac{\xi_i}{\sigma_\xi}\eta^{*(h\cdot)}_{it|t-1}(g)\eta^{*(J\cdot)}_{it|t-1}(g) & \text{for } h=1,\ldots,J-1\\ -\frac{\xi_i}{\sigma_\xi}\eta^{*(J\cdot)}_{it|t-1}(g)[1-\eta^{*(J\cdot)}_{it|t-1}(g)] & \text{for } h=J;\end{cases} \quad (6.90)$$

$$\frac{\partial\pi^*_{(i1)\cdot r}}{\partial\sigma_\xi^2}=\frac{\partial}{\partial\sigma_\xi^2}\begin{cases}\frac{\exp(w^{*\prime}_{i1}\alpha^*_r+\sigma_\xi\xi_i)}{1+\sum_{g=1}^{R-1}\exp(w^{*\prime}_{i1}\alpha^*_g+\sigma_\xi\xi_i)} & \text{for } r=1,\ldots,R-1\\ \frac{1}{1+\sum_{g=1}^{R-1}\exp(w^{*\prime}_{i1}\alpha^*_g+\sigma_\xi\xi_i)} & \text{for } r=R,\end{cases}$$

$$=\begin{cases}\frac{\xi_i}{\sigma_\xi}\pi^*_{(i1)\cdot r}\pi^*_{(i1)\cdot R} & \text{for } r=1,\ldots,R-1\\ -\frac{\xi_i}{\sigma_\xi}\pi^*_{(i1)\cdot R}[1-\pi^*_{(i1)\cdot R}] & \text{for } r=R;\end{cases} \quad (6.91)$$

and

$$\frac{\partial}{\partial\sigma_\xi^2}[\eta_{it|t-1}^{*(\cdot r)}(g)] = \frac{\partial}{\partial\sigma_\xi^2}\begin{cases} \frac{\exp\left[w_{it}^{*'}\alpha_r^*+\lambda_r' y_{i,t-1}^{(g)}+\sigma_\xi\xi_i\right]}{1+\sum_{v=1}^{R-1}\exp\left[w_{it}^{*'}\alpha_v^*+\lambda_v' y_{i,t-1}^{(g)}+\sigma_\xi\xi_i\right]}, & \text{for } r=1,\ldots,R-1 \\ \frac{1}{1+\sum_{v=1}^{R-1}\exp\left[w_{it}^{*'}\alpha_v^*+\lambda_v' y_{i,t-1}^{(g)}+\sigma_\xi\xi_i\right]}, & \text{for } r=R, \end{cases}$$

$$= \begin{cases} \frac{\xi_i}{\sigma_\xi}\eta_{it|t-1}^{*(\cdot r)}(g)\eta_{it|t-1}^{*(\cdot R)}(g) & \text{for } r=1,\ldots,R-1 \\ -\frac{\xi_i}{\sigma_\xi}\eta_{it|t-1}^{*(\cdot R)}(g)[1-\eta_{it|t-1}^{*(\cdot R)}(g)] & \text{for } r=R. \end{cases} \tag{6.92}$$

References

Sutradhar, B. C. (2011). *Dynamic mixed models for familial longitudinal data*. New York: Springer.

Sutradhar, B. C., Prabhakar Rao, R., & Pandit, V. N. (2008). Generalized method of moments versus generalized quasi-likelihood inferences in binary panel data models. *Sankhya B, 70*, 34–62.

Index

A
Algorithm
  iterative,19, 23, 29, 38, 43, 47, 52, 58, 82, 95, 98, 103, 104, 106, 107, 118, 127, 128, 134, 136, 142, 156, 161, 167, 171, 174, 177, 193, 196, 205, 217, 221, 230, 234, 241, 259, 262, 264, 276, 279, 288, 297, 303, 306, 315, 324, 329, 359, 360, 362, 364
ANOVA type
  covariate free multinomial probability model, 284–294
  parameter estimation, 287–294
Aspirin and heart attack data, 39, 40, 45
Asthma data, 97–100, 104, 106, 107, 113, 119, 120, 128, 142
Auto correlations of repeated
  binary responses under dynamic logit model, 64, 79, 114–120
  binary responses under linear dynamic conditional probability model, 94, 100, 107
  multinomial responses under dynamic logit model, 91, 92, 147–148, 248, 339–340
  multinomial responses under linear dynamic conditional probability model, 107, 114, 180–193, 247
Auto regressive order 1
  binary linear conditional model, 91, 321
  binary non-linear conditional model, 91, 114, 248, 265
  multinomial linear conditional model, 138, 171, 243
  multinomial non-linear conditional model, 91, 114, 167, 171, 175, 248

B
Binary dynamic models
  linear conditional probability, 138, 213, 317, 337
  non-linear logit, 114, 119, 120, 167, 248
Binary mapping for ordinal data
  pseudo-likelihood estimation, 78–83, 213–219
  quasi-likelihood estimation, 83–87, 219–223
Binomial
  factorization, 11–12
  marginal distribution, 9
  product binomial, 32, 33, 38, 39, 123
Binomial approximation to the normal distribution of random effects
  cross-sectional bivariate data, 281–284
  longitudinal bivariate data, 339–366
Bivariate multinomial models
  fixed effects model, 114
  mixed effects model, 3, 114

C
Class of autocorrelations, 93–100
  stationary, 93–100, 119
Conditional model
  linear form for repeated binary responses, 94, 115, 152
  linear form for repeated multinomial responses, 2, 4, 89, 91, 92, 147, 148, 152, 154, 168, 248, 256
  logit form for repeated binary responses, 115, 137, 168, 194, 195, 232

B.C. Sutradhar, *Longitudinal Categorical Data Analysis*, Springer Series in Statistics, DOI 10.1007/978-1-4939-2137-9

Conditional model (*cont.*)
logit form for repeated multinomial responses, 3, 147–150
Cumulative logits for ordinal data
cross-sectional setup, 2, 90, 92, 120, 213
longitudinal setup using conditional linear model, 145
longitudinal setup using conditional logit model, 209

D
Data example
aspirin and heart attack data, 39, 40, 45
asthma data, 97–100, 104, 106, 107, 113, 119, 120, 128, 142
diabetic retinopathy data, 310, 331–337
physician visit status data, 47, 49, 52, 62, 71, 77, 78
snoring and heart disease data, 38
three miles island stress level (TMISL) data, 152–154, 167, 175–182, 200–209
Diabetic retinopathy data, 310, 331–337
Dynamic dependence
for repeated binary data, 89, 100, 145, 150
for repeated multinomial data, 89, 145, 154
Dynamic dependence parameter, 115, 137, 138, 140, 142, 150, 156, 166, 168, 170, 173, 175, 177, 195, 199, 205, 207, 265, 270–273, 278, 339–341, 348, 359–363
Dynamic logit models
for repeated binary data, 89, 100, 145, 150
for repeated multinomial data, 89, 145, 154

E
Estimation of parameters
generalized quasi-likelihood estimation, 83–87, 94–97, 105, 107, 111–114, 119, 122–157, 219–223, 256, 294–309, 313–316, 322, 323, 336, 348–360
likelihood estimation, 13, 16–17, 78–83, 100–105, 107–111, 116–120, 219, 260–264, 272–280
moment estimation, 12, 150, 222, 259–260, 359–366
product multinomial likelihood, 45, 48, 71
pseudo-likelihood estimation, 78–83, 213–219
weighted least square estimation, 65–78

F
Fixed and mixed effects model
binary fixed, 120–143
multinomial fixed, 7–20, 179–209
multinomial mixed, 3, 152, 293

G
Generalized estimating equations (GEE), 5, 91, 248–253
Generalized quasi-likelihood (GQL), 91, 107, 157, 175, 220, 262, 293, 322, 325, 333, 336, 348, 349

J
Joint *GQL* estimation (JGQL), 293, 294, 299–303, 312, 322, 325, 326, 329, 330, 333–336

L
Likelihood estimation, 13–16, 78–83, 100–105, 107–111, 116, 131–143, 191, 195, 213–219, 228, 240, 260–264, 272–280, 289–293

M
Marginal *GQL* estimation, 293–303, 312–316, 322–324, 333, 335, 336, 348, 349, 359
Mixed effects model, 3, 114
Moment estimation, 12–13, 150–157, 222–223, 259–260, 359–366

N
Non-stationary
conditional linear dynamic models, 248, 264–280
correlations for multinomial responses, 248, 252–264
dynamic logit models, 247, 248

O
Ordinal data
cross-sectional, 63–87
longitudinal, 209–244

P
Physician visit status data, 47, 49, 52, 62, 71, 77, 78
Product multinomial likelihood, 45, 48, 71
Pseudo-likelihood estimation, 78–83, 213–219

R

Regression models
multinomial with individual specific covariates, 310, 340
multinomial with individual specific time dependent covariates, 247, 248, 251, 253, 264
multinomial with no covariates, 5, 27, 31, 92, 114
multinomial with one categorical covariate, 39–53, 64–78
multinomial with two categorical covariates, 48, 53

S

Snoring and heart disease data, 22, 24, 38, 44
Software
FORTRAN – 90, 5
R, 5
S-PLUS, 5

T

Three miles island stress level (TMISL) data, 152–154, 167, 175–182, 200–209
Transitional counts
for longitudinal binary responses, 98, 99, 121, 128, 129
for longitudinal multinomial responses, 181, 182, 210–212, 214
Two-way *ANOVA* type joint probability model, 284–293

W

Weighted least square (WLS) estimation, 65–78

MIX
Papier aus verantwortungsvollen Quellen
Paper from responsible sources
FSC® C105338

If you have any concerns about our products,
you can contact us on
ProductSafety@springernature.com

In case Publisher is established outside the EU,
the EU authorized representative is:
Springer Nature Customer Service Center GmbH
Europaplatz 3, 69115 Heidelberg, Germany

Printed by Libri Plureos GmbH
in Hamburg, Germany